Anesthesia for Hepatico-Pancreatic-Biliary Surgery and Transplantation

Zoka Milan · Chula Goonasekera
Editors

Anesthesia for Hepatico-Pancreatic-Biliary Surgery and Transplantation

Springer

Editors
Zoka Milan
Department of Anaesthesia
King's College Hospital
London, UK

Chula Goonasekera
King's College Hospital
London, UK

ISBN 978-3-030-51330-6 ISBN 978-3-030-51331-3 (eBook)
https://doi.org/10.1007/978-3-030-51331-3

This Springer imprint is published by the registered company Springer Nature Switzerland AG
The registered company address is: Gewerbestrasse 11, 6330 Cham, Switzerland

Contents

Part IV Pancreas

Part V Paediatric

Part I
Anatomy and Physiology of the Liver

Chapter 1
Anatomy of Hepato-Pancreato-Biliary Surgery and Liver Transplantation

Evangelia Florou, Joe Macmillan and Parthi Srinivasan

Introduction

Surgical procedures for the liver, biliary tract and pancreas have evolved significantly over time. These organs are complex in structure and their function is fundamental in regulating homeostasis of the body. Surgical intervention aims to minimize structural damage, maintain organ function and physiological homeostasis.

A high level of knowledge of anatomy, physiology and pathology in hepato-pancreato-biliary (HPB) procedures and in liver transplantation surgery will enable the anesthetist to manage the perioperative challenges of this demanding and evolving surgical specialty posed to both patient and clinician.

This anatomical review is aided by illustrations and focuses on the most relevant to HPB surgery points in order to simplify and familiarize the reader with surgical approaches, strategies and considerations.

E. Florou (✉)
Clinical Fellow in Hepato-Pancreato-Biliary Surgery and Liver Transplantation,
King's College Hospital, London, UK
e-mail: e.florou@nhs.net

J. Macmillan
Consultant Anaesthetist, King's College Hospital, London, UK
e-mail: jmacmillan1@nhs.net

P. Srinivasan
Consultant Surgeon in Hepato-Pancreato-Biliary Surgery and Liver Transplantation,
King's College Hospital, London, UK
e-mail: parthi.srinivasan@nhs.net

Z. Milan and C. Goonasekera (eds.), *Anesthesia for Hepatico-Pancreatic-Biliary Surgery and Transplantation*, https://doi.org/10.1007/978-3-030-51331-3_1

Arteries

Arterial supply to all abdominal organs arises from the abdominal portion of the descending aorta. The aorta lies in the retroperitoneal space in front of the spine and slightly to the left of the midline, parallel to inferior vena cava, which lies on its right. After entering the abdominal cavity via the aortic foramen, the descending aorta runs down to the pelvis where it branches into right and left iliac arteries to supply pelvic organs and lower limbs [1, 3, 4].

The first large arterial trunk that arises from the anterior surface of the abdominal aorta at the level of T12 is the coeliac axis (CA), a common trunk of the following three arteries: the common hepatic artery (CHA), the left gastric artery (LGA) and the splenic artery (SA). The coeliac axis supplies the abdominal compartment of the embryonic foregut: stomach, duodenum, biliary tree, liver, pancreas and spleen [1, 2]. Thus, the common hepatic artery gives rise to the gastroduodenal artery (GDA) to supply the head of the pancreas and continues its course as the proper hepatic artery in a cephalad direction to supply the liver. High up in the liver hilum it divides into right and left branches to supply right and left hemilivers respectively [1, 3, 4] (Figs. 1.1 and 1.2).

The second arterial branch coming off the anterior aspect of the descending aorta, is the superior mesenteric artery (SMA) that arises at the level of L1 and supplies abdominal viscera corresponding to the embryonic midgut; distal duodenum, small bowel, ceacum, ascending colon and proximal part of transverse colon [1, 2, 4] (Fig. 1.2).

A third artery, the inferior mesenteric artery (IMA), arises at the level of L3 before the aortic bifurcation to the right and left iliac arteries and supplies the rest of the large bowel; distal transverse colon, splenic flexure, descending colon, sigmoid, rectum and upper anus, organs which represent the embryonic hindgut [1, 2] (Fig. 1.2).

The renal arteries (RA) arise from the lateral aspect of the abdominal aorta at the level of L2 usually just below the SMA orifice [1] (Fig. 1.2).

Veins

The whole of the gastrointestinal (GI) tract drains into the liver via the portal system.

The venous drainage follows the previously described arterial supply. Thus, the superior mesenteric vein (SMV) drains the small bowel and part of the large bowel while the inferior mesenteric vein (IMV) drains the rest of the large bowel. The splenic vein (SV) drains the spleen and part of the stomach whereas the left gastric vein (LGV) along with smaller veins drain the rest of the stomach [1, 3, 4] (Fig. 1.3).

The confluence of both the SMV and SV creates the portal vein (PV). The proximal PV lies behind the duodenum and pancreatic head and courses upwards

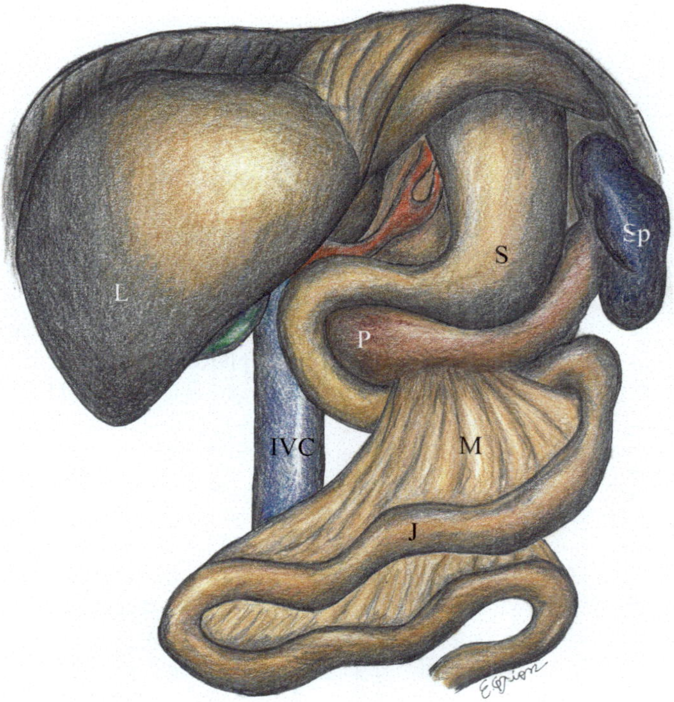

Fig. 1.1 Simplified surgical field view of organs of the upper abdomen; Liver (L), stomach (S), pancreas (P) and spleen (Sp). The pancreas lies retroperitoneally within the lesser sac. This picture depicts part of the jejunum (J) along with the corresponding mesentery (M), while the rest of the small and large bowel as well as the omentum have been removed. Inferior Vena Cava (IVC)

in a cephalad direction to enter the liver hilum where it divides into right and left portal branches. Along its course to enter the liver, the left gastric vein empties into the PV. Smaller veins drain the pancreas via the SMV and the PV. The IMV enters the portal system in a variable position across the PV, SMV course or at the PV/SMV confluence [1, 3, 4] (Fig. 1.3).

The inferior vena cava (IVC) is the outflow trunk of the liver, both kidneys, pelvic organs and lower limbs. The right and left iliac veins join together in the pelvis in front of the sacrum, to create the distal IVC. The latter runs upwards and at the level of the inferior border of the liver both right and left renal veins drain both kidneys into the IVC [1, 3] (Fig. 1.4a, b).

The IVC course continues posteriorly to the liver and multiple small branches drain the liver parenchyma and caudate lobe at this particularly adherent area of both organs.

Higher at the sub-diaphragmatic level, the liver drains via three main hepatic veins into the IVC [1] (Fig. 1.4b). The right hepatic vein drains separately as

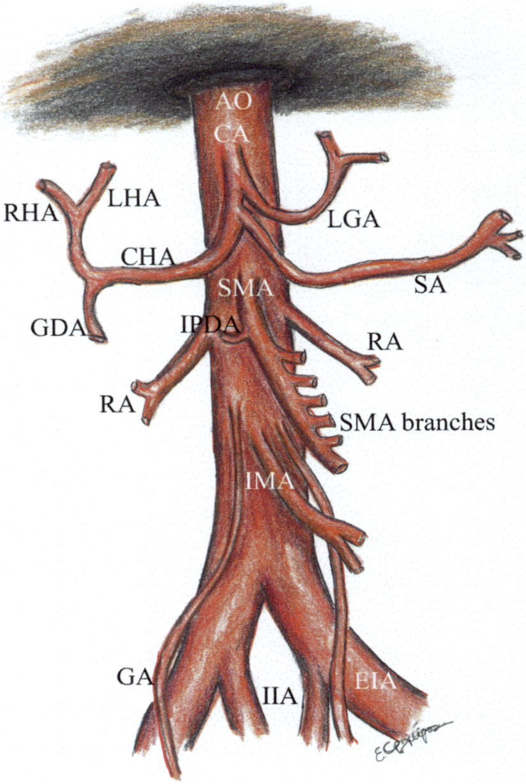

Fig. 1.2 Arteries arising from the abdominal portion of the descending aorta. The Coeliac Axis (CA) branches into; Common Hepatic Artery (CHA), Left Gastric Artery (LGA) and Splenic Artery (SA). The CHA branches into Right (RHA) and Left hepatic (LHA) arteries. The gastroduodenal artery (GDA) supplies the head of the pancreas. Superior Mesenteric Artery (SMA). The first branch of SMA is the Inferior Pancreaticoduodenal Artery (IPDA) which supplies the head of the pancreas. Multiple branches from the SMA supply the small bowel as well as the ascending colon, hepatic flexure and part of the transverse colon. Inferior Mesenteric Artery (IMA) supplies the rest of the large bowel. Gonadal Arteries (GA). On the lateral aspect of the aorta (AO), the renal arteries (RA). Common Iliac Arteries (CIA), Internal (IIA) and External Iliac Arteries (EIA)

opposed to the common drainage trunk of the left and middle hepatic veins. After a short distance of about three to four centimeters, the IVC runs through its diaphragmatic foramen to enter the right atrium (RA). It is important to note this very close proximity between the hepatic vein level and the right atrium [1, 3, 4] (Fig. 1.4a, b).

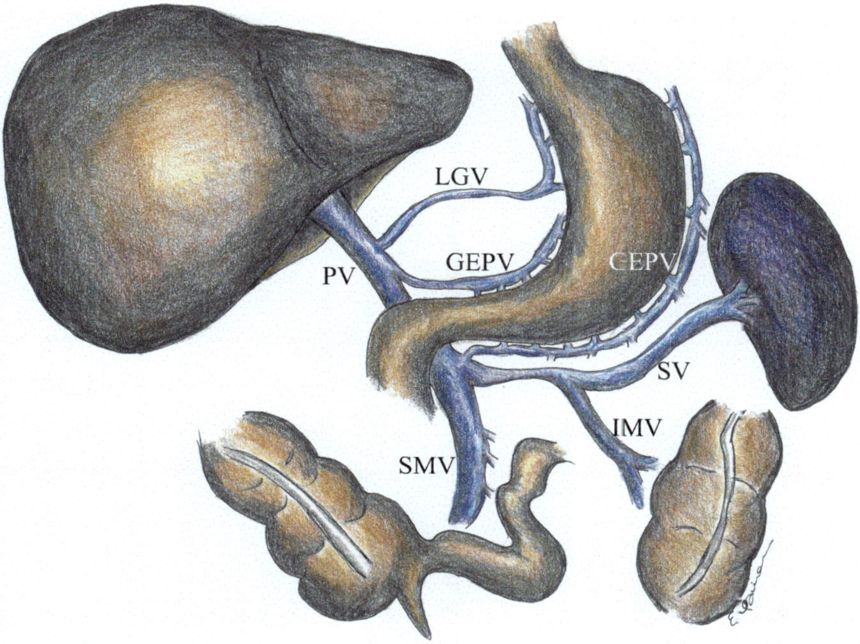

Fig. 1.3 Portal venous system. The portal Vein (PV) is created by the confluence of the Superior Mesenteric Vein (SMV) and the Splenic Vein (SV). The SMV drains the small bowel, ascending colon and part of the transverse colon. The Inferior Mesenteric Vein (IMV) drains the rest of the large bowel. The Left Gastric Vein (LGV), right and left Gastrepiploic Veins (GEPV) and other smaller veins drain the stomach. The pancreas is drained by small branches of PV and SV

Anatomical Variations

Arteries

Arterial anatomy can be variable. Often there is an aberrant left hepatic artery (LHA) arising from LGA or an aberrant RHA arising from SMA. These vessels can have an accessory role, thus contributing to the main blood supply of the left and right liver respectively, or can have a replacing role, meaning that their unconventional position represents the only blood supply to the corresponding liver [1]. These anatomical variations are very important as they can render tumors un-resectable or favour surgical resections that would otherwise not be feasible. These arterial variations can similarly complicate or facilitate liver transplant surgery [1, 5, 6] (Fig. 1.5).

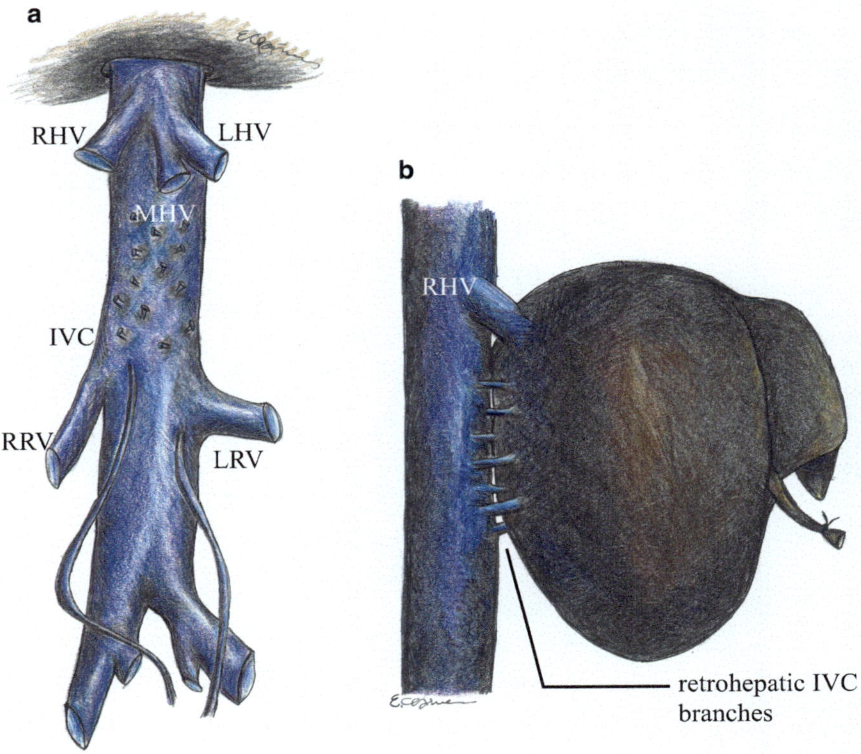

Fig. 1.4 **a** Inferior Vena Cava (IVC) and the three hepatic veins; Right Hepatic Vein (RHV); Middle (MHV) and Left Hepatic Veins (LHV) have common orifice. The liver parenchyma also drains into the IVC via multiple small branches. Right (RRV) and Left Renal Veins (LRV). **b** Profile aspect of inferior vena cava (IVC), liver, Right Hepatic Vein (RHV) and retrohepatic IVC branches

Veins

The hepatic vein anatomy also demonstrates anatomical variations. Most importantly one or more accessory hepatic veins. The existence of these accessory veins is of great significance in liver transplantation using partial grafts [5, 6] (Fig. 1.6).

Portosystemic Shunts

There are areas where communication between portal and systemic circulation naturally occurs in adults and all of them are extra-hepatic. In those areas the portal blood mixes with blood from systemic veins that eventually drain into the systemic circulation [1, 5, 6].

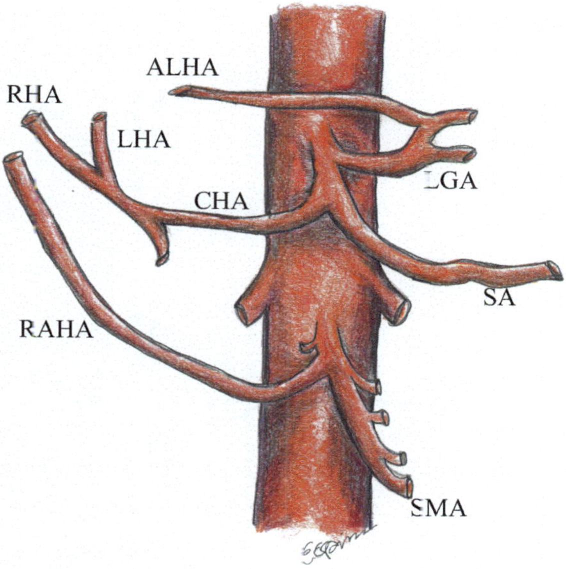

Fig. 1.5 The most common anatomical arterial variations of the liver. Aberrant Left Hepatic Artery (ALHA) arises from Left Gastric Artery (LGA). Aberrant Right Hepatic Artery (ARHA) from Superior Mesenteric Artery (SMA). Their role can be either accessory or replacing, thus the term 'aberrant' is used. One or both may be present with the simultaneous presence of Common Hepatic Artery (CHA). Splenic Artery (SA). Arterial variations play a great role in HPB and Liver transplantion

These anastomotic plexuses exist in four areas:

1. Distal esophagus/gastric fundus
2. Umbilicus
3. Lower rectum
4. Retroperitoneal area around the pancreas, duodenum, spleen, splenic flexure, left kidney.

In the setting of portal hypertension, these areas represent the sites of development of large portosystemic shunts or "varices"; saccular vein structures containing significant amounts of blood, scattered within the abdomen. Variceal formation is a sign of altered haemodynamics and blood flow circulation within the portal system, sign of portal hypertension [1, 5] (Fig. 1.7).

Liver

The liver is the largest solid organ of the body and lies on the right sub-diaphragmatic area, under the lower ribs. Visceral peritoneum surrounds most of the liver surface and peritoneal reflections create several ligaments (left and right triangulars, coronary or hepatophrenic, falciform, hepatorenal and hepatogastric) that support its position and attach it to adjacent organs and structures [1, 3, 4].

The falciform ligament is the landmark for the anatomic division of the liver into right and left lobes. However, surgically speaking the division of the liver into

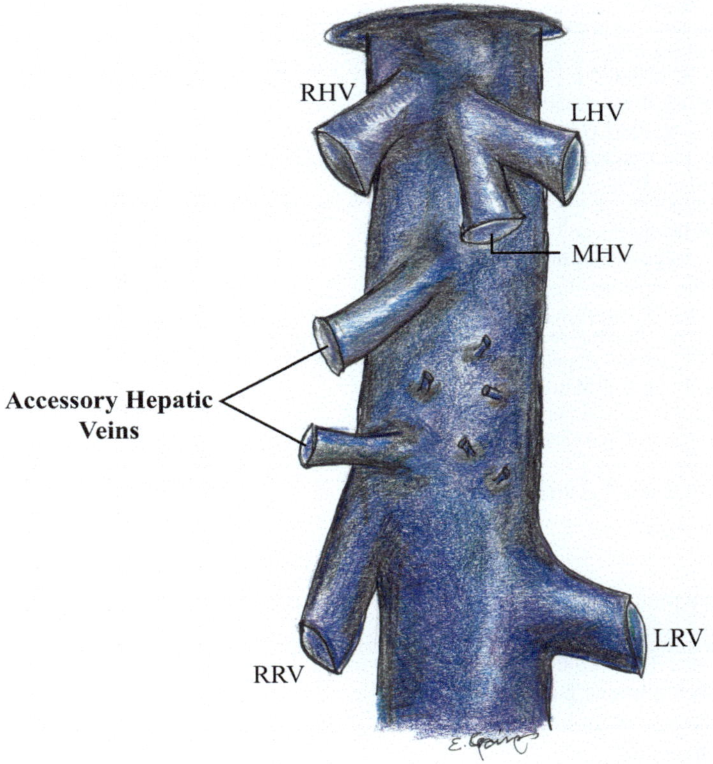

Fig. 1.6 Inferior vena cava (IVC) Right Hepatic Vein (RHV), Middle Hepatic Vein (MHV) and Left Hepatic Vein (LHV). Accessory veins may exist contributing to segmental liver parenchyma drainage. Right Renal Vein (RRV), Left Renal Vein (LRV)

right and left lobes is based on an imaginary line, which runs from the left side of suprahepatic IVC to the middle of the gallbladder bed. This line, often referred to as the Cantlie's line, marks the course of the middle hepatic vein which lies deeper within the liver parenchyma. Thus, liver lying on the right of this line represents the surgical right liver lobe or right liver and liver lying on the left of the line represents left liver lobe or left liver [1, 6] (Fig. 1.8a).

The liver parenchyma is further divided into segments, reflecting the complex infrastructure of the portal pedicles. Each pedicle consists of portal, arterial and bile duct branch and supplies a single anatomical segment dividing the liver in a total of eight segments [6].

Therefore, segments II, III, IVa, IVb constitute the left liver while the segments V, VI, VII, VIII form the right liver. The caudate lobe, which constitutes segment one, has separate inflow and drainage and is not usually included in the terminology of the right and left liver [6] (Fig. 1.8a, b).

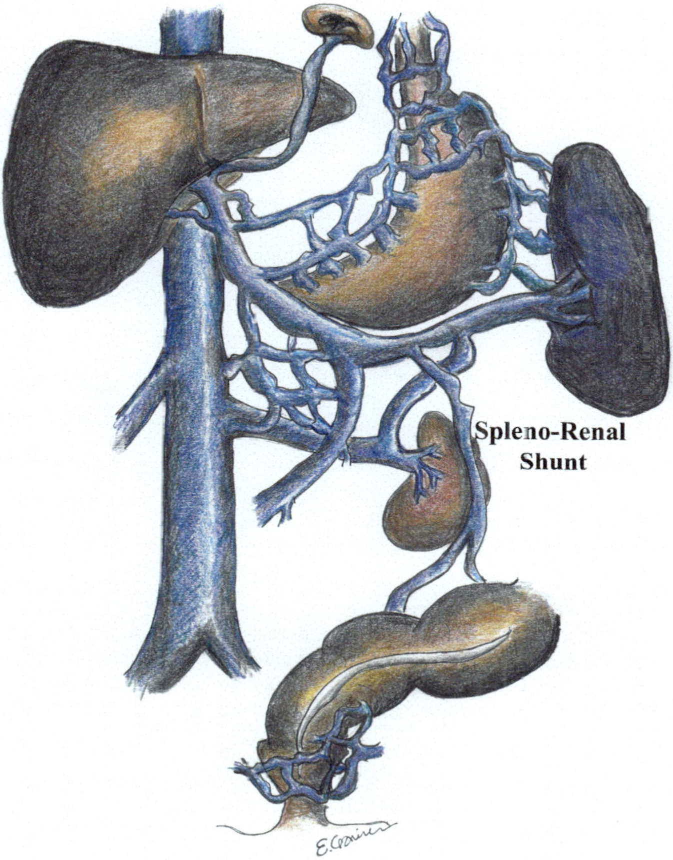

Fig. 1.7 Sites of extrahepatic portosystemic shunts with variceal transformation in the context of portal hypertension; umbilical, esophageal, hemorrhoidal and retroperitoneal. Splenorenal shunt is one of the commonest findings in cirrhotic patients with severe portal hypertension

The liver has dual blood supply from both hepatic artery (HA) and portal vein (PV). The HA, as described above, arises from the CA. At the level of the hilum it branches to right and left HA supplying the right and left liver respectively.

The PV runs from the level of the head of the pancreas into the liver hilum.

The bile duct (BD), the common biliary trunk, is formed by the contribution of bile ducts of the left and right liver lobes, and runs also in the liver hilum in front of the PV, on the right of the HA (Fig. 1.8b) [1, 3, 6].

The three structures bile duct, hepatic artery and portal vein are well surrounded by peritoneal tissue, an extension of the lesser omentum, forming the "hepatoduodenal ligament". Therefore, all three structures can be easily looped by a tape which can be tightened and loosened around the hepatoduodenal ligament

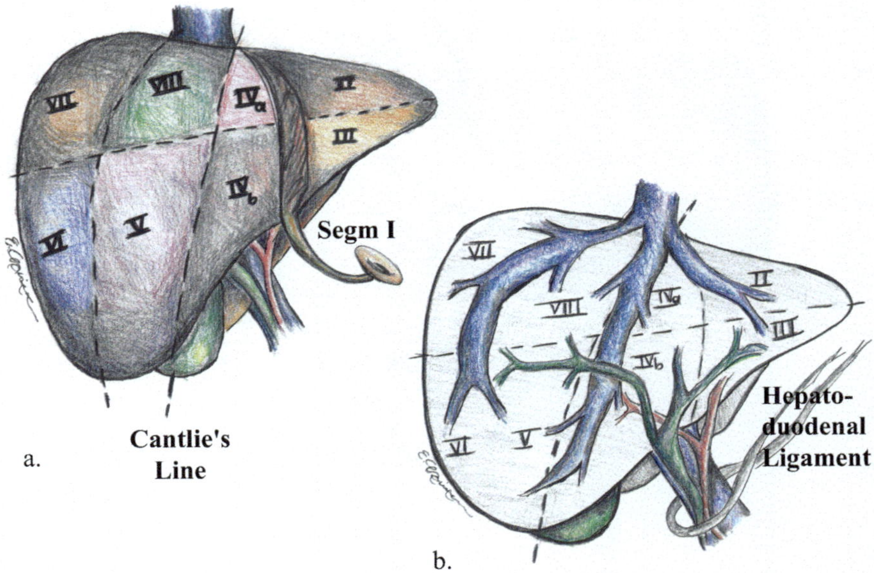

Fig. 1.8 **a** Cantlie's line marks the division of liver in right and left lobes. Arterial, portal and biliary anatomy (portal triads) follow segmental liver anatomy within the liver parenchyma defining surgical division of the liver in eight segments I-VIII. Saegment I, the caudate lobe. **b** The portal vein bile duct and hepatic artery are the structures contained in the hepatoduodenal ligament. Encirclement by tape facilitates intermittent inflow control, the "Pringle maneuver"

therefore achieving control of the blood supply into the liver. This maneuver is commonly used in hepatic resections and liver trauma surgery and is known as the "Pringle maneuver" (Fig. 1.8b) [1, 3, 6].

Biliary Tree

The biliary channels form small and large bile ducts, resembling the branches of a tree expanding into the liver, creating the right and left hepatic ducts. These join into a common channel at the level of the liver hilum, the common bile duct. During the bile duct's course to join the pancreatic duct into the gland's head, the gallbladder's cystic duct joins the former at a variable level [1, 3, 6]. The distal end of bile and pancreatic ducts form a common channel which drains into the bowel. The latter is known as the ampulla of Vater or hepatopancreatic ampulla, located in the second part of the duodenum. The common channel formed by the two ducts is surrounded by a regulating mechanism, the sphincter of Oddi (Fig. 1.9) [1, 3, 6].

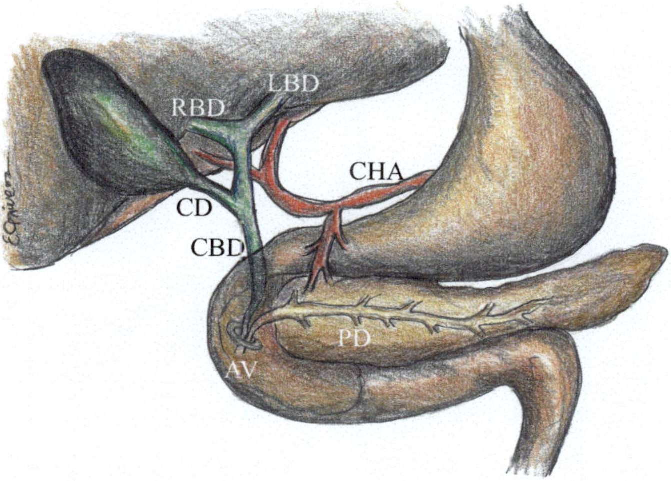

Fig. 1.9 The right bile duct (RBD) and left bile ducts (LBD) join to form the Common Bile Duct (CBD) at the liver hilum. The cystic duct (CD) joins the CBD across its course towards the head of the pancreas. The distal CBD and the pancreatic duct (PD) form a short common channel while entering the second part of the duodenum at the ampulla of Vater (AV)

The ampullary mechanism which includes the junction of the biliary and pancreatic ducts is not amenable to surgical separation. Thus, pathologies at this area require resection of head of the pancreas and duodenum en block [6].

The biliary tree is very oxygen dependent and arterial supply is crucial for its viability. This characteristic is of vital importance in hepatobiliary surgery and liver transplantation [5].

Pancreas

The pancreas is a retroperitoneal organ and lies in front of the spine at the level of L1–L2. Anatomically, the gland is divided into the head, which includes the uncinate process, neck, body and tail. The second and third parts of the duodenum encompass the head of the pancreas while the uncinate process surrounds the orifice of the mesenteric vessels. The rest of the pancreatic parenchyma, expands laterally on the left, across to the splenic hilum [1, 3, 6] (Fig. 1.10). Surgically, pathologies lying on the right side of the SMV/PV axis involve the head of the pancreas, whereas the ones lying on the left side involve the distal pancreas. This anatomical delineation defines the type and the extent of the pancreatic resection required (Fig. 1.10) [6].

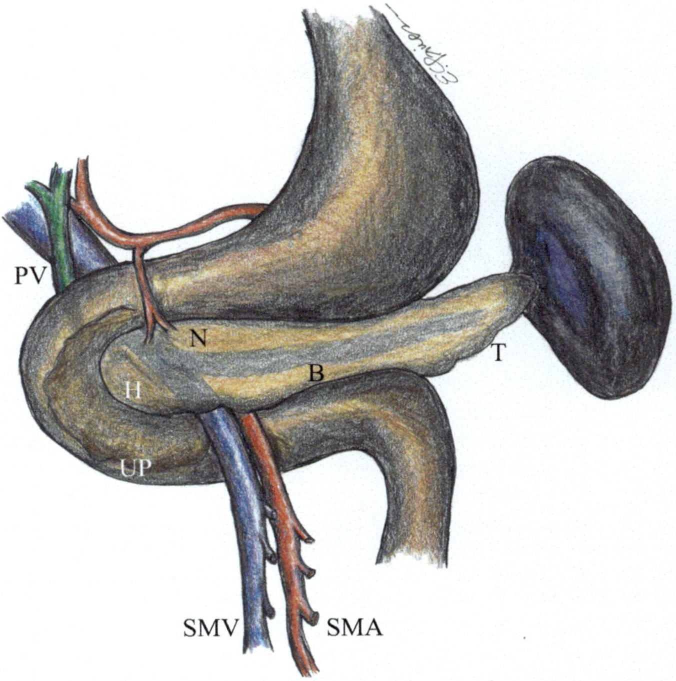

Fig. 1.10 The pancreas; the head (H) of the gland along with uncinate process (UP) is lying on the right of the superior mesenteric vein/ portal vein SMV/PV axis. The body (B) and tail (T) are lying on the left side of the mesenteric vessels. The neck (N) of the gland corresponds to the part of the gland lying anteriorly to the mesenteric vessels. In the background, the superior mesenteric vein (SMV) and splenic vein (SV) confluence to create the portal vein (PV)

References

1. Netter FH. Atlas of human anatomy. 7th ed. Elsevier Health.
2. Sadler TW. Langman' s medical embryology. 14th ed. Walters Kluwer.
3. Standring S. Gray's anatomy: the anatomical basis of clinical practice. 41th ed. Elsevier Health.
4. Snell R. Clinical anatomy by regions. 8th ed. Walters Kluwer.
5. Busuttil R, Klintmalm G. Transplantation of the liver. 3rd ed. Elsevier.
6. Blumgart LH. Surgery of the liver, biliary tract and pancreas. 5th ed. Elsevier.

Chapter 2
Anatomy and Physiology of the Liver

Lucy L. Yang

Introduction

The liver is the largest solid organ in the body with a mass of 1200–1500 g. It develops embryologically as a glandular outgrowth of the primitive gut, forming also the largest gland of the body [1]. It measures roughly 10 cm cranio-caudally with a transverse diameter of approximately 20 cm. Along with the biliary tree and the gall bladder, it lies inferior to the diaphragm, occupying most of the right hypochondrium, protected by the lower ribs 7–12. It is maintained in its position by ligaments formed by the peritoneal layers, intra-abdominal pressure, and attachments to blood vessels and adjacent organs. It has a smooth dome-like surface related to the inferior aspect of the diaphragm, and a visceral surface related to the stomach, the first part of the duodenum, the gall bladder, right colonic flexure, and the right kidney and adrenal glands. The liver is almost entirely covered by the peritoneum, except a small 'bare area' in the postero-cranial aspect, and around the bed of the gallbladder and the porta hepatis; where the vessels and ducts enter and leave the liver.

This chapter will consider liver physiology from the perspective of nutritional modulation, including carbohydrate metabolism, synthesis of important proteins and their metabolism, and lipid metabolism. Furthermore, the liver's ability to process and clear exogenous drugs will be extensively discussed. And finally, the liver's role as a vast storage organ, and its role in regulating the haematological and endocrine systems will be discussed.

L. L. Yang (✉)
Department of Anaesthetics, Royal Free Hospital, Pond Street, London Hampstead NW3 2QG, England
e-mail: Lucyliu.yang@nhs.net

Z. Milan and C. Goonasekera (eds.), *Anesthesia for Hepatico-Pancreatic-Biliary Surgery and Transplantation*, https://doi.org/10.1007/978-3-030-51331-3_2

As background to understanding where the physiological reactions take place, it is helpful to first visualise its macroscopic and microscopic anatomy, mainly from a functional perspective.

Macroscopic Anatomy

The macroscopic anatomy of the liver can be considered structurally or functionally.

Structural Anatomy

Morphologically, the liver is divided into the left and right lobes by the falciform ligament, which connects the diaphragmatic surface of the liver to the inferior aspect of the diaphragm. Anatomically, the right side is approximately 6 times larger than the left. There are two separate smaller lobes which are visible from beneath; the posterior is the caudate lobe and the inferior is the quadrate lobe. However, this anatomical appearance bears no relation to the functions of the liver, and it is generally more clinically relevant to consider the liver in terms of its functional anatomy.

Functional Anatomy

Functionally, the liver is thought of as independent left and right portal lobes, which correspond to the left and right branches of its blood supply. Thus, the functional left and right lobes are approximately equal in size. The left and right lobes are further divided into eight independent segments based on further ramifications of the blood supply. Each segment is supplied by a branch of the hepatic artery and portal vein, and drained by a branch of the bile duct, and the segments are usually numbered by roman numerals I to VIII, beginning with the caudate lobe (Segment I). The left lobe consists of segments I to IV, and the right V to VIII.

Blood Supply to the Liver

The unique feature of the liver is that it receives a dual blood supply; about a third from the hepatic artery and the rest from the portal vein. The liver receives approximately a quarter of cardiac output at rest (1500 mL/min), thus, 500 mL/min comes from the hepatic artery, and the remainder is supplied by the portal vein.

Both vessels enter the liver via the porta hepatis, which is also the region where the common hepatic bile duct exits.

Portal Vein

The portal vein carries poorly-oxygenated, but nutrient rich blood from the capillary network at the gastro-intestinal tract. It is a short wide vein formed by the superior mesenteric and splenic veins posterior to the neck of the pancreas, and it ascends anterior to the inferior vena cava before bifurcating into the left and right branches. In a fasted state, portal blood has an oxygen saturation of approximately 85%, whereas in a fed state, the saturations can be reduced to 70% due to increased oxygen consumption for digestive metabolism.

Hepatic Artery

The hepatic artery carries well-oxygenated blood from the aorta. One of the branches of the coeliac trunk gives rise to the hepatic artery. The initial branch is known as the common hepatic artery, which describes the part from the coeliac trunk to the origin of the gastroduodenal artery, and then it becomes the hepatic artery proper, which is from the gastroduodenal artery to its bifurcation into left and right hepatic branches. Blood from the hepatic arteries is fully saturated with oxygen (98–100%), thus contributing to approximately 50% of the liver's oxygen supply despite only providing a third of the blood flow.

Vascular Segments

Both the portal vein and the hepatic artery divide into left and right branches at or close to the porta hepatis. Within the liver, the left and right branches further ramify to supply each respective segment.

The anatomical classification of the liver based on its eight vascular segments was first described by the French surgeon Claude Couinaud in 1957. The discovery of the completely separate blood supply to the segments allowed surgeons to perform hepatic lobectomies and segmentectomies without excessive bleeding. The intersegmental hepatic veins serve as guides to the interlobular planes, though these can also be major sources of bleeding.

Drainage from the Liver

Venous Drainage

Between the segments lie the hepatic veins, which are formed by the union of central veins of the liver, which drain each of the liver segments. The hepatic veins form tributaries to the inferior vena cava just inferior to the diaphragm.

Bile Drainage

A digestive function of the liver is to produce bile, which is either secreted directly into the duodenum or stored in the gallbladder until required. Bile produced by liver cells drains into bile canaliculi, which merge to form the left and right hepatic ducts. The left and right hepatic ducts drain the left and right lobes of the liver respectively, and eventually form the common hepatic duct. Bile from the gallbladder enters the cystic duct, which joins the common hepatic duct to form the common bile duct that eventually transports bile into the duodenum.

Lymphatic Drainage

The liver produces a huge amount of lymph, contributing to between 25–50% of all the lymph received by the thoracic duct [2]. Lymph from the liver has the highest protein concentration, and drains into the superficial and deep lymphatic vessels of the liver. Superficial vessels lie in the subperitoneal fibrous capsule of the liver and the deep vessels accompany the ramifications of the portal triad and hepatic veins. They carry lymph via several paths; lymph from the anterior aspects of the liver drain into the hepatic lymph nodes, followed by the coeliac lymph nodes, and eventually into the chyle cistern (a dilated sac at the inferior end of the thoracic duct). Lymph from the posterior aspect of the liver drain towards the bare area of the liver into the phrenic lymph nodes and posterior mediastinal lymph nodes, eventually into the right lymphatic and thoracic ducts. Some lymph also drain via the gastric, parasternal, and anterior abdominal wall lymphatics [3].

Nerve Supply of the Liver

Like most visceral organs, the liver receives sympathetic and parasympathetic nervous innervation [4]. The sympathetic supply is from T7-10 via the coeliac plexus, which intermingles with parasympathetic fibres from the vagus and phrenic nerves to form the anterior and posterior hepatic plexus. There is significant anatomical variation in humans [5], but it is thought that the anterior plexus forms a sheath around the hepatic artery and supplies the cystic duct and the gallbladder, and the pancreatico-choledochus nerve and the posterior plexus enters the liver connective tissue and perivascular spaces via the porta hepatis [6].

Microscopic Anatomy

The microscopic anatomy of the liver could be considered in two ways: 1. in the form of thousands of 1–2 mm diameter hexagonal shaped lobules or 2. as functional acini around the portal tracts.

Liver Lobules

The hexagonal shaped arrangements are formed by connective tissue with a branch of the hepatic vein at the centre, and columns of hepatocytes and sinusoids radiating to the six sides (Fig. 2.1). At the corners where the sides meet is the portal triad, made up by a portal venule, hepatic arteriole and a bile duct (Fig. 2.1).

The notion that the liver consists of lobules dates back to as early as the Hippocratic Collections [7]. This concept was adopted by Galen and became the teaching of medieval physicians and anatomy teachers, though there were often disagreements on the number of lobules [8]. In the 16th Century, in his public anatomy in Bologna, Andreas Versalius suggested that the human liver is not made up of distinct lobules, contrary to those observed in animal dissections [7]. In 1833, Kiernan further confirmed distinct lobules in the liver of pigs [8], but it became clearer in the 20th Century that in humans, as connective tissue is sparse compared to that in animals, the hepatocytes form a continuum rather than fixed matrices in a lobular structure. Thus, considering the human liver as acini is more physiologically informative (Fig. 2.1).

Liver Acinus

The microcirculatory acinar structure was first described by Rappaport in 1976 [9]. This was based on earlier observations that liver parenchyma transformed to nodules (cirrhosis) in the areas of microcirculatory periphery, no longer receiving their afferent blood supply. Thus, the acinus is classified according to zones of blood supply and oxygenation. The most oxygen rich region is the area closest to the portal triads (Zone 1). Blood flows from the portal triads towards the central veins. Therefore, the area of lowest oxygen tension is surrounding the central vein (Zone 3) (Fig. 2.1). Zone 2 is an intermediate area between Zones 1 and 3. Zone 3 is the most likely to suffer from hypoxic, toxic, and viral injury.

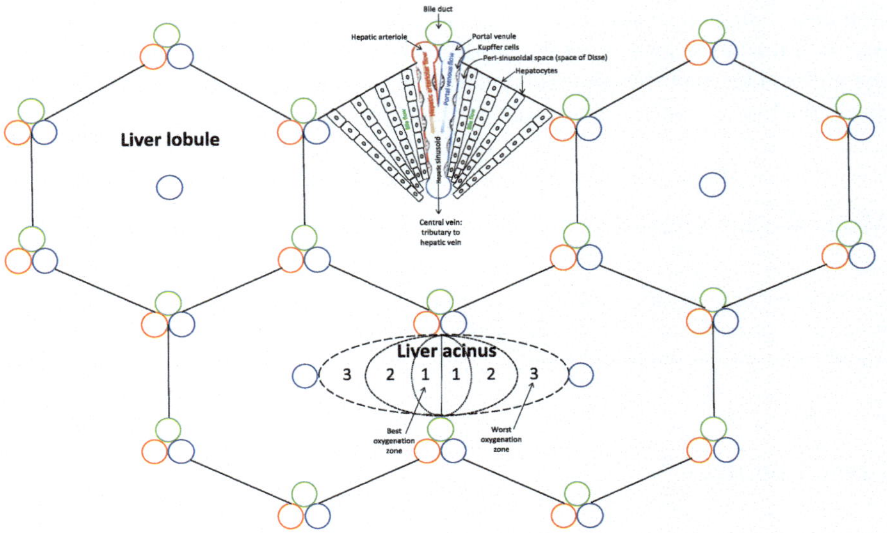

Fig. 2.1 Microscopic anatomy of the liver. Microscopic anatomy of the liver showing the hexagonal liver lobule and functional acinus. Blood flows from the hepatic arterioles and the portal venules towards the central veins, which eventually confluent to form the hepatic vein. Thus, when considering the liver as an acinus, zone 1 is the closest to the oxygenated blood flow, whereas zone 3 is the furthest and is the area most likely to become ischaemic

Cells Within the Liver

Approximately 80% of the volume of the liver is made up by hepatocytes. The rest are sinusoidal cells and peri-sinusoidal cells, which include three main cell types; endothelial cells, specialised macrophages known as Kupffer cells, and stellate cells. Microscopically, hepatocytes form polyhedral anastomosing plates, and the sinusoids run between the cells to carry blood towards the terminal hepatic venule to drain into the hepatic vein. The sinusoids are lined by fenestrated endothelium, with no basement membrane, which is separated from the hepatocytes by a narrow peri-sinusoidal space (space of Disse), where lymphatic drainage takes place.

Hepatocytes

Hepatocytes are highly specialised cells with unusual cellular features. They are large polyhedral cells with round nuclei, which not only vary in size depending on the amount of chromosomes contained in each nuclei, but binucleate hepatocytes are also common in normal liver [1]. It is not unusual for most of the hepatocytes to contain more than twice the normal complement of chromosome in each nucleus, and some even four or eight times this amount. The cytoplasm contains numerous mitochondria, extensive free ribosomes, and smooth and rough endoplasmic reticulum, in order to supply the energy and facilities required for protein synthesis, processing of lipids, lipoproteins, and carbohydrates. Hepatocytes act as a large storage source for glycogen in a well-nourished state. Histologically, hepatocytes with round nuclei can easily be distinguished from the sinusoidal and peri-sinusoidal cells, which have flattened condensed nuclei.

Sinusoidal Cells

Majority of the sinusoidal cells are endothelial cells with a flat nuclei and thin fenestrated cytoplasm. Scattered among them are Kupffer cells, which are large phagocytic cells which form part of the monocyte-macrophage defence system. Stellate cells, also known as Itc cells or hepatic lipocytes are more recently discovered cells. They contain lipid droplets with vitamin A in their cytoplasm and are involved in vitamin A storage and produce extracellular matrix and collagen. These cells become more active during liver injury and produce increased amounts of collagen, leading to the fibrotic appearance that is characteristic of liver cirrhosis.

Liver Function

The physiological function of the liver is complex and affects all systems of the body. The following section will discuss the liver's role in metabolising vital nutrients for the body, metabolising foreign substances such as drugs, and detoxifying and excreting harmful substances. In addition, the liver's role as a large storage organ and in maintaining a healthy immune and haematological system will be discussed.

Nutritional Modulation by the Liver

Large amounts of water-soluble nutrients are absorbed from the intestine and transported to the liver via portal blood. The nutrients include amino acids, monosaccharides, fatty acids, and vitamins. The liver plays a key role in the synthesis, metabolism, and storage of all of these.

Metabolism of Carbohydrates

Glucose is a vital component for supplying the body with energy. Red blood cells and the renal medulla are totally dependent on blood glucose, and glucose is the preferred substrate for the brain. The liver is extensively involved in carbohydrate metabolism and regulates blood glucose by the following mechanisms: 1. the glycolysis pathway converts glucose to pyruvate as a substrate for energy and for the synthesis of fatty acids, 2. the glycogenesis pathway converts glucose to the storage molecule glycogen, and 3. during fasting, gluconeogenesis and glycogenolysis take place, so that glucose can be secreted and used as energy by glucose-dependent tissues.

After a meal, the liver oxidises glucose by glycolysis to meet its immediate energy needs and stores excess glucose as glycogen. Glucose is taken up by hepatocytes via the GLUT 4 transporter and is converted to glucose-6-phosphate; a substrate for glycolysis or glycogenesis. In glycolysis, glucose-6-phosphate converts to fructose-1,6-biphosphate, which enters a multi-step pathway, resulting in the production of 2 mol of adenosine triphosphate (ATP) and pyruvate, which is a vital substrate for producing further energy. Pyruvate can either be converted to acetyl co-enzyme A (acetyl-CoA) to enter the tricarboxylic acid (TCA) cycle and oxidative phosphorylation in order to generate a large amount of ATP, or it can be reduced to lactate under anaerobic conditions (Fig. 2.2).

In glycogenesis, glucose-6-phosphate is converted to glucose-1-phosphate and then to uridine diphosphate glucose (UDP-glucose), eventually resulting in glycogen (Fig. 2.2). Glycogen is the main carbohydrate store and may account for 7–10% of the weight of a healthy liver.

During fasting, glycogenolysis occurs to release glucose molecules. In addition, gluconeogenesis occurs, whereby glucose is synthesized from non-carbohydrate precursors. The three major sources of carbon for gluconeogenesis are lactate, glycerol, and amino acids, particularly alanine, which can all be converted to pyruvate. In this case, pyruvate is an important substrate for gluconeogenesis. Starting from pyruvate, the steps in gluconeogenesis is almost the reverse of glycolysis (Fig. 2.2), though the energy requirements differ. Gluconeogenesis requires 6 moles of ATP, whereas glycolysis releases 2 moles of ATP. This energy deficit is recovered by oxidative means, or obtained from ß-oxidation of fatty acids under fasting conditions [11].

The regulation of glucose is tightly controlled by hormones and depending on the physiological condition, either glycolysis or gluconeogenesis predominates. The pancreas secretes insulin into the portal blood; the liver is extremely sensitive to and is the first organ to respond to changes in insulin levels. Insulin lowers the blood sugar level by stimulating glycolysis and glycogenesis, as well as greatly suppresses gluconeogenesis. In type 1 diabetics, excessive gluconeogenesis occurs as a result of a lack of insulin. Glucagon and adrenaline increase the blood sugar level by stimulating glycogenolysis and gluconeogenesis. The rate limiting

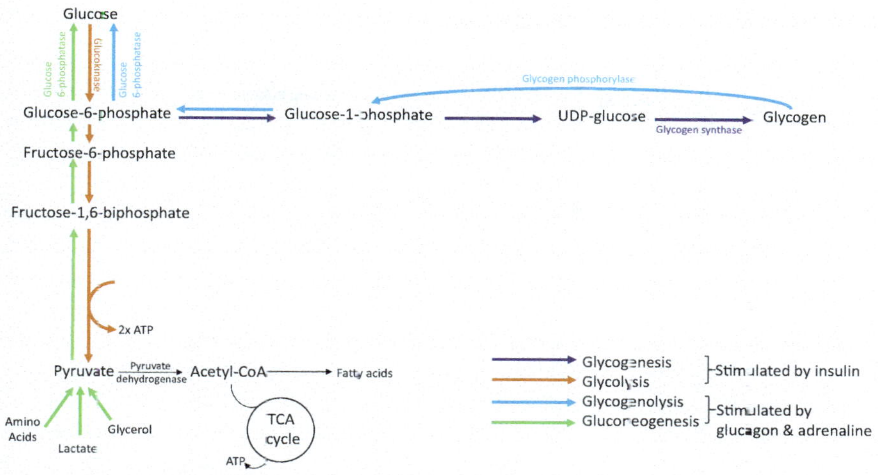

Fig. 2.2 Carbohydrate metabolism. Glucose is taken up by hepatocytes and is converted to glucose-6-phosphate. In glycolysis, glucose-6-phosphate converts to fructose-1,6-biphosphate and eventually to pyruvate. In glycogenesis, glucose-6-phosphate is converted to glucose-1-phosphate, then to UDP-glucose, eventually to glycogen. Pyruvate can be produced from glycolysis, but can also be produced from amino acids, lactate, and glycerol. It is an important substrate for energy (ATP) production and for gluconeogesis. Gluconeogenesis is almost the reverse of glycolysis, and glycogenolysis the reverse of glycogenesis. *Abbreviations* Acetyl-CoA, acetyl coenzyme A; ATP, adenosine triphosphate; TCA, tricarboxylic acid cycle; UDP-glucose, uridine diphosphate glucose

factor of glucose metabolism is usually not liver enzymes but the availability of substrates, hence deranged glucose regulation is usually a late sign of liver failure.

Lactate Metabolism

Whilst the liver is a major site for glycolysis, almost every cell in the body can oxidise glucose for energy [11]. During short periods of intensive work, muscles utilise glycogen stores to generate glucose-6-phosphate and drive the anaerobic production of 2 ATP and pyruvate. However, when there is a lack of substrates for the TCA cycle and oxidative phosphorylation, the pyruvate will be reduced to lactate. Lactate can also be produced by numerous other cells, including red blood cells and skin cells. Built up lactate returns to the liver via the blood stream and is metabolised back into glucose via gluconeogenesis, which requires 6 moles of ATP. Thus, under anaerobic conditions or in liver dysfunction, there is often a deleterious accumulation of lactate in the blood stream. The process of lactate production and metabolism is collectively known as the Cori cycle (Fig. 2.3).

Protein Synthesis and Metabolism

The major protein synthesised in the liver is albumin, which comprises approximately 60% of all plasma proteins. The liver can synthesise about 3 g of albumin a day, which is essential for maintaining the oncotic pressure of plasma and preserving intravascular volume. The importance of this is epitomised in both chronic liver disease and severe long-term starvation, whereby reduced plasma proteins manifests clinically as tissue oedema and ascites. Albumin is also an important carrier protein for transporting many substances, such as fatty acids and certain drugs.

Globulins make up approximately 35% of plasma proteins, of which only alpha and beta globulins are synthesised in the liver and gamma-globulins are produced by plasma cells. The alpha globulins include haptoglobulin which binds to free haemoglobin released from red blood cells after haemolysis, caeruloplasmin which transports copper and oxidises iron, and thyroxine-binding globulin which transports thyroxine. Beta globulins include transferrin which transports iron, and sex hormone-binding globulin which binds androgens and oestrogen.

The other 5% of proteins consist of those involved in inflammation, coagulation, alpha-1-acid glycoprotein for transporting basic and neutrally-charged drugs, enzymes such as pseudocholinesterases, and protease inhibitors.

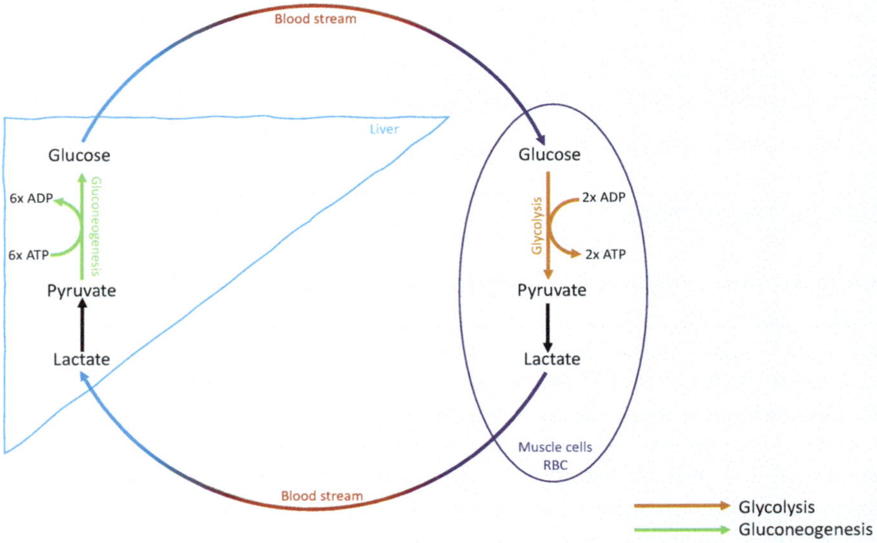

Fig. 2.3 The Cori cycle. Lactate can be produced by numerous cells, including the red blood cells, muscles, and skin cells. Lactate returns to the liver via the blood stream and is metabolised back into glucose via gluconeogenesis. *Abbreviations* ADP, adenosine diphosphate; ATP, adenosine triphosphate; RBC, red blood cells

Inflammatory Proteins and Protease Inhibitors

The liver's Kupffer cells play a major role in modulating immune function. Bacteria, viruses, and parasites ingested into the gastrointestinal tract pass through the liver via the portal circulation before reaching the systemic circulation. Kupffer cells phagocytose these micro-organisms and initiate an inflammatory response by synthesising and secreting pro-inflammatory cytokines and inflammatory proteins. Systemic inflammation can be observed by measuring inflammatory proteins in the blood, such as fibrinogen, ferritin, complement proteins, and C-reactive protein.

The liver also has its own way of attenuating inflammation to protect the body from chronic inflammatory damage. It does this by synthesising protease inhibitors. One important protease inhibitor is alpha-1-antitrypsin. Alpha-1-antitrypsin inhibits enzymes released from activated inflammatory cells such as neutrophils. Neutrophils secrete the protease neutrophil elastase, which could destroy elastic tissue in lungs and in the liver. Alpha-1-antitrypsin inhibits proteases including neutrophil elastase and prevents severe damage to tissues caused by inflammation. When this function is deficient, as seen in the genetic condition alpha-1-antitrypsin deficiency, patients are highly predisposed to chronic obstructive pulmonary disease, and liver cirrhosis.

Synthesis and Regulation of Coagulation Factors

Many clotting factors are synthesised by the liver hepatocytes in the rough endoplasmic reticulum. These include: factors I (fibrinogen), II (prothrombin), V, VII, IX, X, XI, antithrombin III, protein C and protein S. Vitamin-K-catalysed-gamma-carboxylation is involved in the synthesis and activation of factors II, VII, IX and X, protein C and protein S.

The Kupffer cells (monocyte-macrophage system) are involved in the removal of clotting factors and factor-inhibiting complexes. The liver's reserve for this is small, thus liver dysfunction is often associated with ineffective clearance of activated coagulation proteins, resulting in a predisposition to major haemorrhage and disseminated intravascular coagulation.

Amino Acid Metabolism and Nitrogen Balance

In comparison to carbohydrate metabolism, amino acid metabolism is complex. The liver uses amino acids to synthesise proteins and non-essential amino acids, and some amino acids are used for gluconeogenesis (Fig. 2.4). The process of interconverting amino acids and removing nitrogen requires several enzymes including transaminases, glutamate dehydrogenase, and deaminases. The eventual outcome of amino acids is that the carbons are oxidised to carbon dioxide and water, whereas the nitrogen is converted to urea, which can be easily excreted. Various cells in the body and gut bacteria release the nitrogen from amino acids and nucleic acids as ammonia or ammonium ions, which are highly neurotoxic. Ammonia and ammonium ions can be interconverted, thus the two terms are often used interchangeably [11]. In a healthy individual, ammonia and ammonium ions are rapidly removed from the blood and converted to urea by the liver in the urea cycle (Fig. 2.4). In the case of chronic liver disease, insufficient removal of ammonia can lead to severe hepatic encephalopathy.

Lipid Metabolism

The liver plays a key role in the metabolism and recycling of dietary lipids. Dietary lipids enter the body as triglycerides, which exist as a glycerol backbone with 3 fatty acids. Triglycerides are insoluble in water, thus are packaged together with proteins and phospholipids to form chylomicrons, very low density lipoproteins (VLDL), low density lipoproteins (LDL), and high density lipoproteins

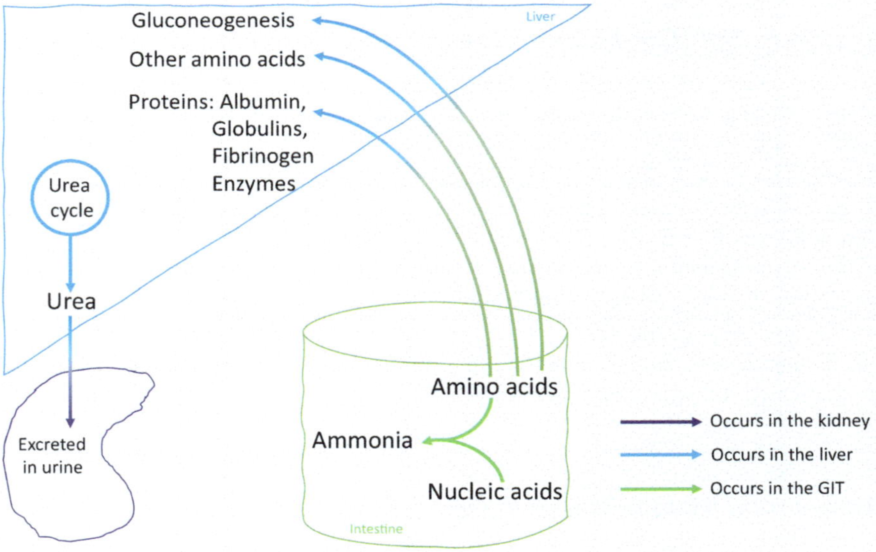

Fig. 2.4 Protein synthesis and amino acid metabolism. The liver uses amino acids to synthesise proteins, synthesise non-essential amino acids, and for gluconeogenesis. Nitrogen is released from amino acids and nucleic acids as ammonia or ammonium ions. Ammonia and ammonium ions enter the urea cycle and are converted to urea, which can be excreted in the urine. *Abbreviations* GIT, gastrointestinal tract

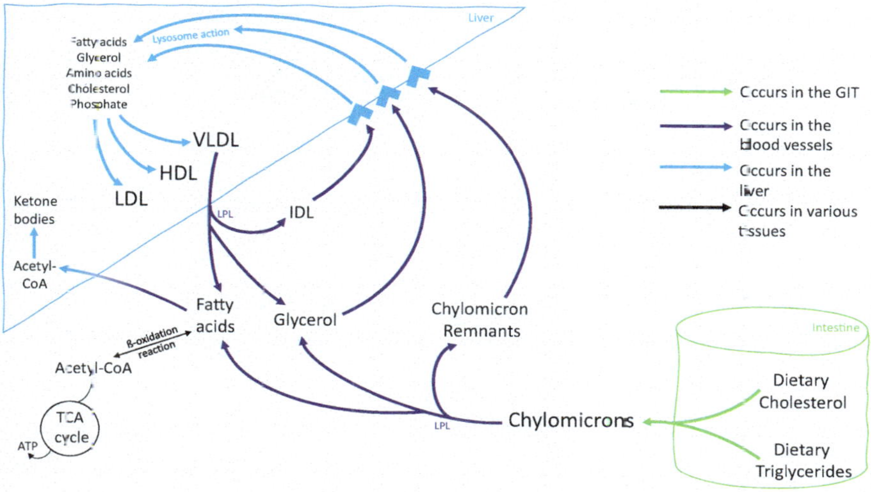

Fig. 2.5 Lipid metabolism. Chylomicrons are produced in the small intestine, whereas VLDL, LDL, and HDL are mainly synthesised in the liver. Dietary cholesterol and triglycerides are packaged into chylomicrons and secreted from the small intestine. Liproprotein lipase in vascular endothelial cells liberate fatty acids and glycerol from chylomicrons and VLDLs, leaving chylomicron remnants and IDL. In the liver, fatty acids, amino acids, glycerol, cholesterol, and phosphate are liberated by lysosomes and re-utilised to synthesise VLDL, LDL, and HDL. *Abbreviations* Acetyl-CoA, acetyl coenzyme A; ATP, adenosine triphosphate, GIT, gastrointestinal tract; HDL, high density lipoprotein; IDL, intermediate density lipoprotein; LDL, low density lipoprotein; LPL, lipoprotein lipase; TCA, tricarboxylic acid cycle; VLDL, very low density lipoprotein

(HDLs) (Fig. 2.5). Aside from chylomicrons, which are produced in the small intestine, the vast majority of the lipoproteins are synthesised in the liver. The protein and phospholipid on the surface of these lipoprotein particles stabilise the hydrophobic triglyceride centre so that it can be transported in blood. Dietary cholesterol is also transported in the blood as these lipoproteins (Fig. 2.5).

The exogenous lipoprotein pathway begins with the incorporation of dietary lipids into chylomicrons (Fig. 2.5), which are the lowest density due to the high triglyceride and low protein content. After they are secreted into the circulation from the small intestine, lipoprotein lipase from vascular endothelial cells acts on them to liberate fatty acids and glycerol, producing chylomicron remnants. These are taken into the liver via a receptor-mediated endocytosis to be used for synthesis of VLDL, LDL, and HDL (Fig. 2.5). VLDL are denser but smaller in size than chylomicrons. They can be produced in the small intestine, but the liver synthesises about 10 times more. VLDL are liberated into glycerol, fatty acids, and intermediate density lipoproteins (IDL), which are either used as fuel for the body, or are re-utilised by the liver to synthesise lipoproteins (Fig. 2.5) [11]. Functionally, VLDLs and LDLs transport cholesterol from the liver to other organs, whereas HDL can remove cholesterol from the peripheral tissue and transport it to the liver (reverse cholesterol transport). Hepatic cholesterol can be

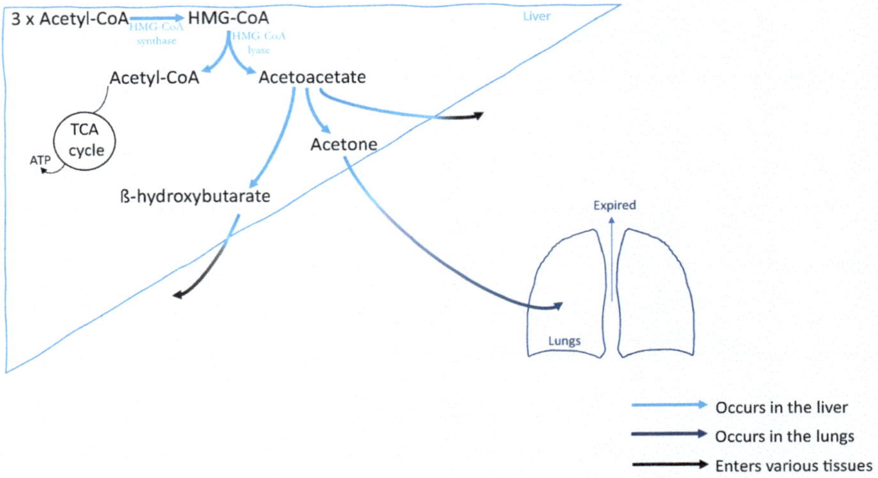

Fig. 2.6 Ketone body generation. Three acetyl-CoA join together to form HMG-CoA. HMG-CoA is then cleaved by HMG-CoA lyase to form acetyl-CoA and acetoacetate. Acetoacetate can enter blood as a ketone body, or it can be converted to ß-hydroxybutarate or acetone, which is expired by the lungs. *Abbreviations* Acetyl-CoA, acetyl coenzyme A; ATP, adenosine triphosphate; HMG-CoA, 3-hydroxy-3-methylglutaryl Coenzyme A; TCA, tricarboxylic acid cycle

recycled by means of forming bile acids, biliary cholesterol secretion, the lipoproteins, and the synthesis of liver membranes.

The group of proteins associated with lipoprotein synthesis is the apolipoproteins, which are also produced in the liver. Apolipoprotein B48 are mainly associated with chylomicron synthesis, whereas B100 are associated with VLDLs. B48 and B100 are encoded by the same gene and are structurally similar. Apolipoprotein E is associated with LDL and A, C, and E with HDLs [11]. In abetalipoproteinemia where apolipoprotein B synthesis is blocked, lipoprotein secretion is impaired and large lipid droplets remain in the hepatocytes.

In the fasted state, stored fatty acids are liberated from adipose tissue and are taken up by the liver cells. Hepatocytes oxidise free fatty acids by ß-oxidation to generate acetyl-CoA. Acetyl-coA can either enter the TCA cycle or produce ketone bodies, and when there is a shortage of substrates for the TCA cycle, the acetyl-CoA is channelled towards producing ketones (Figs. 2.5 and 2.6) [11].

Ketone Body Production

There are three main ketone bodies in humans; acetoacetate, ß-hydroxybutarate, and acetone, but they all originate from acetoacetate. The process of ketone body production begins by three acetyl-CoA joining together to form

3-hydroxy-3-methylglutaryl coenzyme A (HMG-CoA), which is a reaction catalysed by the enzyme HMG-CoA synthase (Fig. 2.6). Subsequently, HMG-CoA is cleaved by HMG-CoA lyase to form acetyl-CoA and acetoacetate (Fig. 2.6). Acetoacetate can enter blood as a ketone body itself, or it can be converted to the secondary ketone bodies ß-hydroxybutarate or acetone, which can be expired by the lungs (Fig. 2.6). The enzymes required to produce ketone bodies are mainly found in the liver mitochondria, and are induced during fasting [11]. This is a useful mechanism during prolonged fasting with low glucose, as the many tissues (brain, muscles, and kidneys) can use ketone bodies for energy. However, the body lacks the necessary enzymes to metabolise ketone bodies, thus in prolonged fasting, or in the case of diabetes mellitus, where the body is not able to utilise glucose, ketosis and ketoacidosis can occur.

Synthesis of Bile

According to Hippocratic physiology, black bile and yellow bile were recognised as cardinal humours that circulated throughout the body and influenced disease [12]. Today, the circulation and function of bile is slightly better understood. The liver uses cholesterol to synthesise bile acids by reactions involving cytochrome P450 enzymes that hydroxylate the steroid nucleus, followed by oxidation and cleavage of the side chain (or less commonly, hydroxylate the steroid side chain and subsequently modify the nucleus) [13]. It produces 0.2–0.4 g of bile acids and secretes approximately 1–1.5 litres of bile per day. This is either secreted into the duodenum or significantly concentrated and stored within the gall bladder (Fig. 2.7) [14]. After a meal, cholecystokinin released from the pancreas stimulates gallbladder contraction and releases stored bile into the gastrointestinal tract, where it serves as a detergent to facilitate the absorption of dietary fats via the gut wall, and transports waste products for elimination and excretion. The pKa of bile acids is about 6, thus in the intestinal lumen (pH 6), about half the molecules are ionised to bile salts (sometimes used interchangeably with bile acids). On average, approximately 85–90% bile circulates in the intestines and 10–15% is stored in the gallbladder [13]. Greater than 95% of bile acids are reabsorbed from the small intestine into the enterohepatic circulation and recycled by the liver. Less than 5% bile acids are excreted via faeces and this is the main route of cholesterol excretion [11]. Although bile is essential for intestinal absorption of dietary fat, the gallbladder is not essential, as humans are still able to digest and absorb fats after a cholecystectomy.

Bile is the primary pathway for the elimination of bilirubin, excess cholesterol, and drug molecules. Bilirubin is a degradation product of haem and the liver plays an important role in its conjugation. When erythrocytes reach their life span (approx. 120 days), they are phagocytosed by the spleen and the reticuloendothelial system (Fig. 2.7). Globin is cleaved to its constituent amino acids and iron is returned to the body's stores or is recycled for erythropoiesis. Haem is oxidised

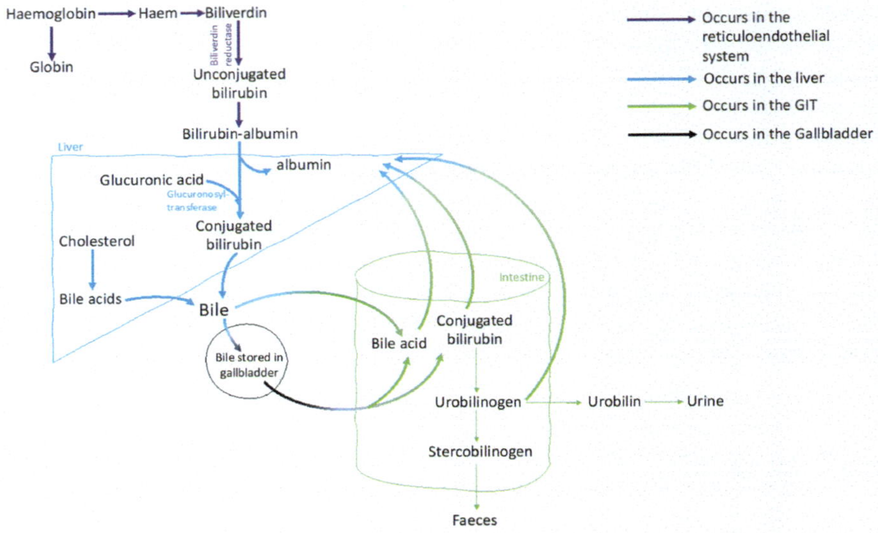

Fig. 2.7 Synthesis of bile and bilirubin metabolism. The liver synthesises bile, which is released into the duodenum and stored in the gallbladder. Bile contains bile acids, which are synthesised from cholesterol, and bile is also an important transport medium for excretion of waste products. Haemoglobin from senescent erythrocytes are broken down to haem and globin. Haem is converted to biliverdin, which is reduced to bilirubin. This unconjugated bilirubin is bound to albumin and transported to the liver. Hepatocytes conjugate bilirubin to glucuronic acid. Conjugated bilirubin is secreted with the bile into the gall bladder. When secreted into the intestine, most bile acids and conjugated bilirubin are reabsorbed are re-excreted in bile. The small amount of conjugated bilirubin that is not reabsorbed passes into the large intestine and is converted to urobilinogen. Some urobilinogen is reabsorbed, and the remainder is either converted to urobilin and excreted by the kidneys, or to stercobilinogen and excreted in faeces. *Abbreviations* GIT, gastrointestinal tract

and cleaved to produce carbon monoxide and biliverdin. Biliverdin is reduced to bilirubin by biliverdin reductase. This unconjugated bilirubin is not water soluble, thus is bound to albumin and transported to the liver for conjugation.

In the liver, the hepatocytes take up bilirubin and conjugate bilirubin to glucuronic acid; a reaction catalysed by glucuronosyltransferase and takes place in the endoplasmic reticulum (Fig. 2.7). Conjugated bilirubin is secreted with the bile into the small intestine. Almost all of the conjugated bilirubin is reabsorbed from the small intestine and enters into the enterohepatic circulation in which it is transported back into the liver, where it is re-excreted into bile. Bilirubin is the main pigment in bile, but the small amount that is not reabsorbed passes into the large intestine and is converted to colourless urobilinogen by colonic bacteria. Approximately 20% urobilinogen is reabsorbed again by the gut entering the enterohepatic circulation. However, hepatic uptake is incomplete, thus some enter the systemic circulation and are converted to urobilin and excreted by the kidneys. The urobilinogen destined for excretion is further oxidised in the large intestine to urobilin or stercobilinogen, which are excreted in faeces (Fig. 2.7). Stercobilinogen gives faeces the brown colour.

Metabolism and Clearance of Drugs

One major role of the liver that is of particular interest to anaesthetists and intensivists is the significant capacity to metabolise and clear drugs. For the purposes of this chapter, drugs can be defined as a chemical substance of known structure, other than a nutrient or an essential dietary ingredient, which when administered to a living organism produces a biological effect [15].

Drugs are introduced to the body through the digestive system, by direct injection into the blood stream, or absorbed into the blood stream via a mucosal membrane or muscle. Some drugs are more hydrophilic and can mostly be eliminated unchanged in the urine (e.g. digoxin and ephedrine). However, drugs which are less hydrophilic are usually transported to the liver, enter the hepatocytes, where they are metabolised with the aim of making the drug more water soluble so that it can eventually be excreted in the urine or bile. Depending on the structure and properties of the drug, it may undergo either phase 1 or phase 2 reaction, but most drugs undergo phase 1 followed by phase 2 reaction to become sufficiently water soluble. Although both phases have the same end goal, they are catalysed by completely different enzymes.

Phase 1

Phase 1 reactions are catabolic, involving oxidation, reduction, or hydrolysis, resulting in the introduction of a hydrophilic group, such as a hydroxyl group (OH), or carboxyl group (COOH) into the molecule. This hydroxyl group can also be the target for conjugation phase 2 reactions. The hydroxyl group is often reactive, thus paradoxically, the products of phase 1 reactions can be more chemically toxic and carcinogenic than the parent drug. Many hepatic drug-metabolising enzymes are intracellular; cytochrome P450 enzymes are mainly embedded in the smooth endoplasmic reticulum of hepatocytes, some enzymes are in the cytoplasm, and others are found in the mitochondria. Thus, to reach these metabolising enzymes, drugs need to cross the plasma membrane. Hydrophilic drugs do so less easily, so these intracellular mechanisms of metabolism are important for more lipid-soluble drugs.

Oxidation Reactions

Many drugs can be oxidised by different cytochrome P450 enzymes. Cytochrome P450 enzymes (CYP) are a superfamily of haemproteins (haem group bonded to a protein) classified into families and subfamilies by their degree of shared amino acid sequences. Subfamilies are further divided into isoforms. Families are labelled CYP1, CYP2, subfamilies CYP1A, CYP1B, and isoforms CYP1A1, CYP1A2. Over seventy CYP gene families have been described, of which CYP1, CYP2, and CYP3 are the three main ones involved in drug metabolism in the liver (Table 2.1).

The mechanism involves a complex cycle resulting in the addition of one atom of oxygen to the drug to form a hydroxyl group, and the other molecule of oxygen being converted to water. The cycle begins when the drug combines with CYP450 in the oxidised state, which is when the iron in the haem group exists in the ferric form (Fe^{3+}) (Fig. 2.8). Subsequently, NADPH-P450 reductase donates an electron and reduces the iron to the ferrous form Fe^{2+}. The reduced complex combines with oxygen to form an oxygenated intermediate (Fig. 2.8). Another proton and electron are added either from NADPH-P450 reductase or cytochrome b5. From this complex, the OH group forms water with H^+, leaving Drug-CYP450Fe^{3+}O. Finally, the drug product is released with the oxygen atom incorporated, freeing up the CYP450Fe^{3+} to enter the cycle again (Fig. 2.8).

Many drugs are metabolised by more than one isozyme; for example, midazolam and diazepam are metabolised by both CYP3A4 and CYP3A5 (Table 2.1). There are also important genetic variations in the expression and regulation of CYP450 enzymes. Polymorphisms found in CYP2D6 are associated with

Table 2.1 Cytochrome P450 enzymes involved in drug metabolism. Cytochrome P450 enzymes are divided into families, subfamilies and isoforms. Families CYP1, CYP2, and CYP3 are the three main families involved in drug metabolism and the specific isoforms are described here

CYP family	CYP isoform	Drug metabolised
CYP1	CYP1A2	Caffeine, paracetamol, theophylline
CYP2	CYP2A6	Warfarin
	CYP2B6	Propofol, cyclophosphamide, methadone
	CYP2C9	Ibuprofen, warfarin, propofol, losartan
	CYP2C19	Losartan, omeprazole, phenytoin, clopidogrel, diazepam
	CYP2D6	Codeine, metoprolol, flecainide
	CYP2E1	Alcohol, paracetamol, sevoflurane, halothane
CYP3	CYP3A4	Diazepam, temazepam, midazolam, fentanyl, alfentanil, lidocaine, vecuronium
	CYP3A5	Diazepam, midazolam

Abbreviation CYP, cytochrome P450 enzymes

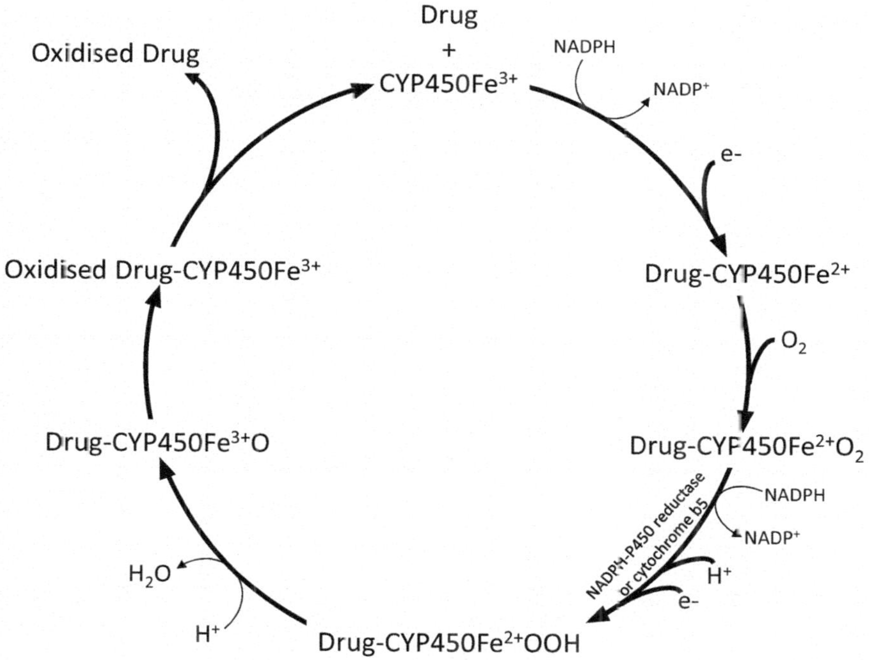

Fig. 2.8 Drug oxidation by CYP450 enzymes. The drug combines with CYP450 in the oxidised state (CYP450Fe^{3+}). NADPH-P450 reductase donates an electron and reduces the iron to Fe^{2+}, forming Drug-CYP450Fe^{2+}. The reduced complex combines with oxygen to form Drug-CYP450$Fe^{2+}O_2$. Another proton and electron are added either from NADPH-P450 reductase or cytochrome b5, to form Drug-CYP450Fe^{2+}OOH. From this complex, the OH group forms water with H^+, leaving Drug-CYP450Fe^{3+}O. Finally, the oxidised drug product is released, freeing up CYP450Fe^{3+} to enter the cycle again. *Abbreviations* CYP450, cytochrome P450 enzyme; Fe^{2+}, ferrous iron; Fe^{3+}, oxidised ferric iron; $NADP^+$, nicotinamide adenine dinucleotide phosphate; NADPH, nicotinamide adenine dinucleotide phosphate in the reduced form

defective metabolism of codeine. Environmental factors and drugs can also inhibit or induce the activity of CYP450 enzymes. A component of grapefruit juice inhibits CYP activity reducing drug metabolism, whereas Brussels sprouts and cigarette smoke induce CYP450 enzymes resulting in faster metabolism of drugs. Ketoconazole and fluconazole inhibit CYP450 enzymes, whereas carbamazepine and rifampicin increase their activity.

Not all drug oxidation reactions involve the CYP450 enzymes. The mitochondrial enzyme monoamine oxidase metabolises the monoamines adrenaline, noradrenaline, and dopamine. Ethanol is metabolised by CYP2E1 as well as a cytosolic enzyme alcohol dehydrogenase, which rapidly converts ethanol to acetaldehyde, which is then further oxidised to acetic acid.

Reduction

Reductive reactions are much less common than oxidations, but some are clinically important. Warfarin is inactivated by conversion of a ketone to a hydroxyl group by CYP2A6.

Hydrolysis

Hydrolytic reactions do not involve CYP450 enzymes. Esterases found in the plasma and cytoplasm of many tissues including liver and muscles hydrolyse esters including aspirin, etomidate, suxamethonium, atracurium and remifentanil.

Phase 2

Phase 2 reactions are anabolic, which involve synthesis or conjugation with a polar group. Although most drugs undergo phase 1 and phase 2 reactions sequentially, if a drug has a suitable 'handle' (e.g. a hydroxyl, thiol or amino group), it is susceptible to conjugation and could directly undergo phase 2 reaction. The polar group may be glucuronyl (morphine, propofol), acetyl (isoniazid, sulphonamides), sulphate (quinol metabolite of propofol), or methyl (cathechols such as noradrenaline) [16]. These reactions mainly occur in the hepatic endoplasmic reticulum, but can also take place in other sites; acetylation also occurs in the lung and spleen. The resulting compound is often inactive, though there are some exceptions, for example morphine-6-glucuronide is an active metabolite of morphine. The compound is usually more water-soluble, ready for excretion in the urine, and high molecular weight or less water-soluble compounds not filtered or secreted by the kidney can be excreted in bile [16].

Hepatic Clearance of Drugs

The manner in which the liver handles drugs is dependent on multiple factors. Drugs administered orally can be extracted during the first pass across the liver (first pass metabolism), this means only a fraction of the drug reaches the systemic circulation and is able to exert its pharmacological effect. The level of extraction is variable and drugs with a high extraction ratio are more dependent on hepatic blood flow (such as morphine and midazolam). In liver disease, particularly in the presence of cirrhosis, the contact between blood and hepatocytes may be altered due to formation of portosystemic shunts, thus reduced extraction of these drugs can lead to a significant increase in its bioavailability [17]. In this case, both the loading and maintenance dose of these drugs should be reduced.

Drugs which have a low extraction ratio during the first pass are less dependent on liver blood flow, but more dependent on the hepatic enzymes for metabolism (e.g. levetiracetam). The bioavailability of these drugs is less affected by portosystemic shunts, but drug clearance is reduced. Thus, these drugs can be started at the normal dose, but maintenance dose of these drugs may need to be reduced. The exception to this rule is low-extraction drugs with high binding to albumin (e.g. phenytoin and valproic acid) [17]. Patients with liver disease often have impaired synthetic function and reduced albumin, resulting in an increased fraction of the unbound drug, which is the one metabolised and excreted by the liver. In this case, the clearance may not be reduced but may in fact be increased [17]. This is significant when considering drug levels; i.e. it would be advisable to look at the free concentration of such drugs rather than total plasma concentration when albumin is reduced.

Unfortunately, there is no naturally occurring substance which could be used to measure hepatic clearance as creatinine is used for the kidney. Liver function can be measured by tests which assess synthetic function (albumin and coagulation) and enzymes associated with hepatocyte inflammatory damage (transaminases). The complexity increases as this does not necessarily correlate with impaired enzymes of drug metabolism. Oxidative metabolism by the cytochrome system is more sensitive to damage in liver disease than phase 2 conjugation reactions, and the enzymes affected are variable. It appears that CYP2C9 and CYP2D6 are less affected by liver disease, whereas CYP2E1 and CYP2C19, and CYP3A4 are significantly impaired [18]. However, this should always be considered in the clinical context. For example, warfarin is metabolised by CYP2C9 (Table 2.1), but patients with liver disease may already exhibit significant coagulopathy.

The presence of hepatic encephalopathy in severe liver failure may be due to the inability to clear ammonia and other molecules. These patients are more susceptible to the effects of benzodiazepines and opioids, thus these drugs should be used sparingly or avoided.

Age and Nutritional Status

It is worth considering the alterations in drug metabolism in liver disease in the context of age and nutritional status. At the extremes of age, capacity to metabolise drugs is reduced regardless of liver disease. In the newborn, the majority of the enzymes involved in drug metabolism are not fully developed, whereas in the elderly, activity of hepatic enzymes is reduced. In addition, patients with severe liver failure are often malnourished due to reduced protein intake and reduced protein synthesis, thus affecting the protein binding of drugs. Presence of ascites due to reduced circulating plasma proteins also changes the fluid compartments and volume of distribution.

Storage and Homeostasis of Iron

The liver acts as a huge reservoir of blood and can release 10–15% of the total blood volume in the form of venous blood into the systemic circulation in response to sympathetic stimulation. The liver contributes to the regulation of red blood cells through iron homeostasis in the following ways: 1. it is a storage site for iron, 2. it produces proteins that balance circulating iron, and 3. it produces proteins which maintain iron transport and metabolism.

Dietary iron is mostly absorbed from the duodenum and the proximal jejunum. At physiological pH, iron exists in the oxidised ferric state (Fe^{3+}), but to be absorbed, iron must be in the ferrous (Fe^{2+}) state. The low pH of gastric acid in the proximal duodenum allows enterocytes to convert ferric ions (Fe^{3+}) to absorbable ferrous (Fe^{2+}) ions [19] (Fig. 2.9). Once Fe^{2+} is absorbed into the enterocyte, it can be released into the circulation via the iron exporter ferroportin. In the circulation,

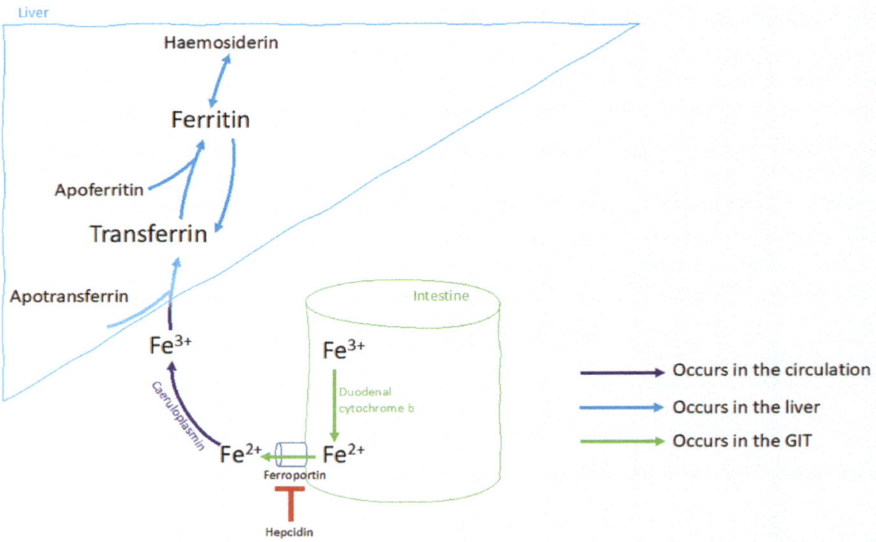

Fig. 2.9 Iron absorption, transport, and storage. Iron exists in the oxidised ferric state (Fe^{3+}) at physiological pH. The low pH of gastric acid in the proximal duodenum allows duodenal cytochrome b enzymes in the enterocytes to convert ferric ions (Fe^{3+}) to absorbable ferrous (Fe^{2+}) ions. The iron exporter ferroportin on enterocytes exports Fe^{2+} into the circulation, where Fe^{2+} is oxidised back to Fe^{3+} by caeruloplasmin. Apotransferrin binds to Fe^{3+} to form the iron-transporting complex transferrin. Apoferritin then binds to transferrin, forming ferritin, which is a storage complex with ferric iron (Fe^{3+}). Excess iron can be added to ferritin to be stored as haemosiderin. The liver also synthesises hepcidin, which inhibits ferroportin, thus inhibiting Fe^{2+} absorption. *Abbreviations* Fe^{2+}, ferrous iron; Fe^{3+}, oxidised ferric iron; GIT, gastrointestinal tract

iron is oxidised back to Fe^{3+} by the copper containing enzyme caeruloplasmin [19] (Fig. 2.9). Free iron is toxic, thus it is transported when bound to proteins such as haem or apotransferrin.

Apotransferrin binds to Fe^{3+} forming a complex known as transferrin (Fig. 2.9), which carries iron in the blood. Transferrin is synthesised by hepatocytes and is normally 20–50% saturated with iron. Storage of iron occurs in most cells, but the majority is in the liver, spleen, and bone marrow. In hepatocytes, the storage protein, apoferritin binds to transferrin and forms the protein ferritin, which is a storage complex with ferric iron (Fe^{3+}) (Fig. 2.9). When excess iron is absorbed, an additional iron can be added to ferritin forming the haemosiderin storage complex. When required, iron can be drawn from ferritin stores, transported in the blood as transferrin, and taken up by the reticulocytes for haemoglobin synthesis. The amount of ferritin in the blood directly correlates to total body iron stores. Clinically, iron overload manifests itself as high serum ferritin level and transferrin saturation, whereas in iron deficiency, ferritin is usually low (in the absence of inflammation), but transferrin may be raised in order to enhance the intestinal absorption of iron [20].

The liver also regulates the systemic balance of iron by synthesising hepcidin. Hepcidin inhibits ferroportin and thus prevents enterocyte Fe^{2+} export and iron absorption. The significance of this is observed in the genetic condition haemochromatosis, where hepcidin deficiency results in un-inhibited ferroportin and excessive Fe^{2+} absorption.

The liver has the capacity to remove old or damaged red blood cells by means of removing haptoglobin bound to free haemoglobin, or haemopexin bound to free haem. Haem oxygenase enzyme in the hepatocytes and Kupffer cells catalyses the release of iron from the haem, which is then recycled and stored as ferritin. Of note, foetal liver is the main site of erythropoiesis in the first trimester [21].

Storage and Regulation of Vitamins

A number of fat soluble vitamins are stored in the liver, including Vitamins A, D, K, B12 and folate. Vitamin A is obtained in the diet from animal fat, fish oils and certain plants. The plant form of vitamin A exist as ß-carotene, which is cleaved to 2 molecules of vitamin A by intestinal cells. In the human body, vitamin A exists in three oxidation states. It is absorbed and transported as retinol, the alcohol. Retinol is oxidised to retinal, the aldehyde, which forms the light-sensing component of the visual cycle. And it is stored in the liver stellate cells as retinyl, the ester [11]. Vitamin K plays an important role in coagulation, and the liver's store of vitamin K is limited, thus significant liver dysfunction often manifests with coagulopathy [22]. The liver is not only involved in the storage of vitamin D, but also in its activation.

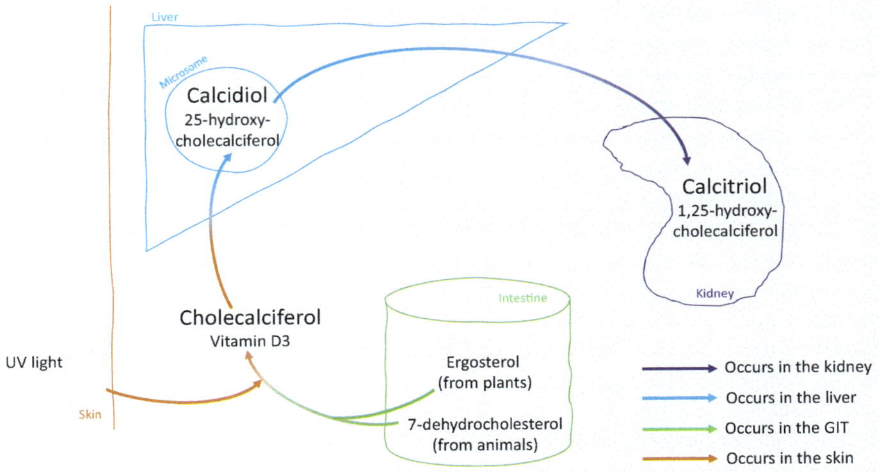

Fig. 2.10 Vitamin D metabolism. Ultraviolet light converts the vitamin D precursors ergosterol and 7-dehydrocholesterol to cholecalciferol. In the liver, cholecalciferol is hydroxylated at carbon 25 to form calcidiol (25-hydroxycholecalciferol). In the kidneys, calcidiol is further hydroxylated at carbon 1 to the active hormone calcitriol (1,25-hydroxycholecalciferol). *Abbreviations* GIT, gastrointestinal tract; UV, ultraviolet

Vitamin D Metabolism

In humans, ultraviolet light in the skin converts vitamin D precursors to cholecalciferol (vitamin D3). The precursors may be obtained in the diet from animals (7-dehydrocholesterol) or plants (ergosterol) (Fig. 2.10). Cholecalciferol travels to the liver, where it is hydroxylated to form calcidiol (25-hydroxycholecalciferol). This is an essential step before calcidiol travels to the kidneys, where it is further hydroxylated to the active hormone calcitriol (1,25-hydroxycholecalciferol) in the proximal convoluted tubules (Fig. 2.10). The renal hydroxylation step is increased when there is a declining level of serum and renal tubular phosphate and calcium. Calcitriol is approximately 100 times more potent than calcidiol, yet the blood concentration of calcidiol is about 100 times greater, thus both hormones play important roles in calcium and phosphorus homeostasis [11].

Regulation of Hormones

Other than the activation of vitamin D, the liver also plays a role in the secretion, transportation, and inactivation of many other important hormones. The liver secretes angiotensinogen, which is a vital component in the renin-angiotensin-aldosterone-system involved in the modulation of systemic blood pressure. Angiotensinogen is a substrate of renin, which converts to angiotensin I in the juxtaglomerular apparatus in the kidneys. Angiotensin I is converted to angiotensin II by angiotensin converting enzyme. Angiotensin II is a potent vasoconstrictor involved in the regulation of vascular tone and blood pressure.

The liver also produces hormones involved in growth and cell differentiation. The hypothalamus produces growth hormone releasing hormone, which stimulates the anterior pituitary to release growth hormone. Growth hormone binds to cell surface receptors and stimulates insulin-like growth factors (IGF). Most cells in the body have mRNA for IGF, but the liver has the greatest concentration, thus is a major site for IGF synthesis and release. The kidney and heart also produce IGF.

The liver synthesises thyroxine-binding globulin which transports thyroxine. The liver is also a major site for the conversion of thyroxine (T4) to the biologically active triiodothyronine (T3), or to the inactive reverse T3.

As already discussed, the liver's role in carbohydrate regulation is sensitive to insulin and glucagon. These hormones are also degraded by the liver and the kidneys. Up to half of insulin is inactivated by the liver (via the portal vein) before it passes into the systemic circulation. Insulin can bind to surface receptors on hepatocytes which leads to the degradation of insulin molecules. Hepatocyte proteases can also degrade insulin without the involvement of the receptor. A number of other hormones are also degraded by the liver, including gastrin, aldosterone, antidiuretic hormone, and oestrogen.

Summary

The liver is an incredible organ extensively involved in nutrition modulation, drug metabolism, excretion of endogenous and exogenous substances, storage, and maintaining haematological and hormonal balance. With physiological pathways that influence so many systems of the body, the liver was thought to be the seat of human emotions by ancient Greeks, reflecting a long-standing recognition of its complexity. In addition to the astonishing regenerative properties of the liver, perhaps this adds insight as to why king Zeus, represented by an eagle, tormented Prometheus for stealing fire by targeting this vital organ. In modern times, it is perhaps more practical to consider the liver resembling a tireless factory with highly specialised workers continuously generating and regenerating, processing, recycling, discarding, and packaging excess material into storage. Though, needless to say, this still greatly underestimates its enormous physiological capacity.

References

1. Young B, Heath JW. Wheater's functional histology. Fourth: Churchill Livingstone; 2000.
2. Ohtani O, Ohtani Y. Lymph circulation in the liver. Anat Rec Hoboken NJ 2007. 2008;291(6):643–52.

3. Moore K, Dalley A, Agur A. Clinically oriented anatomy. 6th ed. Baltimore: Wolters Kluwer|Lippincott Williams & Wilkins; 2010. p. 39.
4. Lautt WW. Hepatic nerves: a review of their functions and effects. Can J Physiol Pharmacol. 1980;58(2):105–23.
5. Skandalakis JE, Gray SW, Soria RE, Sorg JL, Rowe JJ. Distribution of the vagus nerve to the stomach. Am Surg. 1980;46(3):130–9.
6. Sutherland SD. The intrinsic innervation of the liver. Rev Int Hepatol. 1965;15(4):569–78.
7. Sjöstrand NO. The medical illustration as the expression of illusion and imagination–the liver as an example from history. Sven Med Tidskr. 2007;11(1):17–51.
8. History of Liver, Gallbladder, and Spleen [Internet]. [cited 2019 Apr 24]. https://web.stanford.edu/class/history13/earlysciencelab/body1/liverpages/livergallbladderspleen.html.
9. Rappaport AM. The microcirculatory acinar concept of normal and pathological hepatic structure. Beitr Pathol. 1976;157(3):215–43.
10. Chen K-Y, Shen X, Diehl AM. Prometheus revisited. J Clin Invest. 2018;128(6):2192–3.
11. Marks D, Marks A, Smith C. Basic medical biochemistry. Lippincott Williams & Wilkins; 2005.
12. Bullmore E. The inflamed mind. London: Short Books; 2018.
13. Chiang JYL, Ferrell JM. Bile acid metabolism in liver pathobiology. Gene Expr. 2018;18(2):71–87.
14. Chambers D, Huang C, Matthews G. Basic physiology for anaesthetists. First ed. Cambridge: Cambridge University Press; 2015.
15. Rang HP, Dale MM, Ritter JM, Flower RJ, Henderson G. Pharmacology. Seventh ed. London: Elsevier Churchill Livingstone; 2012.
16. Peck TE, Hill SA. Pharmacology for anaesthesia and intensive care. Fourth ed. Cambridge: Cambridge University Press; 2014.
17. Krähenbühl S, Reichen J. Pharmacokinetics and pharmacodynamics in cirrhosis. Med (Baltimore). 2002;30(11):24–7.
18. Rodighiero V. Effects of liver disease on pharmacokinetics. Clin Pharmacokinet. 1999;37(5):399–431.
19. Ems T, Huecker MR. Biochemistry, iron absorption. In: StatPearls [Internet]. Treasure Island (FL): StatPearls Publishing; 2019. http://www.ncbi.nlm.nih.gov/books/NBK448204/.
20. Kelly AU, McSorley ST, Patel P, Talwar D. Interpreting iron studies. BMJ. 2017;15(357):j2513.
21. Congote LF. Regulation of fetal liver erythropoiesis. J Steroid Biochem. 1977;8(5):423–8.
22. Rhoades R, Bell DR. Medical physiology: principles for clinical medicine. Lippincott Williams & Wilkins; 2009.

Part II
Liver Transplantation

Chapter 3
Pathophysiology Behind Cardiopulmonary Complications of Cirrhosis and Portal Hypertension

Søren Møller, Karen V. Danielsen and Flemming Bendtsen

Abbreviations

CABG	Coronary artery by-pass graft
CAD	Coronary artery disease
CCM	Cirrhotic cardiomyopathy
CEE	Contrast-enhanced echocardiography
ECG	Electrocardiography
ET	Endothelin
FEV	Forced expiratory volume
FVC	Forced Vital Capapcity
HH	Hepatic hydrothorax
HPS	Hepatopulmonary syndrome
IL	Interleukine
LVEF	Left ventricular ejection fraction
NAFLD	Non-alcoholic fatty liver disease
NASH	Non-alcoholic steatohepatitis
NOS	Nitrate oxide synthase
PAMPS	Pathogen-associated molecular patterns
PAP	Pulmonary artery pressure
PCI	Percutaneous coronary intervention

S. Møller (✉) · K. V. Danielsen
Department of Clinical Physiology and Nuclear Medicine 260, Center for Functional and Diagnostic Imaging and Research, Copenhagen University Hospital, Faculty of Health Sciences, Kettegaard alle 30, DK-2650 Hvidovre, Denmark
e-mail: soeren.moeller@regionh.dk

F. Bendtsen
Medical Division, Gastro Unit 360, Copenhagen University Hospital, Faculty of Health Sciences, Copenhagen, Denmark

Z. Milan and C. Goonasekera (eds.), *Anesthesia for Hepatico-Pancreatic-Biliary Surgery and Transplantation*, https://doi.org/10.1007/978-3-030-51331-3_3

PoPH	Portopulmonary hypertension
SVR	Systemic vascular resistance
TIPS	Transjugular porto-systemic shunt
TLC	Total lung capacity
TNF	Tumour necrosis factor
VEGF	Vascular endothelial growth factor
vWF	Von Willebrand factor

Introduction

Patients with cirrhosis of the liver during the disease course often develop complications of portal hypertension. These comprise classical complications such as oesophageal varices with risk of bleeding [1, 2], fluid and salt retention resulting in oedema with ascites of various degrees often commencing as mild ascites and progressing to tense and refractory ascites [3]. In the advanced stages of cirrhosis renal function is compromised, which may progress to the hepatorenal syndrome [4]. Clinically, the patients often show signs of vasodilation with characteristic changes in splanchnic as well as in systemic hemodynamics [5–7]. Increased splanchnic inflow and post-sinusoidal resistance are among the splanchnic hemodynamic changes that lead to an increase in portal pressure, which can be assessed by measurement of the hepatic venous pressure gradient [8, 9]. In addition, patients with cirrhosis typically present with a characteristic hyperdynamic circulation with an increased cardiac output, increased heart rate, and low systemic vascular resistance (SVR) and low arterial blood pressure [10–12]. This hyperdynamic syndrome affects most of the organ systems in the body including the heart, the lungs, the kidneys, and adrenal glands referred to as cirrhotic cardiomyopathy (CCM), hepatopulmonary syndrome (HPS), and relative adrenal insufficiency [13–16].

The pathophysiological basis of the hyperdynamic syndrome is a peripheral arterial vasodilatation [17]. An important consequence is an increased portal venous inflow contributing to increased portal pressure [6, 18]. In the systemic circulation the arterial vasodilatation leads to a reduced central blood volume mimicking a physiological effective hypovolemia [19]. Despite intense activation of endogenous vasoconstrictive systems the patients inevitably develop arterial hypotension partly due to reduced vascular responsiveness to vasoconstrictors [20, 21]. Along with the progression of the disease the circulation becomes more and more hyperdynamic until a certain limit. The cardiac output cannot increase further and arterial blood pressure continues to decrease [22].

The pathophysiological consequences for the cardiovascular and respiratory function of the arterial vasodilatation in patients with cirrhosis has become more and more evident during the last decades and the aim of this chapter is in particular to focus on the pathophysiological background behind development of the hyperdynamic circulation, CCM, HPS, porto-pulmonary hypertension (PoPH), and hepatic hydrothorax (HH).

Pathophysiology of Haemodynamic Alterations in Cirrhosis

Cirrhosis of the liver is characterized by hepatic fibrosis and formation of regeneration nodules. Increasing disturbances of the liver architecture is often followed by deterioration of the liver function resulting from reduced capacity of metabolic and excretory functions leading to compromised degradation of vasoactive substances [23]. Development of portal hypertension also represents a significant contribution to the imbalance in vasoactive substances by shunting these through portosystemic collaterals by-passing the liver and thereby degradation. In addition bile acids exert toxic effects on the heart by suppressing myocardial function [24–26]. The results from several experimental studies have pointed to multiple pathogenetic mechanisms for the impaired cardiac contractility in cirrhosis. Among these are defects in the cardiac beta-adrenergic receptor system, and abnormalities in the membrane calcium channels [27]. The pathophysiological effects of humoral factors accentuated by vasodilators such as nitric oxide, cytokines, carbon monoxide, and endocannabinoids escaping hepatic degradation. The combined effect of these vasoactive substances may harmfully affect the contractility of the heart as well as the distribution of flow and volume in the hyperdynamic cirrhotic patient [28, 29]. Finally, recent studies indicate a relationship with the increasing amount of fibrosis in the liver and myocardial fibrosis [30].

Abnormal Haemodynamic Homeostasis

Systemic vasodilatation in cirrhosis is a key element in hemodynamic derangement. Arterial vasodilatation leads to a reduction in SVR and arterial blood pressure and a redistribution of the circulating blood volume with a displacement from central vascular territories to the splanchnic area [5, 31]. In compensated stages of cirrhosis the haemodynamic changes are moderate and the effect of vasodilatation on the SVR and arterial pressure is counterbalanced by the increase in cardiac output [28]. However, in the decompensated stage of cirrhosis the arterial vasodilatation is much more severe with a pronounced decrease in SVR. The cardiac output may no longer be able to compensate the decrease in SVR and central hypovolemia leading to arterial hypotension. At this stage there is an intense activation of sodium and water retaining factors and vasoconstrictive systems such as the sympathetic-, renin-angiotensin-aldosterone-, and vasopressin systems. The resulting hyperdynamic circulation with increased heart rate and cardiac output and activated vasoconstricting mechanisms seeks to maintain the central blood volume and blood pressure at a low/normal level. However, at later stages, the massive renal vasoconstriction together with a fading cardiac output affects kidney function with decreased glomerular filtration rate contributing to cardiorenal syndrome [22, 29, 32, 33].

It is striking that the haemodynamic consequences of sepsis and septic shock very much resemble those of decompensated cirrhosis [34]. Systemic

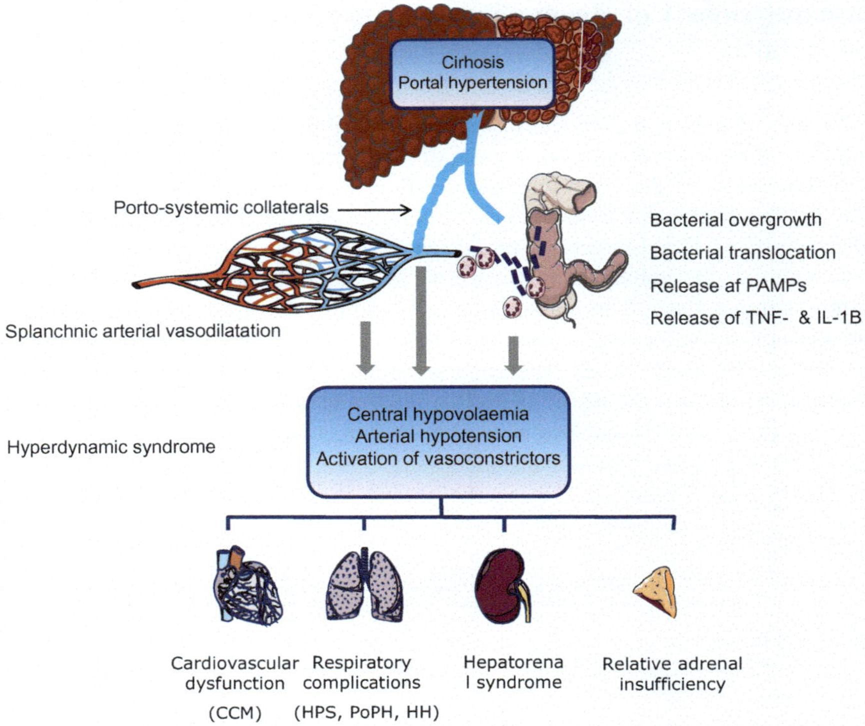

Fig. 3.1 Mechanisms behind the arterial vasodilatation and development of the hyperdynamic syndrome and associated complications in advanced cirrhosis and portal hypertension. Portal hypertension, liver failure, and immunological incompetence facilitate bacterial translocation with release of pathogen-associated molecular patterns (PAMPs), and cytokines (tumor necrosis factor-α (TNF-α, interleukin-1β (IL-1B) and other vasodilators including nitric oxide. A preferential splanchnic vasodilatation leads to activation of vasoconstrictive systems such as the sympathetic nervous system, the renin-angiotensin- aldosterone system and others, central hypovolemia, and arterial hypotension. Complications of the hyperdynamic syndrome include cirrhotic cardiomyopathy (CCM), the hepatopulmonary syndrome (HPS), portopulmonary hypertension (PoPH), hepatic hydrothorax (HH), and others

inflammation also seems to play an important role in the progression to decompensated cirrhosis. Because of impaired immune defence, there is translocation of bacteria and bacterial products from the intestine to extra-intestinal organs. These pathogen-associated molecular patterns (PAMPs) also migrate due to an increased intestinal permeability and thereby activating immune cells that subsequently release cytokines such as TNF, IL-6, IL-8 and NO [35, 36]. Systemic inflammation directly induces cell damage and contributes to the circulatory dysfunction, which may lead to the multi-organ failure in decompensated cirrhosis [28, 32, 37, 38]. Figure 3.1 summarises the relations between the arterial vasodilatation and the hyperdynamic circulation and development of organ failure in cirrhosis and portal hypertension.

Cardiovascular Complications of Cirrhosis

Hyperdynamic Circulation

The physiological consequence of arterial vasodilatation is a reduction in systemic vascular resistance with functional central hypovolemia and arterial hypotension [31, 39]. This is a powerful stimulat of the SNS, RAAS, and the vasopressin system through deactivation of baroreceptors resulting in an increase in heart rate, stroke volume, and cardiac output [40–42]. Nevertheless, arterial hypotension persists because of reduced vascular responsiveness to vasoconstrictors [43, 44]. Increased cardiac output augments flow-mediated endothelial production and liberation of NO and other vasodilators into the systemic circulation [45]. This further augments the vasodilatation with increasing demands on the cardiac output [6, 46]. Therefore, systemic NO overproduction can be considered a result of a primary hyperdynamic circulation [47].

Vasodilatation and impaired vascular reactivity and responsiveness to vasoconstrictors leads to and, increased arterial compliance of the vascular system, which is directly related to the degree of the hyperdynamic circulation and degree of arterial hypotension [48]. Together with altered mechanical properties of large and small arteries this manifests in changed arterial pressure profiles. Thus, the arterial pulsation in cirrhosis seems qualitatively changed with reduced pulse reflections, which may protect against manifest cardiac failure in advanced cirrhosis [49]. This knowledge is utilized in the analysis of the arterial diastolic reflected waveform by calculation of the diastolic augmentation index. The latter seems to predict hyperdynamic circulation, for example, in patients undergoing liver transplantation [50].

Activation of the RAAS and other sodium-water retaining mechanisms subsequently expand plasma volume and increase cardiac preload leading to a further increase in stroke volume and cardiac output [20, 51]. This may in turn lead to an increase in splanchnic flow and portal venous inflow into the liver and tend to further increase the portal pressure [52]. Recently, McAvoy et al. observed increased hepatic arterial flow and increased liver blood flow and reduced renal blood flow by magnetic resonance angiography. This indicated a dysregulated splanchnic vasodilatation causing extrasplanchnic vasoconstriction as part of a splanchnic steal phenomenon [52]. From a pathophysiological point of view, it is unclear, which events that initiate the hyperdynamic circulation are coupling to splanchnic hemodynamics. Thus, in patients with compensated cirrhosis, features of hyperdynamic circulation are more pronounced in patients with clinically significant portal hypertension than in those with a lesser degree of portal hypertension [12]. Recently, in a large patient population comprising 410 cirrhotic patients, we found that a hyperdynamic circulation was independently associated with a higher hepatic venous pressure gradient, a higher hepatic blood flow, and the presence of ascites [10]. Furthermore, the presence of central hypovolemia was associated with hepatic blood flow and hepatic vascular resistance. Therefore, development of the hyperdynamic circulation and central hypovolemia seem mainly explained by changes in portal pressure and hepatic blood flow [10]. Although there seems to be a close correlation between parameters of portal and systemic hemodynamics, it cannot be ruled out what is the chicken and what is the egg. However, the findings support that a backward shear stress on splanchnic resistance vessels lead to splanchnic vasodilatation and consequently systemic vasodilatation and hyperdynamic circulation [53].

Cirrhotic Cardiomyopathy

More than 65 years ago Kowalsky et al. launched the concept of a cardiac dysfunction that was specifically related to the diseased liver [54]. This state of cirrhosis is now recognised as part of the hyperdynamic syndrome [37]. Since then it has been increasingly clear that different pathophysiological mechanisms lead to changes in the filling, strain, volumes, and structure of the heart. Autopsy studies have shown significant changes in cardiac atrial and ventricular volumes and myocardial mass and structure [55]. Recent observations point to the cirrhotic heart as a contributing player, for example, in the development of hepatic nephropathy and the hepatorenal syndrome [32, 56]. The above mentioned assumptions has coined the entity of CCM, which was worded at the World Conference of Gastroenterology in 2005. CCM denotes a triad comprising systolic and diastolic dysfunction and electrophysiological abnormalities of the heart [9, 27].

Pathophysiology

Within the last decades, numerous experimental studies have pointed to different pathogenetic mechanisms for the impaired cardiac contractility in cirrhosis. Among these are defects in the cardiac beta-adrenergic receptor system, and abnormalities in the membrane calcium channels [27]. The pathogenic effects of humoral factors accentuates with the circulation or vasodilators escaping hepatic degradation such as nitric oxide, cytokines, carbon monoxide, and endocannabinoids and may harmfully affect the contractility of the heart as well as the distribution of flow and volume in the hyperdynamic cirrhotic patient [28, 29]. Finally, recent studies indicate a relationship with the increasing amount of fibrosis in the liver and myocardial fibrosis [30]. Bile acids may excert a suppressive effect on the cardiovascular system. Recently, Desai et al. found that high concentrations of bile acids were associated with increased ejection fraction and shortening fraction of the left ventricle but lower heart rate [26]. The same group recently used a double knockout model to show similarities between experimental severe bile acid overload and human cirrhotic cardiomyopathy [57]. They found that electrocardiographic and ultrasonographic features of cardiomyopathy resolved with reversal of liver injury and the authors proposed a new term “Cholecardia” to describe the cardiodepressant effects of bile acids. These results convincingly argue for a direct

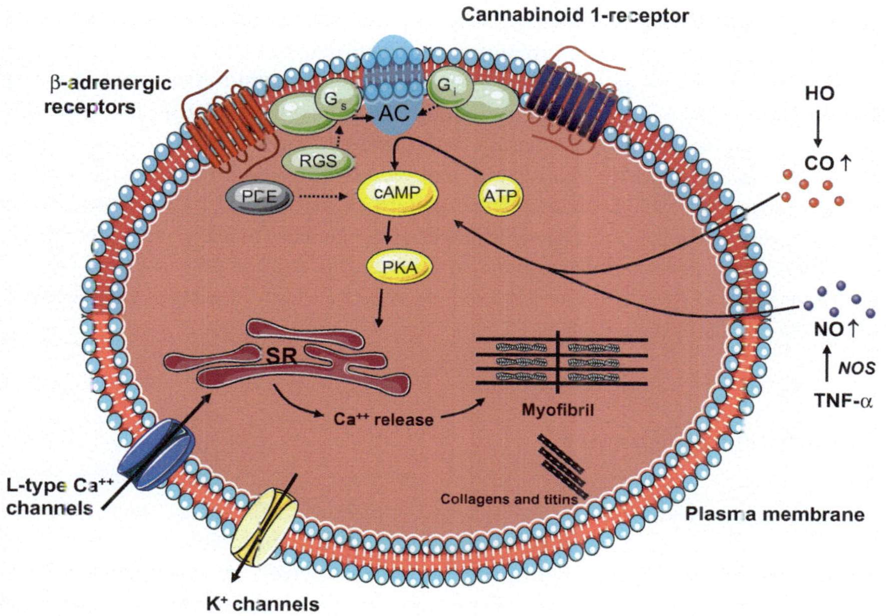

Fig. 3.2 Mechanisms of cirrhotic cardiomyopathy. The figure reviews the most important mechanisms involved in *cirrhotic cardiomyopathy*: Desensitisation and downregulation of β-adrenergic receptors with decreased content of G-protein ($G_{\alpha i}$: inhibitory G protein; $G_{\alpha s}$: stimulatory G protein) and following impaired intracellular signalling; alterations in particular in M2 muscarinic receptors; upregulation of cannabinoid 1-receptor stimulation; altered plasma membrane cholesterol/phospholipid ratio; increased inhibitory effects of haemooxygenase (HO), carbon monoxide (CO), nitric oxide (NO), and tumour necrosis factor-α (TNF-α); reduced density of potassium channels; changed function and fluxes through L-type calcium channels; altered ratio and function of collagens and titins. Many post-receptor effects are mediated by adenylcyclase (AC) inhibition or stimulation. PKA: protein kinase A). From [185]

and reversible effect of bile acids on cardiomyocytes. However, most of the studies on the effects on bile acids on the heart come from experimental studies and more data are needed in relation to human hyperdynamic circulation and cirrhotic cardiomyopathy [24]. Future experiemntal and human studies are likely reveal that differential pathophysiological processes act parallelly in the development of changes of the cirrhotic heart. Figure 3.2 summarizes the pathogenetic mechanisms involved in the CCM.

The Cirrhotic Heart

The cirrhotic heart seems to change in size and structure along with the development of the liver disease. The left ventricular end-diastolic and left atrial volumes tend to be slightly increased, which may be partly explained by a combination of an unrelieved hyperdynamic circulation and diastolic dysfunction [31, 58–60]. The ventricular myocardial mass increases in particular as septal hypertrophy [61–64] and human autopsy studies show frequently cardiomegaly, hypertrophy, and dilatation of the right ventricle correlating with elevated markers of myocardial injury such as pro-BNP [55, 65]. The histological picture from post-mortem myocardial biopsies seems to reveal a characteristic pattern of myocardial hypertrophy, fibrosis, and cardiomyocytes of varied diameter [66]. Newer findings from our group and others have demonstrated increased myocardial extracellular volume (ECV) as measured by magnetic resonance imaging (MRI), which may reflect myocardial fibrosis as a structural element of CCM [30].

Coronary Artery Disease

The prevalence of coronary artery disease (CAD) in cirrhosis has been debated and reports of several studies have been divergent [67, 68]. Newer studies, however, have evidenced a high prevalence of atherosclerotic manifestations with a high frequency of high-grade coronary sclerosis in cirrhotic patients compared to healthy individuals [55]. Similar results have been achieved by cardiac CT where Danielsen et al. found increased coronary artery calcium-score compared with adjusted reference values. The coronary artery calcium-score in alcohol-related cirrhosis was significantly higher than in non-alcohol-related cirrhosis and was moreover associated with diastolic dysfunction [69]. These results show that coronary artery lesions are more common in alcoholic cirrhosis than previously anticipated, results that have been confirmed in a recent meta-analysis [70].

Definition of Cirrhotic Cardiomyopathy (CCM)

CCM is defined by a combination of systolic dysfunction, impaired diastolic relaxation and electrophysiological disturbance*s* such as prolonged QT_C interval. Systolic dysfunction is defined by a blunted increase in cardiac output during exercise or pharmacological stimuli, or a resting ejection fraction < 55%. Diastolic dysfunction is defined from tissue Doppler measurements as E/é > 14, septal e´velocity < 7 cm/s and lateral e´velocity < 10 cm/s, tricuspid velocity > 2.8 m/s, or left atrial volume index (LAVI) > 34 ml/m^2. In addition, supportive criteria include electrophysiological abnormalities in particular a prolonged QT_C interval, heart chamber alterations (enlarged left atrium and myocardial hypertrophy), and humoral changes (elevated BNP, ANP and hs-Troponin-1, Table 3.1) [9, 14, 27, 71]. These definitions were first worded at the World Congress of Gastroenterology in Montreal 2005 [9, 27], but are still under revision.

Table 3.1 Diagnostic and supportive criteria for cirrhotic cardiomyopathy. A working definition

Diagnostic criteria
Systolic dysfunction (one of following)
– Blunted increase in cardiac output on exercise, volume challenge or pharmacological stimuli – Resting left ventricular ejection fraction (LVEF) <55%
Diastolic dysfunction (one of following)
– Average E/é >14 – Septal e´velocity <7 cm/s – Lateral e´velocity < 10 cm/s – Tricuspid velocity >2.8 m/s – Left atrial volume index (LAVI) >34 ml/m^2
Supportive criteria
– Electromechanical abnormalities including the following:
Abnormal chronotropic response to stress Electromechanical uncoupling/dyssynchrony Prolonged QTc interval Heart chamber alterations: enlarged left atrium (LA) and increased left ventricular wall thickness Increased pro–brain-type natriuretic peptide (BNP) and BNP Increased troponin I

Systolic Dysfunction

Systolic dysfunction is often latent but becomes manifest only under conditions of haemodynamic stress [72]. During exercise, the left ventricular end-diastolic pressure increases simultaneously, but the expected increases in cardiac stroke index and left ventricular ejection fraction (LVEF) are blunted indicating an inadequate response of the ventricular reserve to a rise in filling pressure [72]. Pharmacological cardiac strain by use of vasoconstrictors such as dobutamin or glypressin may also reveal a systolic dysfunction with increases in left ventricular end-diastolic volume and pressure and reduced LVEF [73, 74]. A somewhat comparable response is seen after insertion of a transjugular intrahepatic portosystemic shunt (TIPS) and about 12% of the patients develop manifest heart failure [75]. However, the cardiac pressures usually normalise over time [75, 76]. Recently, it has been shown that systolic dysfunction also can be revealed at rest by tissue-Doppler imaging and speckle tracking echocardiography. By these techniques it is possible to measure abnormal peak systolic tissue velocity and strain rate at rest [77]. The reduced cardiac performance may be attributed a combination of blunted heart rate response to exercise, reduced myocardial reserve, and profound skeletal muscle wasting. With the progression of the liver failure the systemic circulation becomes more and more hyperdynamic with an increase in cardiac output owing to increased left ventricular preload [31]. Incapacity to further increase cardiac output, despite increased ventricular filling pressure, indicates that normalisation of the afterload impairs cardiac performance. Moreover, at this point the increase in cardiac output is no longer able to compensate for the effective arterial hypovolemia [63]. This unmasked left ventricular dysfunction may play a role in the development of complications such as the hepatorenal syndrome as part of a cardiorenal syndrome [22, 33]. Recently, Turco et al. described the importance of the cardiodynamic state for prediction of outcomes such as ascites and death with a progressive loss of inotropic performance throughout prognostic stages [38]. The effects of liver transplantation on systolic function are complex and relates to peri- and immediate postoperative periods [27]. Six to 12 months after the liver transplantation there is a significant improvement in cardiac performance and response to physical stress and normalisation of the cardiac output and myocardial mass [78].

Diastolic Dysfunction

The pathophysiological substrate for the diastolic dysfunction in cirrhosis is increased left ventricular myocardial mass, subendothelial oedema, and myocardial fibrosis, which changes composition of collagen and increased ECV of the myocardium [30, 63, 66, 79]. The pathophysiological consequences of the decreased left ventricular compliance and relaxation are an abnormal filling pattern of the ventricles with a delayed trans-mitral blood flow despite an increased atrial contribution to the late ventricular filling. These hemodynamic changes are mirrored in the echocardiogram with a decreased E/A or increased E/é ratios. Newer definitions of diastolic dysfunction are primarily based on measurements by tissue-Doppler echocardiography according to the guidelines of the European Association of Cardiovascular Imaging (Table 3.1) [80].

Diastolic dysfunction precedes systolic dysfunction and is more prevalent than systolic dysfunction ranging from 35–60% independent of aetiology [27, 63, 81, 82]. There seems to be some association between the degree of diastolic dysfunction and severity of liver dysfunction as evaluated by Child or MELD scores [62, 63, 83, 84]. In particular patients with ascites may have a marked diastolic dysfunction that improves after paracentesis [62]. In addition diastolic dysfunction is associated with poor survival [82]. By stratifying according to the degree of diastolic dysfunction (E/é) the mortality seems to be clearly related to the degree of diastolic dysfunction [59, 63, 85]. In these studies the Child or MELD scores as well as E/é turned out to be independent predictive factors. Diastolic dysfunction implies a higher sensitivity to volume changes as seen following TIPS insertion [86]. These changes include a further increase in the left atrial diameter and pulmonary capillary wedged pressure, which indicates that the cirrhotic heart is unable adequately to adapt to the increased preload. This may result in a poorer outcome in patients with diastolic dysfunction after TIPS insertion [87]. The increase in diastolic volumes after TIPS seems, however, to normalise after months but with persistence of a mild left ventricular hypertrophy [88]. After a liver transplantation, a certain degree of the hyperdynamic circulation may persist for some years. The hemodynamic changes immediately after the liver transplantation may result in an accentuation of the diastolic dysfunction and development of heart failure for up to three months post-transplant [89, 90], but hereafter the, diastolic function seems to improve [78].

Prolonged QT Interval

The most important electrophysiological abnormality in cirrhotic cardiomyopathy is the prolonged QT interval, which is one of the supportive criteria in the definition of CCM [14]. The QT interval is prolonged by 30–50% of the cirrhotic patients and it is significantly related to the severity of the liver disease, portal hypertension, and portosystemic shunts [91]. From a pathophysiological point of view the prolonged QT-interval is related to myocardial dysfunction, activation of the sympathetic nervous system, and autonomic dysfunction as reflected by increased pro-BNP, plasma noradrenaline, and decreased heart rate variability [92, 93]. Prolonged QT-interval is also related to poor survival in particular in patients suffering from complications such as bleeding oesophageal varices [94]. The prolongation of the QT interval is partly reversible after liver transplantation [27, 78, 95, 96] and acute as well as chronic treatment with non-selective beta-blockers improve the prolonged QT-interval [97, 98].

Treatment and Evaluation of Cardiac Function in Liver Disease

Liver transplantation reverses most of the features of cirrhotic cardiomyopathy [78]. At present, there is no specific pharmacological therapy for CCM. However, once cardiac failure becomes evident, management should follow common principles for treatment of heart failure for patients without cirrhosis including treatment with diuretics. Non-selective, but not selective β-blockers apart from improving the prolonged QT interval might reduce the hyperdynamic load in patients with cirrhosis [97–99]. However, whether this correction of the QT interval has any beneficial effect on prognosis remains unclear. Aldosterone antagonists are used to counteract the known effects of secondary hyperaldosteronism, which induces myocardial fibrosis, activation of the sympathetic nervous system, and baroreceptor dysfunction.

In general, major surgical procedures including a liver transplantation represent a severe challenge to the cardiovascular system and cardiovascular complications are common in association with the procedure [27]. Within the last decades the population of liver transplant candidates has changed towards a higher proportion of patients with non-alcoholic fatty liver disease (NAFLD) and non-alcoholic steatohepatitis (NASH) as the aetiology of cirrhosis [100]. These patients have a

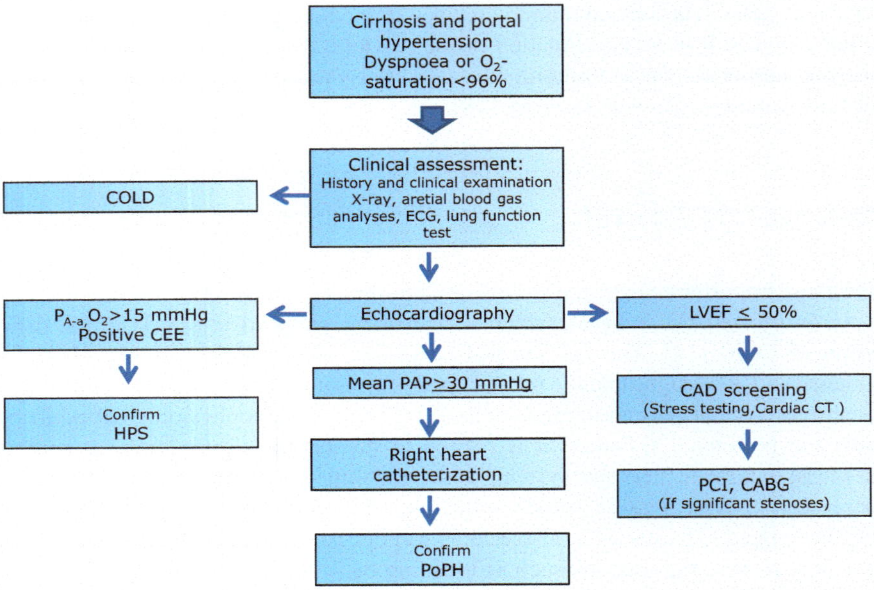

Fig. 3.3 The figure presents a proposal for an algorithm for evaluation and management of cardiopulmonary symptoms in patients with cirrhosis and portal hypertension. CABG: Coronary by-pass graft; CAD: Coronary artery disease; CEE: Contrast-enhanced echocardiography; CT: Computerized tomography; ECG: Electrocardiogram; HPS: Hepatopulmonary syndrome; LVEF: left ventricular ejection fraction; $P_{A\text{-}a}O_2$: Alveolar-arterial oxygen gradient; PAP: Pulmonary Artery Pressure; PCI: Percutaneous Coronary Intervention; PoPH: Portopulmonary hypertension

higher risk of CAD and the need of a careful cardiovascular evaluation prior to liver transplantation is therefore pertinent [101]. This evaluation should take into account aspects such as reduced physical activity, severity of the liver disease, and concurrent morbidity, in particular presence of CAD.

The evidence of the full programme of a cardiovascular wrap-up prior to liver transplantation is not yet fully established, but it is recommended that a detailed functional cardiac characterisation is part of the assessment for liver transplantation and insertion of a TIPS [71]. A proposal for a flow chart taking into account the definition of CCM is shown in Fig. 3.3. By echocardiography left ventricular ejection fraction, pulmonary artery pressure (PAP), and presence of HPS can be evaluated (see below). Depending on the results, successive investigations should be performed to rule out clinically significant PoPH by right heart catheterisation [102]. In case of low ejection fraction and presence of risk factors such as age>50 years, diabetes mellitus, smoking, family history of CAD, arterial hypertension, and hyperlipidemia, CAD-screening should follow. However, the predictive value of non-invasive functional testing for ischaemia is hampered in patients with advanced cirrhosis who cannot undergo exercise and Dobutamine stress tests. This is partly due to chronotropic incompetence and reduced vascular responsiveness to vasoconstrictors and in these patients myocardial perfusion imaging is more appropriate [103]. In case of obstructive CAD coronary revascularization should be performed before transplantation.

In conclusion, CCM is now a well-established entity independent of the aetiology of cirrhosis. Patients with cirrhosis on the basis of NASH suffer an additional risk of developing cardiovascular complications and in general the risk of coronary artery disease is increased in cirrhosis. The pathogenic mechanisms are complex and often interrelated at the molecular and cellular level. The definition includes a systolic as well as diastolic dysfunction and prolonged QT interval. CCM may be present in up to 50% of patients with cirrhosis, and may be implicated in renal complications of cirrhosis, complicate invasive procedures such as TIPS insertion and liver transplantation. Therefore a careful cardiovascular evaluation including Doppler/echocardiography is recommended in all liver transplant candidates to assess myocardial and valvular functions and to rule out HPS and porto-pulmonary hypertension (PoPH). Since cardiomyopathy prior to transplantation and an increasing incidence of CAD among NAFLD-patients tends to increase the risk of heart failure after liver transplantation, these patients should be managed properly before transplantation including revascularisation [27, 102].

Respiratory Complications in Patients with Liver Disease

Patients with cirrhosis often complain of breathlessness and a considerable number presents with clinical signs of respiratory insufficiency such as cyanosis, digital clubbing, and tachypnoea with hyperventilation [104]. Arterial oxygenation may be impaired and depend on the patients' position. The dynamic lung functions, such as forced expiratory volumes and capacities (FEV_1 and FVC) are largely normal, in the absence of obstructive airway disease. The aetiology of abnormal lung function and ventilation in cirrhosis is multifarious and is often a combination of cardiac dysfunction, interstitial lung disease, heavy smoking, and chronic obstructive air way disease, which is particular common in patients with alcoholic cirrhosis [105]. In decompensated patients, tense ascites may affect the pulmonary mechanics and increase the intra-abdominal and intrapulmonary pressures and reduce thoracic volumes but after paracentesis, the total lung capacity (TLC) is often normalised [106]. Specific liver-related pulmonary complication includes HPS, a condition with reduced diffusing capacity, ventilation/perfusion inequality, and intrapulmonary vascular dilatations and PoPH. In some patients with severe portal hypertension, ascites may cross the diaphragm into the intrapleural space as HH [107]. These three entities are separately discussed below.

Hepatopulmonary Syndrome

HPS denotes a condition with reduced diffusing capacity, abnormal ventilation/perfusion ratio and intrapulmonary vascular dilatations, and low arterial oxygen saturation in association with liver disease [108, 109]. Arterial deoxygenation is reflected by an increased alveolar-arterial oxygen gradient, $P_{A\text{-}a'}$ O_2, which is one of the earliest and most sensitive signs of HPS. Patients with the syndrome are also characterised by hyperventilation, hypocapnia, and respiratory alkalosis [110, 111]. From a practical point of view HPS is defined by arterial hypoxaemia ($PaO_2 < 70$ mmHg (or 9.3 kPa)), an age-adjusted increase in $P_{A\text{-}a'}$ $O_2 > 15$ mmHg (or 2.0 kPa) and presence of intrapulmonary vasodilatations [108, 109]. From a clinical point, a large proportion of patients with HPS present with insidious onset of dyspnoea, plathypnoea (upon standing), orthodeoxia, clubbing, and cyanosis [112]. Currently, the following criteria for HPS are: 1. Presence of liver disease; 2. $P_{A\text{-}a'}$ $O_2 \geq 15$ mmHg (2.0 kPa); and 3. a positive CEE (see Table 3.2). The prevalence of HPS in patients with cirrhosis may vary dependent on the severity of the liver disease, aetiology, and geography [113–115]. Different reports have given different frequencies of HPS in cirrhotic patients varying from about 10% to as high as 70% [116–118].

Pathophysiology of the Hepatopulmonary Syndrome

The precise link between the liver dysfunction and portal hypertension and HPS has not been fully established. However, the pathophysiological characteristic of HPS with dilatation of capillaries, shunting of blood, changes in blood flow, and fibromembraneous thickening have correlates in the liver. However, most of our

Table 3.2 Diagnostic criteria for the hepatopulmonary syndrome (HPS) and portopulmonary hypertension (PoPH)

HPS	PoPH
Presence of liver disease	Presence of liver disease and portal hypertension
$P_{A\text{-}a,}$ $O_2^* > 15$ mmHg (>2 kPa)	Mean pulmonary arterial pressure > 25 mmHg
Positive contrast enhanced echocardiography$^+$	Pulmonary vascular resistance > 240 dyn•s•cm$-^5$ Left atrial pressure < 15 mmHg

$P_{A\text{-}a,}O_2$: Alveolar-arterial oxygen gradient

$^+$Visualisation of microbubbles in the left heart chambers within three or more cardiac cycles implies definite intrapulmonary vascular dilatation

$^*P_{A\text{-}a,}$ O_2 can be calculated from the alveolar gas equation

$P_{A\text{-}a,}$ $O_2 = (FIO_2\ (PB - 47) - (PACO_2/R) + FIO_2(1 - R)(PACO_2/R)) - PaO_2$, where FIO_2 is the O_2 inspiratory fraction set to 0.21 breathing room air and 1.00 during 100% oxygen inhalation. PB is the barometric pressure, $PACO_2$ is the alveolar PCO_2, assumed to be equal to $PaCO_2$ and R is the respiratory quotient estimated to 0.80 [110, 117]

understanding of the pathophysiology of HPS is based on animal and experimental studies and it needs to be verified whether it also holds true in human HPS.

HPS is partly a consequence of the arterial vasodilatation in cirrhosis and the imbalance between vasodilating and vasoconstricting forces. Release of the potent vasoconstrictor endothelin-1 (ET-1) from cholangiocytes activates pulmonary endothelial NO-synthase (eNOS) resulting in NO-mediated vasodilatation through stimulation of endothelin-B receptors in the lungs [119–121]. Bacterial translocation with increased endotoxin levels activates pulmonary macrophages to release pro-inflammatory cytokines such as TNF-α, which triggers NO-release by iNOS-activation [122]. Experimental NO-dependent vasodilatation is supported by clinical studies showing increased NO in exhaled air from cirrhotic patients [123, 124]. A recent paper has shown increased carboxyhaemoglobin levels that correlate with arterial oxygen tension and alveolar-arterial oxygen gradient in patients with HPS [125].

Development of intrapulmonary shunts is another important feature of HPS. An important mechanism is angiogenesis, which is development of new blood vessels from preexisting vessels. Angiogenesis is mediated by angiogenic growth factors in particular placental growth factor and vascular endothelial growth factor-A (VEGF-A) produced by intravascular monocytes [126]. Increased expression of von Willebrand factor (vWF) is associated with HPS and increased circulating concentrations of vWF is seen in cirrhosis and HPS [15, 126, 127].

A hallmark of the respiratory pathophysiology in cirrhosis is the reduced diffusing capacity. The diffusing capacity expresses the rate by which a gas crosses the membrane between the alveoli and the lung capillary. Independently of concomitant conditions, patients with cirrhosis have a compromised diffusing capacity and ventilation/perfusion (V_A/Q) abnormalities [105, 109]. A V_A/Q ineqality is arterial hypoxaemia, which is seen in 10–70% of patients with chronic liver disease, depending on severity [110, 128]. In addition to the above mentioned mechanisms, reduced diffusing capacity can be attributed to abnormal V_A/Q, changes in the pulmonary blood volume, presence of arterial venous shunts, and biochemical changes in the alveolar-capillary membrane [129].

Thickening of the alveolar-capillary membrane may limit the diffusion of oxygen from the alveolar gas to the capillary blood. However, the membrane is largely normal in cirrhosis, although it may increase in thickness in some patients with tense ascites and fluid in the intrapleural space. Figure 3.4 reviews essential pathophysiological factors of HPS.

Diagnosis of the Hepatopulmonary Syndrome

Progressive dyspnoea is the most prominent symptom of HPS [130]. Platypnoea, is the condition of worsening dyspnoea when changing the position from supine to erect position and considered pathognomonic for HPS [130]. This is a result of orthodeoxia with increased perfusion of the lung bases with augmented V_A/Q

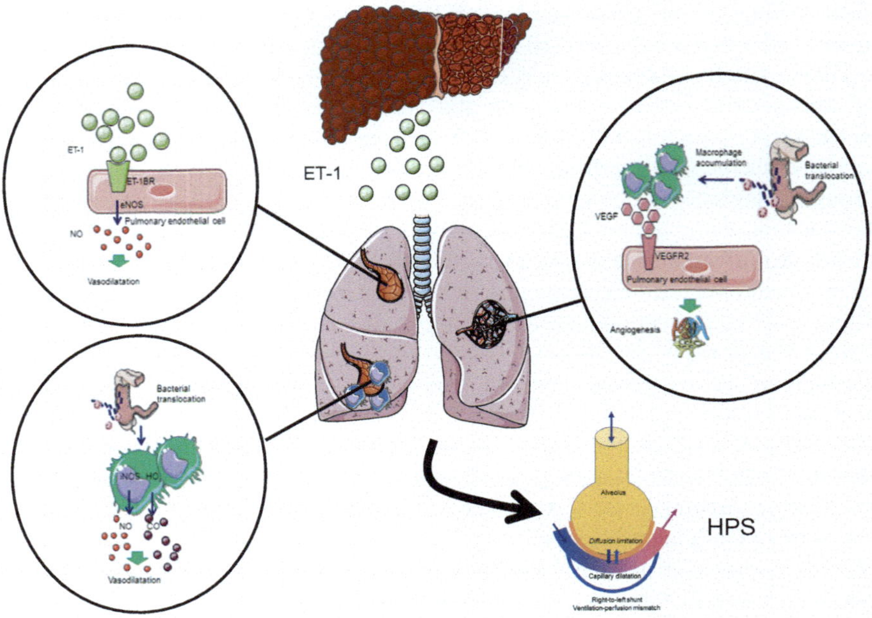

Fig. 3.4 The figure reviews some basic pathophysiological proposals for development of the hepatopulmonary syndrome (HPS) as derived from experimental studies. Cirrhosis and portal hypertension lead to generation of endothelin-1 (ET-1), which acts on ET-1B receptors on pulmonary endothelial cells. Activation endothelial nitric oxide synthase (eNOS) generates NO leading to pulmonary vasodilatation. Bacterial translocation with generation of cytokines accumulates pulmonary macrophages and monocytes and generate NO and carbon monoxide (CO) through iNOS and haemoxygenase, respectively, which additionally augment the pulmonary vasodilatation. The accumulation of macrophages triggers production of vascular endothelial growth factor (VEGF). Interaction with the VEGF2-receptor stimulates to angiogenesis. The overall result of several pathophysiological processes are development of HPS comprising intrapulmonary vascular dilatations and shunting and ventilation/perfusion mismatch (V_A/Q) leading to an increased alveolar-arterial oxygen gradient and arterial hypoxaemia

inequality in the up-right position [131]. Other clinical findings include cyanosis, digital clubbing, and spider naevi. The diagnosis of HPS requires demonstration of the presence of liver disease, elevated age-adjusted alveolar arterial oxygen gradient ($P_{A\text{-}a}$, $O_2 > 15$ mmHg) in room air, and intrapulmonary vascular dilatations (Table 3.2) [109, 132].

The degree of arterial deoxygenation is determined from arterial blood gas analyses and the arterial oxygen tension is part of the definition of HPS as shown in Table 3.2. Arterial hypoxaemia is seen in 10–70% of patients with chronic liver disease, depending on severity and the reference level of the laboratory [110, 133]. However, calculation of the alveolar-arterial oxygen gradient ($P_{A\text{-}a},O_2$) appears to be a more sensitive indicator than solely PaO_2. This relates to the fact that $PaCO_2$

is part of the equation for the calculation of the alveolar-arterial oxygen gradient. Pulse oximetry with the assessment of oxygen saturation has been proposed as a screening tool for HPS [134], but recent studies have evidenced that this method is not sufficiently sensitive neither in adults nor in children evaluated for liver transplantation [135, 136].

The increase in the alveolar-arterial oxygen gradient is associated with impaired diffusing capacity. The diffusing capacity expresses the rate by which a gas crosses the membrane between the alveoli and the lung capillary. Independent of concomitant conditions, patients with cirrhosis have a compromised diffusing capacity and ventilation/perfusion abnormalities. Various pathophysiological factors may be involved in the reduced diffusing capacity, including an abnormal ventilation/perfusion ratio (V_A/Q), changes in the pulmonary blood volume, the presence of arterial venous shunts, and changes in the alveolar-capillary membrane, see Fig. 3.4. We have previously found direct relations between the diffusing capacity and the degree of hyperdynamic circulation, central and pulmonary hypovolemia, and pulmonary transit times [117, 137].

Prognosis

There are only a few studies on the prognosis of HPS. In a retrospective study, Krowka et al. found a mortality rate of 41% over a period of 2–5 years [138]. In general, patients with HPS and cirrhosis have a poorer 5-year survival (23%) compared to cirrhotic patients without HPS (63%) [139, 140]. However, new results with application of a standard exception policy to prioritise patients with severe HRS indicate that the overall pre-and post-transplant survival is similar in HPS compared to non-HPS patients [141].

Intrapulmonary Vascular Dilatation

Macroscopic and microscopic intrapulmonary arteriovenous shunts are hallmarks in the pathophysiology of HPS and different experimental observations support that vascular remodeling, endothelial dysfunction, as well as angiogenesis is involved [15]. The intrapulmonary vascular dilatation can be visualized by pulmonary angiography and by measuring a short pulmonary transit time<3.55 s [137, 142]. A recent case–control study has evidenced that presence of HPS is moreover associated with significant intrahepatic vascular changes and signs of portal hypertension [143]. From a practical point of view the intravascular dilatations can be detected by a contrast-enhanced echo-cardiography (CEE). CEE is today considered the method of choice and gold standard in the diagnosis of HPS [109, 117]. Agitated saline (microbubbles) is injected into a brachial vein and the bolus is shortly seen in the right heart chambers. A positive test for intrapulmonary vasodilatation is visualisation of the microbubbles in the left heart chambers after more than three heart beats. In addition, a grading of the intrapulmonary vascular dilatations with good correlations to Child classification and gas exchange abnormalities is possible by this technique [117, 144]. Alternatively, a lung perfusion scintigraphy with injection of macroaggregated albumin and estimation of the extra-pulmonary shunt fraction has been used [145, 146]. The shunt fraction can be calculated from counts over lungs and brain and a value>6% is considered positive with a sensitivity of 85% [132, 145]. However, the lung perfusion scan is considered less sensitive than CEE and does not distinguish intracardiac from intrapulmonary shunting and is in general not well-suited for the purposes of screening [109, 147].

Treatment of Hepatopulmonary Syndrome

No specific treatment is available for HPS. Liver transplantation efficiently reverse HPS with significant improvement in gas exchange in the majority of the patients [128, 140, 148]. Insertion of TIPS in patients with HPS may also improve gas exchange, but can only be considered as a bridge towards liver transplantation [149–151]. Concerns relate to the fact that TIPS insertion increases pulmonary artery pressure and cardiorespiratory complications are not unusual [152, 153]. Because HPS is reversible after liver transplantation, it has become an indication for urgent liver transplantation [154].

Potential new targets for medical treatment of HPS relate to reversion of the intrapulmonary vascular dilatation. Theoretically, this can be achieved by inhibition of NO production by L-Nitroarginine methyl ester inhibitors, ET receptor antagonists, or by angiogenesis inhibition (see Fig. 3.4) [126, 155, 156]. Amelioration of pulmonary inflammation by TNF-α inhibitors, chemokine antagonists, and antibiotics such as norfloxacin has been studied with variable results [157, 158].

Porto-Pulmonary Hypertension

As mentioned previously, portal hypertension is defined as the presence of a hepatic venous pressure gradient above 5 mmHg. The association between portal hypertension and pulmonary hypertension is termed PoPH. PoPH is defined as a mean pulmonary artery pressure>25 mmHg and pulmonary vascular resistance>240 dyn•s•cm^{-5} (>3 Wood units) and normal left atrial pressure (pulmonary capillary wedge pressure<15 mmHg) in the presence of portal hypertension, see Table 3.2 [132, 159, 160]. The prevalence of PoPH ranges between 1–5% and somewhat higher in liver transplant candidates [160, 161].

Clinical Signs and Diagnosis

Symptoms are typically progressive and include dyspnoea on exertion and fatigue, chest pain, oedema, dyspnoea at rest, and syncope [112]. Pulmonary function tests often exhibit reduced lung volumes, forced vital capacity, and lung diffusing capacity. In advanced cases cardiomegaly, enlarged pulmonary arteries, right ventricular hypertrophy and dilatation of the right atrium and ventricle are common. Right heart catheterization remains the gold standard for diagnosis with a quantification of cardiac and pulmonary pressures. Recently, Raevens et al. demonstrated that a systolic pulmonary artery pressure cut-off value of 38 mmHg was associated to a negative predictive value of 100% and a specificity of 82%. By adding presence or absence of right ventricular dilatation the specificity even increased to 93% [162]. In patients with advanced cirrhosis and portal hypertension the pulmonary artery pressure may be increased mildly in 20–50% of the patients owing to the hyperdynamic circulation ("false" PoPH) [31]. "True" PoPH is characterised by an increase in pulmonary vascular resistance and the transpulmonary gradient. Measurement of these parameters has been suggested for the differentiation between true or false PoPH [112, 163].

The median survival in patients with porto-pulmonary hypertension is considered low about six months, and lower than in patients with idiopathic pulmonary hypertension [161, 164]. The 5-year survival of patients with PoPH ranges from 14–40% [160, 165, 166].

Pathophysiology of Porto-Pulmonary Hypertension

The histological appearance of pulmonary vessels is similar to that seen in primary pulmonary artery hypertension, and includes smooth muscle proliferation, hypertrophy, and fibrosis [132]. Various pathophysiological aspects seem to be involved in the development of PoPH, including angiogenesis, genetics, humoral changes, and inflammation with increased pulmonary phagocytosis [132]. For example female gender and oestrogen metabolism with increased levels oestrogens have been associated with development of PoPH [167]. Of particular interest is the activation of potent local vasoconstrictor systems, like serotonin and the endothelin system. ET-1 is produced in the pulmonary endothelium and binding to ET_A and ET_B receptors on the pulmonary smooth muscle cells leads to vasoconstriction [120]. In other conditions, as in chronic heart failure, ET-1 has also been shown to correlate with the degree of pulmonary hypertension [168, 169]. Portal hypertension leads to development of portosystemic shunts. A relation between the presence of large portosystemic shunts, > 1 cm in diameter and the degree of PoPH has been demonstrated [170]. This has led to the hypothesis that increased portosystemic shunting exposes the pulmonary vascular system to additional shear stress and mediators that elicit pulmonary arterial vasoconstriction [109].

Treatment of Portopulmonary Hypertension

Treatment of PoPH is in general non-specific and palliative, and includes diuretics, cardiac glycosides, vasodilators, such as nitrates, and prostacyclins and long-term oxygen therapy [132]. Intravenous epoprostenol have been used to ameliorate the haemodynamic profile in the waiting for an eventual liver transplantation. Also inhaled iloprost has been associated with improvement in symptoms [160]. Results of treatment with endothelin antagonists have proved promising in a few patients. For example administration of the mixed ET antagonist Bosentan showed beneficial effects on exercise capacity and haemodynamics in PoPH [171, 172]. Phosphodiesterase-5 inhibitors (Sildenafil) has been used in PoPH with improvements in pulmonary artery pressure and pulmonary vascular resistance and in 6-min walk test [173].

Liver transplantation in patients with PoPH with a mean pulmonary arterial pressure > 35 mmHg is associated with increased mortality. Liver transplantation is therefore contraindicated in patients with severe PoPH [154, 159, 174]. Insertion of a TIPS leads to acute porto-systemic shunting and may further deteriorate cardiopulmonary haemodynamics and should therefore be avoided. Also use of non-selective beta-blockers should be avoided due to the deleterious effects on central haemodynamics [112, 175].

Hepatic Hydrothorax

Hepatic hydrothorax (HH) is defined as a transudative pleural effusion in patients with portal hypertension. It is seen in 5–15% of the patients with cirrhosis most often with concomitant ascites [176, 177]. Approximately 20% of the patients with HH have no clinical significant ascites [104].

HH is the most frequent cause of pleural effusion in cirrhosis and is typically right-sided (70%) and left-sided and bilateral in 18% and 17%, respectively [176]. Patients with HH present with respiratory symptoms such as cough, dyspnea, chest pain, hypoxia, and fever in case of spontaneous bacterial pleuritis. In 80% of the patients increasing amounts of ascites contributes to the respiratory discomfort [178].

Cirrhosis complicated with portal hypertension is a key element in the development of HH. Tense ascites from the peritoneal cavity may translocate through diaphragmatic defects into the pleural cavity. These pleuroperitoneal communications have been visualized by ^{99m}Tc-fluor colloid, are often < 1 cm, and mainly located in the right diaphragmatic half [179, 180]. In addition, the negative intra-thoracic pressure during inspiration facilitates a one-way movement of fluid from the peritoneal to the pleural cavities.

The diagnosis of HH is based on chest radiography and a diagnostic thoracocenthesis. Biochemical factors indicative of HH include a serum-to-pleural fluid albumin gradient>1.1, a total pleural fluid protein content<25 g/l, and a polymorphnuclear cell count<250 cells/μl [178]. A higher polymorphnuclear cell count (>500 cells/μl) is diagnostic for spontaneous bacterial pleuritis. Pleural infection develops in 10–15% of cirrhotic patients with HH and is characterized by fever and pleural chest pain [109, 181].

Occurrence of HH is often part of the clinical picture of hepatic decompensation and radical treatment strategies such as referral to TIPS or liver transplantation should be considered. Treatment with diuretics and sodium restriction as for ascites may be effective in some patients. However, thoracocentesis with percutaneous drainage of the peritoneal fluid is often necessary, but should be limited to 1–2 l to minimize risk of pulmonary edema [109, 182]. Prior to liver transplantation, insertion of a TIPS is often efficient for HH [107, 183, 184].

In conclusion, patients with cirrhosis and portal hypertension often present with respiratory symptoms and biochemical and physiological signs of pulmonary insufficiency. A considerable number of the patients present with reduced pulmonary vascular resistance, impaired ventilation, and hypoxaemia as part of HPS. A subset of portal hypertensive patients develops PoPH with increased pulmonary vascular resistance or HH. However, the prevalence varies with the severity of the hepatic dysfunction. A timely diagnosis of the particular respiratory complication to portal hypertension is essential to initiate the appropriate treatment when possible.

Conclusive Remarks

The recent years have considerably improved our knowledge on the mechanisms of disease processes in chronic liver disease and portal hypertension. Extra-hepatic complications include changes in numerous organ systems as a multi-organ failure syndrome. The function of the heart in cirrhosis is disturbed, with a hyperdynamic circulation with increased cardiac output and heart rate. Cardiac performance and the systolic and diastolic functions are clearly impaired as part of a cirrhotic cardiomyopathy, which may contribute to other complications such as the hepatorenal syndrome as part of a cardio-renal syndrome. The arterial vasodilatation and reactive vasoconstriction are also linked to changes in pulmonary haemodynamics and function. In HPS and PoPH a preferential vasodilatation and reactive and counter-regulatory vasoconstriction is prevailing, respectively. Future research in this area should add to refine the diagnosis of cardiorespiratory complications to portal hypertension and to reveal new therapeutic targets for improvement of the prognosis of the individual subsets of patients.

Acknowledgments Professor Søren Møller was supported by a grant from the Novo Nordisk Foundation and The University of Copenhagen.

References

1. Vorobioff JD, Groszmann RJ. Prevention of portal hypertension: From variceal development to clinical decompensation. Hepatology. 2015;61(1):375–81.
2. Bosch J, Iwakiri Y. The portal hypertension syndrome: etiology, classification, relevance, and animal models. Hepatol Int. 2018;12(Suppl 1):1–10.
3. Piano S, Tonon M, Angeli P. Management of ascites and hepatorenal syndrome. Hepatol Int 2017;10–9815.
4. Sole C, Pose E, Sola E, Gines P. Hepatorenal syndrome in the era of Acute Kidney injury. Liver Int. 2018;38(11):1891–901.
5. Fernandez M. Molecular pathophysiology of portal hypertension. Hepatology. 2015;61(4):1406–15.
6. Bolognesi M, Di Pascoli M, Verardo A, Gatta A. Splanchnic vasodilation and hyperdynamic circulatory syndrome in cirrhosis. World J Gastroenterol. 2014;20(10):2555–63.
7. Møller S, Henriksen JH, Bendtsen F. Extrahepatic complications to cirrhosis and portal hypertension: haemodynamic and homeostatic aspects. World J Gastroenterol. 2014;20(42):15499–517.
8. Bosch J. Vascular deterioration in cirrhosis: the big picture. J Clin Gastroenterol 2007;41(Suppl 3):S247–53. S247–S253.
9. Møller S, Henriksen JH. Cardiovascular complications of cirrhosis. Gut. 2008;57(2):268–78.
10. Møller S, Hobolth L, Winkler C, Bendtsen F, Christensen E. Determinants of the hyperdynamic circulation and central hypovolaemia in cirrhosis. Gut. 2011;60:1254–9.
11. Siniscalchi A, Aurini L, Spedicato S, Bernardi E, Zanoni A, Dante A, et al. Hyperdynamic circulation in cirrhosis: predictive factors and outcome following liver transplantation. Minerva Anestesiol. 2013;79(1):15–23.
12. Villanueva C, Albillos A, Genesca J, Abraldes JG, Calleja JL, Aracil C, et al. Development of hyperdynamic circulation and response to beta-blockers in compensated cirrhosis with portal hypertension. Hepatology. 2016;63(1):197–206.
13. Fede G, Privitera G, Tomaselli T, Spadaro L, Purrello F. Cardiovascular dysfunction in patients with liver cirrhosis. Ann Gastroenterol. 2015;28(1):31–40.
14. Møller S, Lee SS. Cirrhotic cardiomyopathy. J Hepatol. 2018;69:958–60.
15. Raevens S, Fallon MB. Potential clinical targets in hepatopulmonary syndrome: lessons from experimental models. Hepatology. 2018;68(5):2016–28.
16. Acevedo J, Fernandez J, Prado V, Silva A, Castro M, Pavesi M, et al. Relative adrenal insufficiency in decompensated cirrhosis. relationship to short-term risk of severe sepsis, hepatorenal syndrome and death. Hepatology 2013;58(5):1757–1765.
17. Schrier RW, Arroyo V, Bernardi M, Epstein M, Henriksen JH, Rodés J. Peripheral artery vasodilatation hypothesis: a proposal for the initiation of renal sodium and water retention in cirrhosis. Hepatology. 1988;5:1151–7.
18. Bosch J, Groszmann RJ, Shah VH. Evolution in the understanding of the pathophysiological basis of portal hypertension: how changes in paradigm are leading to successful new treatments. J Hepatol. 2015;62(1 Suppl):S121–30.
19. Lenz K. Hepatorenal syndrome–is it central hypovolemia, a cardiac disease, or part of gradually developing multiorgan dysfunction? Hepatology. 2005;42(2):263–5.
20. Møller S, Bendtsen F, Henriksen JH. Determinants of the renin-angiotensin-aldosterone system in cirrhosis with special emphasis on the central blood volume. Scand J Gastroenterol. 2006;41:451–8.
21. Jimenez W, Rodes J. Impaired responsiveness to endogenous vasoconstrictors and endothelium-derived vasoactive factors in cirrhosis. Gastroenterology. 1994;107:1201–3.
22. Krag A, Bendtsen F, Burroughs AK, Møller S. The cardiorenal link in advanced cirrhosis. Med Hypotheses. 2012;79(1):53–5.
23. Wiese S, Bendtsen F, Møller S. Cardiovascular biomarkers in cirrhosis and portal hypertension—relation to cardiac and circulatory dysfunction. In: Patel VC, Preedy VR, editors. Biomarkers in cardiovascular disease. 1st ed. Dordrecht: Springer; 2016. p. 573–99.

24. Voiosu A, Wiese S, Voiosu T, Bendtsen F, Møller S. Bile acids and cardiovascular function in cirrhosis. Liver Int. 2017;37(10):1420–30.
25. Vasavan T, Ferraro E, Ibrahim E, Dixon P, Gorelik J, Williamson C. Heart and bile acids—clinical consequences of altered bile acid metabolism. Biochim Biophys Acta Mol Basis Dis 2018;1864(4 Pt B):1345–1355.
26. Desai MS, Mathur B, Eblimit Z, Vasquez H, Taegtmeyer H, Karpen SJ, et al. Bile acid excess induces cardiomyopathy and metabolic dysfunctions in the heart. Hepatology. 2016;65(1):189–201.
27. Liu H, Jayakumar S, Traboulsi M, Lee SS. Cirrhotic cardiomyopathy: implications for liver transplantation. Liver Transpl. 2017;23(6):826–35.
28. Bernardi M, Caraceni P. Novel perspectives in the management of decompensated cirrhosis. Nat Rev Gastroenterol Hepatol. 2018. https://doi.org/10.1038/s41575-018-0045-2.:10-0045.
29. Gines P, Sola E, Angeli P, Wong F, Nadim MK, Kamath P. Hepatorenal syndrome. Nat Rev Dis Primers. 2018;4(1):23–0022.
30. Wiese S, Hove J, Mo S, Mookerjee RP, Petersen CL, Vester-Andersen MK, et al. Myocardial extracellular volume quantified by magnetic resonance is increased in cirrhosis and related to poor outcome. Liver Int. 2018;38(9):1614–23.
31. Møller S, Bendtsen F. The pathophysiology of arterial vasodilatation and hyperdynamic circulation in cirrhosis. Liver Int. 2018;38(4):570–80.
32. Ruiz-Del-Arbol L, Monescillo A, Arocena C, Valer P, Gines P, Moreira V, et al. Circulatory function and hepatorenal syndrome in cirrhosis. Hepatology. 2005;42:439–47.
33. Kazory A, Ronco C. Hepatorenal syndrome or hepatocardiorenal syndrome: revisiting basic concepts in view of emerging data. Cardiorenal Med. 2018;9(1):1–7.
34. Lipcsey M, Castegren M, Bellomo R. Hemodynamic management of septic shock. Minerva Anestesiol. 2015;81(11):1262–72.
35. Arroyo V. Microalbuminuria, systemic inflammation, and multiorgan dysfunction in decompensated cirrhosis: evidence for a nonfunctional mechanism of hepatorenal syndrome. Hepatol Int. 2017;11(3):242–4.
36. Coenraad MJ, Porcher R, Bendtsen F. Hepatic and cardiac hemodynamics and systemic inflammation in cirrhosis: it takes three to tango. J Hepatol. 2018;68(5):887–9.
37. Møller S, Bendtsen F. Cirrhotic multiorgan syndrome. Dig Dis Sci. 2015a;60:3209–25.
38. Turco L, Garcia-Tsao G, Magnani I, Bianchini M, Costetti M, Caporali C, et al. Cardiopulmonary hemodynamics and c-reactive protein as prognostic indicators in compensated and decompensated cirrhosis. J Hepatol. 2018;68(18):949–58.
39. Iwakiri Y, Shah V, Rockey DC. Vascular pathobiology in chronic liver disease and cirrhosis—current status and future directions. J Hepatol. 2014;61(414):912–24.
40. Møller S, Iversen JS, Henriksen JH, Bendtsen F. Reduced baroreflex sensitivity in alcoholic cirrhosis:relations to hemodynamics and humoral systems. Am J Physiol Heart Circ Physiol 2007;292. H2966–H2972.
41. Møller S, Mortensen C, Bendtsen F, Jensen LT, Gotze JP, Madsen JL. Cardiac sympathetic imaging with mIBG in cirrhosis and portal hypertension: Relation to autonomic and cardiac function. Am J Physiol Gastrointest Liver Physiol. 2012;303:G1228–35.
42. Di SC, Milazzo V, Milan A, Veglio F, Maule S. The role of autonomic dysfunction in cirrhotic patients before and after liver transplantation. Review of the literature. Liver Int. 2016;36(8):1081–9.
43. Tazi KA, Moreau R, Heller J, Poirel O, Lebrec D. Changes in protein kinase C isoforms in association with vascular hyporeactivity in cirrhotic rat aortas. Gastroenterology. 2000;119(1):201–10.
44. Ferlitsch A, Pleiner J, Mittermayer F, Schaller G, Homoncik M, Peck-Radosavljevic M, et al. Vasoconstrictor hyporeactivity can be reversed by antioxidants in patients with advanced alcoholic cirrhosis of the liver and ascites. Crit Care Med. 2005;33(9):2028–33.
45. Greuter T, Shah VH. Hepatic sinusoids in liver injury, inflammation, and fibrosis: new pathophysiological insights. J Gastroenterol. 2016;51(6):511–9.

46. Wiest R, Groszmann RJ. Nitric oxide and portal hypertension: its role in the regulation of intrahepatic and splanchnic vascular resistance. Semin Liver Dis. 1999;19(4):411–26.
47. Tazi KA, Barriere E, Moreau R, Heller J, Sogni P, Pateron D, et al. Role of shear stress in aortic eNOS up-regulation in rats with biliary cirrhosis. Gastroenterology. 2002;122(7):1869–77.
48. Henriksen JH, Fuglsang S, Bendtsen F, Møller S. Arterial hypertension in cirrhosis: arterial compliance, volume distribution, and central haemodynamics. Gut. 2006;2006:380–7.
49. Henriksen JH, Fuglsang S, Bendtsen F. Arterial pressure profile in patients with cirrhosis: Fourier analysis of arterial pulse in relation to pressure level, stroke volume, and severity of disease: on the reduction of afterload in the hyperdynamic syndrome. Scand J Gastroenterol. 2012;47(5):580–90.
50. Kim SK, Shin WJ, Kim JW, Park JY, Hwang GS. Prediction of hyperdynamic circulation by arterial diastolic reflected waveform analysis in patients undergoing liver transplantation. Blood Press Monit. 2016;21(1):9–15.
51. Paternostro R, Reiberger T, Mandorfer M, Schwarzer R, Schwabl P, Bota S, et al. Plasma renin concentration represents an independent risk factor for mortality and is associated with liver dysfunction in patients with cirrhosis. J Gastroenterol Hepatol. 2017;32(1):184–90.
52. McAvoy NC, Semple S, Richards JM, Robson AJ, Patel D, Jardine AG, et al. Differential visceral blood flow in the hyperdynamic circulation of patients with liver cirrhosis. Aliment Pharmacol Ther. 2016;43(9):947–54.
53. Rossle M. Hyperdynamic circulation and portal hypertension: chicken or egg? Gut. 2011;60(9):1167–9.
54. Kowalski HJ, Abelmann WH. The cardiac output at rest in Laennecs cirrhosis. J Clin Invest. 1953;32:1025–33.
55. Wehmeyer MH, Heuer AJ, Benten D, Puschel K, Sydow K, Lohse AW, et al. High rate of cardiac abnormalities in a postmortem analysis of patients suffering from Liver cirrhosis. J Clin Gastroenterol. 2015;49(10):866–72.
56. Krag A, Bendtsen F, Henriksen JH, Møller S. Low cardiac output predicts development of hepatorenal syndrome and survival in patients with cirrhosis and ascites. Gut. 2010;59(1):105–10.
57. Desai MS, Mathur B, Eblimit Z, Vasquez H, Taegtmeyer H, Karpen SJ, et al. Bile acid excess induces cardiomyopathy and metabolic dysfunctions in the heart. Hepatology. 2017;65(1):189–201.
58. Wong F, Liu P, Lilly L, Bomzon A, Blendis L. Role of cardiac structural and functional abnormalities in the pathogenesis of hyperdynamic circulation and renal sodium retention in cirrhosis. Clin Sci. 1999;97(3):259–67.
59. Cesari M, Frigo AC, Tonon M, Angeli P. Cardiovascular predictors of death in patients with cirrhosis. Hepatology. 2018;68(1):215–23.
60. Junge N, Junge C, Schroder J, Pfister ED, Leiskau C, Hohmann D, et al. Pediatric cirrhotic cardiomyopathy: impact on liver transplant outcomes. Liver Transpl. 2018;24(6):820–30.
61. Gunay N, Erdem S, Guvenc TS, Bulur A, Ozdil K, Hasdemir H, et al. Morphologic and functional changes in right-sided cardiac chambers in patients with chronic liver disease and normal pulmonary artery pressure. J Ultrasound Med. 2018;37(7):1681–91.
62. Pozzi M, Carugo S, Boari G, Pecci V, de Ceglia S, Maggiolini S, et al. Evidence of functional and structural cardiac abnormalities in cirrhotic patients with and without ascites. Hepatology. 1997;26(5):1131–7.
63. Ruiz-Del-Arbol L, Achecar L, Serradilla R, Rodriguez-Gandia MA, Rivero M, Garrido E, et al. Diastolic dysfunction is a predictor of poor outcomes in patients with cirrhosis, portal hypertension and a normal creatinine. Hepatology. 2013;58(5):1732–42.
64. Merli M, Torromeo C, Giusto M, Iacovone G, Riggio O, Puddu PE. Survival at 2 years among liver cirrhotic patients is influenced by left atrial volume and left ventricular mass. Liver Int. 2017;37(5):700–6.

65. Henriksen JH, Gøetze JP, Fuglsang S, Christensen E, Bendtsen F, Møller S. Increased circulating pro-brain natriuretic peptide (proBNP) and brain natriuretic peptide (BNP) in patients with cirrhosis. Relation to cardiovascular dysfunction and severity of disease. Gut 2003;52:1511–1517.
66. Saner FH, Neumann T, Canbay A, Treckmann JW, Hartmann M, Goerlinger K, et al. High brain-natriuretic peptide level predicts cirrhotic cardiomyopathy in liver transplant patients. Transpl Int. 2011;24:425–32.
67. Kazankov K, Munk K, Ovrehus KA, Jensen JM, Siggaard CB, Gronbaek H, et al. High burden of coronary atherosclerosis in patients with cirrhosis. Eur J Clin Invest. 2017;47(8):565–73.
68. Patel SS, Nabi E, Guzman L, Abbate A, Bhati C, Stravitz RT, et al. Coronary artery disease in decompensated patients undergoing liver transplantation evaluation. Liver Transpl. 2018;24(3):333–42.
69. Danielsen KV, Wiese S, Hove J, Bendtsen F, Møller S. Pronounced coronary arteriosclerosis in cirrhosis: influence on cardiac function and survival? Dig Dis Sci. 2018;63(5):1355–62.
70. Zhao J, Li N, Sun H, Liang C. The prevalence of coronary artery disease in patients with liver cirrhosis: a meta-analysis. Eur J Gastroenterol Hepatol. 2018;30(1):118–20.
71. EASL Clinical Practice Guidelines for the management of patients with decompensated cirrhosis. J Hepatol 2018;69(2):406–460.
72. Wong F, Girgrah N, Graba J, Allidina Y, Liu P, Blendis L. The cardiac response to exercise in cirrhosis. Gut. 2001;49(2):268–75.
73. Krag A, Bendtsen F, Mortensen C, Henriksen JH, Møller S. Effects of a single terlipressin administration on cardiac function and perfusion in cirrhosis. Eur J Gastroenterol Hepatol. 2010;22(9):1085–92.
74. Sampaio F, Lamata P, Bettencourt N, Alt SC, Ferreira N, Kowallick JT, et al. Assessment of cardiovascular physiology using dobutamine stress cardiovascular magnetic resonance reveals impaired contractile reserve in patients with cirrhotic cardiomyopathy. J Cardiovasc Magn Reson. 2015;17(1):61–0157.
75. Busk TM, Bendtsen F, Møller S. Cardiac and renal effects of a transjugular intrahepatic portosystemic shunt in cirrhosis. Eur J Gastroenterol Hepatol. 2013;25(5):523–30.
76. Merli M, Valeriano V, Funaro S, Attili AF, Masini A, Efrati C, et al. Modifications of cardiac function in cirrhotic patients treated with transjugular intrahepatic portosystemic shunt (TIPS). Am J Gastroenterol. 2002;97(1):142–8.
77. Kazankov K, Holland-Fischer P, Andersen NH, Torp P, Sloth E, Aagaard NK, et al. Resting myocardial dysfunction in cirrhosis quantified by tissue doppler imaging. Liver Int. 2011;31(4):534–40.
78. Torregrosa M, Aguade S, Dos L, Segura R, Gonzalez A, Evangelista A, et al. Cardiac alterations in cirrhosis: reversibility after liver transplantation. J Hepatol. 2005;42(1):68–74.
79. Glenn TK, Honar H, Liu H, ter Keurs HE, Lee SS. Role of cardiac myofilament proteins titin and collagen in the pathogenesis of diastolic dysfunction in cirrhotic rats. J Hepatol. 2011;55(6):1249–55.
80. Nagueh SF, Smiseth OA, Appleton CP, Byrd BF III, Dokainish H, Edvardsen T, et al. Recommendations for the evaluation of left ventricular diastolic function by echocardiography: An update from the american society of echocardiography and the European Association of Cardiovascular Imaging. Eur Heart J Cardiovasc Imaging. 2016;17(12):1321–60.
81. Wong F, Villamil A, Merli M, Romero G, Angeli P, Caraceni P, et al. Prevalence of diastolic dysfunction in cirrhosis and its clinical significance., 54 ed 2011. p. 475A.
82. Karagiannakis DS, Vlachogiannakos J, Anastasiadis G, Vafiadis-Zouboulis I, Ladas SD. Diastolic cardiac dysfunction is a predictor of dismal prognosis in patients with liver cirrhosis. Hepatol Int. 2014;8(4):588–94.
83. Karagiannakis DS, Vlachogiannakos J, Anastasiadis G, Vafiadis-Zouboulis I, Ladas SD. Frequency and severity of cirrhotic cardiomyopathy and its possible relationship with bacterial endotoxemia. Dig Dis Sci. 2013;58(10):3029–36.

84. Nazar A, Guevara M, Sitges M, Terra C, Sola E, Guigou C, et al. Left ventricular function assessed by echocardiography in cirrhosis: relationship to systemic hemodynamics and renal dysfunction. J Hepatol. 2013;58(1):51–7.
85. Lee SK, Song MJ, Kim SH, Ahn HJ. Cardiac diastolic dysfunction predicts poor prognosis in patients with decompensated liver cirrhosis. Clin Mol Hepatol. 2018;24(4):409–16.
86. Busk TM, Bendtsen F, Poulsen JH, Clemmesen JO, Larsen FS, Goetze JP, et al. Transjugular intrahepatic portosystemic shunt: impact on systemic hemodynamics and renal and cardiac function in patients with cirrhosis. Am J Physiol Gastrointest Liver Physiol. 2018;314(2):G275–86.
87. Cazzaniga M, Salerno F, Pagnozzi G, Dionigi E, Visentin S, Cirello I, et al. Diastolic dysfunction is associated with poor survival in cirrhotic patients with transjugular intrahepatic portosystemic shunt. Gut. 2007;56(6):869–75.
88. Rabie RN, Cazzaniga M, Salerno F, Wong F. The use of E/A ratio as a predictor of outcome in cirrhotic patients treated with transjugular intrahepatic portosystemic shunt. Am J Gastroenterol. 2009;104:2458–66.
89. Therapondos G, Flapan AD, Plevris JN, Hayes PC. Cardiac morbidity and mortality related to orthotopic liver transplantation. Liver Transpl. 2004;10(12):1441–53.
90. Dowsley TF, Bayne DB, Langnas AN, Dumitru I, Windle JR, Porter TR, et al. Diastolic dysfunction in patients with end-stage liver disease is associated with development of heart failure early after liver transplantation. Transplantation. 2012;94(6):646–51.
91. Bernardi M, Maggioli C, Dibra V, Zaccherini G. QT interval prolongation in liver cirrhosis: innocent bystander or serious threat? Expert Rev Gastroenterol Hepatol. 2012;6(1):57–66.
92. Ytting H, Henriksen JH, Fuglsang S, Bendtsen F, Møller S. Prolonged Q-T(c) interval in mild portal hypertensive cirrhosis. J Hepatol. 2005;43(4):637–44.
93. Henriksen JH, Gulberg V, Fuglsang S, Schifter S, Bendtsen F, Gerbes AL, et al. Q-T interval (QT(C)) in patients with cirrhosis: relation to vasoactive peptides and heart rate. Scand J Clin Lab Invest. 2007;67:643–53.
94. Trevisani F, Di Micoli A, Zambruni A, Biselli M, Santi V, Erroi V, et al. QT interval prolongation by acute gastrointestinal bleeding in patients with cirrhosis. Liver Int. 2012;32(10):1510–5.
95. Adigun AQ, Pinto AG, Flockhart DA, Gorski JC, Li L, Hall SD, et al. Effect of cirrhosis and liver transplantation on the gender difference in QT interval. Am J Cardiol. 2005;95(5):691–4.
96. Shin WJ, Kim YK, Song JG, Kim SH, Choi SS, Song JH, et al. Alterations in QT interval in patients undergoing living donor liver transplantation. Transplant Proc. 2011;43(1):170–3.
97. Henriksen JH, Bendtsen F, Hansen EF, Møller S. Acute non-selective beta-adrenergic blockade reduces prolonged frequency-adjusted Q-T interval (QTc) in patients with cirrhosis. J Hepatol. 2004;40(2):239–46.
98. Zambruni A, trevisani F, Di Micoli A, Savelli F, Berzigotti A, Bracci E, et al. Effect of chronic beta-blockade on QT interval in patients with liver cirrhosis. J Hepatol 2008;48(3):415–421.
99. Silvestre OM, Farias AQ, Ramos DS, Furtado MS, Rodrigues AC, Ximenes RO, et al. beta-Blocker therapy for cirrhotic cardiomyopathy: a randomized-controlled trial. Eur J Gastroenterol Hepatol. 2018;30(8):930–7.
100. Khan RS, Newsome PN. Non-alcoholic fatty liver disease and liver transplantation. Metabolism. 2016;65(8):1208–23.
101. Møller S, Bendtsen F. NAFLD: cardiovascular complications of NAFLD–they do matter. Nat Rev Gastroenterol Hepatol. 2015b;12(8):434–6.
102. Ripoll C, Yotti R, Bermejo J, Banares R. The heart in liver transplantation. J Hepatol. 2010;54:810–22.
103. Harinstein ME, Iyer S, Mathier MA, Flaherty JD, Fontes P, Planinsic RM, et al. Role of baseline echocardiography in the preoperative management of liver transplant candidates. Am J Cardiol. 2012;110(12):1852–5.

104. Ramalingam VS, Ansari S, Fisher M. Respiratory complication in liver disease. Crit Care Clin. 2016;32(3):357–69.
105. Møller S, Krag A, Henriksen JH, Bendtsen F. Pathophysiological aspects of pulmonary complications of cirrhosis. Scand J Gastroenterol. 2007;42(4):419–27.
106. Duranti R, Laffi G, Misuri G, Riccardi D, Gorini M, Foschi M, et al. Respiratory mechanics in patients with tense cirrhotic ascites. Eur Resp J. 1997;10:1622–30.
107. Rossle M, Gerbes AL. TIPS for the treatment of refractory ascites, hepatorenal syndrome and hepatic hydrothorax: a critical update. Gut. 2010;59(7):988–1000.
108. Rodriguez-Roisin R, Krowka MJ. Hepatopulmonary syndrome–a liver-induced lung vascular disorder. N Engl J Med. 2008;358(22):2378–87.
109. Machicao VI, Balakrishnan M, Fallon MB. Pulmonary complications in chronic liver disease. Hepatology. 2014;59(4):1627–37.
110. Møller S, Hillingsø J, Christensen E, Henriksen JH. Arterial hypoxaemia in cirrhosis: fact or fiction? Gut. 1998;42(6):868–74.
111. Henriksen JH, Bendtsen F, Møller S. Acid-base disturbance in patients with cirrhosis: relation to hemodynamic dysfunction. Eur J Gastroenterol Hepatol. 2015;27(8):920–7.
112. Raevens S, Geerts A, Van Steenkiste C, Verhelst X, Van Vlierberghe H, Colle I. Hepatopulmonary syndrome and portopulmonary hypertension: recent knowledge in pathogenesis and overview of clinical assessment. Liver Int. 2015;35(6):1646–60.
113. Gaines DI, Fallon MB. Hepatopulmonary syndrome. Liver Int. 2004;24(5):397–401.
114. Deibert P, Allgaier HP, Stefanie L, Mueller C, Olschewski M, Hamm H, et al. Hepatopulmonary syndrome in patients with chronic liver disease: role of pulse oximetry. BMC Gastroenterol. 2006;6:15.
115. Yigit IP, Hacievliyagil SS, Seckin Y, Oner RI, Karincaoglu M. The relationship between severity of liver cirrhosis and pulmonary function tests. Dig Dis Sci. 2008;53(7):1951–6.
116. Schenk P, Fuhrmann V, Madl C, Funk G, Lehr S, Kandel O, et al. Hepatopulmonary syndrome: prevalence and predictive value of various cut offs for arterial oxygenation and their clinical consequences. Gut. 2002;51(6):853–9.
117. Møller S, Krag A, Madsen JL, Henriksen JH, Bendtsen F. Pulmonary dysfunction and hepatopulmonary syndrome in cirrhosis and portal hypertension. Liver Int. 2009;29:1528–37.
118. Voiosu AM, Daha IC, Voiosu TA, Mateescu BR, Dan GA, Baicus CR, et al. Prevalence and impact on survival of hepatopulmonary syndrome and cirrhotic cardiomyopathy in a cohort of cirrhotic patients. Liver Int. 2015;35(12):2547–55.
119. Zhang M, Luo B, Chen SJ, Abrams GA, Fallon MB. Endothelin-1 stimulation of endothelial nitric oxide synthase in the pathogenesis of hepatopulmonary syndrome. Am J Physiol. 1999;277(5 Pt 1):G944–52.
120. Luo B, Liu L, Tang L, Zhang J, Stockard CR, Grizzle WE, et al. Increased pulmonary vascular endothelin B receptor expression and responsiveness to endothelin-1 in cirrhotic and portal hypertensive rats: a potential mechanism in experimental hepatopulmonary syndrome. J Hepatol. 2003;38(5):556–63.
121. Luo B, Tang L, Wang Z, Zhang J, Ling Y, Feng W, et al. Cholangiocyte Endothelin 1 and transforming growth factor beta1 production in rat experimental hepatopulmonary syndrome. Gastroenterology. 2005;129(2):682–95.
122. Zhang J, Ling Y, Luo B, Tang L, Ryter SW, Stockard CR, et al. Analysis of pulmonary heme oxygenase-1 and nitric oxide synthase alterations in experimental hepatopulmonary syndrome. Gastroenterology. 2003;125(5):1441–51.
123. Söderman C, Leone A, Furst V, Persson MG. Endogenous nitric oxide in exhaled air from patients with liver cirrhosis. Scand J Gastroenterol. 1997;32:591–7.
124. Afzelius P, Bazeghi N, Bie P, Bendtsen F, Vestbo J, Møller S. Circulating nitric oxide products do not solely reflect nitric oxide release in cirrhosis and portal hypertension. Liver Int 2011;10–3231.

125. Arguedas MR, Drake BB, Kapoor A, Fallon MB. Carboxyhemoglobin levels in cirrhotic patients with and without hepatopulmonary syndrome. Gastroenterology. 2005;128(2):328–33.
126. Raevens S, Geerts A, Paridaens A, Lefere S, Verhelst X, Hoorens A, et al. Placental growth factor inhibition targets pulmonary angiogenesis and represents a therapy for hepatopulmonary syndrome in mice. Hepatology. 2018;68(2):634–51.
127. Horvatits T, Drolz A, Roedl K, Herkner H, Ferlitsch A, Perkmann T, et al. vWF, a screening tool for detection of hepatopulmonary syndrome in patients with liver cirrhosis. J Hepatol. 2014;61:544–9.
128. Martinez GP, Barbera JA, Visa J, Rimola A, Pare JC, Roca J, et al. Hepatopulmonary syndrome in candidates for liver transplantation. J Hepatol. 2001;34(5):651–7.
129. Cotes JE, Chinn DJ, Quanjer PH, Roca J, Yernault JC. Standardization of the measurement of transfer factor (diffusing capacity). Eur Respir J. 1993;6(Suppl 16):41–52.
130. Fallon MB, Krowka MJ, Brown RS, Trotter JF, Zacks S, Roberts KE, et al. Impact of hepatopulmonary syndrome on quality of life and survival in liver transplant candidates. Gastroenterology. 2008;135(4):1168–75.
131. Gomez FP, Martinez-Palli G, Barbera JA, Roca J, Navasa M, Rodriguez-Roisin R. Gas exchange mechanism of orthodeoxia in hepatopulmonary syndrome. Hepatology. 2004;40:660–6.
132. Rodriguez-Roisin R, Krowka MJ, Herve P, Fallon MB. Pulmonary-hepatic vascular disorders (PHD). Eur Respir J. 2004;24(5):861–80.
133. Voiosu AM, Voiosu TA, Smarandache B, Radoi A, Mateescu RB, Baicus CR, et al. The impact of hypoxaemia on the outcome in liver cirrhosis. J Gastrointestin Liver Dis. 2016;25(4):481–487.
134. Arguedas MR, Singh H, Faulk DK, Fallon MB. Utility of pulse oximetry screening for hepatopulmonary syndrome. Clin Gastroenterol Hepatol. 2007;5(6):749–754.
135. Hoerning A, Raub S, Neudorf U, Muntjes C, Kathemann S, Lainka E, et al. Pulse oximetry is insufficient for timely diagnosis of hepatopulmonary syndrome in children with liver cirrhosis. J Pediatr. 2014;164(3):546–52.
136. Forde KA, Fallon MB, Krowka MJ, Sprys M, Goldberg DS, Krok KL, et al. Pulse oximetry is insensitive for detection of hepatopulmonary syndrome in patients evaluated for liver transplantation. Hepatology. 2019;69:270–81.
137. Møller S, Burchardt H, Ogard CG, Schiodt FV, Lund JO. Pulmonary blood volume and transit time in cirrhosis: relation to lung function. Liver Int. 2006;26(9):1072–8.
138. Krowka MJ, Dickson ER, Cortese DA. Hepatopulmonary syndrome—clinical observations and lack of therapeutic response to somatostatin analogue. Chest. 1993;104:515–21.
139. Schenk P, Schoniger-Hekele M, Fuhrmann V, Madl C, Silberhumer G, Muller C. Prognostic significance of the hepatopulmonary syndrome in patients with cirrhosis. Gastroenterology. 2003;125(4):1042–52.
140. Swanson KL, Wiesner RH, Krowka MJ. Natural history of hepatopulmonary syndrome: impact of liver transplantation. Hepatology. 2005;41(5):1122–9.
141. Raevens S, Rogiers X, Geerts A, Verhelst X, Samuel U, van RM, et al. Outcome of liver transplantation for hepatopulmonary syndrome: a eurotransplant experience. Eur Respir J. 2019;53(2). https://doi.org/10.1183/13993003.01096-2018.
142. Zhao H, Tsauo J, Zhang X, Ma H, Weng N, Wang L, et al. Pulmonary transit time derived from pulmonary angiography for the diagnosis of hepatopulmonary syndrome. Liver Int. 2018;38(11):1974–81.
143. Lejealle C, Paradis V, Bruno O, de RE, Francoz C, Soubrane O, et al. Evidence for an association between Iitrahepatic vascular changes and the development of hepatopulmonary syndrome. Chest 2019;155(1):123–136.
144. Aller R, Moya JL, Moreira V, Garcia-Lledo A, Sanroman AL, Paino C, et al. Diagnosis and grading of intrapulmonary vascular dilatation in cirrhotic patients with contrast transesophageal echocardiography. J Hepatol. 1999;31(6):1044–52.

145. Abrams GA, Nanda NC, Dubovsky EV, Krowka MJ, Fallon MB. Use of macroaggregated albumin lung perfusion scan to diagnose hepatopulmonary syndrome: a new approach. Gastroenterology. 1998;114:305–10.
146. Krishnamurthy GT, Krishnamurthy S. Nuclear hepatology. a textbook of hepatobiliary diseases. Berlin: Springer;2000.
147. Fragaki M, Sifaki-Pistolla D, Samonakis DN, Koulentaki M, Koukouraki S, Stathaki M, et al. Screening for hepatopulmonary syndrome in cirrhotic patients using Technetium 99m-macroaggregated Albumin Perfusion Lung Scan (Tc-MAA): diagnostic approach and clinical correlations. J Clin Gastroenterol. 2018;52(9):828–34.
148. Arguedas MR, Abrams GA, Krowka MJ, Fallon MB. Prospective evaluation of outcomes and predictors of mortality in patients with hepatopulmonary syndrome undergoing liver transplantation. Hepatology. 2003;37(1):192–7.
149. Allgaier HP, haag K, Ochs A, Haenstein KH, Jeserich M, Krause T, et al. Hepatopulmonary syndrome: succesful treatment by transjugular intrahepatic portosystemic stent-shunt (TIPS). J Hepatol. 1995;23:102.
150. Paramesh AS, Husain SZ, Shneider B, Guller J, Tokat I, Gondolesi GE, et al. Improvement of hepatopulmonary syndrome after transjugular intrahepatic portasystemic shunting: case report and review of literature. Pediatr Transplant. 2003;7(2):157–62.
151. Tsauo J, Zhao H, Zhang X, Ma H, Jiang M, Weng N, et al. Effect of transjugular intrahepatic portosystemic shunt creation on pulmonary gas exchange in patients with hepatopulmonary syndrome: a prospective study. J Vasc Interv Radiol. 2019;30(2):170–7.
152. Schwartz JM, Beymer C, Althaus SJ, Larson AM, Zaman A, Glickerman DJ, et al. Cardiopulmonary consequences of transjugular intrahepatic portosystemic shunts: role of increased pulmonary artery pressure. J Clin Gastroenterol. 2004;38(7):590–4.
153. Boyer TD, Haskal ZJ. The role of transjugular intrahepatic portosystemic shunt in the management of portal hypertension. Hepatology. 2005;41(2):386–400.
154. Murray KF, Carithers RL Jr. AASLD practice guidelines: evaluation of the patient for liver transplantation. Hepatology. 2006;41(6):1407–32.
155. Brussino L, Bucca C, Morello M, Scappaticci E, Mauro M, Rolla G. Effect on dyspnoea and hypoxaemia of inhaled N(G)-nitro-L-arginine methyl ester in hepatopulmonary syndrome. Lancet. 2003;362(9377):43–4.
156. Gomez FP, Barbera JA, Roca J, Burgos F, Gistau C, Rodriguez-Roisin R. Effects of nebulized N(G)-nitro-L-arginine methyl ester in patients with hepatopulmonary syndrome. Hepatology 2006;1084–1091.
157. Gupta S, Faughnan ME, Lilly L, Hutchison S, Fowler R, Bayoumi AM. Norfloxacin therapy for hepatopulmonary syndrome: a pilot randomized controlled trial. Clin Gastroenterol Hepatol. 2010.
158. Liu L, Liu N, Zhao Z, Liu J, Feng Y, Jiang H, et al. TNF-alpha neutralization improves experimental hepatopulmonary syndrome in rats. Liver Int. 2012;32(6):1018–26.
159. Rodriquez-Roisin R, Krowka MJ, Herve P, Fallon MB. Highlights of the ERS task force on pulmonary-hepatic vascular disorders (PHD). J Hepatol. 2005;42(6):924–7.
160. AbuHalimeh B, Krowka MJ, Tonelli AR. Treatment barriers in portopulmonary hypertension. Hepatology. 2019;69(1):431–43.
161. Kawut SM, Taichman DB, Ahya VN, Kaplan S, Archer-Chicko CL, Kimmel SE, et al. Hemodynamics and survival of patients with portopulmonary hypertension. Liver Transpl. 2005;11(9):1107–11.
162. Raevens S, Colle I, Reyntjens K, Geerts A, Berrevoet F, Rogiers X, et al. Echocardiography for the detection of portopulmonary hypertension in liver transplant candidates: an analysis of cutoff values. Liver Transpl. 2013;19(6):602–10.
163. Krowka MJ. Evolving dilemmas and management of portopulmonary hypertension. Semin Liver Dis. 2006;26(3):265–72.
164. Krowka MJ. Portopulmonary hypertension and the issue of survival. Liver Transpl. 2005a;11(9):1026–7.

165. Swanson KL, Wiesner RH, Nyberg SL, Rosen CB, Krowka MJ. Survival in portopulmonary hypertension: mayo clinic experience categorized by treatment subgroups. Am J Transplant. 2008;8(11):2445–53.
166. Sithamparanathan S, Nair A, Thirugnanasothy L, Coghlan JG, Condliffe R, Dimopoulos K, et al. Survival in portopulmonary hypertension: outcomes of the United Kingdom National Pulmonary Arterial Hypertension Registry. J Heart Lung Transplant. 2017;36(7):770–9.
167. Roberts KE, Fallon MB, Krowka MJ, Brown RS, Trotter JF, Peter I, et al. Genetic risk factors for portopulmonary hypertension in patients with advanced liver disease. Am J Respir Crit Care Med. 2009;179(9):835–42.
168. Cody RJ, Haas GJ, Binkley PF, Capers Q, Kelly R. Plasma endothelin correlates with the extent of pulmonary hypertension in patients with chronic congestive heart failure. Circulation. 1993;87:1064.
169. Barnes PJ. Endothelins and pulmonary diseases. J Appl Physiol. 1994;77:1051–9.
170. Talwalkar JA, Swanson KL, Krowka MJ, Andrews JC, Kamath PS. Prevalence of spontaneous portosystemic shunts in patients with portopulmonary hypertension and effect on treatment. Gastroenterology. 2011;141(5):1673–9.
171. Kuntzen C, Gulberg V, Gerbes AL. Use of a mixed endothelin receptor antagonist in portopulmonary hypertension: a safe and effective therapy? Gastroenterology. 2005;128(1):164–8.
172. Hoeper MM, Halank M, Marx C, Hoeffken G, Seyfarth HJ, Schauer J, et al. Bosentan therapy for portopulmonary hypertension. Eur Respir J. 2005;25(3):502–8.
173. Reichenberger F, Voswinckel R, Steveling E, Enke B, Kreckel A, Olschewski H, et al. Sildenafil treatment for portopulmonary hypertension. Eur Respir J. 2006;28(3):563–7.
174. Krowka MJ. Hepatopulmonary syndrome and portopulmonary hypertension: implications for liver transplantation. Clin Chest Med. 2005b;26(4):587–97.
175. Provencher S, Herve P, Jais X, Lebrec D, Humbert M, Simonneau G, et al. Deleterious effects of beta-blockers on exercise capacity and hemodynamics in patients with portopulmonary hypertension. Gastroenterology. 2006;130(1):120–6.
176. Malagari K, Nikita A, Alexopoulou E, Brountzos E, Papathanasiou M, Mitromaras J, et al. Cirrhosis-related intrathoracic disease. Imaging features in 1038 patients. Hepatogastroenterology 2005;52(62):558–562.
177. Badillo R, Rockey DC. Hepatic hydrothorax: clinical features, management, and outcomes in 77 patients and review of the literature. Medicine (Baltimore). 2014;93(3):135–42.
178. Gurung P, Goldblatt M, Huggins JT, Doelken P, Nietert PJ, Sahn SA. Pleural fluid analysis and radiographic, sonographic, and echocardiographic characteristics of hepatic hydrothorax. Chest. 2011;140(2):448–53.
179. Benet A, Vidal F, Toda R, Siurana R, De Virgala CM, Richart C. Diagnosis of hepatic hydrothorax in the absence of ascites by intraperitoneal injection of 99m-Tc-Fluor colloid. Postgrad Med J. 1992;68(796):153.
180. Rajnish A, Sudhakar P. Diagnosis of hepatic hydrothorax by Tc-99m sulfur colloid peritoneal scintigraphy. Clin Nucl Med. 2001;26(10):888.
181. Cardenas A, Kelleher T, Chopra S. Review article: hepatic hydrothorax. Aliment Pharmacol Ther. 2004;20(3):271–9.
182. Xiol X, Castellote J, Cortes-Beut R, Delgado M, Guardiola J, Sese E. Usefulness and complications of thoracentesis in cirrhotic patients. Am J Med. 2001;111(1):67–9.
183. Siegerstetter V, Deibert P, Ochs A, Olschewski M, Blum HE, Rossle M. Treatment of refractory hepatic hydrothorax with transjugular intrahepatic portosystemic shunt: long-term results in 40 patients. Eur J Gastroenterol Hepatol. 2001;13(5):529–34.
184. Wilputte JY, Goffette P, Zech F, Godoy-Gepert A, Geubel A. The outcome after transjugular intrahepatic portosystemic shunt (TIPS) for hepatic hydrothorax is closely related to liver dysfunction: a long-term study in 28 patients. Acta Gastroenterol Belg. 2007;70(1):6–10.
185. Møller S, Henriksen JH. Cirrhotic cardiomyopathy. J Hepatol. 2010;53(1):179–90.

Chapter 4
Liver Transplantation: Graft Variables

Shirin Elizabeth Khorsandi

Graft Types

Donor After Brain Stem Death (DBD)

The introduction of criteria to define brain stem death in 1968 by the Harvard Medical School made a significant impact on the developing field of liver transplantation [1–3]. As previously the only available livers for transplantation were from donors after cardiac death (DCD) (see Sect. "Donor After Cardiac Death (DCD)"). In countries where brain stem death definition was accepted, an expansion in liver transplantation occurred as DBD livers became the main organ utilized. However, globally there are variations in the testing and acceptance of brain stem death and in infants less than 2 months modifications are required [2, 4, 5]. In countries where DBD is accepted physiological optimization of the donor in the Intensive Care environment is to be encouraged by the application of care bundles designed to address the events that occur on brain stem death such as hypovolemia, diabetes insipidus and the systemic inflammation of the associated cytokine storm [6].

From the DBD procurement aspect, the operation undertaken to remove organs from the donor, will in general have the appearance of a "conventional" operation with the donor coming to theatre on full life support. The majority of the dissection is peformed in the warm phase (i.e. the donor has a cardiac output) enabling anatomy to be identified and vessels prepared to facilitate cannulation. Before cross clamp of the thoracic aorta the donor is systemically heparinized, life support stops and the systemic circulation vented into the chest. Perfusion with chilled preservation fluid (University of Wisconsin (UW)) then commences (see

S. E. Khorsandi (✉)
Kings College Hospital & Kings College London, London, UK
e-mail: shirinelizabethkhorsandi@nhs.net

Z. Milan and C. Goonasekera (eds.), *Anesthesia for Hepatico-Pancreatic-Biliary Surgery and Transplantation*, https://doi.org/10.1007/978-3-030-51331-3_4

Sect. "Cold Static Storage") via cannulas that have been inserted in the infra-renal aorta or iliac artery and cross clamp applied. For liver preservation the portal vein/superior mesenteric vein is also cannulated to allow for dual aortic and portal perfusion in situ, though some donor teams elect to do this at a later stage and perform ex situ portal perfusion on the back bench. Procurement now enters the cold phase, where organs accepted for transplant are removed from the donor and packed appropriately for transportation.

Donor After Cardiac Death (DCD)

With liver transplantation becoming an established treatment for a range of liver diseases, disparity between the waiting list and available donor pool has become more evident and this is a determinant of death on the waiting list. To address this imbalance, the use of "marginal" livers such as the DCD liver has been revisited. Earlier reports on DCD liver transplantation demonstrated poorer outcomes compared to DBD, attributed to the higher rate of primary non function, hepatic artery thrombosis and primary ischemic cholangiopathy [7, 8] leading to a reluctance to utilize these grafts.

Critical determinants of DCD outcome are primarily related to the sequence of donor warm ischemia followed by a period of cold ischemia that drives tissue damage (see Sect. "Ischemic Times of Note"). The biliary epithelium is especially vulnerable leading to the development of a primary ischemic cholangiopathy. However, in high volume units with an established experience in DCD liver transplantation, outcomes in DCD and DBD liver transplantation can become equivalent [9, 10]. DCD liver transplantation has not been adopted by all countries and the proportion of DCD contributing to the donor pool vary according to each country. In the UK DCD donors account for 30–40% of the donor pool (Fig. 4.1).

The Maastricht classification is used to group the DCD donors as follows [12]:

I Brought in dead (uncontrolled).
II Unsuccessful resuscitation (uncontrolled).
III Awaiting cardiac arrest (controlled).
IV Cardiac arrest after brain-stem death (controlled/uncontrolled).

Typically, Category III DCD are used in liver transplantation with a smaller contribution from Category IV [13]. In contrast to the events of DBD procurement, withdrawal of life support occurs in the anesthetic room or in Intensive Care Unit, according to donor hospital preference. In the UK, the donor team will be scrubbed and on standby in the operating room while receiving regular updates on the donor's observations (blood pressure, heart rate, and oxygen saturation). On declaration of circulatory death, a 5-min standoff period is observed before

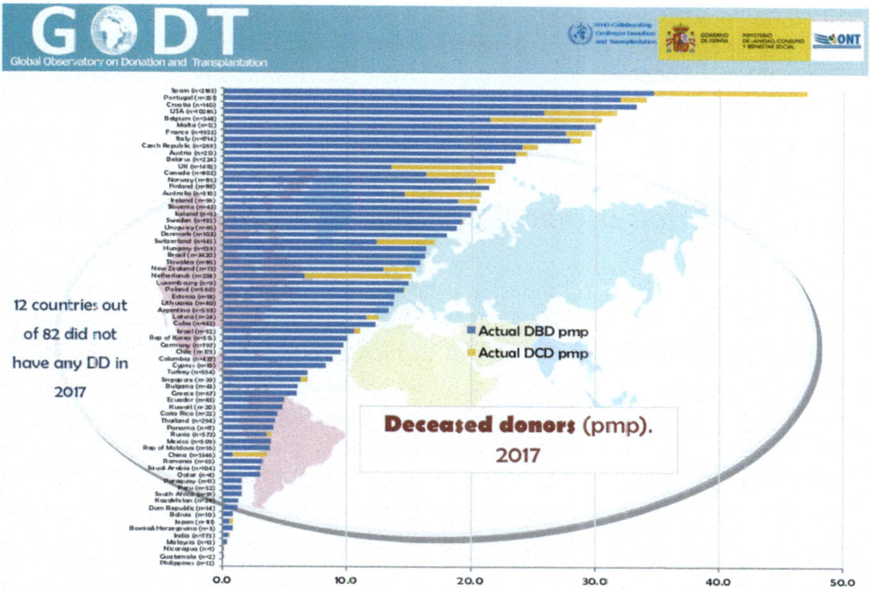

Fig. 4.1 Summary of Global Transplant Donor Activity in 2017, demonstrating country variation in the adoption in Donor After Brain Stem Death (DBD) and Donor After Cardiac Death (DCD). This 2017 data is based on the Global Observatory on Donation and Transplantation (GODT) data, produced by the WHO-ONT (Spanish Transplant Organization) collaboration [11]

the donor is transferred into the operating room. A superfast procurement is advocated.

In brief, a thoraco-abdominal incision is made with caval venting typically into the chest, followed in sequence by aortic cannulation, cross-clamp in the chest and portal or superior mesenteric vein cannulation. On commencement of perfusion with UW that initially contains heparin, the gallbladder and bile duct are promptly and copiously flushed with chilled UW. Single center, and nationwide studies have demonstrated a negative impact on DCD liver transplant outcomes if hepatectomy time is longer than 60 minutes [14, 15] so a rapid donor hepatectomy is encouraged. Cold static storage is presently the standard, with the organ stored in UW, triple bagged and packed in ice for transportation. Though in the last 5 years, selected cases according to local preference have been managed with ex-situ normothermic perfusion, hypothermic machine perfusion or in situ regional normothermic perfusion (see Sect. "Machine Perfusion: Normothermic/Hypothermic").

In general, best practice is to decide on the use of a DCD graft in a given recipient at time of listing, with the recipient consented in advance of transplant. Recipients selected for a DCD liver are typically primary transplants for chronic liver disease with or without Hepatocellular Carcinoma (HCC), with a low MELD/

UKELD, not in acute liver failure or where a prolonged/difficult recipient hepatectomy is anticipated such as redo transplantation, young adult extrahepatic biliary atresia or the presence of extensive portomesenteric thrombosis. Thereby helping to minimize the cold ischemic time.

Partial Liver Grafts (Reduced, Split and Living Related)

The use of partial grafts provides a solution to both organ shortage and size restriction in transplanting young children and small adults <40Kg. Liver reduction techniques were initially developed to increase the donor pool available for children and was made possible by the introduction of UW solution, which allows for up to 20 hours of cold preservation time [16]. Reduction techniques are based on the segmental anatomy of the liver and typically produce three grafts of varying size. The left lateral segment (LLS) (segments II and III), which comprises 25–30% of the whole liver and allows a size reduction from donor to recipient of 10:1. Use of a left lobe (segments 1–4), provides a size reduction of 3:1 and the right lobe (segments 5–8), of 1.5:1. Partial grafts account for 80% and 52% of all LT performed among patients aged 0–2 and 2–15 years old, respectively (Fig. 4.2).

Liver reduction is performed as a bench procedure in the operating theatre on DBD grafts. Outcomes of DCD reduction are presently poor and is avoided. The liver is kept in cold (4 °C) UW solution throughout the procedure. The extent of

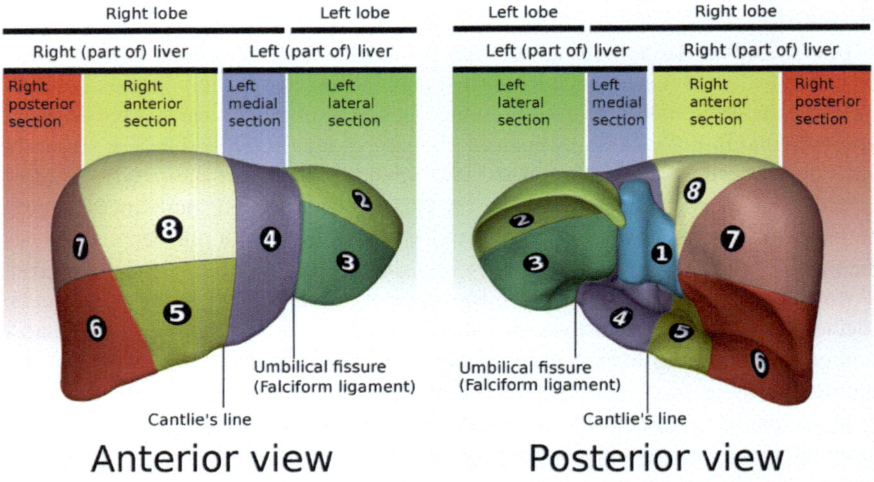

Fig. 4.2 Graphical summary of the segmental anatomy of the liver that determine transection lines for partial graft preparation [17]

reduction is determined by visual comparison between the donor liver and the recipient hepatic fossa. Reduction produces one section of liver to be transplanted, with the donor vena cava remaining with the lobe (left or right) to be transplanted while the residual liver is discarded or offered for hepatocyte isolation.

Early experience of reduced grafts, either left lobe or left lateral segment (LLS) in pediatric practice [18] led to the evolution of split and living donor liver transplantation with both these techniques being incorporated into routine clinical practice from 1991 onwards. Split transplantation is where a whole DBD adult liver is divided into two grafts, allowing the transplantation of two recipients, classically one child that receives the LLS and one adult who receives the right lobe. Split transplantation can either be done in situ at time of initial procurement or ex situ on the back bench as for the process of a reduction. Advantages of an in situ split are shorter cold ischemic times and a cut surface that is less likely to bleed on reperfusion [19]. Donors that are typically considered for split are DBD, less than 40 years of age, less than 5 days on Intensive Care Unit, have good liver function and the liver is non steatotic.

The feasibility of deceased split liver transplantation and the increased safety of conventional liver surgery led to the concept of removing part of the liver, initially the left lateral segment (LLS), from a living adult donor and transplanting the graft into a pediatric recipient. The drive for the development of this procedure was the shortage of organs for children during the early 1990′s that was producing a waiting list mortality upto 25%. Living donor liver transplantation (LDLT) has become an important source of grafts for children worldwide following its first description in 1989 [20]. The success of LDLT in pediatrics led to the establishment of adult to adult LDLT that has become main graft type in countries where deceased donation has not been widely adopted (21). The LLS is the most commonly used graft in pediatric LDLT while full left or right lobe grafts tend to be reserved for adults [22]. The main priority in LDLT is there should be no compromise in donor safety (Fig. 4.3).

Auxiliary Partial Liver Transplantation (APOLT)

Auxiliary Partial Liver Transplantation (APOLT) is a where a partial liver graft is transplanted into an anatomically correct position (orthotopic) while leaving a section of native liver behind. This can be done in adult or pediatrics in the context of acute liver failure (ALF) in order to support liver function. After recovering from the critical illness, immunosuppression can be slowly weaned so that the graft gradually involutes while the native liver regenerates. Thereby allowing the recipient to have an immunosuppression free life in the future. Recipients for this type of transplantation need to be reasonably stable in the context of ALF, in order to tolerate native hepatectomy that is needed to provide the space for the partial graft and the native liver is anticipated to have regenerative capacity [23].

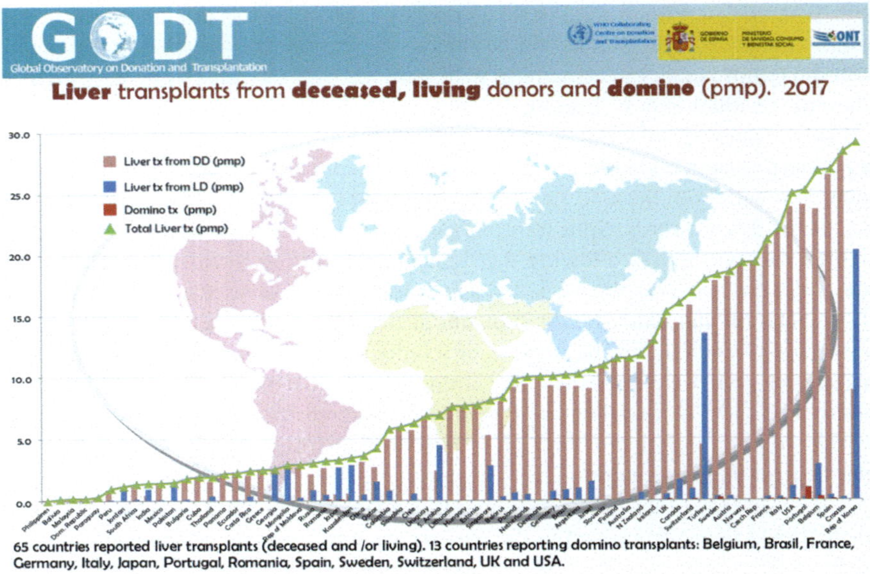

Fig. 4.3 Summary of Global Transplant Donor Activity in 2017, demonstrating country variation in graft usage for liver transplantation from deceased (DBD and DCD), living donor and domino. This 2017 data is based on the Global Observatory on Donation and Transplantation (GODT) data, produced by the WHO-ONT collaboration [11]

The other clinical scenario where APOLT can be considered is in selected cases of non cirrhotic monogenetic metabolic disease with the aim to improve quality of life but allowing the potential of gene therapy to the native liver and immunosuppression withdrawal in the future [24]. When performing APOLT in this scenario, a ligature is placed around the portal branch to the native liver to ensure sufficient portal flow to the graft. In contrast APOLT for ALF, the native liver will be "stiff" ensuring sufficient portal flow to the graft. The partial grafts used in APOLT can be from living or DBD donors applying the same selection criteria when a partial graft is used to replace the whole liver. Typically, children will receive a left lateral segment or left lobe while adults receive a right lobe.

Domino

The shortage in organ availability continually drives the exploration of alternative strategies to find suitable livers for transplantation. One such approach is domino transplantation where selected liver transplant recipients can donate their explanted liver to another patient. There are a number of hereditary diseases caused by aberrant or deficient protein production in the liver, and presently liver transplantation is used to treat these conditions until gene therapy becomes established. Apart from a well-defined gene defect, these explanted livers will be otherwise structurally and functionally normally.

However, there can be the risk of de novo disease in the domino liver recipient. The biggest domino experience is in Familial amyloid polyneuropathy (FAP), an autosomal dominant hereditary disease, where a mutation in the transthyretin (TTR) gene leads to the deposition of misfolded amyloid resulting in a range of neurologic, gastrointestinal and cardiac symptoms ([25], see Fig. 4.3). The Val30Met is the most common mutation but has the highest risk of de novo amyloidosis in the recipient, occurring at approximately 10 years after transplant [26, 27]. As a consequence, many centres will select older recipients with hepatocellular cancer, as the risk benefit of de novo systemic amyloidosis versus death/going outside cancer listing criteria is appropriate and the recipient will be accordingly counselled before giving informed consent.

Ischemic Times of Note

Cold Ischemic Time

The Cold ischemia time (CIT) is widely acknowledged as a donor related risk factor in liver transplantation and is defined as the time from cross-clamping in the donor to removal of the liver from cold static storage solution prior to transplantation. The CIT is often determined by transportation times but can also be influenced by other variables such as logistical factors at the receiving transplant unit or a technically difficult recipient hepatectomy. The CIT is often incorporated into scoring systems such as the donor risk index (DRI) or DCD-DRI, which are used to try and quantify the risk of graft failure [14, 28]. Ideally, in DBD liver transplantation the CIT is kept under 12 hours and for DCD under 8 hours, as beyond these times outcome becomes poorer. Minimizing the CIT in marginal grafts (e.g. elderly donors, steatosis) is of increasing importance as it will reduce the degree of ischemic reperfusion injury and subsequent risk of initial poor graft function or primary non function.

Warm Ischemic Time (WIT)

In the context of DCD liver transplantation, the warm ischemic time (WIT) has a significant impact on outcome, being associated with the occurrence of cholangiopathy, initial poor graft function and primary non function. In the literature, varying ways of defining the WIT has been used. In the USA, the donor warm ischemic time (dWIT) is often defined as the time from withdrawal of life support to the start of in situ cold aortic perfusion. While other units prefer to use the donor agonal time (DAT), also known as the functional dWIT, which is defined as a time from a specific donor blood pressure or oxygen saturation (SaO_2) after the withdrawal of life support to the start of aortic perfusion [29]. However, different Units use different hemodynamic parameters to define the start of the functional dWIT. In the United Network for Organ Sharing data, the agonal phase starts when the donor systolic blood pressure drops below 80 mm Hg and/or donor SaO2 drops below 80% [30]. At King's College Hospital, the functional dWIT is defined from a SaO2 below 70% or systolic of 50 mmHg, dependent on which agonal observation occurs first. A dWIT or DAT longer than 30 minutes is considered to increase the risk of graft loss [31, 32] and stringency to this time is thought to be the basis of cholangiopathy rates and the need for retransplantation [33].

The Marginal Graft

The lack of suitable donors for liver transplantation has driven the use of marginal or extended criteria livers. To assess the risk of using such grafts led to the development of the Donor Risk Index (DRI) [28] that included variables such as DBD/DCD, donor age, donor cause of death, CIT or split. Since the introduction of the DRI, additional donor variables have been added such as BMI>30, liver steatosis>40%, serum sodium>165 mmol/L and serum liver function tests [34]. Classically, marginal grafts or grafts from extended criteria donors can be prone to ischemia—reperfusion injury, which can result in early graft dysfunction and biliary complications [35]. In addition, these grafts increase the risk of post-reperfusion syndrome, a decrease in systemic mean BP>30% below baseline for at least 1 minute during the first 5 minutes of liver reperfusion, which negatively impacts both graft and patient outcome [36].

Donor Recipient Matching

To produce good outcome in liver transplantation it is important to balance the risk between the donor and the recipient, as epitomized by using a high risk graft (e.g DCD) in a low risk recipient that has a low MELD, typically these will be recipients where Hepatocellular Carcinoma is the primary indication for transplant. The ability to balance the risk of the donor with that of the recipient variables has often been based on clinical experience. However, a number of scoring systems have been developed to assist in the decision making on using a DBD or DCD graft in a given recipient [37]. In the context of a donor/recipient DCD risk index, important variables to be considered are the functional dWIT, donor hepatectomy time, CIT, MELD and indication for liver transplantation [14, 38]. While the continued refinement in algorithms to match the donor liver to the recipient for best outcome, has led to the clinical application of the Transplant Benefit

Score (TBS) that has become the basis for the UK National Liver Offering System (NLOS) for DBD grafts in adults [39].

Liver Preservation

Cold Static Storage (CSS)

Cold static storage is the traditional method of donor liver preservation i.e. the liver is flushed with chilled preservation fluid and stored on ice. Working on the principle of reducing cellular metabolism to slow down ATP depletion and accumulation of metabolites. Initial preservation fluids used came from the field of kidney transplantation [40, 41], with the introduction of UW in the late 1980s [16] changing the field of liver transplantation by prolonging the cold ischemic time. Subsequent, alternatives to UW are histidine-tryptophan-ketoglutarate solution (HTK), Celsior solution (CE) and Institute Georges Lopez solution (IGL-1) [42] but for many, UW remains the gold standard. Of note, preservation fluid can be rich in potassium (i.e. UW and IGL-1) and therefore before reperfusion in the recipient, the graft must be flushed to avoid hyperkalemic cardiac arrest.

Machine Perfusion: Normothermic/Hypothermic

Over the past 5–10 years the utility of machine perfusion to recondition/resuscitate marginal grafts and/or extend preservation times has been increasingly explored. It can be subdivided into normothermic machine perfusion at 37 °C (NMP) using oxygenated blood or hypothermic machine perfusion at 4 °C (HMP) using oxygenated preservation fluid. Furthermore, normothermic machine perfusion can be applied to the liver while it remains in situ or ex situ.

Normothermic machine perfusion "in situ" is otherwise known as normothermic regional perfusion (NRP) and involves cannulating the donor to allow an "ECMO" circuit to be applied to the liver. Proponents of this approach advocate its use in the context of a DCD only, in order to minimize the ischemic damage and to improve outcomes compared to that of an expedited donor hepatectomy [43, 44]. In contrast, NMP can be applied to the donor liver (DBD/DCD) after hepatectomy with commencement of machine perfusion either starting in the donor hospital or at the recipient hospital (back to base/back to hub). The safety and feasibility of NMP has been clinically demonstrated, with a randomized control study demonstrating a benefit over CSS in terms of reducing recipient peak serum aspartate aminotransferase (AST) and potentially reducing liver discard rate [45]. NMP also allows a period of viability assessment eg lactate clearance, glucose metabolism, pH maintenance [46]. However, NMP viability criteria are yet to be validated.

Hypothermic Machine Perfusion also has data demonstrating that it can reduce biliary complications and shorten hospital stay in DCD liver transplantation [47]. Randomized control trials are presently running to demonstrate the benefit of HMP over CSS for both DBD and DCD grafts. But studies in the future are ultimately needed to compare the benefits of normothermic over hypothermic machine perfusion in liver transplantation.

References

1. A definition of irreversible coma: report of the Ad Hoc Committee of the Harvard Medical School to Examine the Definition of Brain Death. JAMA. 1968;205(6):337–40.
2. https://aomrc.org.uk/wp-content/uploads/2016/04/Code_Practice_Confirmation_Diagnosis_Death_1008-4.pdf. Accessed March 2020.
3. https://nhsbtdbe.blob.core.windows.net/umbraco-assets-corp/1354/neurological-death-dnc-guide-final.pdf. Accessed 2020.
4. Gardiner D, Shemie S, Manara A, Opdam H. International perspective on the diagnosis of death. Br J Anaesth. 2012;108(Suppl 1):i14–28.
5. Wijdicks EF. Brain death worldwide: accepted fact but no global consensus in diagnostic criteria. Neurology. 2002;58(1):20–5.
6. https://www.odt.nhs.uk/deceased-donation/best-practice-guidance/donor-optimisation/. Accessed March 2020.
7. Foley DP, Fernandez LA, Leverson G, Chin LT, Krieger N, Cooper JT, et al. Donation after cardiac death: the University of Wisconsin experience with liver transplantation. Ann Surg. 2005;242(5):724–31.
8. Mathur AK, Heimbach J, Steffick DE, Sonnenday CJ, Goodrich NP, Merion RM. Donation after cardiac death liver transplantation: predictors of outcome. Am J Transplant. 2010a;10(11):2512–9.
9. Croome KP, Lee DD, Keaveny AP, Taner CB. Improving national results in liver transplantation using grafts from donation after cardiac death donors. Transplantation. 2016;100(12):2640–7.
10. Khorsandi SE, Yip VS, Cortes M, Jassem W, Quaglia A, O'Grady J, Heneghan M, Aluvihare V, Agarwal K, Menon K, Vilca-Melendez H, Prachalias A, Srinivasan P, Suddle A, Rela M, Heaton N. Does donation after cardiac death utilization adversely affect hepatocellular cancer survival? Transplantation. 2016;100(9):1916–24.
11. https://www.transplant-observatory.org. Accessed March 2020.
12. Kootstra G, Daemen JH, Oomen A. Categories of non-heart-beating donors. Transpl Proc. 1995;27(5):2893–4.
13. Davila D, Ciria R, Jassem W, et al. Prediction models of donor arrest and graft utilization in liver transplantation from maastricht-3 donors after circulatory death. Am J Transplant. 2012;12:3414–24.
14. Khorsandi SE, Giorgakis E, Vilca-Melendez H, O'Grady J, Heneghan M, Aluvihare V, et al. Developing a donation after cardiac death risk index for adult and pediatric liver transplantation. World J Transplant. 2017;7(3):203–12.
15. Jochmans I, Fieuws S, Tieken I, Samuel U, Pirenne J. The impact of hepatectomy time of the liver graft on post-transplant outcome: a eurotransplant cohort study. Ann Surg. 2019;269(4):712–7.
16. Kalayoglu M, Hoffmann RM, D'Alessandro AM, et al. Results of extended preservation of the liver for clinical transplantation. Transplant Proc. 1989;21:3487–8.
17. https://commons.wikimedia.org/w/index.php?curid=45604146. Accessed March 2020.

18. Broelsch CE, Emond JC, Thistlethwaite JR, Whitington PF, Zucker AR, Baker AL, Aran PF, Rouch DA, Lichtor JL. Liver transplantation, including the concept of reduced-size liver transplants in children. Ann Surg. 1988;208(4):410–20.
19. Reyes J, Gerber D, Mazariegos GV, Casavilla A, Sindhi R, Bueno J, Madariaga J, Fung JJ. Split-liver transplantation: a comparison of ex vivo and in situ techniques. J Pediatr Surg. 2000;35(2):283–9.
20. Raia S, Nery JR, Mies S. Liver transplantation from live donors. Lancet. 1989;2:49.
21. Chan SC, Fan ST. Historical perspective of living donor liver transplantation. World J Gastroenterol. 2008;14(1):15–21.
22. Tanaka K, Uemoto S, Tokunaga Y, Fujita S, et al. Surgical techniques and innovations in living donor liver transplantation. Ann Surg. 1992;140:82–91.
23. Rela M, Kaliamoorthy I, Reddy MS. Current status of auxiliary partial orthotopic liver transplantation for acute liver failure. Liver Transplant. 2016;22(9):1265–74.
24. Reddy MS, Rajalingam R, Rela M. Revisiting APOLT for metabolic liver disease: a new look at an old idea. Transplantation. 2017;101(2):260–6.
25. Familial Amyloidotic Polyneuropathy World Transplant Registry. https://www.fapwtr.org. Accessed March 2020.
26. Llado L, Baliellas C, Casasnovas C, et al. Risk of transmission of systemic transthyretin amyloidosis after domino liver transplantation. Liver Transplant. 2010;16:1385.
27. Vollmar J, Schmid JC, Hoppe-Lotichius M, Barreiros AP, Azizi M, Emrich T, Geber C, Schad A, Weyer V, Otto G, Heise M, Mittler J, Birklein F, Lang H, Galle PR, Zimmermann T. Progression of transthyretin (TTR) amyloidosis in donors and recipients after domino liver transplantation-a prospective single-center cohort study. Transpl Int. 2018;31(11):1207–1215.
28. Feng S, Goodrich NP, Bragg-Gresham JL, Dykstra DM, Punch JD, DebRoy MA, Greenstein SM, Merion RM. Characteristics associated with liver graft failure: the concept of a donor risk index.
29. Coffey JC, Wanis KN, Monbaliu D, Gilbo N, Selzner M, Vachharajani N, et al. The influence of functional warm ischemia time on DCD liver transplant recipients' outcomes. Clin Transplant. 2017;31:e13063.
30. https:// optn.transplant.hrsa.gov/resources/glossary. Accessed March 2020.
31. Foley DP. Impact of donor warm ischemia time on outcomes after donation after cardiac death liver transplantation. Liver Transplant. 2014;20:509–11.
32. Mathur AK, Heimbach J, Steffick DE, Sonnenday CJ, Goodrich NP, Merion RM. Donation after cardiac death liver transplantation: predictors of outcome. Am J Transplant. 2010b;10:2512–9.
33. DeOliveira ML, Jassem W, Valente R, Khorsandi SE, Santori G, Prachalias A, Srinivasan P, Rela M, Heaton N. Biliary complications after liver transplantation using grafts from donors after cardiac death: results from a matched control study in a single large volume center. Ann Surg. 2011;254(5):716–22.
34. Flores A, Asrani SK. The donor risk index: a decade of experience. Liver Transplant. 2017;23(9):1216–25.
35. Busuttil RW, Tanaka K. The utility of marginal donors in liver transplantation. Liver Transplant. 2003;9:651–63.
36. Paugam-Burtz C, Kavafyan J, Merckx P, Dahmani S, Sommacale D, Ramsay M, Belghiti J, Mantz J. Postreperfusion syndrome during liver transplantation for cirrhosis: outcome and predictors. Liver Transplant. 2009;15:522–9.
37. Haydon GH, Hiltunen Y, Lucey MR, Collett D, Gunson B, Murphy N, Nightingale PG, Neuberger J. Self-organizing maps can determine outcome and match recipients and donors at orthotopic liver transplantation. Transplantation. 2005;79:213–8.
38. Schlegel A, Kalisvaart M, Scalera I, Laing RW, Mergental H, Mirza DF, Perera T, Isaac J, Dutkowski P, Muiesan P. The UK DCD risk score: a new proposal to define futility in donation-after-circulatory-death liver transplantation. J Hepatol. 2018;68(3):456–64.

39. https://www.odt.nhs.uk/odt-structures-and-standards/odt-hub-programme/national-liver-offering-scheme/. Accessed March 2020.
40. Collins GM, Bravo-Shugarman M, Terasaki PI. Kidney preservation for transportation. Initial perfusion and 30 hours ice storage. Lancet. 1969;2:1219–1222.
41. Belzer FO, Ashby BS, Dunphy JE. 24-hour and 72-hour preservation of canine kidneys. Lancet. 1967;2:536–8.
42. Adam R, Delvart V, Karam V, Ducerf C, Navarro F, Letoublon C, Belghiti J, Pezet D, Castaing D, Le Treut YP, Gugenheim J, Bachellier P, Pirenne J. Muiesan P ELTR contributing centres, the European Liver, Intestine Transplant Association (ELITA) compared efficacy of preservation solutions in liver transplantation: a long-term graft outcome study from the European Liver Transplant Registry. Am J Transplant. 2015;15:395–406.
43. Oniscu GC, Randle LV, Muiesan P, et al. In situ normothermic regional perfusion for controlled donation after circulatory death–the United Kingdom experience. Am J Transplant. 2014;14:2846.
44. Watson CJE, Hunt F, Messer S, et al. In situ normothermic perfusion of livers in controlled circulatory death donation may prevent ischemic cholangiopathy and improve graft survival. Am J Transplant. 2019;19(6):1745–58.
45. Nasralla D, Coussios CC, Mergental H, et al A randomized trial of normothermic preservation in liver transplantation. Nature. 2018;557:50.
46. Watson CJE, Kosmoliaptsis V, Pley C, et al. Observations on the ex situ perfusion of livers for transplantation. Am J Transplant. 2018;18:2005.
47. Dutkowski P, Polak WG, Muiesan P, et al. First comparison of hypothermic oxygenated perfusion versus static cold storage of human donation after cardiac death liver transplants: an international-matched case analysis. Ann Surg. 2015;262:764.

Chapter 5
Surgical Aspects of Liver Transplantation

Evangelia Florou, Joe Macmillan and Andreas Prachalias

Introduction

Over the past 30 years there have been significant advancements and improvements in the surgical technique, perioperative care and outcomes in patients undergoing liver transplant (LT) surgery [1–3].

A greater understanding of chronic liver disease and of the physiological impact of liver failure, as well as improvements in the knowledge of liver anatomy, have all contributed to significant conceptual and technical advances in liver transplantation [2, 3].

Liver transplantation is the standard treatment for end stage liver disease. The current national survival rate in the UK following a first liver transplant is 94% at one year and 80% at 5 years [4]. Cadaveric and living donor liver transplants between adults or between adult and child are now routinely performed in high volume transplant centers worldwide.

Liver pathophysiology is reviewed and a thorough description of both the caval replacement and the piggyback techniques are described in a comprehensive manner supported by multiple illustrations. Additionally, key complications related to liver transplant surgery are described and their causes discussed.

E. Florou (✉)
Clinical Fellow in Hepato-Pancreato-Biliary Surgery and Liver Transplantation, King's College Hospital, London, UK
e-mail: e.florou@nhs.net

J. Macmillan
Consultant Anaesthetist, King's College Hospital, London, UK
e-mail: jmacmillan1@nhs.net

A. Prachalias
Consultant Surgeon in Hepato-Pancreato-Biliary Surgery and Liver Transplantation, King's College Hospital, London, UK
e-mail: andreas.prachalias@nhs.net

Z. Milan and C. Goonasekera (eds.), *Anesthesia for Hepatico-Pancreatic-Biliary Surgery and Transplantation*, https://doi.org/10.1007/978-3-030-51331-3_5

Basic Liver Pathophysiology and Haemodynamics

The liver has a dual blood supply; the hepatic artery provides 25%, while the portal vein provides the remaining 75% of hepatic inflow. The arterial supply provides 50–70% of the oxygen requirements of the liver, while portal inflow provides the remaining 30–50% of oxygenated blood rich in nutrients from gut absorption [5, 6]. The liver parenchyma is highly vascularized with blood representing 25% of its volume [6, 7]. The total blood liver inflow is approximately 1500 ml/ 29 min for a 70 kg adult, representing 25% of the cardiac output (CO) [6, 7, 8].

The arterial system is both a high pressure and high resistance system and its regulation is subjected to systemic arterial pressure changes. Conversely, the portal system is a very low pressure, low resistance and valveless system. Normal portal vein pressure is 5–8 mmHg. The pressure in the hepatic veins is 1–2 mmHg and the normal estimated wedge pressure (pressure within liver sinusoids) is 2–4 mmHg [6].

The large blood volume retained within the liver is indicative of its high capacitance: 40% of the intraparenchymal blood volume is contained within the hepatic veins (HV), portal vein (PV) and hepatic artery (HA), while the remaining 60% is held within the hepatic sinusoids [5, 6].

Therefore, the liver is also acting as a blood reservoir. Almost half of the hepatic blood volume can be released from the liver in response to active or passive stimuli [5, 8, 9]. Splanchnic vasoconstriction following haemorrhage leads to a passive decrease in portal flow and intrahepatic pressure, resulting in the release of blood from the liver into the systemic circulation. Cardiac output increases by virtue of the Frank-Starling Law, due to an increase in preload which results in an improvement of splanchnic circulation and eventually restores portal inflow [5–10].

The hepatic vascular bed is also very compliant giving the liver the ability to accommodate changes in intravasular blood volume in response to changes in intrahepatic pressure [5, 8]. Moreover, the blood flow within the portal system is only indirectly regulated by a combination of extrahepatic and intrahepatic mechanisms [5, 6, 8]. The hepatic resistance is naturally very low and the portal blood flow is affected by portal pressure changes in a complex manner. The resistance at pre- and post- sinusoidal vasculature sites has been found to be passively distensible [5, 6, 8, 9]. If vascular resistance to the portal flow is increased up to a level, for example by stimulation of sympathetic nerve system, the portal pressure will rise, however, the flow will not drop [5, 7]. The physiology of the hepatic vascular bed is more complex and both its microcirculation and flow regulation mechanisms remain poorly understood.

The hepatic compliance in liver cirrhosis has not been studied, however, it is considered to be impaired due to fibrosis causing limited distensibility of the liver parenchyma [5, 6, 8, 9].

Portal hypertension (PHTN) is a term describing high pressure across the portal system and is defined by elevation of the hepatic venous pressure gradient (HVPG) [11–13].

$$\text{HVPG} = \text{WHVP} - \text{FHVP}$$

(Hepatic Venous Pressure Gradient) = (Wedge Hepatic Venous Pressure−Free Hepatic Venous Pressure).

PHTN develops progressively in the setting of liver disease and is evident in cases of cirrhotic liver parenchyma. Portal hypertension is defined by a HVPG > 5 mmHg. An HVPG that is > 10 mmHg is clinically significant PHTN and is predictive of variceal formation. An HVPG > 12 mmHg denotes a severe risk for variceal bleeding and ascites [11, 12].

The elevated pressure in portal circulation found in end stage liver disease (ESLD) is the result of a combination of changes within the vascular bed. These are mostly structural changes such as extensive parenchymal fibrosis leading to cirrhosis. The resulting accumulation of metabolic products affects the systemic vascular tone, causing a hyperdynamic circulation [13, 14].

When it comes to liver transplantation, altered haemodynamics due to cirrhosis need to be reversed by the new liver graft. Portal hyperperfusion can have deleterious effects to the newly transplanted liver since the liver itself is unable to accommodate the increased portal flow immediately. These implications can be profound when marginal or partial grafts are used.

The hepatic arterial buffer response (HABR) refers to the change of hepatic arterial inflow due to changes in portal flow and represents the hepatic parenchyma mechanism of coping with variations in portal flow. With a drop in splanchnic flow, portal inflow decreases and adenosine accumulates in the peri-portal spaces causing arterial vasodilation [5, 7, 15, 16]. This arterial dilatation increases liver inflow restoring the overall blood supply. Conversely, when portal flow increases, adenosine is rapidly washed out, causing hepatic artery constriction, thereby limiting the hepatic inflow [5, 15].

Surgical interference to portal or arterial flow can provoke or prevent HABR respectively. Manipulation of portal flow is achieved by splenic artery ligation or portocaval shunt creation, both surgical approaches used in liver transplantation and extended liver resections [15, 16]. Surgical manipulation of portal flow is sometimes required to alleviate the graft from portal hyperperfusion and the subsequent portal hypertension in order to avoid post-transplant complications.

Liver cirrhosis and PHTN not only have a physiological effect, but also a physical effect on intra-abdominal anatomy. These alterations may be subtle or have such an affect as to compromise graft survival and in rare cases render a patient un-transplantable [13].

Preoperative surgical evaluation of LT candidates includes triple phase, contrast enhanced computed tomography (CT). The extent of liver cirrhosis and underlying

PHTN can be assessed indirectly by radiological features. CT findings confirm feasibility of LT from a surgical perspective and help identify surgical limitations or interventions that may be needed intraoperatively [16, 13].

Important radiological features of portal hypertension for liver transplant surgery include:

- Portal vein diameter
- Evidence of portal vein thrombosis and its extent within the portal system, particularly extension to the superior mesenteric vein
- The extent of splenomegaly
- The extent and location of retroperitoneal shunting via variceal formation.

Other anatomical features also need to be addressed in the preoperative setting including hepatic artery anatomy, celiac axis and aortic atheromatosis and hepatic veins anatomy.

Cadaveric Liver Graft Anatomy

A cadaveric liver graft is presented on Fig. 5.1.

Liver Tranplantation

The concept of the procedure is simply to remove the failed liver and replace it with a new one, the donor liver graft. The procedure is completed in three phases:

Phase I
The 'pre-anhepatic' or 'explantation' phase; describing the time period in which removal of the cirrhotic liver takes place.
Phase II
The 'anhepatic' or 'implantation' phase; the interval time period when the donor graft is connected to the recipient's vasculature.
Phase III
The 'reperfusion phase'; this period starts upon reperfusion of the implanted graft.

1. **Caval Replacement**

Surgery starts with a transverse incision above the level of the umbilicus, extending bilaterally to the anterior axillary lines to allow wide exposure of the upper abdomen. An extension to the midline is common practice, allowing an even wider surgical field, known as the Mercedes incision.

In order to achieve explantation, all hepatic vasculature (inflow and outflow) needs to be divided in addition to the division of the biliary system. The liver is

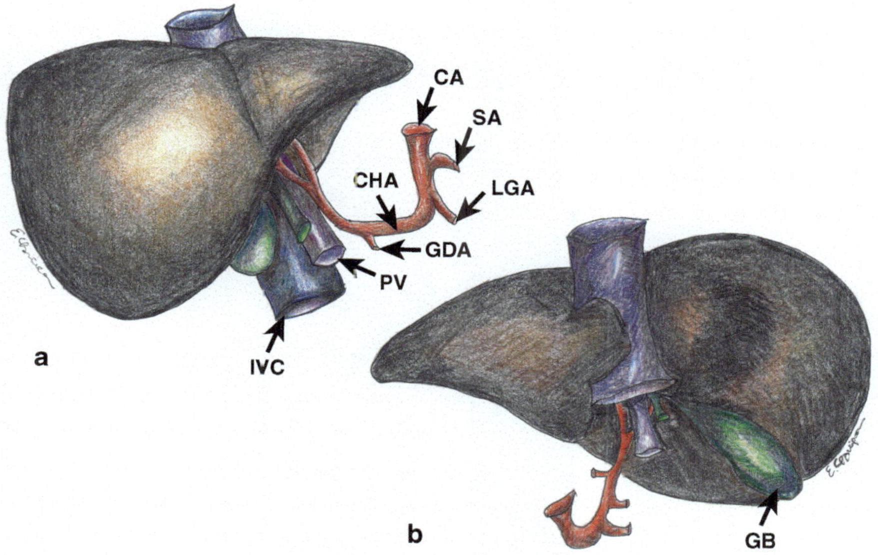

Fig. 5.1 Cadaveric whole liver graft: front and back. The native inferior vena cava (IVC) along with the hepatic veins, the gallbladder and hilar structures: the bile duct, the portal vein and the hepatic artery. The hepatic artery (HA) is retrieved along with the coeliac axis (CA), carrying the gastroduodenal artery (GDA), left gastric artery (LGA) and splenic artery (SA) stumps

intimately attached to the inferior vena cava, therefore resection of the native cava is required. The latter will be replaced by the donor's cava [17, 18] (Fig. 5.2).

The procedure starts at the liver hilum where the structures within the hepatoduodenal ligament are identified. In the context of PHTN, varices commonly surround hilar structures which can lead to significant bleeding even in this initial part of the procedure.

The hepatic artery and bile duct are ligated and divided, meanwhile the portal vein maintains blood inflow to the liver (Fig. 5.3).

Surgery continues with separation of the liver from all surrounding organs. Division of all ligaments (triangular, hepatorenal, hepatogastric and hepatophrenic) allows identification and isolation of the IVC axis. The suprahepatic IVC is isolated to allow enough space for clamp application. Similarly, the infrahepatic portion of the IVC is isolated above the level of both right and left renal veins. The final step remaining to complete explantation, is the clamping of all structures; the portal vein, the infrahepatic and suprahepatic IVC (Fig. 5.3).

Once the liver is ready to be explanted a test clamping takes place (Fig. 5.3).

Clamps are applied to the portal vein, suprahepatic cava and infrahepatic cava. Communication between the surgical and anesthetic teams is crucial at this point. Haemodynamic stability of the recipient is confirmed by the anesthetist and the surgeon proceeds to division of all clamped structures and removal of the diseased liver. The recipient has now entered the anhepatic phase.

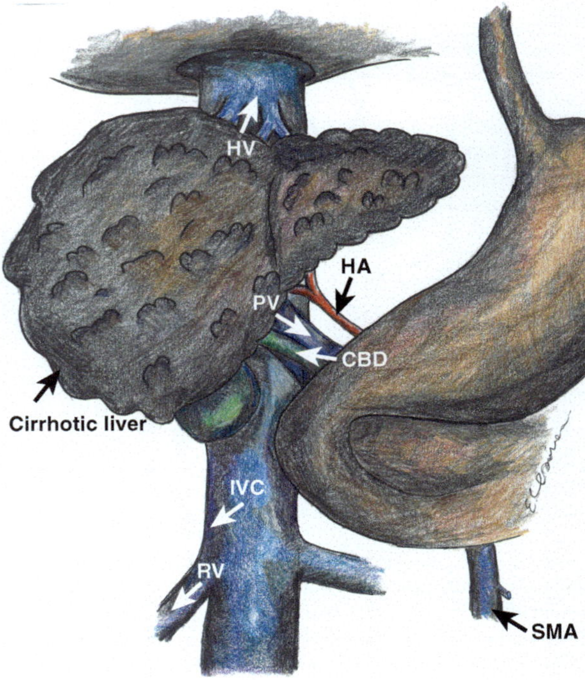

Fig. 5.2 The cirrhotic liver. The suprahepatic and infrahepatic portion of the IVC. The three hepatic veins (HV) are also depicted in this picture; note their close proximity to the liver and the diaphragm. In the liver hilum, the three structures that need to be divided are the hepatic artery (HA), the common bile duct (CBD) and the portal vein (PV). The stomach, duodenum and pancreas are lying anterior to the vascular structures; PV, HA. Note the relationship of the pancreas, PV and superior mesenteric vein (SMV). The aorta is lying on a deeper level and is not depicted in the picture

If the patient demonstrates cardiovascular instability, the trial clamping has failed and the clamps are removed immediately. Hemodynamic stability is re-established and the surgical strategy changes. In this situation, the surgical approach should be changed to either veno-venous bypass or piggyback technique [19].

The donor liver graft is removed from cold storage and the implantation phase begins. Implantation starts with fashioning of the suprahepatic caval anastomosis, which represents the outflow of the liver graft. The donor's suprahepatic cava is anastomosed to the recipient's suprahepatic cava (Fig. 5.4).

The infrahepatic caval anastomosis follows. The donor's infrahepatic cava is anastomosed to the recipient's suprarenal cava. Before completion of this anastomosis the graft needs to be flushed to wash out the preservation fluid. A cannula is inserted into the donor's portal vein and the graft is flushed with one litre of

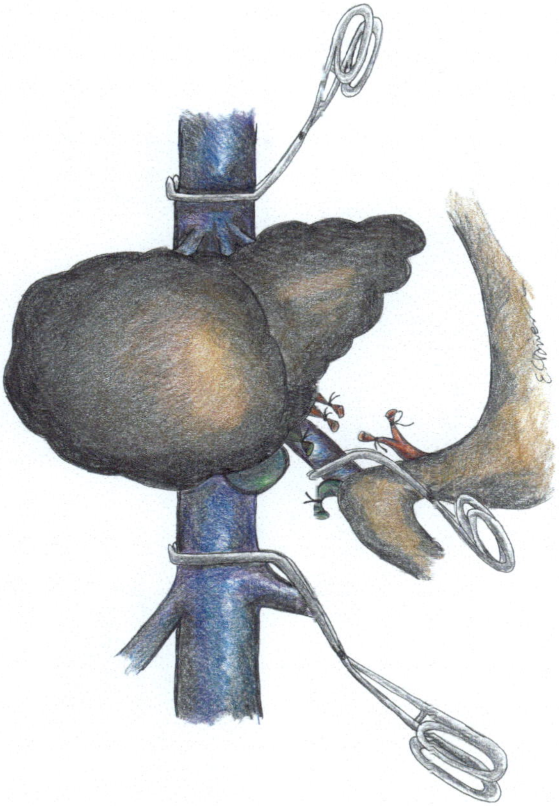

Fig. 5.3 Caval replacement type liver transplantation (LT); Explantation involves resection of the native inferior vena cava (IVC). The common bile duct and the hepatic artery are divided. The portal vein is proximally clamped. At the suprahepatic portion of IVC, a clamp is applied above the level of the hepatic veins while infrahepatically another clamp is applied above the level of the renal veins. Application of clamps is tested via a 'trial clamping period' for a few minutes to assess hemodynamic stability of the recipient before the cirrbotic liver is removed

normal saline. The saline flush drains into the abdomen via the incomplete infrahepatic caval anastomosis flushing the graft of the preservation fluid which has a high potassium concentration. This step is vital to avoid potentially significant hyperakalemia during reperfusion, as the preservation solution is rich in potassium (Fig. 5.5).

The infrahepatic caval anastomosis is completed and the anastomosis of the portal vein is then fashioned.

Upon completion of all three anastomoses, the clamps are removed and the graft is reperfused. This can result in a period of extreme cardiovascular instability as a result of reperfusion injury and the graft acting as a blood reservoir.

After careful preparation of the recipient's common hepatic artery, the arterial anastomosis is performed. Clamps are removed and arterial reperfusion takes place, completing the graft's reperfusion. It is worth noting that reperfusion injury following arterial anastomosis can also have severe cardiovascular and systemic effects.

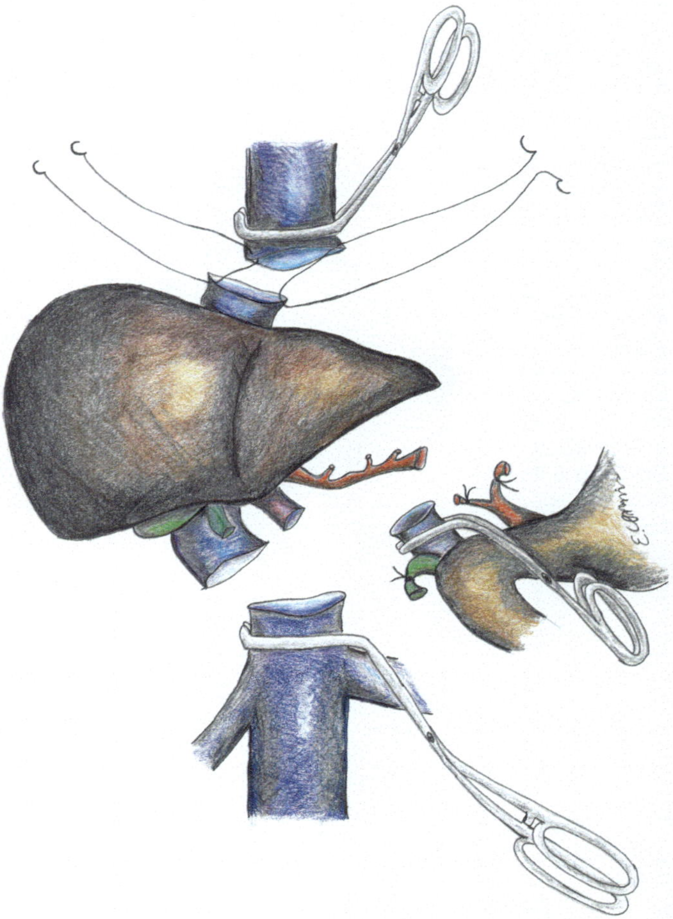

Fig. 5.4 Caval replacement type LT; Liver Transplantation; Fashioning of the outflow anastomosis of the graft between recipient 's and donor 's suprahepatic IVC

Upon the graft's reperfusion, the anesthetist's main focus is now on correcting any coagulapathy in addition to the optimization of homeostasis. Simultaneously the surgical team should aim for meticulous haemostasis. There are numerous suture lines and dissected areas, each site a potential bleeding point. Coagulopathy may be apparent in the surgical field and continued communication and teamwork between the anaesthetist and surgeon is vital. Haemostasis takes place in several rounds with interval breaks for the administration of blood products. This strategy is good practice although it may prolong the procedure.

To complete the procedure, anastomosis of the biliary system is required. The graft's gallbladder is removed and the bile duct of the graft is anastomosed to the

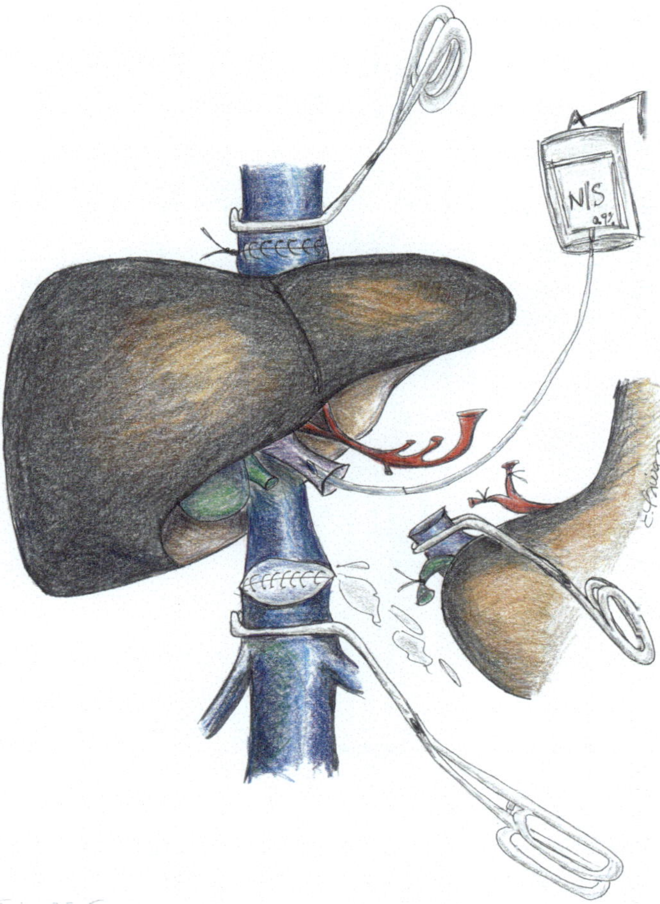

Fig. 5.5 Caval replacement type LT; The infrahepatic caval anastomosis left incomplete. A cannula is inserted into graft's portal vein and the graft is flushed with normal saline washing away the potassium rich preservation fluid

recipient's. Signs of bile production draining from the graft's bile duct at this stage is an indicative sign of good early function of the transplanted liver.

Finally, surgical drains are inserted followed by closure of all the abdominal wall layers; muscles and fasciae, subcutaneous fat and skin (Fig. 5.6).

2. **Piggyback**

In this type of transplantation the recipient's cava remains in situ and is prepared to carry the new liver 'on its shoulders', thus, the graft is 'piggybacked' onto the native cava [19, 20].

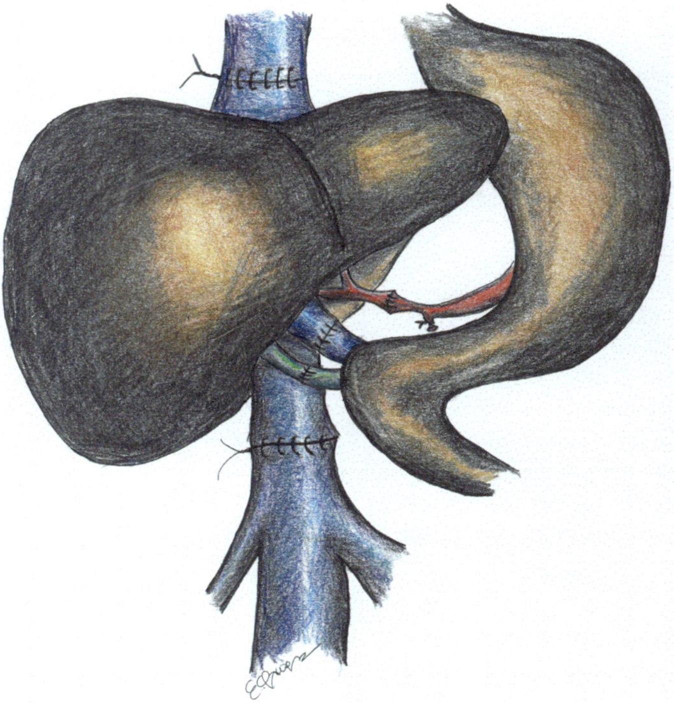

Fig. 5.6 Caval Replacement liver transplantation completed

Piggyback liver transplantation requires dissection of the liver from the recipient's IVC. This is a time-consuming process, leading to a more prolonged explantation phase. However, preservation of the native cava, permits only partial clamping during graft implantation and thus has significant advantages in terms of maintaining hemodynamic stability. The venous return to the right atrium from lower limbs, pelvis and kidneys is only partially compromised as opposed to being completely disrupted as occurs with the caval replacement technique. Nowadays, the piggyback technique is the preferred mode of liver transplantation worldwide.

Surgical incision and liver dissection are identical to the caval replacement technique. The structures in the liver hilum are ligated and divided. Now the remaining structure, the portal vein, is divided and its proximal end is clamped (Fig. 5.7).

The portal circulation is now occluded and the procedure can potentially continue, however, this carries the risk of bowel edema and congestion. In addition the systemic circulation is now deprived of the portal component and this can potentially lead to hemodynamic instability. To minimize the risks associated with the loss of portal vein venous return the a temporary portacaval shunt (TPCS) can be used.

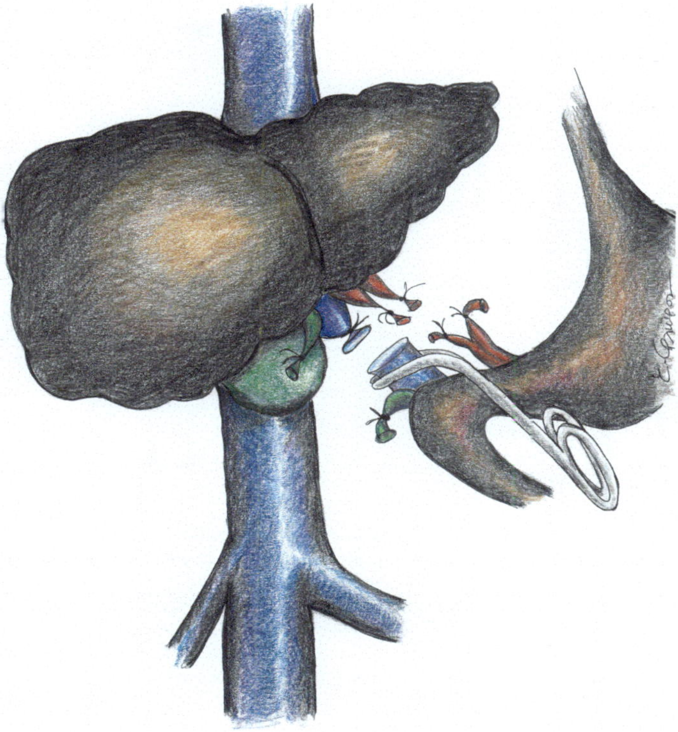

Fig. 5.7 Piggyback LT; Explantation phase in process for a piggyback liver transplantation. The structures in liver hilum, hepatic artery and bile duct, are both ligated and divided. The proximal portal vein is clamped and its distal end is ligated

Temporary Porto-Caval Shunt (TPCS)

The portal circulation is altered in cirrhotic patients. Part of the portal blood flow via collateral pathways returns to the systemic circulation bypassing the cirrhotic liver. The extent of shunting in cirrhosis can vary from minimal to extensive [14, 21]. Moreover, despite the extensive shunting, hepatopetal[1] portal flow still exists and is of higher pressure due to the mechanisms that contribute to the underlying hyperdynamic circulation [13, 14].

The abrupt occlusion of the portal circulation by clamping, has been found to cause an increase in the systemic vascular resistance via a reflex mechanism [6, 21]. This helps to maintain the mean arterial pressure, despite the fall in the cardiac output caused by the exclusion of portal return to the right atrium. However, this is a temporary effect [6, 21]. Once the reflex fades away and given the

---

[1]hepatopetal; portal flow towards the liver.
hepatofugal or non-forward portal flow; portal flow away from the liver (reversed portal flow).

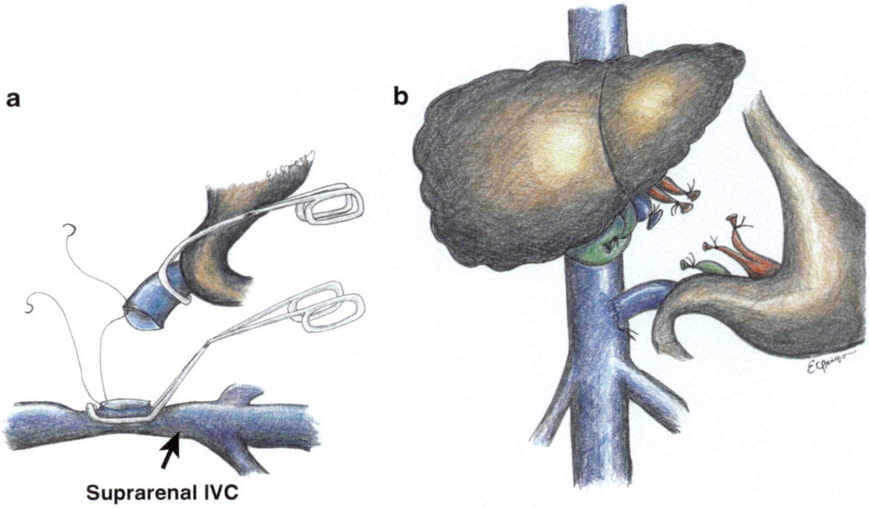

Fig. 5.8 **a.** Piggyback LT; The IVC is partially clamped to facilitate fashioning of the TPCS. **b.** The TPCS is completed and the explantation phase continues to dissect the liver from the retrohepatic IVC

prolonged explantation phase of the procedure, the portal flow occlusion can lead to splanchnic venous congestion and bowel edema which in addition to the compromised preload, can lead to hemodynamic instability [18, 19]. To avoid these issues, a portocaval shunt is fashioned, forming a direct communication between the proximal native portal vein with the IVC as described below [20, 21].

Upon completion of hilar dissection, the suprarenal IVC is partially clamped in a tangential fashion (Fig. 5.8a). An opening on the IVC is created and the recipient's portal vein is anastomosed to the IVC in an end-to-side fashion. Clamps are removed and the gastrointestinal (GI) tract drains directly into the systemic circulation (Fig. 5.8b).

The TPCS is essentially a bypass of the portal flow into the systemic circulation which prevents bowel congestion and edema whilst retaining and improving venous return. Hence, even in the setting of caval preserving LT, haemodynamic stability during the explantation phase is well supported [21–23].

Retrospective studies have failed to consistently demonstrate the beneficial effect of the TPCS in patients undergoing cava preserving LT. The beneficial effects reported in literature are: reduced intraoperative blood loss and blood transfusions, reduced liver injury and improved haemodynamics intraoperatively as well as reduced severity of kidney injury [22, 24–26]. One retrospective study demonstrated that the TPCS improves graft's survival and initial graft function in marginal grafts [23]. A recent large metanalysis demonstrated that TPCS prevented primary non function (PNF), decreased hospital length of stay and intensive care unit stay and also reduced mortality rate [27].

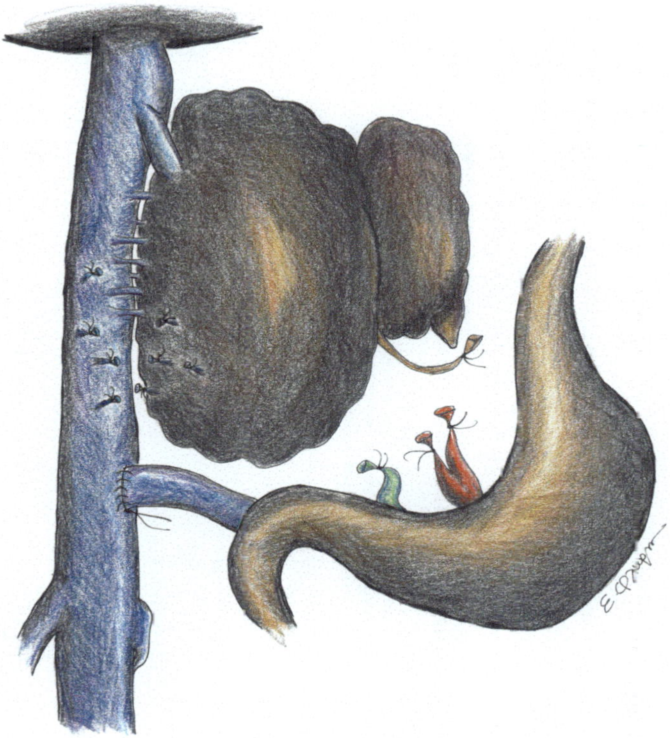

Fig. 5.9 Piggyback LT; Explantation phase: The liver is rotated towards the left to expose the retrohepatic aspect of IVC. All small branches are ligated and divided, disconnecting the liver from the IVC. Eventually, the cirrhotic liver will remain remotely hanging from the three hepatic veins

After completing the TPCS, the liver is mobilized, by dividing all surrounding ligaments. Now the liver can be lifted and rotated towards the left side. This manouver allows visualization of the retrohepatic IVC where multiple small branches drain the liver parenchyma. These are ligated and divided, thus disconnecting the liver completely from the retrohepatic aspect of the cava. This process accounts for the prolonged explantation period on piggyback LT which on average takes one to two hours to be completed (Fig. 5.9).

There is high risk of bleeding during this phase; while the liver is rotated towards the left, the retrohepatic vein branches can tear, as can also the right hepatic vein. Special care is taken to minimize blood loss during this time-consuming phase of the procedure. Upon completion of this stage, the native IVC is left intact and the liver is free with its only remaining connection to the body being its outflow via the three hepatic veins.

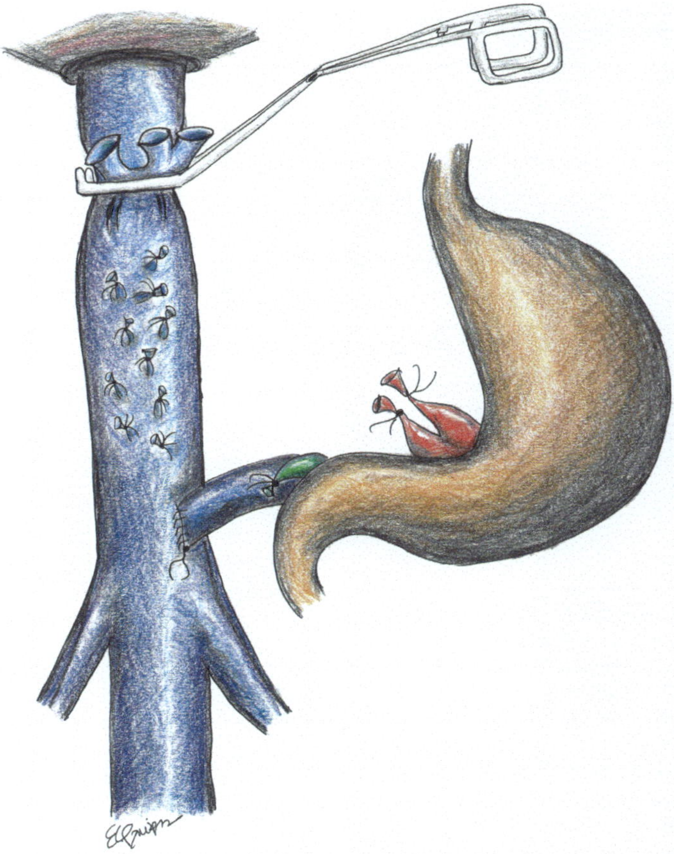

Fig. 5.10 Piggyback LT; Anhepatic phase: The cirrhotic liver has been removed. A clamp has been applied across all three hepatic veins. The circumference of inferior vena cava (IVC) is compromised but is not completely occluded allowing venous flow running through to the right atrium underneath the clamp. The portocaval shunt adds the portal flow component to the systemic circulation

The cirrhotic liver is now ready to be removed. The surgeon applies one clamp across all three hepatic veins, in a way to cause partial occlusion of IVC. This allows continued venous flow to the right atrium (Fig. 5.10).

A trial clamp test is once again needed and is a crucial and compulsory step. The clamp is applied for few minutes and the anesthetist confirms hemodynamic stability of the recipient in order the surgeon to proceed to the division of the hepatic veins and removal of the cirrhotic liver. The position of the clamp deeper than appropriate can result in a significant drop in venous return and hypotension.

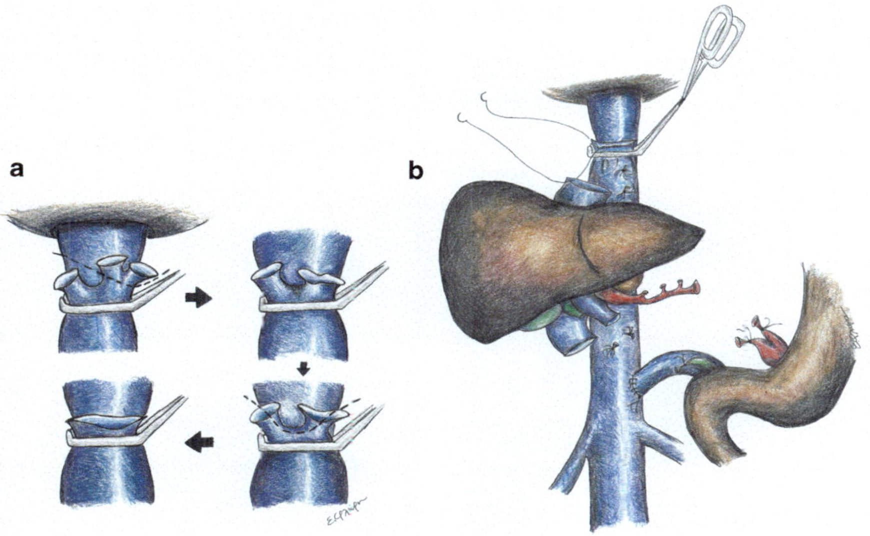

Fig. 5.11 Piggyback LT; **a.** The three hepatic veins are unified to one common orifice. Unification is important to ensure wide adequate outflow to the graft. The size matches in both the anastomosed parts; donor's caval with recipient's caval opening. **b.** Piggyback LT; Fashioning of graft's outflow anastomosis. The clamp is partially occluding the IVC

In case the trial fails, repositioning of the clamp is necessary. Alternatively, surgical strategy changes and a veno-venous by-pass may be needed.

The implantation begins. The first anastomosis performed is the outflow of the graft. The donor's suprahepatic IVC is anastomosed to the recipient's three hepatic veins that have previously been unified to one common orifice (Fig. 5.11a, b).

After completion of this anastomosis, the surgeon re-applies a new clamp proximal to it but towards the graft this time thus releasing the initial clamp that was partially occluding the IVC, allowing again the venous return to the right atrium (Fig. 5.12).

The portocaval shunt is then taken down, the cavotomy is closed and the proximal portal vein is clamped. The graft is flushed with normal saline via its portal vein. The flush drains from the donor's infrahepatic IVC which remains open until flushing is complete (Fig. 5.12).

After flushing, the graft's infrahepatic cava is ligated and the portal vein anastomosis is performed. The clamps from the PV and the IVC are removed and the graft is reperfused.

The arterial anastomosis is then fashioned followed by arterial reperfusion. After reperfusion, surgical time is spent on meticulous haemostasis since there are numerous anastomotic sites and dissected areas in the surgical field. One of the markers of initial good graft function is the assessment of clotting during this period of haemostasis.

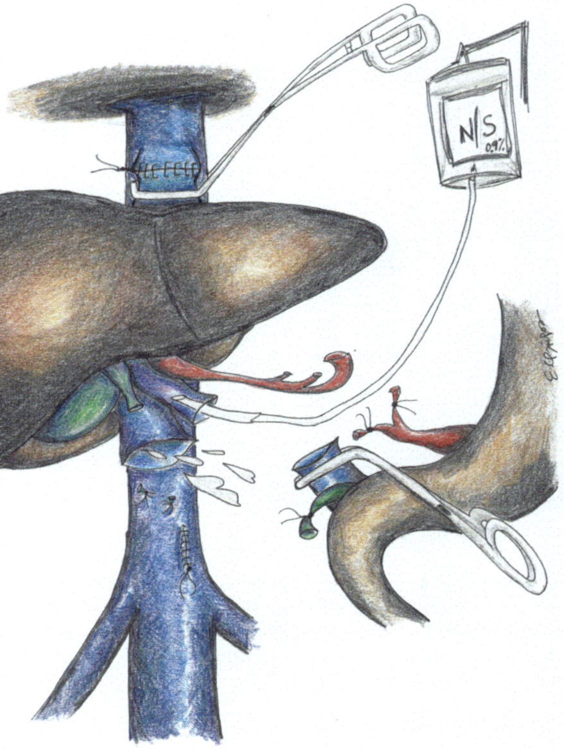

Fig. 5.12 Piggyback LT; The suprahepatic IVC anastomosis is completed and the clamp is reapplied proximally to the graft to release the native IVC restoring the systemic return to the heart. The portocaval shunt has been reversed and the graft is flushed with normal saline

The bile duct anastomosis is the final stage of graft's implantation. Haemostasis is confirmed once again before abdominal closure. Drain insertion is considered mandatory. Formal abdominal wall closure completes the procedure (Fig. 5.13).

The concept of implanting a liver graft onto the recipient's native cava was a significantly evolutionary step in LT. A living donor graft which carries its own hepatic veins could be implanted to the recipient using the piggyback technique.

Piggyback Liver Transplantion–Types of Outflow Anastomosis

There are a number of different ways to fashion an anastomosis between the graft's suprahepatic cava and the recipient's native cava using the piggyback technique. The type of the anastomosis used needs to ensure adequate outflow of the

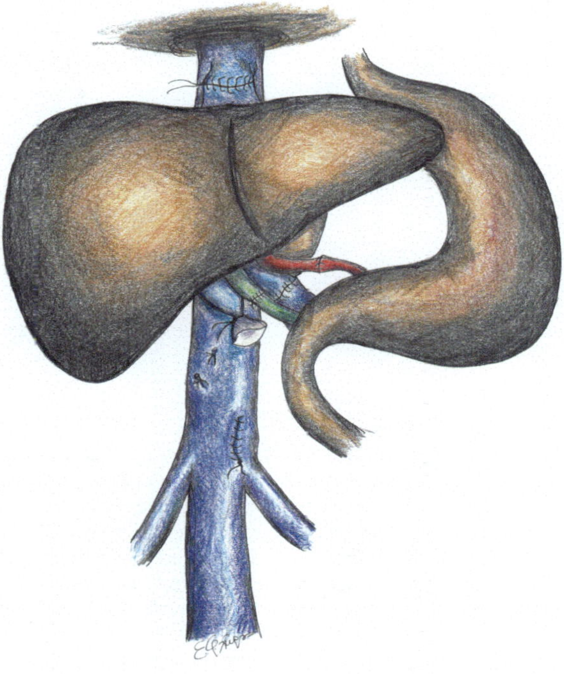

Fig. 5.13 Piggyback LT is complete

graft. This is a surgical issue and is dependent on factors such as technical or anatomical limitations. In the text, the 'three hepatic veins' technique was described, as it is considered the simplest one. Other commonly used ways of piggybacking a graft are shown in (Fig. 5.14) [20, 28, 29].

Technical Considerations

1. **Arterial Conduit**

The complications from the arterial anastomosis pose the greatest risk of graft loss, morbidity and mortality [30, 31]. The arterial supply is also important for the viability of the biliary tree [30, 31]. The quality and vigor of blood flow of the recipient's artery is always evaluated intraoperatively during the fashioning of the arterial anastomosis. On occasions that the native artery is assessed as one of poor quality and poor flow, it cannot be used for the anastomosis and an alternative source of arterial supply needs to be persued.

This alternative arterial source is the aorta itself and the most favorable area anatomically and technically is the infrarenal portion of it. An interpositional arterial graft (usually cadaveric), of the same blood group with the recipient's, is used.

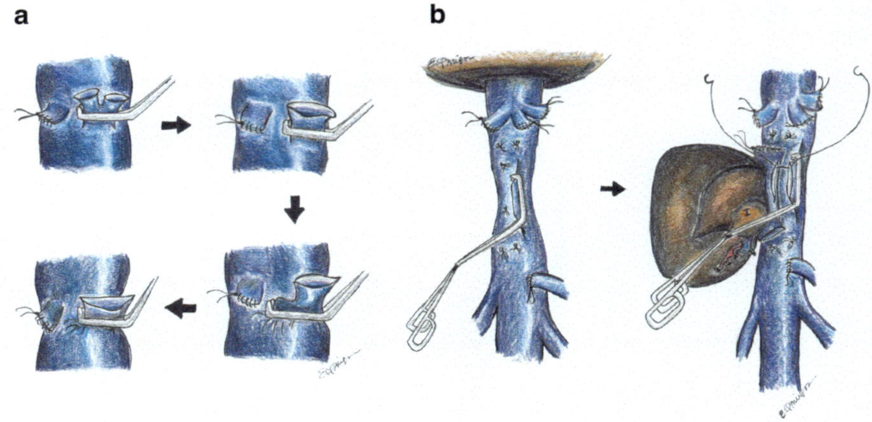

Fig. 5.14 Piggyback LT; Piggy back—types of outflow anastomosis. **a.** 'Two Hepatic Veins with extension'; The Right Hepatic Vein (RHV) is closed. The Middle (MHV) and Left Hepatic Veins (LHV) are unified in one common wider orifice. Subsequently the clamp is reapplied on a deeper level this time in order to include the anterior caval wall compromising partially its diameter. The gained tissue (anterior caval wall) is used to further extend the previously widened MHV/LHV unified orifice. Finally a wide opening is available to size match graft 's superior vena cava opening and provide an anastomosis adequate for graft's outflow. **b.** 'Side to side cavoplasty'; In this type all three hepatic veins are oversewn. The native inferior vena cava (IVC) is partially clamped in a tangential fashion to provide a good in length opening for the outflow anastomosis that follows. The superior end of donor cava is oversewn. A size matched cavotomy is created in the donor cava to correspond to the one created in the recipient's cava. Upon completion of cavoplasty, the graft will be flushed prior to the closure of donor's inferior cava

One end of the cadaveric graft is connected to the aorta, whilst the other end is anastomosed to the graft's hepatic artery. This interpositional graft is known as an 'arterial conduit' (Fig. 5.15).

The challenging step, for both surgeon and anesthetist, is the need for the aortic clamping. The aorta itself needs to be clamped on its whole circumference in order to allow the fashioning of the anastomosis with the interpositional cadaveric graft. Complications in the postoperative setting include bleeding, pseudoaneurysm formation, conduit thrombosis, bile duct complications, pancreatitis, ileus, renal failure [32, 33].

The group of patients that may need an arterial conduit includes cases of severe atherosclerotic disease, intimal dissection of the native hepatic arterial wall, re-transplantation, previous hepatic artery thrombosis, living donor and auxiliary liver transplantations [32, 33].

2. **Portal Vein Thrombosis/Superior Mesenteric Vein Thrombosis/Cavernous Transformation of the Portal Vein**

Portal vein thrombosis is encountered in cirrhotic patients in the context of PHTN. Pre-transplant assessment and imaging studies can demonstrate and assess the extent of a thrombosis and allow surgical planning [34–36].

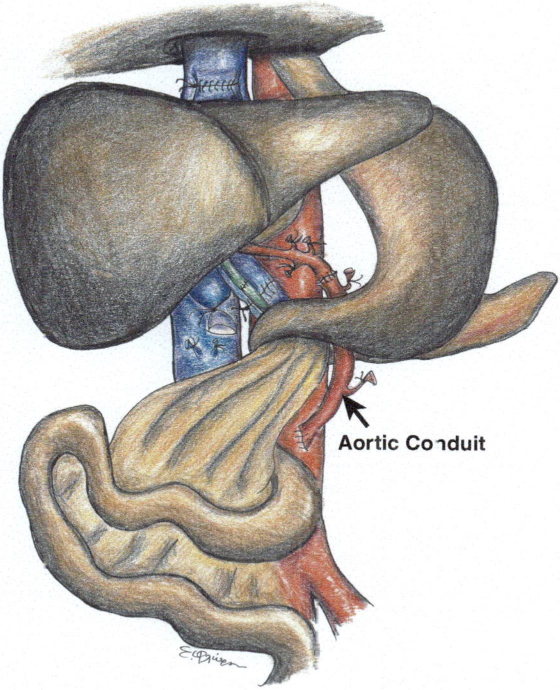

Fig. 5.15 Piggyback LT with aortic conduit. The aortic conduit lies between the stomach and pancreas and needs to be of adequate length in order to facilitate a tension free anastomosis with the donor's hepatic artery

Intraoperatively, the portal vein is isolated and thrombectomy is attempted. If the thrombus is successfully removed in its entirety, then conventional portal vein anastomosis is performed. If thrombectomy is incomplete or not feasible, then an interpositional cadaveric vein graft is implanted. This is anastomosing the recipient's SMV and the graft's PV bypassing the thrombosed section of the latter, ensuring adequate portal flow to the graft [37, 38]. This is known as a 'jump -graft' (Fig. 5.16).

Cavernous transformation of the portal vein is a condition where there is no actual portal vein structure per se present. It is encountered in cirrhotic patients and is a sequela of previous chronic PV occlusion. The portal vein is essentially absent and multiple varices have developed to provide portal blood flow, into the cirrhotic liver [34, 39]. In such cases, a jump-graft is used to bypass the variceal area.

3. **Bilio-enteric anastomosis**

The biliary anastomosis is performed between the bile duct of the graft and the recipient's bile duct. However, when partial liver grafts are used and more than one bile duct is present, or when there are technical and anatomical limitations (e.g. significant distance between the native and graft's bile duct, previous surgery, previous transplantation, cases of primary sclerosing cholangitis), a duct-to-duct anastomosis may not be feasible.

Fig. 5.16 Piggyback LT with Jump-graft; An interpositional cadaveric vein graft is used to bypass the thrombosed part of the porto-mesenteric confluence

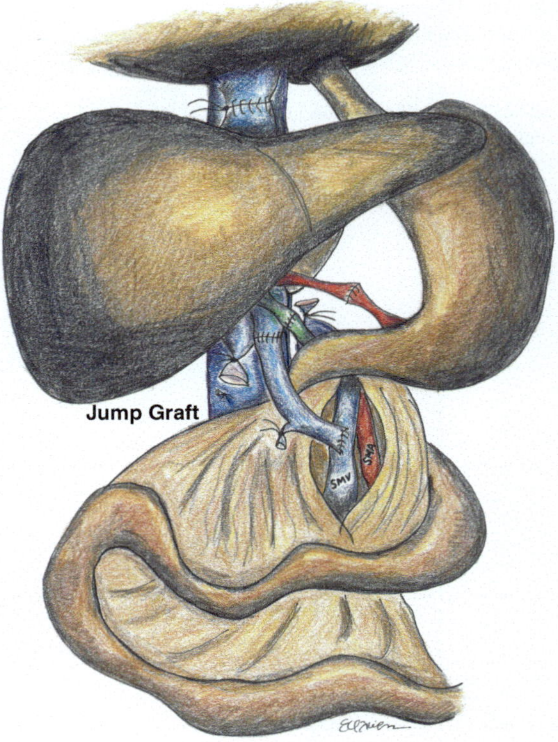

In such cases a bilio-enteric anastomosis is performed, commonly referred to as a hepaticojejunostomy. The proximal jejunum is divided and the distal end is used for the anastomosis between the graft's bile duct and recipient's jejunum, forming the hepaticojejunostomy. The remnant jejunal end is then anastomosed again, further down on to the same jejunal limb to restore continuity of gastrointestinal tract (Fig. 5.17). The reconstruction mentioned is widely used in surgery and is known as the 'Roux en Y' reconstruction.

4. **Partial Abdominal closure/Open Abdomen**

The closure of the abdominal wall following LT is not always feasible or prudent. Occasionally the position or the size of the graft may preclude formal closure due to the risk of pressure induced ischemia in the newly transplanted liver and the potential for abdominal compartment syndrome [40, 41]. Also critically ill recipients often develop significant soft tissue edema and abdominal wall closure is not possible [42, 41].

Depending on the clinical circumstances, partial closure meaning closure of the skin only leaving the underlying muscle layers apart, is an option. Alternatively, the abdomen is left wide open and a synthetic mesh is temporarily stitched across the skin edges. Once the recipient has recovered from their initial LT surgery they return to theatre for reconstruction of the abdominal wall [42].

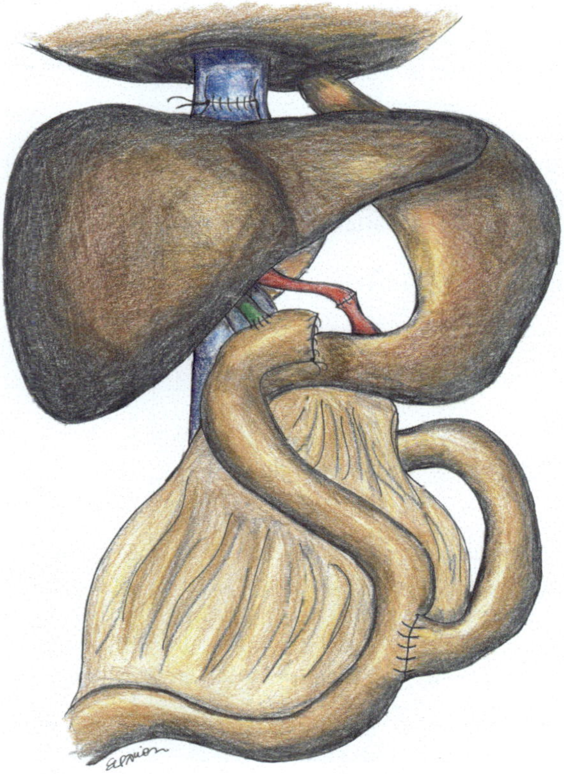

Fig. 5.17 Piggyback LT with bilio-enteric anastomosis via Roux-en-Y. The first part of the jejunum is divided and the distal end is used for the hepaticojejunostomy while the proximal jejunal stump is joined lower down to the jejunal limb that carries the hepaticojejunostomy, to restore GI continuation

Post-transplant Complications

The complications after a liver transplantation can be classified into surgical and non-surgical. The surgical complications that require return to theatre on an urgent basis or those which pose the risk for re-transplantation are described below.

Vascular Complications

1. **Hepatic Artery Thrombosis**

There are several risk factors for hepatic artery thrombosis, presented in Table 5.1 [30, 31].

Irrespective of the causative risk factor, arterial thrombosis poses a great risk of mortality and morbidity to both the recipient and graft. Early or late

Table 5.1 Risk factors for hepatic artery thrombosis

Surgical and anatomical factors
Injury at the time of organ procurement
Small calibre artery
Variant anatomy requiring arterial reconstruction
Multiple attempts for arterial anastomosis and angulation of the anastomotic site
Partial grafts
Recipient related factors
Procoagulant states
Episode of acute rejection
Hypotension
Infection
Polycythaemia rubra vera
ABO incompatibility
Trans arterial chemo embolization (TACE) prior to liver transplantation
High concentration of vassopressors use

re-transplantation is required in most cases [30]. In the UK, hepatic artery thrombosis within day 0 to 21 after LT meets the criteria for super-urgent listing [43].

In cases where the arterial thrombosis is estimated to have happened within a few hours and the recipient is hemodynamically stable, return to theatre for thrombectomy and attempt for anastomotic revision or reconstruction with aortic conduit is considered [30, 31].

2. **Portal Vein Thrombosis**

This is a rare complication post LT. The major predisposing factor is thrombectomy at the time of transplant due to previous PV thrombosis and/or SMV thrombosis and can be attributed to recurrent thrombosis or an incomplete thrombectomy [35, 36].

3. **Hepatic Venous Outflow Obstruction (HVOO)**

The term HVOO is used to describe a reduced/impaired hepatic venous outflow of the graft. It is a relatively rare complication and can occur after LT with whole liver or partial grafts. Living donor grafts are partial grafts deprived of a cava and carry their own hepatic veins. Usually there are more than one hepatic veins that need to be anastomosed to the recipient's cava. Due to the complexity encountered during the reconstruction of partial grafts, HVOO may occur [44, 45]. Overall HVOO occurs mostly after a piggyback liver transplantation [44–46].

The clinical manifestations can be subtle or profound and involve graft dysfunction and intractable ascites [44, 45]. Management includes non-surgical options such as observation and medical management of the ascites and radiological intervention for stent insertion to restore graft's outflow [45, 47]. Surgical management includes re-operation for a technically challenging re-fashioning of the outflow anastomosis, Re-transplantation is often needed at a later stage [44–46].

4. **Biliary Complications**

Biliary complications are a common problem in LT and can occur at an early or late stage post-transplantation. In the early postoperative setting, a biliary anastomotic leak requires reoperation. Biliary complications late post transplantation are anastomotic and non-anastomotic biliary strictures [48, 49].

Risk factors for developing biliary complications are: ischemic graft injury, prolonged cold ischemia time, reperfusion injury, hepatic artery thrombosis and episodes of acute rejection [50–52]. Grafts from non-heart beating donors, partial liver grafts are considered to have higher rates of biliary complications [49, 51, 52].

Recipients with biliary anastomotic strictures may experience repeated episodes of cholangitis and graft dysfunction. Initial management involves endoscopic treatment which usually leads to resolution of symptoms. Surgical treatment is reserved for a later stage and patients return to theatre for biliary reconstruction and gastrointestinal tract restoration with hepaticojejunostomy [49, 51, 52].

All illustrations are made by the first author and are under rights.

References

1. Calne RY, Williams R, Lindop M, et al. Improved survival after orthotopic liver grafting. Br Med J. 1981;283:115–8.
2. Starzl TE. The saga of liver replacement, with particular reference to the reciprocal influence of liver and kidney transplantation (1955–1967). J Am Coll Surg. (2002):195:587–610.
3. Starzl TE, Fung JJ. Themes of liver transplantation. Hepatology. 2010;51:1869–84.
4. NHSBT annual report on liver transplantation 2017/2018. https://nhsbtdbe.blob.core.windows.net/umbraco-assets-corp/16782/nhsbt-liver-transplantation-annual-report-2018-19.pdf. Accessed 12 Jan 2020.
5. Lautt WW. Regulatory processes interacting to maintain hepatic blood flow constancy: vascular compliance, hepatic arterial buffer response, hepatorenal reflex, liver regeneration, escape from vasoconstriction. Hepatology Res. 2007;37:891–903.
6. Feng AC, Fan HL, Chen TW, Hsieh CB. Hepatic hemodynamic changes during liver transplantation: a review. World J Gastroenterol. 2014;20:11131–41.
7. Lautt WW. The 1995 Ciba-geigy award lecture. Intrinsic regulation of hepatic blood flow. Can J Physiol Pharmacol. (1996);74:223–33.
8. Lautt WW, Greenway CV. Hepatic venous compliance and role of liver as a blood reservoir. J Physiol. 1976;231:292–5.
9. Lautt WW, Legare DJ. Passive autoregulation of portal venous pressure: distensible hepatic resistance. Am J Physiol. 1992;263:702–8.
10. Lautt WW, Brown LC, Durham JS. Active and passive control of hepatic blood volume responses to hemorrhage at normal and raised hepatic venous pressure in cats. Can J Physiol Pharmacol. 1980;58:1049–57.

11. Reiberger T, Püspök A, Schoder M, Baumann-Durchschein F, Bucsics T, et al. Austrian consensus guidelines on the management and treatment of portal hypertension (Billroth III). Wien Klin Wochenschr. 2017;129(Suppl 3):S135–58.
12. Gjeorgjievski M, Cappell MS. Portal hypertensive gastropathy: a systematic review of the pathophysiology, clinical presentation, natural history and therapy. World J Hepatol. 2016;8:231–62.
13. Hackl C, Schlitt HJ, Renner P, Lang SA. Liver surgery in cirrhosis and portal hypertension. World J Gastroenterol. 2016;22:2725–35.
14. Møller S, Henriksen JH, Bendtsen F. Extrahepatic complications to cirrhosis and portal hypertension: haemodynamic and homeostatic aspects. World J Gastroenterol. 2014;20:15499–517.
15. Eipel C, et al. Regulation of hepatic blood flow: the hepatic arterial buffer response revisited. World J Gastroenterol. 2010;16:6046–57.
16. Kim PTW, Klintmalm GB. Importance of Hepatic Flows in Liver Transplantation. J Hepatol Gastroint Dis. 2016;2:1–14.
17. Starzl TE, Iwatsuki S, Van Thiel DH, Gartner JC, Zitelli BJ, Malatack RR, et al. Evolution of liver transplantation. Hepatology. 1982;2:614–36.
18. Starzl TE, Marchioro TL, Porter KA, Brettschneider L. Homotransplantation of the liver in humans. Surg Gynecol Obstet. 1963;117:659–76.
19. Fonouni H, Mehrabi A, Soleimani M, Muller SA, Buchler MW, Schmidt J. The need for venovenous bypass in liver transplantation review. HPB (Oxford). 2008;10:196–203.
20. Tzakis A, Todo S, Starzl TE. Orthotopic liver transplantation with preservation of the inferior vena cava. Ann Surg. 1989;210:649–52.
21. Arzu GD, De Ruvo N, Montalti R, Masetti M, Begliomini B, Di Benedetto F, et al. Temporary porto-caval shunt utility during orthotopic liver transplantation. Transplant Proc. 2008;40:1937–40.
22. Davila D, Barlett A, Heaton N. Temporary portocaval shunt in orthotopic liver transplantation: need for a standardized approach? Liver Transpl. 2008;14:1414–9.
23. Rayar M, Levi Sandri GB, Cusumano C, et al. Benefits of temporary porto-caval shunt during orthotopic liver transplantation with vena cava preservation: a propensity score analysis. Liver Transpl. 2017;23:174–83.
24. Muscari F, Suc B, Aguirre J, Di Mauro GL, Bloom E, Duffas JP, et al. Orthotopic liver transplantation with vena cava preservation in cirrhotic patients: is systematic temporary portacaval anastomosis a justified procedure? Transplant Proc. 2005;37:2159–62.
25. Figueras J, Llado L, Ramos E, Jaurrieta E, Rafecas A, Febregat J et al. Temporary portocaval shunt during liver transplantation with vena cava preservation. Results of a prospective randomized study. Liver Transplant. (2001);7:904–11.
26. Pratschke S, Meimarakis G, Bruns CJ, et al. Temporary intraoperative portocaval shunt: useless or beneficial in piggy back liver transplantation? Transpl Int. 2012;26:90–8.
27. Nacif LS, Zanini LY, Sartori VF, Kim V, Rocha-Santos V, Andraus W, et al. Intraoperative surgical portosystemic shunt in liver transplantation: systematic review and meta-analysis. Ann Transplant. 2018;23:721–32.
28. Belghiti J, Panis Y, Sauvanet A, Gayet B, Fedeke F. A new technique of side to side caval anastomosis during orthotopic hepatic transplantation without inferior vena caval occlusion. Surg Gynecol Obstet. 1992;175:270–2.
29. Ringe B, Pichlmayr R, Burdelski M. A new technique of hepatic vein reconstruction in partial liver transplantation. Transp Int. 1988;1:30–5.
30. Heaton ND. Hepatic artery thrombosis: conservative management or retransplantation? Liver Transpl. 2013;19(Suppl 2):S14–6.
31. Piardi T, Lhuaire M, Bruno O, Memo R, Pessaux P, Kianmanesh R et al. Vascular complications following liver transplantation: a literature review of advances in 2015. World J Gastroenterol. (2016);8:36–57.

32. Nikitin D, Jennings LW, Khan T, et al. Twenty years of follow-up of aortohepatic conduits in liver transplantation. Liver Transpl. 2008;14:1486–90.
33. Denecke C, Weiss S, Biebl M, et al. An arterial conduit is not a risk factor for survival following orthotopic liver transplantation: an analysis of 20 years of liver transplantation in Innsbruck. Ann Transplant. 2016;21:321–8.
34. Stieber A, Zetti G, Tzakis A, et al. The spectrum of portal vein thrombosis in liver transplantation. Ann Sur. 1991;213:199–206.
35. Duffy JP, Hong JC, Farmer DG, Ghobrial RM, Yersiz H, et al. Vascular complications of orthotopic liver transplantation: experience in more than 4,200 patients. J Am Coll Surg. 2009;208:896–903.
36. Kadry Z, Selzner N, Handschin A, Müllhaupt B, Renner EL, Clavien PA. Living donor liver transplantation in patients with portal vein thrombosis: a survey and review of technical issues. Transplantation. 2002;74:696–701.
37. Tzakis A, Todo S, Stieber A, Starzl T. Venous jump grafts for liver transplantation in patients with portal vein thrombosis. Transplantation. 1989;48:530–1.
38. Hibi T, Nishida S, Levi DM et al. When and why portal vein thrombosis matters in liver transplantation. A critical audit of 174. Cases Ann Surg. 2014;259:706–766.
39. Chawla Yogesh K, Bodh Vijay. Portal vein thrombosis. J Clin Exp Hepatol. 2015;5:22–40.
40. Hobeika C, Allard MA, Bucur PO, et al. Management of the open abdomen after liver transplantation. World J Surg. 2017;41:3199–204.
41. Bressan AK, Ball CG. Intra-abdominal hypertension and abdominal compartment syndrome in acute pancreatitis, hepato-pancreato-biliary operations and liver transplantation. Anaesthesiol Intensive Ther. 2017;49:159–66.
42. Arai M, Kim S, Ishii H, Hagiwara J, Kushimoto S, Yokota H. The long-term outcomes of early abdominal wall reconstruction by bilateral anterior rectus abdominis sheath turnover flap method in critically ill patients requiring open abdomen. World J Emerg Surg. 2018;13:39–45.
43. http://odt.nhs.uk/pdf/liver_selection_policy.pdf. Accessed 20 Feb 2020.
44. Ye Q, Zeng C, Wang Y, Fang Z, Hu X, Xiong Y, et al. Risk factors for hepatic venous outflow obstruction in piggyback liver transplantation: the role of recipient's pattern of hepatic veins drainage into the inferior vena cava. Ann Transplant. 2017;22:303–8.
45. Khorsandi SE, Athale A, Vilca-Melendez H, Jassem W, Prachalias A, Srinivasan P, Rela M, Heaton N. Presentation, diagnosis, and management of early hepatic venous outflow complications in whole cadaveric liver transplant. Liver Transpl. 2015;21:914–21.
46. Sommovilla J, Doyle MM, Vachharajani N, et al. Hepatic venous outflow obstruction in pediatric liver transplantation: technical considerations in prevention, diagnosis, and management. Pediatr Transplant. 2014;18:497–502.
47. Wang SL, Sze DY, Busque S, et al. Treatment of hepatic venous outflow obstruction after piggyback liver transplantation. Radiology. 2005;236:352–9.
48. Rao HB, Prakash A, Sudhindran S, Venu RP. Biliary stricture complicating living donor liver transplantation: problems, novel insights and solutions. World J Gastroenterol. 2018;24:2061–72.
49. Moy BT, Birk JW. A review on the management of biliary complications after orthotopic liver transplantation. J Clin Transl Hepatol. 2019;7:61–71.
50. Nemes B, Gaman G, Polak WG, Gelley F, Hara T, Ono S, et al. Extended-criteria donors in liver transplantation Part II: reviewing the impact of extended-criteria donors on the complications and outcomes of liver transplantation. Expert Rev Gastroenterol Hepatol. 2016;10:841–59.
51. Nemes B, Gámán G, Doros A. Biliary complications after liver transplantation. Expert Rev Gastroenterol Hepatol. 2015;9:447–66.
52. Feier FH, Seda-Neto J, da Fonseca EA, Candido HL, Pugliese RS, Neiva R, et al. Analysis of factors associated with biliary complications in children after liver transplantation. Transplantation. 2016;100:1944–54.

Chapter 6
Pre-assessment for Hepato-Pancreato-Biliary and Liver Transplant Surgery

Marina Gitman

Preoperative Assessment of Liver Transplant Candidates

Liver transplantation (LT) is a common treatment option for end-stage liver disease (ESLD). LT is a complex surgical procedure that involves complete excision of the patient's diseased liver and its replacement with either a cadaveric or a live-donor graft. This operation carries a high potential for blood loss requiring large volume resuscitation. In addition to the fluid shifts that arise from massive blood transfusion, LT recipients also suffer the physiologic stresses and hemodynamic instability associated with portal and vena-caval clamping and subsequent organ reperfusion. Furthermore, because today's LT recipients are older and have more comorbidities, preoperative assessment before LT is paramount for safe and favorable outcomes. This includes careful diagnosis and optimization of all systemic manifestations of ESLD.

Assessment of the Severity of ESLD

Child-Turcotte-Pugh (CTP) Classification

First introduced by Child and Turcotte in 1964 and later revised by Pugh in 1973, the CTP classification predicts mortality of patients with ESLD. It is calculated using the patient's albumin and bilirubin level, the prothrombin time (PT), the severity of hepatic encephalopathy and the extent of ascites [1]. Each component receives a score from 1–3, and the total of all scores defines each class—Class A (5–6), Class B (7–9), Class C (10–15) with the corresponding predicted 3-month

M. Gitman (✉)
University of Illinois, Chicago, IL, USA
e-mail: marina_gitman@yahoo.com

Z. Milan and C. Goonasekera (eds.), *Anesthesia for Hepatico-Pancreatic-Biliary Surgery and Transplantation*, https://doi.org/10.1007/978-3-030-51331-3_6

mortality rates of 4, 14, and 51% [2] (Table 6.1). More current data show that, with recent advances in surgical and anesthetic techniques, these rates may actually be as low as 2, 12, and 12% in some abdominal surgical cases [3]. Although the CTP score has been used for more than five decades as a tool for preoperative planning for patients with cirrhosis, it has significant limitations. For example, two of its components—encephalopathy and ascites—are very subjective measures and can have significant inter-provider variability, which may easily skew the score towards a different CPT classification. Furthermore, even the objective values such as the albumin level and the PT can be influenced by albumin infusions and the variations among hospital laboratory measurement standards [4]. This proved problematic when the CTP score, along with ABO blood type and transplant list waiting time, was used for organ allocation.

Model for End-Stage Liver Disease (MELD) Score

The MELD score was developed at the Mayo Clinic and first described by Malinchoc and colleagues in 2000. It is calculated using the levels of total

Table 6.1 Assessment of the severity of end-stage liver disease

	Child-Turcotte-Pugh classification				Model for end-stage liver disease score	
Calculation		1 point	2 points	3 points	$\boldsymbol{MELDScore} = 10 * ((0.957 * ln(Creatinine)) + (0.378 * ln(Bilirubin)) + (1.12 * ln(INR))) + 6.43$ $\boldsymbol{MELD\ Na} = MELD - Na - [0.025 \times MELD \times (140 - Na)] + 140$	
	Bilirubin	<2	2–3	>3		
	INR	<1.7	1.8–2.2	>2.2		
	Albumin	<3.5	2.8–3.5	<2.8		
	Ascites	None	Mild/ Moderate	Moderate/ Severe		
	Encephalopathy	None	Grade 1–2	Grade 3–4		
	Class	Points				
	A	5–6				
	B	7–9				
	C	10–45				
Prognosis	Mortality after hepatic and nonhepatic surgery				90-day pre-transplant mortality	
	Class	% mortality			MELD score	% mortality
	A	4			6–9	1.9
	B	14			10–19	6
	C	51			21–29	19.6
					30–39	52.6
					≥40	71.3

References (Abbas, Farnsworth, Malinchoc, Wiesner, https://optn.transplant.hrsa.gov/resources/allocation-calculators/meld-calculator/)

bilirubin, creatinine and the international normalized ratio (INR) of the PT. The Meld score was originally designed and later validated to predict the 3-month mortality of patients undergoing a transjugular intrahepatic portosystemic shunt (TIPS) procedure [5]. The reported mortality rates of a national cohort shortly after the introduction of the MELD score were the following: 1.9% (MELD<9), 6% (MELD 10–19), 19.6% (MELD 20–29), 52.6% (MELD 30–39), 71.3% (MELD>40) [4] (Table 6.1). Numerous studies have demonstrated that the MELD score is better than the CTP score at estimating short-term mortality [6]. The elements of the MELD score are completely objective and easily reproducible, and it has since been utilized to prioritize patients on the liver transplant waiting list of many countries.

Modifications of the MELD Score

While the MELD score consistently estimates 3-month pre-transplant mortality, it may not always be the best predictor of mortality after liver transplantation. As a result, there have been several amendments to the original MELD score in an attempt to improve its accuracy. One of the major adjustments to the MELD score is the addition of the sodium level to the calculation. Hyponatremia is present in up to 20% of patients with ESLD, and it has long been known to correlate with a higher rate of complications (refractory ascites and hepatorenal syndrome) and death [6]. Similarly, the sodium MELD score (MELD-Na) predicts 90-day mortality better than the regular MELD score. [7] The inclusion of the serum sodium level can increase the MELD score by up to 13 points, expediting transplantation and decreasing overall waitlist mortality of this patient population. The use of the MELD-Na score for liver allocation was initiated in 2016 and has contributed to an increase in survival of patients with hyponatremia [8]. This benefit is significant for LT recipients whose MELD before the sodium modification is less than 11 [9].

Other modifications include the presence of hepatocellular carcinoma (HCC), specific cases of hilar cholangiocarcinoma, portopulmonary hypertension (POPH), hepatopulmonary syndrome (HPS), cystic fibrosis, primary hyperoxaluria, and familial amyloid polyneuropathy. For example, patients whose HCC tumor characteristics fit within the Milan (size- and number-based) criteria are awarded additional (exception) MELD points, because the diagnosis of cancer increases the urgency for transplantation. Patients with HPS and severe hypoxemia (PaO_2<60 mm Hg) and patients with proven moderate POPH (mean pulmonary arterial pressure (mPAP)>35 mmHg, transpulmonary gradient (TPG)>12 mmHg, and pulmonary vascular resistance (PVR)>400 dyn/s/$cm-^5$) that improves with treatment can also receive exception points for their MELD score [6, 10].

Recently, much attention has turned to LT candidates' overall disability, including the need for objective assessment of the physical and nutritional status, which can have significant bearing on pre- and post-transplant course. Muscle wasting (sarcopenia) is associated with increased wait-list mortality, especially in patients with lower MELD scores [11]. Although not yet validated in all patient populations, the addition of sarcopenia to the MELD score may come in the near future. In order to do so, there must be an objective and reproducible method of assessing LT candidate frailty. Furthermore, because extreme deconditioning is not only a result of ESLD but also a predictor of poor post-transplant outcomes, transplant centers may require intervention programs to improve the overall pre-transplant status.

Future Improvements in Severity Scoring

Artificial intelligence (AI) systems are already in use for some organ allocation practices. Recently, AI systems have been introduced to improve organ allocation. For example, one computer-based method called optimized prediction of mortality (OPOM) predicts 3-month mortality on the transplant wait-list better than the MELD score in computer simulations [12].

Neurological Disorders of ESLD

Hepatic Encephalopathy

The 2014 Practice Guideline by the American Association for the Study of Liver Diseases (AASLD) and the European Association for the Study of the Liver (EASL) define hepatic encephalopathy (HE) as "brain dysfunction caused by liver insufficiency and/or portosystemic shunting (PSS)" resulting in a "spectrum of neurological or psychiatric abnormalities ranging from subclinical alteration to coma" [13]. Caused by excess ammonia and inflammation, HE occurs in 30–40% of patients with cirrhosis and presents as a wide range of neuropsychiatric disturbances such as personality changes, agitation, headache, vomiting, hyperreflexia, asterixis, and coma [13–15]. Risk factors for developing HE include diabetes mellitus (DM), renal dysfunction, and hyponatremia [13].

HE can be classified based on several factors: underlying etiology, severity (West Haven criteria, Table 6.2), time-course and precipitating factors. Pre-transplant management is geared towards reducing the ammonia burden. Oral lactulose aids in the conversion of ammonia to ammonium and speeds up its excretion via the gut. Rifaximin, an antibiotic with poor oral bioavailability, has good activity against ammonia-producing gut bacteria and is used in conjunction with lactulose. The combination of the two drugs is synergistic [14]. Other adjuncts include oral branched-chain amino acids (BCAAs), L-ornithine L-aspartate (LOLA), neomycin and metronidazole [13]. Before treatment, it is prudent to exclude other causes of an altered neurological exam such as stroke,

Table 6.2 Grading of hepatic encephalopathy

West-Haven criteria	
Grade	Clinical manifestations
Unimpaired	No encephalopathy
Minimal	No clinical signs of altered mental state Abnormalities detected on psychometric or neuropsychological tests
I	Mild difficulties with attention, awareness, simple tasks, sleep cycle, euphoria, anxiety
II	Asterixis, personality changes, disorientation, apathy, lethargy
III	Confusion, somnolence, incoherent speech
IV	Coma

References (Feltracco, Vilstrup)

seizure, encephalitis, drug toxicity, hypoglycemia or thiamine deficiency. LT usually resolves the symptoms of HE.

Acute liver failure and Grades 3–4 HE are associated with increased intracranial pressure (ICP), cerebral edema and requirement for respiratory support with mechanical ventilation [13, 15]. In these situations, accurate assessment of neurological status (including imaging, if necessary), tight control of ICP with patient positioning, diuretics, and renal replacement therapy (RRT) as well as maintenance of systemic mean arterial pressure (MAP) with vasopressors is crucial for preservation of adequate cerebral perfusion pressure (CPP).

Cerebral Edema

Cerebral edema is almost exclusively seen in the context of acute liver failure (ALF) but, as mentioned earlier, can be seen with high-grade HE. Risk factors comprise hyper-acute liver failure, younger age, renal dysfunction, vasopressor requirement, hyponatremia and ammonia level above 200 mmol/L [16]. Cerebral edema may lead to intracranial hypertension with its myriad of clinical sequelae, including cerebral herniation and brain death. Serial neurological exams do not reliably diagnose acute elevations in ICP. Invasive ICP monitoring provides the best information on which to base treatment, but may not affect outcomes and, while feasible and safe in certain settings, carries the added risk of intracranial hemorrhage [17, 18]. Imaging is only indicated if intracranial bleeding or cerebral herniation is suspected [15]. A non-invasive method of estimating ICP by measuring the optic nerve sheath diameter with ultrasound provides a low-risk method of diagnosis and can guide therapy of intracranial hypertension before and during LT. This particular technique uses a linear ultrasound probe with a preset frequency of 7 MHz. The probe is placed on the superolateral aspect of the closed eyelid, and the optic nerve sheath diameter is measured 3 mm below the retina (Fig. 6.1). The measurement is repeated for a total of 3 times, and the average value is used to

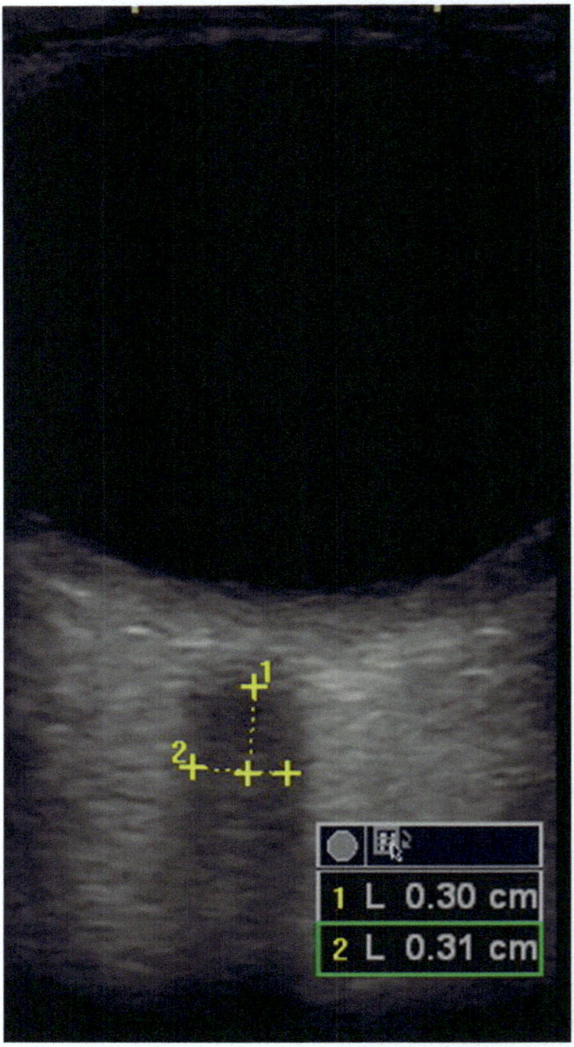

Fig. 6.1 Optic nerve sheath diameter measurement for estimation of intracranial pressure. The optic nerve sheath diameter is measured 3 mm below the optic disk. An average of 3 measurements is taken, and a value of > 0.48 cm corresponds to an ICP > 20 mmHg. Reference (Krishnamoorthy)

estimate ICP. An optic nerve sheath diameter larger than 0.48 cm corresponds to ICP > 20 mm Hg [19] (Fig. 6.1).

Management of increased ICP includes the elevation of the head of the bed to thirty degrees, mild hypothermia, sedation, diuresis and renal replacement therapy (RRT) in order to keep ICP in the range of 20–25 mmHg and CPP above 50 mmHg. Acute elevations in ICP may be treated with intravenous (IV) mannitol, IV indomethacin, hypertonic saline and, in a worst-case scenario a hepatectomy can be attempted while awaiting transplantation [15, 20]. CPP support may require the use of vasopressors. Most of these preoperative tactics may be continued in the operating room. Correction of hyponatremia must be careful and slow to prevent osmotic demyelination syndrome [21]. Cerebral edema with CPP<40 mmHg for longer than two hours or other indication of irreversible neurological damage or medical instability may collectively signal a contraindication to LT [22].

Cautious evaluation, diagnosis and treatment of neurological disorders before LT can provide valuable postoperative prognosis and may improve perioperative management [21].

Cardiovascular Diseases in ESLD

Hyperdynamic Circulation and Cirrhotic Cardiomyopathy

The hyperdynamic state observed in patients with ESLD is typically accompanied by an increased cardiac output with a decreased systemic vascular resistance [23]. This often manifests clinically as a combination of mild tachycardia and hypotension. Cirrhotic cardiomyopathy (CCM) is defined as a diminished contractile response to stress with a reduction in ejection fraction (EF), diastolic dysfunction (DD) and electrophysiological disturbances such as QT prolongation [24]. Although CCM typically resolves after LT, it is an independent risk factor for postoperative systolic heart failure, [25] and its severity corresponds to the degree of liver disease and MELD [26]. Accordingly, echocardiographic evidence of DD during preoperative assessment warrants close postoperative monitoring. In the absence of coronary artery disease (CAD), the presence of elevated preoperative biomarkers such as Troponin I and brain natriuretic peptide (BNP) may be associated with a more severe type of CCM and may also predict worse postoperative outcomes [23]. A 12-lead ECG and a resting echocardiogram are almost ubiquitous initial tests of pre-LT cardiac assessment. Some transplant centers now include random levels of Troponin I and BNP.

Coronary Artery Disease

The prevalence of coronary artery disease (CAD) in LT candidates is similar to that of the general population and may even be higher in older patients [23, 24]. Although the presence of clinically significant CAD is associated with increased post-LT morbidity and mortality, if it is adequately treated, survival rates are comparable to those without severe CAD [27].

Preoperative assessment of CAD includes a careful history, including evaluation of functional status and the presence of traditional CAD risk factors such as hypertension (HTN), diabetes mellitus (DM), smoking, dyslipidemia, and family history of early CAD. In addition to the traditional CAD risk factors, nonalcoholic steatohepatitis (NASH) and renal dysfunction convey additional risk [28]. Patients with 2 or more (this is center dependent) cardiac risk factors should have a noninvasive pharmacological stress test [22, 29, 30]. Most common noninvasive stress tests are dobutamine stress echocardiography (DSE) and nuclear single-photon emission computed tomography (SPECT). DSE provides the value of a combined stress test and an echocardiogram but depends largely on the patient's ability to achieve 85% of the age-predicted maximum heart rate and has variable predictive values [24]. SPECT validity does not depend on the achievement of a certain heart rate and does not require patients to discontinue a beta-blocker. SPECT has a 92% NPV for postoperative cardiovascular (CV) complications, but it may have low sensitivity in already maximally vasodilated LT candidates [24, 28]. Clinically, a negative DSE or SPECT is associated with a low rate of perioperative CV events; [31] therefore, they are good screening tests for LT candidates. Other noninvasive modalities include cardiac magnetic resonance imaging (MRI) and coronary computer tomography (CT), where a coronary artery calcium score>400 Hounsefield units is associated with clinically significant CAD [32]. A pharmacologic stress test with evidence of stress-induced ischemia or clinical suspicion of severe CAD (exertional angina, multiple CAD risk factors, severe coronary artery calcifications seen on CT, etc.) warrant referral to a cardiologist for a coronary angiogram.

The gold standard for diagnosis of CAD is coronary angiography (CA). It carries a risk of bleeding and worsening renal dysfunction due to contrast-induced nephropathy; however, it allows for simultaneous diagnosis and treatment of stenotic lesions with either angioplasty or placement of a coronary stent. CA is associated with a higher rate of percutaneous interventions and also with a reduction in post-LT myocardial infarctions [24]. In fact, the severity of CAD is irrelevant if revascularized before LT [27]. In other words, LT recipients with severe CAD do not do worse than those without severe CAD as long as their disease is appropriately treated before transplantation. Bare metal stents are favored over drug-eluting stents due to a shorter duration for administration of dual anti-platelet therapy (one month versus 6 months) [22, 33]. Simultaneous coronary artery bypass grafting (CABG) and LT has been described as a reasonable option for the treatment of CAD not amenable to percutaneous intervention as CABG alone is associated with increased mortality in patients with ESLD [24]. Non obstructive CAD should be treated with lifestyle modifications, beta blockade and statins [24, 34].

Functional assessment modalities such as metabolic equivalents of tasks (METs), the 6-minute walk distance (6MWD) test or cardiopulmonary exercise testing (CPET) can be used to evaluate the overall functional status. Although they are not diagnostic for a specific disease process, their results correlate with the incidence of cardiac disease and with post transplant outcomes [23, 24]. Inability to walk up two flights of stairs (4 METS), a 6MWD of less than 250 meters, or an anaerobic threshold (AT) of less than 9.0 mL/min/kg are associated with increased postoperative morbidity and mortality [24, 35, 36]. Unfortunately, many LT candidates are deconditioned and cannot participate in CPET. A rehabilitation program can be used to improve functional status and allow select patients to undergo CPET; however, many may still require other modalities to better assess cardiac function.

Heart Failure

Heart failure (HF) in LT candidates may be systolic or diastolic with either preserved or reduced ejection fraction (EF). Echocardiography is used to evaluate for the presence and extent of preoperative heart failure. CPEX may also show reduced aerobic capacity in patients with HF [28]. There is no universally accepted EF threshold that serves as an absolute contraindication to LT. However, since preoperative HF is associated with worse post-LT outcomes, most centers will not commonly transplant patients with an EF < 40%.

Valvular Diseases

Aortic stenosis (AS), especially if severe (mean gradient > 40 mmHg, aortic valve are (AVA) < 1 cm [2], peak aortic jet velocity > 4 m/s), may be a strong relative contraindication to LT as the fixed cardiac output associated with hemodynamically significant AS can result in catastrophic hemodynamic instability during portal and caval clamping or during episodes of acute hemorrhage, endangering the survival of the patient and/or the graft. In fact, severe aortic stenosis is associated with an increased risk of perioperative complications and death in non-cardiac surgery [37]. Preoperative echocardiography is used for diagnosis and grading of AS. Surgical aortic valve repair or replacement (AVR) in the context of ESLD is associated with similarly increased perioperative mortality as CABG. Less invasive modalities such as trans-catheter aortic valve replacement (TAVR) or balloon aortic valvuloplasty provide less risky pre-transplant treatment options [38–40]. Successful simultaneous LT and AVR have been reported and may be a good option for those not amenable to percutaneous interventions [41, 42].

Tricuspid regurgitation (TR), especially if severe, is frequently associated with volume overload and/or severe pulmonary hypertension and may cause deleterious venous congestion of the new liver graft [23]. Preoperative optimization includes diuresis, RRT, and treatment of pulmonary hypertension.

Infiltrative Cardiomyopathies

Most common infiltrative cardiomyopathies include amyloidosis, sarcoidosis, and hemochromatosis. The pathophysiology involves the collection of abnormal material within cardiac tissue eventually causing either diastolic or systolic dysfunction [43].

In amyloidosis, the deposition of amyloid fibrils can cause right and left heart failure, heart block and coronary artery ischemia. Cardiac MRI can diagnose early stages of cardiac amyloidosis, and treatment is largely based on the management of heart failure with diuretics [44]. The type of amyloidosis is important in patient selection for LT, as the etiology is associated with projected survival. Amyloid Light chain (AL) amyloidosis with cardiac involvement corresponds to a median survival of 4 months whereas, for hereditary transthyretin-derived (ATTR), LT may be curative [43]. LT does not alter the course of cardiac involvement; therefore LT should be performed while cardiac disease is mild [22].

Cardiac involvement in sarcoid is rare (less than 5%) but can be associated with heart failure and sudden cardiac death. As with amyloid, cardiac echocardiography or MR is used to evaluate patients with systemic sarcoidosis for the presence of cardiac involvement. Treatment involves glucocorticoids and implantation of a cardiac defibrillator [43].

With hemochromatosis, the deposition of excess iron results in diastolic and systolic heart failure and increased risk of dysrhythmias. Echocardiography and MR can assess the extent of the disease. Phlebotomy and chelating agents are used for treatment [43]. Simultaneous heart and liver transplantation may be considered for selected patients with certain subtypes of infiltrative cardiomyopathies whose cardiac function is not salvageable.

Atrial Fibrillation

Atrial fibrillation (AF) is the most common dysrhythmia among LT candidates. When appropriately rate-controlled and hemodynamically stable, it does not preclude LT. However, if it is new-onset, not rate controlled or hemodynamically unstable, it warrants an evaluation by a cardiologist prior to transplant in order to rule out other cardiac pathology and to achieve heart rate or rhythm control before transplantation. Patients with pre-existing rate-controlled AF are at an increased risk for perioperative cardiovascular complications [45]. In addition to that, AF with a rapid ventricular response during LT can lead to significant hemodynamic instability resulting in poor graft perfusion and an increased risk for perioperative acute cardiac events. Furthermore, LT candidates with AF and who take warfarin for thromboembolic prophylaxis may require rapid correction of INR with either fresh frozen plasma (FFP) or prothrombin complex concentrate (PCC) should they receive an offer for an organ.

Comprehensive Assessment of Cardiovascular Risk in Liver Transplant Candidates

Evaluation of each individual cardiovascular disease can help risk stratify and guide optimization of LT candidates with respect to that disease process (Fig. 6.2). Unfortunately, the diagnosis of CAD does not necessarily mean that a patient will have an acute perioperative cardiac event. Likewise, a negative stress test or

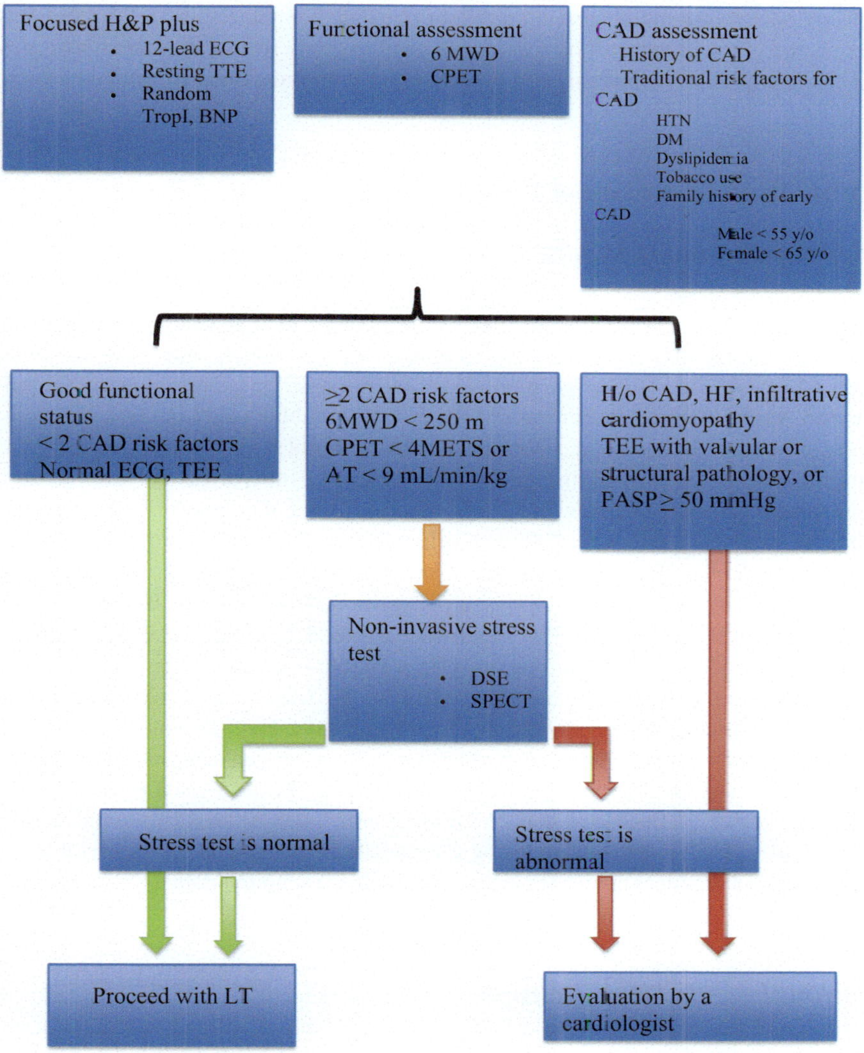

Fig. 6.2 Cardiac evaluation of liver transplant candidates

a coronary angiogram showing a hemodynamically insignificant coronary artery lesion does not guarantee that a patient will not have an event. The Cardiovascular Risk in Orthotopic Liver Transplantation (CAR-OLT) score was developed to help estimate the risk of cardiovascular events during and after LT [30] Variables used in its calculation include age, sex, race, working status, education level, and the presence of atrial fibrillation, respiratory failure, pulmonary hypertension, hepatocellular carcinoma, hypertension, diabetes, and heart failure. The CAR-OLT predicts 1-year risk of acute cardiovascular events, and it can be accessed online at https://carolt.us [46]. Although this model was derived from a patient population at one specific transplant center and may not translate completely to all LT recipients across the globe, it can still be reasonably used to guide risk stratification, and may be easily explained to patients and their families when obtaining informed consent.

Pulmonary Disorders of ESLD

Hepatopulmonary Syndrome

Hepatopulmonary syndrome (HPS) is defined by abnormal oxygenation (alveolar-arterial oxygen gradient ≥ 15 mmHg or ≥ 20 mmHg for patients older than 64 years) in the sitting position at rest on room air and the presence of a pulmonary vascular dilatation (diagnosed either with a bubble study on an echocardiogram or a tagged albumin scan) in the setting of portal hypertension due to ESLD and absence of other lung disease [47]. Changes at a microvascular level cause a ventilation/perfusion mismatch and an anatomic shunt that results in hypoxemia. HPS is graded as mild ($PaO_2 \geq 80$ mmHg), moderate ($PaO_2 = 60$–79 mmHg), severe ($PaO_2 = 50$–59 mmHg), and very severe ($PaO_2 < 50$ mmHg). Diagnosis includes identification of symptoms such as dyspnea, platypnea and orthodeoxia. Initial screening with pulse oximetry (O_2sat < 92%) and arterial blood sampling ($PaO_2 < 80$ mmHg) [48] is followed by an echocardiogram with a bubble study or a lung perfusion scan to evaluate for the presence of an extra cardiac shunt. The extent of liver disease does not always correlate with the severity of hypoxemia [10]. Hypoxemia associated with HPS is treated with supplemental oxygen for a target oxygen saturation higher than 88%. Pulmonary angiography and embolization may be necessary to treat severe refractory cases, defined as PaO2 < 50 mmHg with poor response to supplemental oxygen [48]. HPS is an indication for and usually resolves with LT. Severe hypoxemia (PaO_2 of less than 60 mmHg) allows for MELD exception points.

Portopulmonary Hypertension

Portopulmonary hypertension (POPH) is defined by a mean pulmonary arterial pressure (mPAP) of > 25 mmHg, pulmonary capillary wedge pressure

(PCWP) < 15 mmHg and pulmonary vascular resistance (PVR) > 3 wood units (or 240 dynes/s/cm^{-5}) in the setting of portal hypertension due to ESLD [47]. It is caused by multifactorial obstruction to blood flow in the pulmonary capillaries and is graded based on severity—mild 25 mmHg ≤ mPAP < 35 mmHg; moderate 35 mmHg ≤ mPAP < 45 mmHg; severe mPAP > 45 mmHg. Pulmonary artery systolic pressure (PASP) greater than 50 mmHg or right ventricular dilatation/dysfunction even with a normal PASP seen on screening echocardiography warrants a right heart catheterization to measure mean pulmonary arterial pressures. Treatment includes the use of various pulmonary vasodilators such as phosphodiesterase inhibitors, endothelin receptor antagonists, and prostacyclin analogues in patients with mPAP ≥ 35 mmHg [47, 49]. Because POPH is irreversible and, when severe, is associated with unpredictable outcomes and an increased risk for perioperative mortality, [10] POPH is currently not a universal indication for LT, and mPAP > 45 mmHg is considered an absolute contraindication to transplantation [47]. Some transplant centers will list and transplant patients with moderate-severe POPH if there is a sustained reduction of mPAP to less than 35 mmHg and a reduction of PVR to less than 5 Wood units with pulmonary vasodilators [10, 49].

Diagnosis, grading and treatment strategies for HPS and POPH are highlighted in Table 6.3.

Table 6.3 Pulmonary disorders of end-stage-liver-disease

	Portopulmonary hypertension		Hepatopulmonary syndrome	
Diagnostic criteria	1. Portal hypertension 2. mPAP ≥ 25 mmHg 3. PAOP < 15 mmHg 4. PVR > 240 dynes/s/cm^5 (3 Wood units)		1. Portal hypertension 2. Arterial hypoxemia a. A-a gradient > 15 mmHg (> 20 for patients > 64 y/o 3. Intrapulmonary vascular dilatation diagnosed by a. Echocardiography or b. ^{99m}TC albumin perfusion scan	
Grading	Mild	mPAP = 25–34 mmHg	Mild	$PaO_2 \geq 80$ mmHg
	Moderate	mPAP = 35–44 mmHg	Moderate	$PaO_2 = 60$-79 mmHg
	Severe	mPAP ≥ 45	Severe	$PaO_2 < 59$ mmHg
treatment before LT	Target mPAP < 35 mmHg, PVR < 5 Woods units with: 1. Prostacyclin analogues (epoprostenol, treprostinil) 2. Phosphodiesterase-5 inhibitors (sildenafil) 3. Endothelin receptor antagonists (bosentan, ambrisentan) 4. Guanylate cyclase stimulator (riociguat) 5. Tyrosine kinase inhibitor (imatinib)		Target oxygen saturation > 88–90% with: 1. Supplemental oxygen 2. Pulmonary angiography and embolization for refractory cases	

References AbuHalimeh [10, 47, 48]

Gastrointestinal Disorders of ESLD

Gastrointestinal Hemorrhage

Intrahepatic resistance to portal blood flow associated with cirrhosis frequently results in portal hypertension that can cause the development of portosystemic collaterals, varices (esophageal, gastric, duodenal or colonic) and subsequent gastrointestinal hemorrhage [50]. Almost 90% of patients with ESLD will eventually develop esophageal varices. The degree of portal hypertension as measured by the hepatic venous pressure gradient (HPVG) predicts the risk of bleeding more accurately than conventional coagulation tests such as the international normalzied ratio (INR) [51]. Non-selective beta-blockers such as propranolol or carvedilol are used to prevent variceal hemorrhage, which is usually managed with volume resuscitation, vasopressor agents (octreotide, terlipressin) and endoscopic intervention [50–52]. Transjugular intrahepatic portosystemic shunt (TIPS) is reserved for patients that re-bleed despite therapy and is the treatment of choice for hemorrhage from cardio-fundal varices [50].

Ascites

In addition to the formation of varices, portal hypertension and the accompanying increase in hydrostatic pressure, together with a decrease in the oncotic pressure from hypoalbuminemia cause the transudation of fluid into the peritoneum and the development of ascites. Ascites carries a worse overall prognosis [53]. Complications of ascites include hyponatremia and spontaneous bacterial peritonitis (SBP). Treatment options focus on fluid removal with diuretics and paracentesis as well as sodium restriction [54]. Large volume paracentesis (LVP), defined as the removal of more than 5 L of ascites, can improve symptoms such as dyspnea and nausea; however, it can also cause circulatory dysfunction that is usually prevented by infusion of 8 g/L of ascitic fluid of albumin [53].

Severe hyponatremia (< 125 mmol/L) can present a unique problem intraoperatively as both, fresh frozen plasma (FFP) and sodium bicarbonate, given during LT contain a large amount of sodium and may cause an acute elevation of plasma sodium level increasing the risk for osmotic demyelination syndrome [55]. Severe hyponatremia must either be slowly corrected prior to transplantation or, if not possible, arrangements must be made to prevent acute intraoperative elevations of sodium either with limiting products with a high sodium load (FFP, sodium bicarbonate, albumin) or with a carefully titrated infusion of free water.

SBP, defined as a leucocyte count of more than 250 cells/mm^3, is caused by bacterial translocation from the intestinal tract, bacteremia and subsequent peritonitis. It is the most common bacterial infection in patients with cirrhosis [56]. Associated with increased in-hospital mortality due to concurrent renal injury and worsening liver failure, SBP must be treated in a timely manner with broad-spectrum antibiotics such as cefotaxime [53]. The addition of intravenous albumin may decrease the risk of death and development of hepatorenal syndrome (HRS) [56]. Patients who are at high-risk for recurrence may require secondary prevention with chronic antibiotic therapy.

Renal Disorders of ESLD

Hepatorenal Syndrome (HRS)

Splanchnic arterial vasodilatation (due to increased nitric oxide production) [50] and increased splanchnic blood flow cause a decrease in systemic mean arterial pressure resulting in marked renal arterial vasoconstriction and the development of HRS [57]. Diagnostic criteria for HRS include the presence of cirrhosis, ascites and a concurrent diagnosis of acute kidney injury (AKI) with no improvement within 48 hours after administration of albumin and termination of diuretics in the absence of nephrotoxic drugs, structural kidney damage or shock [58, 59]. The actual creatinine level is not indicative of renal function in the context of ESLD, because ESLD is often accompanied by muscle wasting and an increased volume of distribution. HRS is frequently complicated by ascites and hyponatremia. Classically, HRS is grouped into type I HRS (doubling of serum creatinine and fast deterioration within two weeks often leading to death) and Type II (slow decline in renal function and refractory ascites)after administration of albumin [60]. Frontline treatment is volume expansion with albumin, followed by various combinations of vasopressors such as terlipressin, midodrine/octreotide, low-dose dopamine, and norepinephrineafter administration of albumin [57]. The combination of terlipressin and albumin appears to be a better alternative to the combination of octreotide, midodrine and albumin for improving renal function in the setting of HRS, [61] and it is the standard of care in those countries where terlipressin is available [57].

Acute Kidney Injury (AKI)

Renal dysfunction is present in up to 50% of LT candidates and significantly increases morbidity and mortality [58, 62, 63]. AKI (acute increase in serum creatinine > 50% from baseline or a rise of > 0.3 mg/dL in < 48 hrs or a chronic eGFR < 60 mL/min) can occur in the presence or absence of HRS. Cirrhotic cardiomyopathy with a decreased cardiac output, further worsened by non-selective beta-blockers, can increase the risk for HRS with acute kidney injury (AKI) [59, 62, 63]. Non-HRS-AKI etiologies include hypovolemia, bile acid nephropathy and inflammatory and drug-induced tubular damage. Non-HRS-AKI is associated with acute-on-chronic liver failure [63]. As with HRS-AKI, treatment is mainly supportive with the goal of carefully titrated volume resuscitation and maintenance of mean arterial pressure for adequate renal perfusion. Because the MELD score is heavily weighted by the serum creatinine, its use for organ allocation has increased the numbers of LT recipients with AKI and even renal failure requiring RRT. Some transplant centers also use RRT to help manage intraoperative electrolyte disturbances, acid-base status and fluid overload. (Agopian 2014) (S.D. Baek 2017). Preoperative considerations for intraoperative RRT and include creatinine level, presence of oliguria/anuria, the need for preoperative RRT, hyperkalemia, hyponatremia, and pulmonary edema [59, 64].

Although the definitive treatment of renal dysfunction in the setting of liver failure is LT, renal function may or may not return after transplant. In fact, patients with HRS have better overall survival when they receive a simultaneous liver and kidney transplant (SLK) [65] Indications for SLK include CKD with GFR < 30 mL/min, acute kidney injury with renal replacement therapy for > 8 weeks, or in the presence of extensive glomerulosclerosis [22, 66]. Ultimately, the decision for SLK depends on the practice of each individual transplant center.

Coagulation Disorders of ESLD

Pathophysiology

The previously held belief that coagulopathy and hemorrhage in patients with ESLD is a simple result of reduced numbers of clotting factors and platelets is only a small piece of the puzzle. While extremely decreased levels of clotting factors and severe thrombocytopenia may certainly increase the risk for hemorrhage, especially during invasive procedures, they alone do not explain the complex rebalancing of the coagulation system in liver failure. Under normal circumstances, the coagulation cascade is a carefully orchestrated chemistry of endothelial injury, platelet activation and clotting factors—all controlled by an appropriate degree of fibrinolysis. In liver disease, there is a decrease in some procoagulant clotting factors (factors II, V, VII, IX, X, XI, fibrinogen) as well as a decrease in some anticoagulant factors (proteins C and S, antithrombin, heparin cofactor II) [67]. The levels of Factor VIII and vWF are also increased [68]. Additionally, there may be marked thrombocytopenia and thrombocytopathia. And while altogether, these variations in factors can theoretically predispose to bleeding, the overall rebalancing of the coagulation cascade usually results in adequate clotting even during invasive procedures. On the other hand, severe portal hypertension and acute perturbations in homeostasis such as infection, surgical stress, large fluid shifts and transfusion of blood products may result in concurrent bleeding and clotting when the balance is tipped to either side. Portal hypertension, in particular, is a risk factor for spontaneous and periprocedural hemorrhage. Accordingly, efforts to reduce portal pressure either with the use of non-selective beta-blockers or with portosystemic shunting comprise the most effective way to reduce the risk of bleeding [69]. Conversely, a hypercoagulable state in liver disease may manifest as perioperative portal vein thrombosis, pulmonary embolism or deep venous thrombosis.

Diagnostic Laboratory Tests

Conventional coagulation tests such as international normalized ratio (INR) and partial thromboplastin time (PTT) do not accurately reflect the coagulation disturbances of ESLD. First, these tests were originally designed to monitor the effects of anticoagulants. Second, they use fractionated blood and are rarely performed in real-time as they frequently must be sent for processing to a laboratory outside of the operating room. As expected, the ability of INR to predict intraoperative transfusion requirements is quite limited. In fact, studies show that patients with ELSD may have adequate levels of thrombin for clotting. Therefore, prophylactic or empiric correction of the INR with blood products may not be necessary and may actually tip the coagulation cascade towards a hypercoagulable state [67].

Viscoelastic tests such as thromboelastography (TEG) and thromboelastometry (ROTEM) assess coagulation of whole blood in real-time and may be easily performed at bedside as point-of-care testing. Both provide a pictographic analysis of cloth formation, strength and fibrinolysis. Moreover, they offer a differential diagnosis, may help guide transfusion efforts with targeted transfusion protocols and, in some cases, have been shown to decrease the use of blood products [68].

Metabolic Disorders of ESLD

Obesity

Severe obesity (Body Mass Index (BMI) > 40) and the associated comorbidities of metabolic syndrome (cardiovascular disease, DM) can adversely affect post-LT outcomes [22]. Although there are favorable results of simultaneous bariatric surgery and LT, [70] pre-LT weight loss with diet and exercise is first-line strategy for treatment of obesity prior to transplantation.

Non-alcoholic Fatty Liver Disease (NAFLD)

NAFLD is a spectrum of diagnoses from steatosis to steatohepatitis that can manifest as both, fibrosis and cirrhosis [71]. The prevalence of both, NAFLD and nonalcoholic steatohepatitis (NASH) has increased, and NASH has moved into the top three indications for LT [22]. Risk factors for development of NAFLD include obesity, type 2 diabetes, and dyslipidemia [72]. Because NAFLD carries the added burden of metabolic syndrome and, with it, an increased incidence of cardiovascular disease, carotid artery disease, kidney disease, new-onset AF and AS, LT candidates with NAFLD require a more thorough preoperative assessment in order to better optimize their status before transplantation. This may include more thorough cardiac and carotid artery studies and/or interventions, careful use of statins, metformin, and supervised diet and exercise programs [73].

Malnutrition, Sarcopenia and Frailty in ESLD

Malnutrition

Malnutrition in ESLD is common and frequently caused by anorexia, nausea, and decreased oral intake due to ascites, hepatic encephalopathy, dietary restrictions and malabsorption. To assess the overall nutritional status, hospitals use the combination of BMI, triceps skin fold thickness, mid-arm circumference, and other center-specific surveys [74].

Sarcopenia

Sarcopenia, or loss of muscle mass, is a natural process of aging, but can also be seen in the setting of malnutrition and chronic disease such as ESLD and is assessed by measuring the cross-sectional area of the psoas muscle at the level of the third or fourth lumbar vertebra. Sarcopenia strongly correlates with post-LT morbidity and mortality [74] and is used as an objective marker of frailty [75].

Frailty

Frailty is a multifaceted syndrome comprised of a deteriorating functional status and a decrease in physiological reserve leading to a diminished response to stress and increased susceptibility to complications [76]. It affects almost half of patients with ESLD and predicts pre- and post-LT mortality. Multiple tools such as the Karnofsky Performance Status scale and Fried frailty index are used to assess frailty [75, 76]. In fact, the Karnofsky score has been shown to be a good predictor of pre- and post-LT mortality [77]. Some transplant centers also use a battery of physical tests (grip strength, gait speed, timed repeated chair stands, etc.)

to further gauge deconditioning [78]. Frailty scores correlate with mortality independent of the MELD score whereas the combination of the MELD score and the frailty score more accurately predict survival. Preoperative treatment with exercise, nutrition and cognitive interventions improves frailty scores and decreases morbidity [76, 79].

Substance Abuse in ESLD

Alcohol Abuse

Because alcoholic cirrhosis is the second most common cause of ESLD requiring liver transplantation and, because the rate of relapse can be as high as 95% in some cases, [80] most transplant centers require that potential candidates abstain from alcohol use for a specific amount of time and complete some sort of formal alcohol detox program. The 2013 Practice Guideline by the American Association for the Study of Liver Diseases and the American society of Transplantation mentions a "6-month minimum period of abstinence to allow addiction issues to be addressed or to allow for spontaneous recovery" [22]. Special situations in which the patient's condition does not allow the time for the completion of such requirements are discussed among each individual center's transplant committee members.

Tobacco Abuse

Approximately a quarter of LT candidates smoke tobacco, which is one of the most common preventable causes of death. Donnadieu-Rigole et al. [80] And, although smoking has not been shown to definitively affect graft survival, tobacco use increases the risk for cardiovascular disease and de novo malignancies and may significantly impact long-term survival [81]. The 2013 Practice Guideline by the American Association for the Study of Liver Diseases and the American society of Transplantation recommends prohibition of tobacco consumption in LT candidates (Level of evidence 1-A) [22]. Currently, individual transplant center practices vary when it comes to requiring smoking cessation prior to listing for transplantation, but the number of transplant centers that require it has increased in the last fifteen years [81]. All LT candidates who are active smokers should be offered enrollment in a smoking cessation program since tobacco abstinence of four weeks decreases the risk of surgical site infections, and postoperative respiratory and cardiovascular complications [82]. Furthermore, because there is a higher rate of alcohol recidivism in smokers, tobacco use should be strongly discouraged [81].

Illicit Drug Abuse

Little data exists about the use of illicit drugs in LT candidates. Several limited studies looking at the effects of marijuana on LT outcomes failed to provide any convincing evidence regarding increased postoperative complications or waitlist mortality [83]. As with tobacco use, the decision to list patients who either used illicit drugs (marijuana, cocaine, etc.) in the past or are still actively using depends on each individual transplant center. Of course, many transplant recognize the association between illicit drug use, alcohol use and recidivism and may be less inclined to consider those patients for transplantation.

Preoperative Assessment of Patients for Non-transplant, Hepatico-Pancreatic-Biliary Surgery

Common hepatico-pancreatic-biliary (HPB) procedures include pancreaticoduodenectomy, distal or total pancreatectomy, and various types of liver resections. These operations may be open, laparoscopic, or robotic-assisted laparoscopic. The majority of HPB operations are classified as moderate-risk procedures. The preoperative anesthetic evaluation for these types of surgeries should begin with a focused history and physical exam, targeting chronic systemic diseases (hypertension, diabetes mellitus, chronic obstructive pulmonary disease, etc.) that may require optimization. Dementia is associated with worse postoperative outcomes; therefore, patients with dementia should undergo some form of mental status testing [84]. But because cardiac and liver-related complications comprise the majority of post-HPB surgical morbidity, the assessment of the cardiovascular system and liver function require special attention.

Assessment of Cardiovascular Status

Some HPB procedures are more invasive and technically complex and may require high volume resuscitation leading to large intraoperative fluid shifts with increased hemodynamic stress that is further amplified in patients with pre-existing cardiovascular disease. Accordingly, patients should be assessed for a history of coronary artery disease, heart failure, cerebrovascular disease, and chronic kidney disease—all of which are risk factors for perioperative major acute cardiac events (MACE). The patient's overall risk of perioperative MACE and other complications may be estimated using several validated risk-assessment tools. Available risk calculators include the Revised Cardiac Risk Index, [85] and the American College of Surgeons National Quality Improvement Program (NSQIP) Surgical Risk Calculator [86].

According to the *2014 European Society of Cardiology (ESC)/the European Society of Anesthesiology (ESA) Guidelines on non-cardiac surgery: cardiovascular assessment and management* and the *2014 American College of Cardiology (ACC)/American Heart Association (AHA) Guideline for cardiac evaluation for noncardiac surgery*, for patients at low-risk (<1%) for MACE, no further cardiac evaluation is necessary [34, 87]. Patients at elevated risk should be further stratified according to their functional status, which can be assessed using various activity scales, such as the Duke Activity Status Index [34]. Correlation of preoperative functional capacity with postoperative MACE is not uniform among different studies; however, excellent exercise tolerance (>10 METS) corresponds with a low likelihood of postoperative cardiovascular complications [87]. Difficult to assess or poor functional status (less than 4 METS) warrants further cardiac evaluation with some type of a pharmacologic stress test [34].

Assessment of Liver Function

Patients scheduled to undergo a liver resection (either for an excision of a mass or for a donor hepatectomy) must be evaluated for expected postoperative liver function. Projected percentage of functional liver should be more than 20, and even greater in patients with preoperative hepatic dysfunction [88]. Patients with cirrhosis are at increased risk for postoperative complications, with approximate mortality of 1–10% (Childs A) 9.5–20% (Childs B), and 36–60% (Childs C) or 3.6% (MELD<19), 12.5% (MELD 20–24), 36% (MELD>25) after nonhepatic surgery [89, 90]. The risk of mortality is even higher for cirrhotic patients that undergo liver resection. Colon cancer metastatic to the liver is a common indication for liver resection. Surgical resection frequently follows systemic chemotherapy. Chemotherapeutic agents containing irinotecan can cause chemotherapy-associated steatohepatitis (CASH), [91] which is linked to postoperative liver failure and higher mortality [92]. Assessment of liver function should include routine laboratory tests such as a complete metabolic panel, a platelet count, and coagulation tests (INR, PTT).

References

1. Abbas N, Makker J, Abbas H, Balar B. Perioperative care of patients with liver cirrhosis: a review. Health Serv Insights. 2017;10:1178632917691270.
2. Farnsworth N, Fagan SP, Berger DH, Awad SS. Child-Turcotte-Pugh versus MELD score as a predictor of outcome after elective and emergent surgery in cirrhotic patients. Am J Surg. 2004;188:580–3.
3. Telem DA, Schiano T, Goldstone R, et al. Factors that predict outcome of abdominal operations in patients with advanced cirrhosis. Clin Gastroenterol Hepatol. 2010;8:451–7, quiz e58.

4. Wiesner R, Edwards E, Freeman R, et al. Model for end-stage liver disease (MELD) and allocation of donor livers. Gastroenterology. 2003;124:91–6.
5. Malinchoc M, Kamath PS, Gordon FD, Peine CJ, Rank J, ter Borg PC. A model to predict poor survival in patients undergoing transjugular intrahepatic portosystemic shunts. Hepatology. 2000;31:864–71.
6. Machicao VI. Model for end-stage liver disease-sodium score: the evolution in the prioritization of liver transplantation. Clin Liver Dis. 2017;21:275–87.
7. Kim WR, Biggins SW, Kremers WK, et al. Hyponatremia and mortality among patients on the liver-transplant waiting list. N Engl J Med. 2008;359:1018–26.
8. Nagai S, Chau LC, Schilke RE, et al. Effects of allocating livers for transplantation based on model for end-stage liver disease-sodium scores on patient outcomes. Gastroenterology. 2018;155(1451–62):e3.
9. Sharma P, Schaubel DE, Goodrich NP, Merion RM. Serum sodium and survival benefit of liver transplantation. Liver Transpl. 2015;21:308–13.
10. Krowka MJ, Wiesner RH, Heimbach JK. Pulmonary contraindications, indications and MELD exceptions for liver transplantation: a contemporary view and look forward. J Hepatol. 2013;59:367–74.
11. van Vugt JLA, Alferink LJM, Buettner S, et al. A model including sarcopenia surpasses the MELD score in predicting waiting list mortality in cirrhotic liver transplant candidates: a competing risk analysis in a national cohort. J Hepatol. 2018;68:707–14.
12. Bertsimas D, Kung J, Trichakis N, Wang Y, Hirose R, Vagefi PA. Development and validation of an optimized prediction of mortality for candidates awaiting liver transplantation. Am J Transplant. 2019;19:1109–18.
13. Vilstrup H, Amodio P, Bajaj J, et al. Hepatic encephalopathy in chronic liver disease: 2014 practice guideline by the American association for the study of liver diseases and the european association for the study of the liver. Hepatology. 2014;60:715–35.
14. DellaVolpe JD, Garavaglia JM, Huang DT. Management of complications of end-stage liver disease in the intensive care unit. J Intensive Care Med. 2016;31:94–103.
15. European Association for the Study of the Liver. Electronic address eee. EASL clinical practice guidelines: liver transplantation. J Hepatol. 2016;64:433–85.
16. Bernal W, Hall C, Karvellas CJ, Auzinger G, Sizer E, Wendon J. Arterial ammonia and clinical risk factors for encephalopathy and intracranial hypertension in acute liver failure. Hepatology. 2007;46:1844–52.
17. Fortea JI, Banares R, Vaquero J. Intracranial pressure in acute liver failure: to bolt or not to bolt-that is the question. Crit Care Med. 2014;42:1304–5.
18. Rajajee V, Fontana RJ, Courey AJ, Patil PG. Protocol based invasive intracranial pressure monitoring in acute liver failure: feasibility, safety and impact on management. Crit Care. 2017;21:178.
19. Krishnamoorthy V, Beckmann K, Mueller M, Sharma D, Vavilala MS. Perioperative estimation of the intracranial pressure using the optic nerve sheath diameter during liver transplantation. Liver Transpl. 2013;19:246–9.
20. Bernal W, Wendon J. Acute liver failure. N Engl J Med. 2013;369:2525–34.
21. Feltracco P, Cagnin A, Carollo C, Barbieri S, Ori C. Neurological disorders in liver transplant candidates: pathophysiology and clinical assessment. Transplant Rev (Orlando). 2017;31:193–206.
22. Martin P, DiMartini A, Feng S, Brown R Jr, Fallon M. Evaluation for liver transplantation in adults: 2013 practice guideline by the American association for the study of liver diseases and the american society of transplantation. Hepatology. 2014;59:1144–65.
23. Wray CL. Liver transplantation in patients with cardiac disease. Semin Cardiothorac Vasc Anesth. 2018;22:111–21.
24. Hogan BJ, Gonsalkorala E, Heneghan MA. Evaluation of coronary artery disease in potential liver transplant recipients. Liver Transpl. 2017;23:386–95.

25. Sonny A, Govindarajan SR, Jaber WA, Cywinski JB. Systolic heart failure after liver transplantation: Incidence, predictors, and outcome. Clin Transplant. 2018;32:e13199.
26. Ruiz-del-Arbol L, Serradilla R. Cirrhotic cardiomyopathy. World J Gastroenterol. 2015;21:11502–21.
27. Satapathy SK, Vanatta JM, Helmick RA, et al. Outcome of Liver transplant recipients with revascularized coronary artery disease: a comparative analysis with and without cardiovascular risk factors. Transplantation. 2017;101:793–803.
28. VanWagner LB, Harinstein ME, Runo JR, et al. Multidisciplinary approach to cardiac and pulmonary vascular disease risk assessment in liver transplantation: an evaluation of the evidence and consensus recommendations. Am J Transplant. 2018;18:30–42.
29. Gitman M, Albertz M, Nicolau-Raducu R, Aniskevich S 3rd, Pai SL. Cardiac diseases among liver transplant candidates. Clin Transplant. 2018;32:e13296.
30. VanWagner LB, Ning H, Whitsett M, et al. A point-based prediction model for cardiovascular risk in orthotopic liver transplantation: The CAR-OLT score. Hepatology. 2017;66:1968–79.
31. Snipelisky D, Ray J, Vallabhajosyula S, et al. Usefulness for predicting cardiac events after orthotopic liver transplantation of myocardial perfusion imaging and dobutamine stress echocardiography preoperatively. Am J Cardiol. 2017;119:1008–11.
32. Kong YG, Kang JW, Kim YK, et al. Preoperative coronary calcium score is predictive of early postoperative cardiovascular complications in liver transplant recipients. Br J Anaesth. 2015;114:437–43.
33. Levine GN, Bates ER, Bittl JA, et al. 2016 ACC/AHA guideline focused update on duration of dual antiplatelet therapy in patients with coronary artery disease: a report of the American college of cardiology/American heart association task force on clinical practice guidelines: an update of the 2011 ACCF/AHA/SCAI guideline for percutaneous coronary intervention, 2011 ACCF/AHA Guideline for coronary artery bypass graft surgery, 2012 ACC/AHA/ACP/AATS/PCNA/SCAI/STS guideline for the diagnosis and management of patients with stable ischemic heart disease, 2013 ACCF/AHA guideline for the management of ST-elevation myocardial infarction, 2014 AHA/ACC guideline for the management of patients with non-ST-elevation acute coronary syndromes, and 2014 ACC/AHA guideline on perioperative cardiovascular evaluation and management of patients undergoing noncardiac surgery. Circulation. 2016;134:e123–55.
34. Fleisher LA, Fleischmann KE, Auerbach AD, et al. 2014 ACC/AHA guideline on perioperative cardiovascular evaluation and management of patients undergoing noncardiac surgery: executive summary: a report of the American college of cardiology/American heart association task force on practice guidelines. Developed in collaboration with the American college of surgeons, American society of anesthesiologists, American society of echocardiography, American society of nuclear cardiology, heart rhythm society, society for cardiovascular angiography and interventions, society of cardiovascular anesthesiologists, and society of vascular medicine endorsed by the society of hospital medicine. J Nucl Cardiol 2015;22:162–215.
35. Bernal W, Martin-Mateos R, Lipcsey M, et al. Aerobic capacity during cardiopulmonary exercise testing and survival with and without liver transplantation for patients with chronic liver disease. Liver Transpl. 2014;20:54–62.
36. Prentis JM, Manas DM, Trenell MI, Hudson M, Jones DJ, Snowden CP. Submaximal cardiopulmonary exercise testing predicts 90-day survival after liver transplantation. Liver Transpl. 2012;18:152–9.
37. Kertai MD, Bountioukos M, Boersma E, et al. Aortic stenosis: an underestimated risk factor for perioperative complications in patients undergoing noncardiac surgery. Am J Med. 2004;116:8–13.
38. Kalarickal P, Liu Q, Rathor R, Ishag S, Kerr T, Kangrga I. Balloon aortic valvuloplasty as a bridge to liver transplantation in patients with severe aortic stenosis: a case series. Transplant Proc. 2014;46:3492–5.

39. Coverstone E, Korenblat K, Crippin JS, Chapman WC, Kates AM, Zajarias A. Aortic balloon valvuloplasty prior to orthotopic liver transplantation: a novel approach to aortic stenosis and end-stage liver disease. Case Rep Cardiol. 2014;2014:325136.
40. Silvestre OM, Bacal F, Ramos DS, et al. Transcatheter aortic valve implantation as rescue therapy for liver transplant candidates with aortic valve stenosis. Liver Transpl. 2014;20:1277–9.
41. Parker BM, Mayes JT, Henderson JM, Savage RM. Combined aortic valve replacement and orthotopic liver transplantation. J Cardiothorac Vasc Anesth. 2001;15:474–6.
42. Gologorsky E, Tabar KR, Krupa K, et al. Emergency aortic valve replacement combined with liver and kidney transplantation: case report and literature review. J Cardiothorac Vasc Anesth. 2018.
43. Bejar D, Colombo PC, Latif F, Yuzefpolskaya M. Infiltrative cardiomyopathies. Clin Med Insights Cardiol. 2015;9:29–38.
44. Tuzovic M, Yang EH, Baas AS, et al. Cardiac amyloidosis: diagnosis and treatment strategies. Curr Oncol Rep. 2017;19:46.
45. Bargehr J, Trejo-Gutierrez JF, Patel T, et al. Preexisting atrial fibrillation and cardiac complications after liver transplantation. Liver Transpl. 2015;21:314–20.
46. VanWagner LB. A simple clinical calculator for assessing cardiac event risk in liver transplant candidates: the cardiovascular risk in orthotopic liver transplantation score. Clin Liver Dis (Hoboken). 2018;11:145–8.
47. Krowka MJ, Fallon MB, Kawut SM, et al. International liver transplant society practice guidelines: diagnosis and management of hepatopulmonary syndrome and portopulmonary hypertension. Transplantation. 2016;100:1440–52.
48. Krowka MJ. Management of pulmonary complications in pretransplant patients. Clin Liver Dis. 2011;15:765–77.
49. AbuHalimeh B, Krowka MJ, Tonelli AR. Treatment barriers in portopulmonary hypertension. Hepatology. 2019;69:431–43.
50. Garcia-Tsao G, Abraldes JG, Berzigotti A, Bosch J. Portal hypertensive bleeding in cirrhosis: risk stratification, diagnosis, and management: 2016 practice guidance by the American association for the study of liver diseases. Hepatology. 2017;65:310–35.
51. Biecker E. Portal hypertension and gastrointestinal bleeding: diagnosis, prevention and management. World J Gastroenterol. 2013;19:5035–50.
52. Brunner F, Berzigotti A, Bosch J. Prevention and treatment of variceal haemorrhage in 2017. Liver Int. 2017;37(Suppl 1):104–15.
53. Pericleous M, Sarnowski A, Moore A, Fijten R, Zaman M. The clinical management of abdominal ascites, spontaneous bacterial peritonitis and hepatorenal syndrome: a review of current guidelines and recommendations. Eur J Gastroenterol Hepatol. 2016;28:e10–8.
54. Adebayo D, Neong SF, Wong F. Refractory ascites in liver cirrhosis. Am J Gastroenterol. 2019;114:40–7.
55. Crismale JF, Meliambro KA, DeMaria S Jr, Bronster DB, Florman S, Schiano TD. Prevention of the osmotic demyelination syndrome after liver transplantation: a multidisciplinary perspective. Am J Transplant. 2017;17:2537–45.
56. Marciano S, Diaz JM, Dirchwolf M, Gadano A. Spontaneous bacterial peritonitis in patients with cirrhosis: incidence, outcomes, and treatment strategies. Hepat Med. 2019;11:13–22.
57. Acevedo JG, Cramp ME. Hepatorenal syndrome: update on diagnosis and therapy. World J Hepatol. 2017;9:293–9.
58. Angeli P, Gines P, Wong F, et al. Diagnosis and management of acute kidney injury in patients with cirrhosis: revised consensus recommendations of the International club of ascites. J Hepatol. 2015;62:968–74.
59. Cheng XS, Tan JC, Kim WR. Management of renal failure in end-stage liver disease: a critical appraisal. Liver Transpl. 2016;22:1710–9.

60. Thorat A, Jeng LB. Management of renal dysfunction in patients with liver cirrhosis: role of pretransplantation hemodialysis and outcomes after liver transplantation. Semin Vasc Surg. 2016;29:227–35.
61. Cavallin M, Kamath PS, Merli M, et al. Terlipressin plus albumin versus midodrine and octreotide plus albumin in the treatment of hepatorenal syndrome: a randomized trial. Hepatology. 2015;62:567–74.
62. Wong F, Nadim MK, Kellum JA, et al. Working party proposal for a revised classification system of renal dysfunction in patients with cirrhosis. Gut. 2011;60:702–9.
63. Davenport A, Sheikh MF, Lamb E, Agarwal B, Jalan R. Acute kidney injury in acute-on-chronic liver failure: where does hepatorenal syndrome fit? Kidney Int. 2017;92:1058–70.
64. Zimmerman MA, Selim M, Kim J, et al. Outcome analysis of continuous intraoperative renal replacement therapy in the highest acuity liver transplant recipients: a single-center experience. Surgery. 2017;161:1279–86.
65. Doyle MB, Subramanian V, Vachharajani N, et al. Results of simultaneous liver and kidney transplantation: a single-center review. J Am Coll Surg. 2016;223:193–201.
66. Nadim MK, Sung RS, Davis CL, et al. Simultaneous liver-kidney transplantation summit: current state and future directions. Am J Transplant. 2012;12:2901–8.
67. Northup P, Reutemann B. Management of coagulation and anticoagulation in liver transplantation candidates. Liver Transpl. 2018;24:1119–32.
68. Forkin KT, Colquhoun DA, Nemergut EC, Huffmyer JL. The coagulation profile of end-stage liver disease and considerations for intraoperative management. Anesth Analg. 2018;126:46–61.
69. Valla DC, Rautou PE. The coagulation system in patients with end-stage liver disease. Liver Int. 2015;35(Suppl 1):139–44.
70. Heimbach JK, Watt KD, Poterucha JJ, et al. Combined liver transplantation and gastric sleeve resection for patients with medically complicated obesity and end-stage liver disease. Am J Transplant. 2013;13:363–8.
71. Targher G, Byrne CD, Lonardo A, Zoppini G, Barbui C. Non-alcoholic fatty liver disease and risk of incident cardiovascular disease: a meta-analysis. J Hepatol. 2016;65:589–600.
72. Chalasani N, Younossi Z, Lavine JE, et al. The diagnosis and management of nonalcoholic fatty liver disease: practice guidance from the American association for the study of liver diseases. Hepatology. 2018;67:328–57.
73. Lonardo A, Sookoian S, Pirola CJ, Targher G. Non-alcoholic fatty liver disease and risk of cardiovascular disease. Metabolism. 2016;65:1136–50.
74. Kalafateli M, Mantzoukis K, Choi Yau Y, et al. Malnutrition and sarcopenia predict post-liver transplantation outcomes independently of the model for end-stage liver disease score. J Cachexia Sarcopenia Muscle. 2017;8:113–21.
75. Dolgin NH, Smith AJ, Harrington SG, Movahedi B, Martins PNA, Bozorgzadeh A. Association between sarcopenia and functional status in liver transplant patients. Exp Clin Transplant. 2018.
76. Laube R, Wang H, Park L, et al. Frailty in advanced liver disease. Liver Int. 2018;38:2117–28.
77. Thuluvath PJ, Thuluvath AJ, Savva Y. Karnofsky performance status before and after liver transplantation predicts graft and patient survival. J Hepatol. 2018;69:818–25.
78. Lai JC, Dodge JL, Sen S, Covinsky K, Feng S. Functional decline in patients with cirrhosis awaiting liver transplantation: results from the functional assessment in liver transplantation (FrAILT) study. Hepatology. 2016;63:574–80.
79. Duarte-Rojo A, Ruiz-Margain A, Montano-Loza AJ, Macias-Rodriguez RU, Ferrando A, Kim WR. Exercise and physical activity for patients with end-stage liver disease: Improving functional status and sarcopenia while on the transplant waiting list. Liver Transpl. 2018;24:122–39.

80. Donnadieu-Rigole H, Perney P, Ursic-Bedoya J, Faure S, Pageaux GP. Addictive behaviors in liver transplant recipients: the real problem? World J Hepatol. 2017;9:953–8.
81. Fleetwood VA, Hertl M, Chan EY. Liver transplantation to the active smoker: transplant provider opinions and how they have changed: transplantation in smokers: a survey. J Gastrointest Surg. 2015;19:2223–7.
82. Cote DR, Chirichella TJ, Noon KA, et al. Abdominal organ transplant center tobacco use policies vary by organ program type. Transplant Proc. 2016;48:1920–6.
83. Kotwani P, Saxena V, Dodge JL, Roberts J, Yao F, Hameed B. History of marijuana use does not affect outcomes on the liver transplant waitlist. Transplantation. 2018;102:794–802.
84. De Pietri L, Montalti R, Begliomini B. Anaesthetic perioperative management of patients with pancreatic cancer. World J Gastroenterol. 2014;20:2304–20.
85. Lee TH, Marcantonio ER, Mangione CM, et al. Derivation and prospective validation of a simple index for prediction of cardiac risk of major noncardiac surgery. Circulation. 1999;100:1043–9.
86. Bilimoria KY, Liu Y, Paruch JL, et al. Development and evaluation of the universal ACS NSQIP surgical risk calculator: a decision aid and informed consent tool for patients and surgeons. J Am Coll Surg. 2013;217(833–42):e1–3.
87. Kristensen SD, Knuuti J, Saraste A, et al. 2014 ESC/ESA Guidelines on non-cardiac surgery: cardiovascular assessment and management: the joint task force on non-cardiac surgery: cardiovascular assessment and management of the European society of cardiology (ESC) and the European society of anaesthesiology (ESA). Eur J Anaesthesiol. 2014;31:517–73.
88. Egger ME, Gottumukkala V, Wilks JA, et al. Anesthetic and operative considerations for laparoscopic liver resection. Surgery. 2017;161:1191–202.
89. Neeff H, Mariaskin D, Spangenberg HC, Hopt UT, Makowiec F. Perioperative mortality after non-hepatic general surgery in patients with liver cirrhosis: an analysis of 138 operations in the 2000s using Child and MELD scores. J Gastrointest Surg. 2011;15:1–11.
90. Cho HC, Jung HY, Sinn DH, et al. Mortality after surgery in patients with liver cirrhosis: comparison of Child-Turcotte-Pugh, MELD and MELDNa score. Eur J Gastroenterol Hepatol. 2011;23:51–9.
91. Kinkhabwala M, V M. Hepatobiliary surgery: indications, evaluation, and outcomes. In: Wagener G, editor. Liver anesthesiology and critical care medicine. New York, Heiderlberg, Dordrecht, London: Springer; 2012. p. 285–97.
92. Zhao J, van Mierlo KMC, Gomez-Ramirez J, et al. Systematic review of the influence of chemotherapy-associated liver injury on outcome after partial hepatectomy for colorectal liver metastases. Br J Surg. 2017;104:990–1002.

Chapter 7
The Role of Cardiopulmonary Exercise Testing (CPET) in the Preoperative Assessment of Patients for Hepatico-Pancreatic-Biliary (HPB) Surgery and Liver Transplantation (LT)

Alice Loughnan, Shrijit Nair and Stephen James

Introduction

Cardiopulmonary exercise testing (CPET) is a dynamic, non-invasive assessment of the cardiopulmonary system at rest and during exercise [1]. The test measures oxygen uptake at increasing levels of work and predicts cardiopulmonary performance under other conditions of stress, such as after surgery, where post-operative VO_2 can also climb 2–3 fold [2]. It is being used increasingly as part of a comprehensive perioperative assessment of high-risk patients undergoing extensive surgery [3]. CPET can help to better inform patients of their individual perioperative risk, support multidisciplinary decision-making, and plan peri-operative management [2]. More recently CPET has a role in guiding prehabilitation programmes for patients having major HPB surgery and LT [4–6].

The Physiology of Exercise

The performance of exercise or muscular work requires integration of the physiological response of the cardiovascular and ventilatory system coupled with an increase in metabolic activity. For the body to do this efficiently the following must be present:

A. Loughnan (✉) · S. Nair · S. James
Kings College Hospital, Denmark Hill, London, UK
e-mail: a.loughnan@nhs.net

Z. Milan and C. Goonasekera (eds.), *Anesthesia for Hepatico-Pancreatic-Biliary Surgery and Transplantation*, https://doi.org/10.1007/978-3-030-51331-3_7

- Suitable lung and ventilatory mechanics.
- Appropriate functioning ventilatory control mechanisms, able to cope with changes in arterial blood gas and hydrogen ion concentrations.
- A pulmonary circulation where perfusion and ventilation are appropriately matched.
- Blood with a normal haemoglobin concentration.
- Effective pump to deliver oxygenated blood to respiring tissues.
- Neurovascular system capable of selectively distributing blood to tissue units with higher gas exchange requirements.
- Available energy substrate and enzyme concentrations.

A reduction in exercise efficiency and capacity occurs when there is a failure in one or more of these systems [7]. Energy for muscular contraction predominantly occurs through aerobic glycolysis of glucose to produce pyruvate, resulting in the production of high yielding adenosine triphosphate (*ATP*) molecules via oxidative phosphorylation, with production of carbon dioxide (CO_2) and water (H_2O) [1]. Under conditions where the availability of oxygen is insufficient for aerobic glycolysis to keep up with cellular demand, some energy substrate does not go down the aerobic pathway but still produces some *ATP*. This is known as anaerobic glycolysis, and it is through this process that lactic acid is produced. The start of anaerobic *ATP* production does not signal the end of aerobic *ATP* production, both mechanisms work together to generate energy. The lactic acid produced, is first mainly buffered by circulating bicarbonate but when this mechanism becomes saturated there will be a further increase in CO_2 production [1].

As work (exercise) increases, initially so does the volume of oxygen (VO_2) consumed and therefore taken up at the mouth as well as the volume of carbon dioxide (VCO_2) exhaled at the mouth. When VO_2 is plotted against VCO_2 the slope is 1.0. Beyond the anaerobic threshold (AT) the VCO_2 will increase disproportionately to VO_2, due to the relatively higher increase in CO_2 production from anaerobic respiration, resulting in the slope of $VCO_2{:}VO_2$ being greater than 1.0.

Conducting the Cardiopulmonary Exercise Test

Before any test is carried out, patients should be informed about the manner, risks and benefits of the test. On the day of the CPET, they should avoid caffeine, alcohol, smoking and strenuous exercise before the test. They should be asked to not eat 2 hours before the test and to only drink water during this time. We believe that they should continue the medication that they would be expected to take on the day of surgery as this allows the CPET to reflect their likely peri-operative haemodynamic changes. Despite numerous concerns, the majority of HPB and LT patients are capable of performing a CPET test.

CPET is a relatively safe investigation, the incidence of complications requiring hospital admissions is <2 per 1000 tests [8], 1.2 major cardiac events per 10,000 tests [9] and 2–5 deaths per 100,000 tests. At the time of writing there have been no deaths reported during perioperative CPET in the UK [1, 2].

CPET is conducted on an electromagnetically braked cycle ergometer, with each test taking 20–30 minutes to perform. Breath by breath analysis using a rapid gas analyser and a pressure differential pneumotachograph is attached to a tight-fitting face mask giving measurements of VO_2, VCO_2, respiratory rate (*RR*), tidal volume (*VT*), end tidal oxygen ($PETO_2$) and end tidal CO_2 ($PETCO_2$). Continuous oxygen saturation (SpO_2), 12 lead ECG and intermittent non-invasive blood pressure (*NIBP*) are monitored during the test (Fig. 7.1).

Prior to the test commencing, the equipment is calibrated to ambient temperature, pressure and humidity. The patient's baseline demographics and spirometry measurements are recorded which allows the prediction of normal values of peak VO_2, work rate and maximum voluntary ventilation to be calculated.

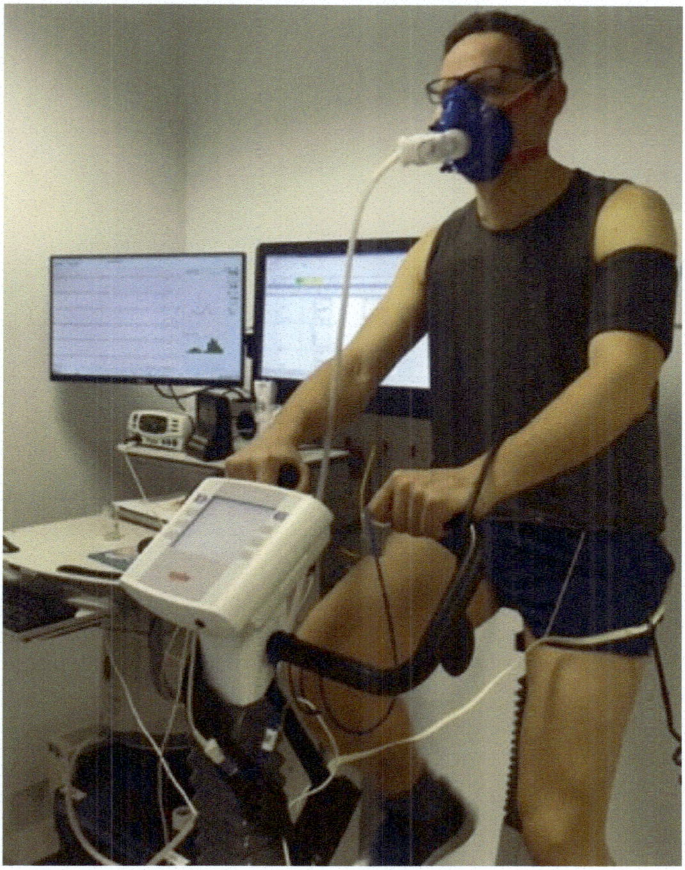

Fig. 7.1 Equipment set up for conducting CPET test

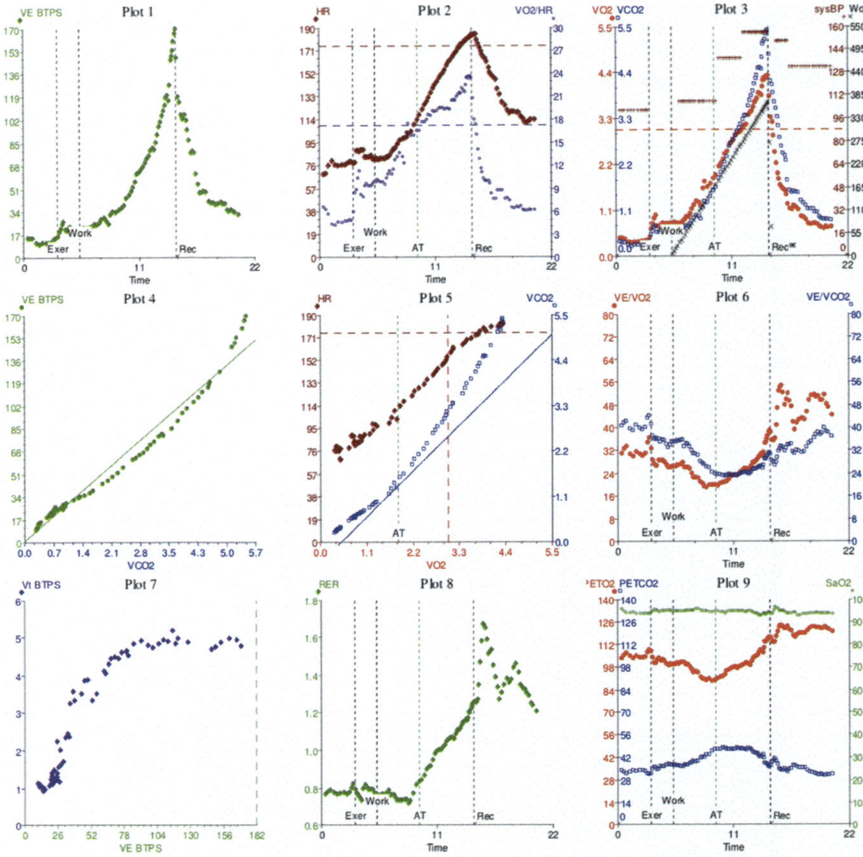

Fig. 7.2 9 panel plot of normal healthy male. Demonstrating a maximal effort test, stopping due to leg fatigue. Peak VO_2 was above predicted range. Heart rate response, VO_2 pulse and VO_2/WR slopes are normal. Normal pattern of $PETCO_2$ in response to exercise, with VE/VCO_2 values normal. **Normal CPET test**

The test starts with recording data at rest for 3 minutes and progresses to unloaded cycling (no resistance) for a further 3 minutes. The work phase follows with pedalling against a continuously increasing workload, for example 10–30 W/min, for 8 to 12 minutes before a recovery phase where values are within 10–20% of baseline.

The CPET produces several recorded and derived variables, which can be categorised as:

- Work done: (i) Work rate (*WR*) in Watts, (ii) Change in VO_2/Change work rate ($\Delta VO_2/\Delta WR$)
- Metabolic gas exchange measurements: VO_2, VCO_2, Respiratory exchange ratio (*RER*)

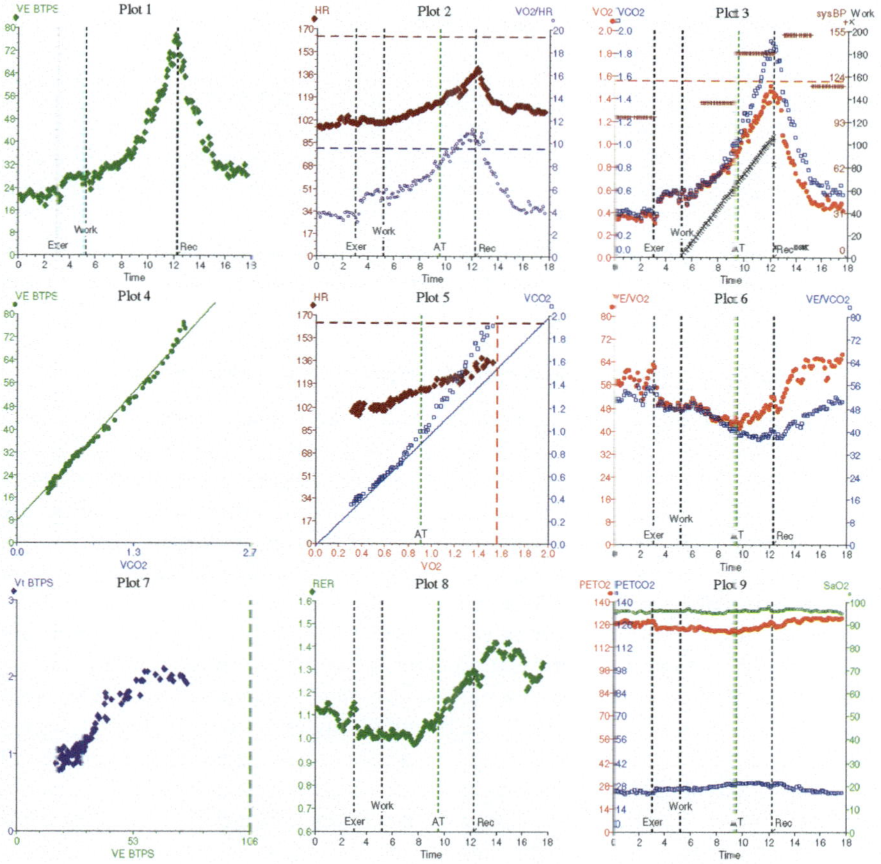

Fig. 7.3 56 year old for liver transplant assessment. This shows a maximal effort test, the patient stopped due to leg fatigue, normal pre-test spirometry. Peak VO_2 achieved was 18.3 ml/min/kg (97% of predicted) with AT of 10.9 ml/min/kg. Slightly reduced heart rate response due to beta blocker therapy is seen. Normal VO_2 pulse and VO_2/WR slopes. Evidence of chronic hyperventilation seen in panel 9 ($PETCO_2$ stays below 30 mmHg for duration of test). Hyperventilation being the likely cause of a raised VE/VCO_2 value at AT, which indicates ventilatory inefficiency. **Otherwise illustrating good status for a liver failure patient**

- Ventilatory measurements: SpO_2, *VE* (minute ventilation), *VT*, *RR*, VE/VO_2 (ventilatory equivalent for oxygen), VE/VCO_2 (ventilatory equivalent for CO_2), $PETCO_2$, $PETO_2$
- Cardiovascular variables: Heart Rate (*HR*), *ECG ST*-segment changes, *NIBP* and VO_2 pulse (VO_2/HR).

These variables are represented graphically in a standard format called the nine-panel plot (Figs. 7.2 and 7.3)..

Nine Panel Plot and Interpretation

The panels in a 9-panel plot are numbered 1 to 9 from top left to bottom right. In the classic Wasserman 9 panel plot [7] the cardiovascular system is represented by panels 2, 3, and 5. Ventilation is represented by panels 1, 4, 7 and 9. The metabolic system is shown in panel 8. Panel 6 shows ventilation perfusion relationships.

A systematic approach to reviewing nine panel plots is recommended as this helps to identify normal and abnormal patterns and aids in interpretation of the physiological response to exercise.

Is this a maximal effort test and can a limiting system be identified?

It is important to know why the patient stopped the test and whether the patient achieved "maximal effort" as this is relevant to the validity of the values such as VO_2 peak. Most patients will stop the test due to leg fatigue, generalised fatigue or breathlessness. Variables will help determine if maximal effort was achieved are peak *HR*, peak *WR, peak respiratory rate* and *RER* prior to stopping exercise. In some cases, the operator will need to terminate the test due to ST changes seen on ECG or a drop in systolic BP > 20 mmHg.

The maximal predicted heart rate is calculated as 220 bpm – age. Achieving within 80–90% of predicted *HR* and predicted peak *WR* helps to ascertain a maximal effort test. However, it is important to consider medications that could cause a reduction in peak heart rate. *RER* is a breath by breath ratio of VCO_2/VO_2 and is displayed on panel 8. A value of < 1.15 at peak exercise suggests the patient did not achieve maximal effort. The maximum voluntary ventilation (MVV) is calculated as 40 times the FEV1. Comparing the peak minute ventilation with the MVV gives an indication of whether the patient was close to their maximal respiratory capacity and therefore a maximal effort test. This can be seen in panel 7 or by looking at the breathing reserve (BR) in the summary page. If the BR is less than 20% of MVV or < 11L/min at peak exercise, there is considered to be a ventilatory limitation to exercise.

What is the exercise capacity? (panel 3)

The VO_2 peak is the highest VO_2 achieved, this is normally when exercise is terminated. It is measured in ml/min but usually indexed to the patient's weight. Commonly liver failure patients will have a peak VO_2 which falls well below their predicted value [10]. Care should be taken when interpreting the indexed VO_2 value in extremes of weight.

Is the $\Delta VO_2/\Delta WR$ slope normal? (panel 3)

The slope of $VO_{2,}$ as a function of work rate increase, is normally 10.6 ml/min/W and is consistent across age, sex, weight and level of fitness [7]. Where VO_2 is plotted in panel 3, it is scaled in such a way that the VO_2 slope should be parallel to the *WR* increase. A reduced gradient or sudden blunting of the VO_2 slope implies a significant cardiovascular abnormality, typically heart failure or ischaemic heart disease [7] (Fig. 7.4). In cases where the VO_2 slope is reduced an oxygen debt is accumulating, thus in recovery it may be noted that the VO_2 returns more slowly to resting values.

Can AT be determined and what is VO_2 at AT? (panel 5 and 6)

AT is most reliably determined on panel 5, where there is a change in the gradient of the slope of VCO_2 vs VO_2. When anaerobic respiration occurs, the VCO_2 will increase disproportionality in relation to VO_2, causing a steepening of this relationship. AT can also be seen in panel 6, at the point where VE/VO_2 begins a steady increase and VE/VCO_2 continues to decrease or is constant. This is due to *VE* increasing disproportionately to VO_2 but remaining in proportion to VCO_2.

The VO_2 at AT can be assessed as an absolute value, an indexed value or as a percentage of predicted peak VO_2. The AT is normally 40–60% of the predicted or actual peak VO_2. Higher AT values reflect better cardiopulmonary conditioning. If peak VO_2 is reduced there is usually a proportional decrease in AT.

In liver failure and HPB patients, the AT is often low due to deconditioning or diseased states, [11–13] (Figs. 7.5 and 7.6) which will be discussed later.

Is there a normal *HR* response? (panel 2)

Heart rate normally increases linearly with increasing work rate but often with little change at very low work rates. The trajectory of *HR* and with VO_2 on panel 5 should track towards the cross point of the two predicted values. This may help in the assessment of chronotropic response and effort. Immediately after cessation of exercise, a reduction in heart rate of 15–25 bpm should be seen with values < 12 bpm considered abnormal. Heart rate may increase by a factor of 2–3 fold while stroke volume typically increases by 50% at peak. Therefore even small reductions in heart rate by drugs may significantly inhibit cardiac output increase in response to stress [14].

A substantially reduced *HR* response is common in liver patients and is seen on CPET as the presence of a large heart rate reserve at peak (Figs. 7.5 and 7.6) for two main reasons: (1) Beta-blockers are used in patients with portal hypertension awaiting LT and (2) autonomic neuropathy is common in patients with end-stage liver disease.

Does the O_2 pulse increase with *WR*? (panel 2)

O_2 pulse (VO_2/HR) is the product of stroke volume (SV) and arteriovenous O_2 difference $C(a\text{-}v)\ O_2$. This can be understood from a re-arrangement of the Fick equation:

$$VO_2 = Cardiac\ Output\ x\ C(a-v)O_2 \ \rightarrow\ VO_2/HR = SV\ x\ C(a-v)\ O_2$$

O_2 pulse is displayed with *HR* in panel 2. O_2 pulse normally increases but with a gradually decreasing rate to the predicted normal value. O_2 pulse fails to increase

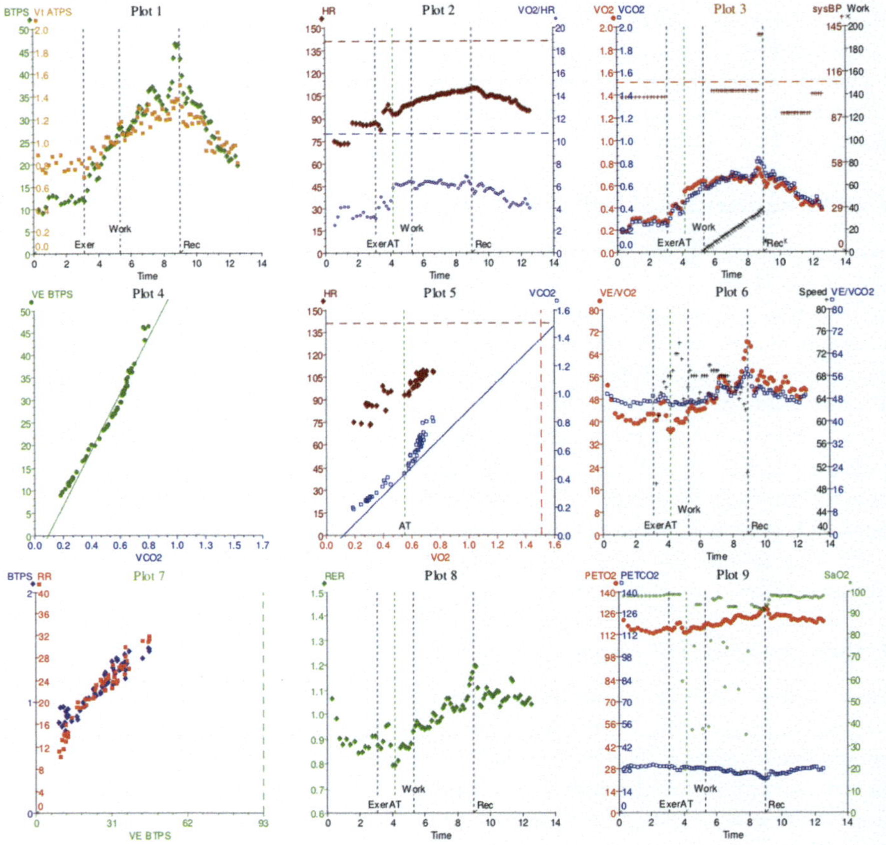

Fig. 7.4 79 year old male for elective Whipples. History of IHD with previous CABG, Diabetic on Insulin, Chronic kidney disease stage 3. Normal pre-test spirometry. Maximal effort test, patient stopped due to leg fatigue. Peak VO_2 was 9.5 ml/min/kg (52% predicted) with AT of 6.7 ml/min/kg. Poor chronotropic response, the VO_2 pulse is low and plateaus early and the VO_2/WR slope is reduced. The ventilatory equivalents for CO_2 are raised, VE/VCO_2 at AT is 46 and slope is 54. **This suggests a cardiac limitation for reduced exercise capacity and high risk of post-operative cardiopulmonary complications**

normally in patients with ischemic heart disease or cardiac failure where increase in stroke volume is impaired (Figs. 7.4 and 7.7). It can also be reduced where $C(a\text{-}v)\ O_2$ is reduced, as in anaemia, which is commonly seen in the liver cirrhosis and HPB patients. Here the $C(a\text{-}v)O_2$ reduction is due to decreased CaO_2, which is offset by a compensatory increase in cardiac output, primarily from *HR* increase. The raised *HR* at rest however leaves less reserve for peak exercise. A precipitous drop in haemoglobin can also occur silently in this group of patients and be the cause for a reduction in exercise capacity in this patient group, it is therefore essential to have a current haemoglobin level prior to the test.

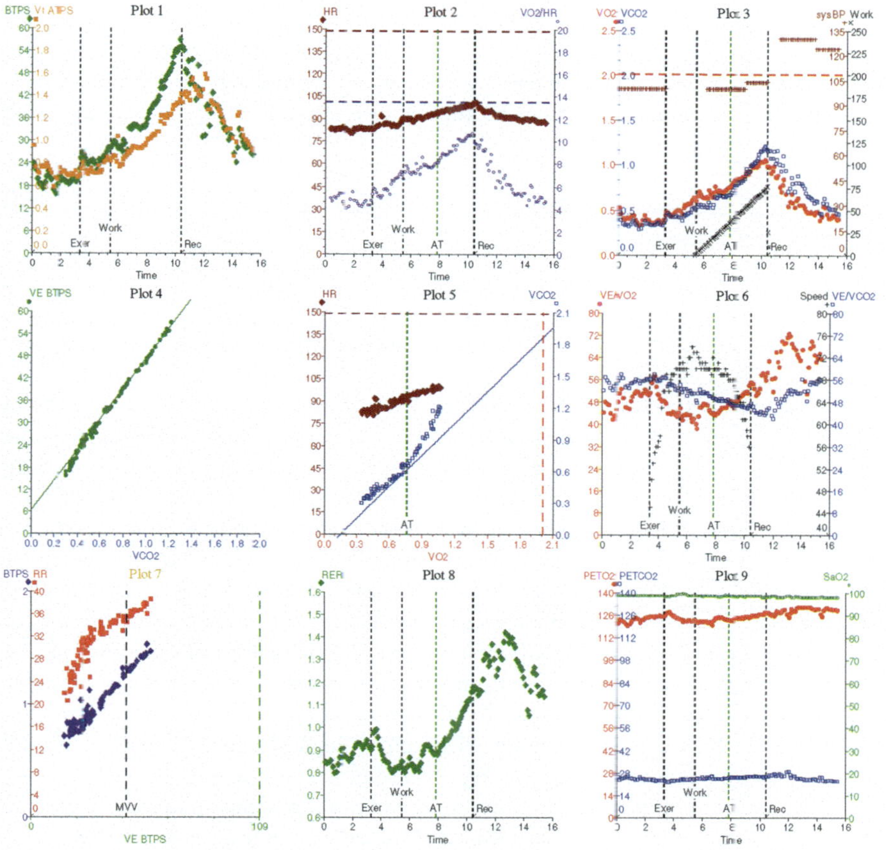

Fig. 7.5 72-year-old for liver transplant assessment. This is maximal effort test, patient stopped due to shortness of breath. Pre-test spirometry values are FEV1 1.14 (37% predicted), FEV 1.79 (44% predicted). Peak VO_2 achieved was 10 ml/min/kg (53% of predicted) with AT of 7.2 ml/min/kg. There is a poor chronotropic response as heart rate fails to increase above 100 bpm. VO_2 pulse is reduced due to a reduction in VO_2. The cause of limitation is respiratory as patient has reached and gone beyond his MVV (plot 7). There is evidence of chronic hyperventilation throughout the test and VE/VCO_2 at AT is significantly raised above 40, which in view of his respiratory limitation is the likely cause of raised ventilatory equivalents. **This demonstrates a poor status liver failure patient**

Is there any ventilatory limitation? (panel 7)

Tidal volume is plotted as a function of minute ventilation (*VE*) on panel 7. At low intensity exercise, tidal volume increases preferentially to respiratory rate. Further into the test as tidal volume reaches a maximal value the respiratory rate is the primary variable to increase *VE*. At peak exercise there is normally a breathing reserve of 10–15 L/min or 20% of the maximal voluntary ventilation (MVV). Breathing reserve is calculated as the difference between the maximal MVV and VE at peak exercise. The MVV is predicted as $40 \times$ FEV1 and may be shown as a vertical dashed line on panel 7. Peak *VE* is normally < 80% of MVV, where *VE* encroaches towards the predicted MVV, this is suggestive of respiratory limitation (Fig. 7.5). Peak respiratory rate usually reaches a maximal value of around 40–42 breaths/minute although this may be higher in restrictive lung disease and with tachypnoeic respiratory patterns.

Is there a limitation in ventilation perfusion matching or ventilatory efficiency (panel 4 and 6)

Ventilatory efficiency is represented using the ratio of minute ventilation (*VE*) to VCO_2 and VO_2. This gives the derived value known as the ventilatory equivalent for associated gas, VE/VCO_2 and VE/VO_2 respectively, which is plotted against time in panel 6.

The normal pattern of VE/VO_2 and VE/VCO_2 during exercise shows an initial decrease in both with increasing workload, as ventilation and perfusion become more efficient with exercise due to recruitment of pulmonary vessels and lung units as well as a relative decrease in dead space. Once AT is reached, VE/VO_2 increases as lung units hyperventilate with respect to O_2 due to the increased CO_2 production from anaerobic respiration and thus efficiency relative to oxygen worsens. The VE/VCO_2 ratio however continues to decrease as *VE* is proportional to VCO_2. However, as the buffering capacity for increased CO_2 is utilised blood lactate levels rise and blood pH will decrease causing activation of chemoreceptors. This is the point where respiratory compensation occurs and ventilation increases with respect to VCO_2, and a rise in VE/VCO_2 is seen.

The VE/VCO_2 value is increased when physiological dead space is increased and $PaCO_2$ is decreased (e.g.: acute hyperventilation). Ventilatory equivalents give an indication of the efficiency of ventilation and perfusion matching, and therefore of gas exchange. When values are raised it indicates either an issue with ventilation perfusion matching such as heart failure, respiratory disease such as chronic obstructive pulmonary disease, pulmonary thromboembolic disease or pulmonary hypertension, or it represents an inefficient use of the alveoli capillary interface secondary to hyperventilation or hypoventilation.

In panel 4, minute ventilation (*VE*) is plotted as a function of VCO_2. *VE* normally increases linearly with VCO_2 at a slope of 23 to 28. At the respiratory compensation point, around 80% of peak, the slope increases. Where the slope of the initial part of the plot has an increased gradient, this represents ventilation perfusion mismatch [2] (Figs. 7.4, 7.7 and 7.8).

Evidence Base for Risk Prediction of Mortality and Morbidity

Accurate prediction of perioperative risk is important for guiding meaningful informed consent and clinical decision making in the perioperative period. Risk assessment is multifactorial and complex although numerous scoring systems have

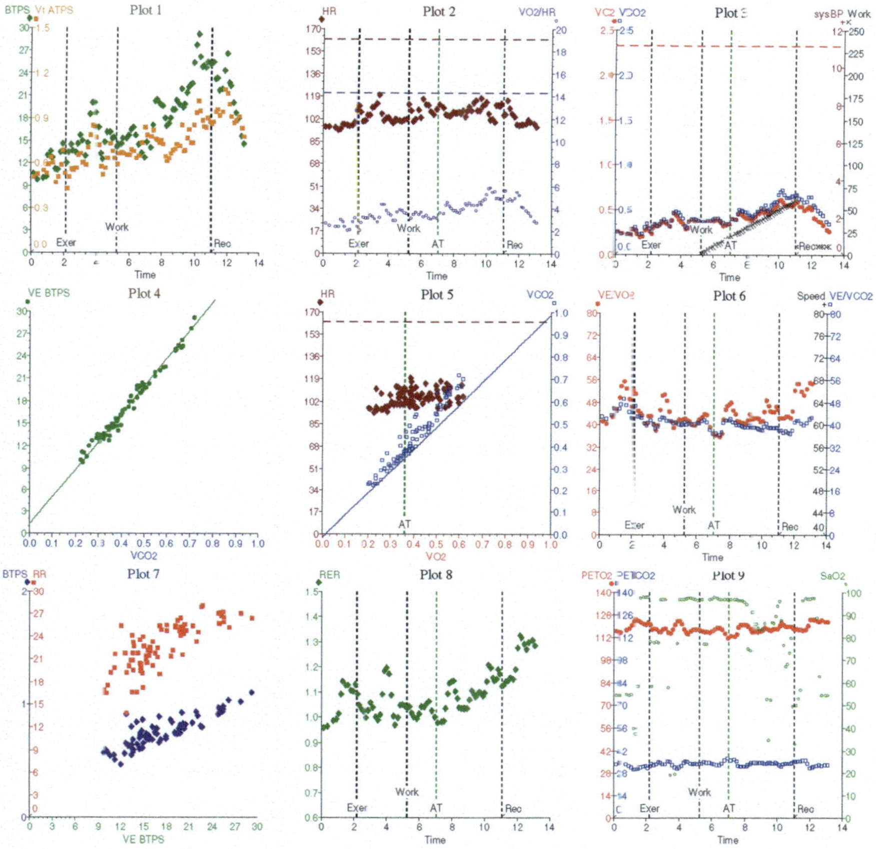

Fig. 7.6 **58-year-old for liver transplant assessment**. This is maximal effort test, patient stopped due leg fatigue. Normal pre-test spirometry. Peak VO_2 achieved was 7.4 ml/min/kg (28% of predicted) with AT of 4.1 ml/min/kg. There is a poor chronotropic response, with a resting tachycardia of 110 bpm. VO_2 pulse is reduced and unchanging due to a reduction in VO_2. **This demonstrates a poor status liver failure patient**

been developed to quantify and predict risk [15]. These tools place patients on a scale, they do not provide information on individualised risk prediction of adverse outcome and scoring can be dependent on subjective variables [16].

For Liver transplant specifically, the Model of End-stage Liver Disease (MELD) score has revolutionised the prognostication in liver transplant patients, [17] but it still underestimates post-transplant mortality [18]. Factors used in prediction of post-transplant mortality include; indication for liver transplant, centre activity, donor characteristics and graft quality and type [19].

CPET has been shown to have the capacity to identify high risk patients in a number of surgical groups [20]. The optimal CPET derived variables differs between surgery types, for example AT has been shown to be the best predictor

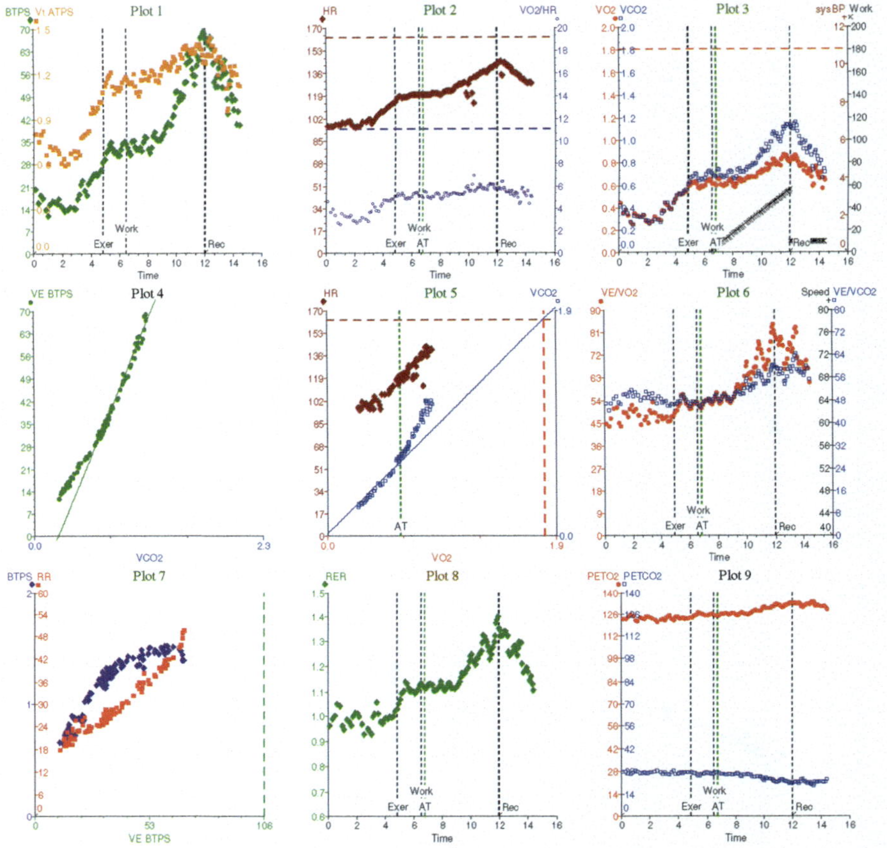

Fig. 7.7 57 year-old assessment for liver transplant. This is a maximal effort test. Normal pre-test spirometry. Pre-test echo: right ventricular pressures 40–50 mmHg, moderate tricuspid regurgitation, left ventricular ejection fraction > 54%. Peak VO_2 achieved was 12.4 ml/min/kg (49% predicted), with AT 8.5 ml/min/kg, occurring just after commencement of the loaded phase. Heart rate response was 85% of predicted. VO_2/WR gradient is reduced and VO_2 pulse is low and unchanging, with an early plateau. $PETCO_2$ is reduced at the start and continues to decrease during exercise. VE/VCO_2 is raised throughout the test, with significantly elevated values at AT (46), along with a markedly increased VE/VCO_2 gradient (72). **These features are suggestive of significant ventilatory perfusion mismatching, consistent with a diagnosis of pulmonary hypertension**

of high-risk patients in intrabdominal surgery, [21] whereas VE/VCO_2 values are more predictive in patients undergoing abdominal aortic aneurysm repair [22]. In addition to providing individualised objective data on a patient's functional capacity, CPET outperforms several commonly used risk prediction tools [20]. However, risk prediction using CPET derived variables should always be evaluated in the context of the whole clinical picture.

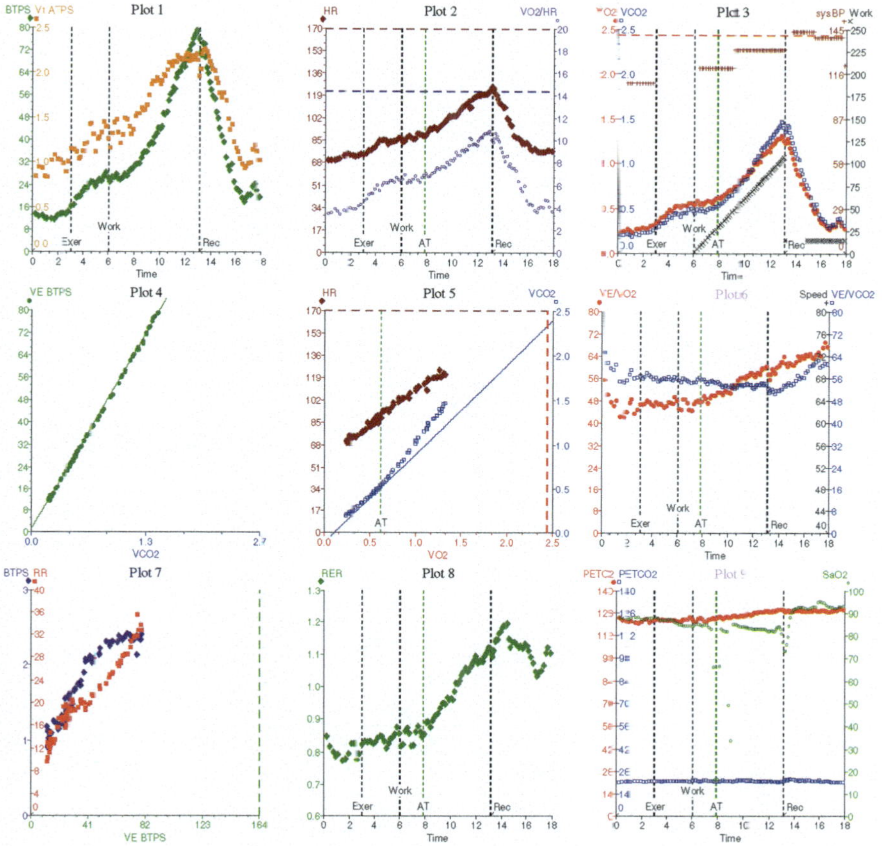

Fig. 7.8 50-year-old assessment for liver transplant. This is a maximal effort test. Pre-test spirometry FEV1 2.43 (63% predicted), FEV 3.76 (75% predicted). Peak VO_2 achieved was 17.5 ml/min/kg (55% of predicted), with AT 8.2 ml/min/kg. There is a reduced heart rate response, VO_2/WR slope is normal, with the VO_2 pulse a normal shape but reduced peak. $PETCO_2$ is low and unchanging throughout the test, suggesting chronic hyperventilation. The VE/VCO_2 is raised throughout, and a value of 53 at AT is profoundly elevated, raised VE/VCO_2 slope and low resting SpO_2 with decreasing values to below 80% during exercise **This patient went on to be diagnosed with hepatopulmonary syndrome**

Given that post-operative morbidity is dependent on multiple, often unrelated factors, CPET alone is unable to completely stratify perioperative risk The use of CPET variables in conjunction with validated risk scoring systems or biomarkers has been suggested to improve accuracy of risk prediction [23].

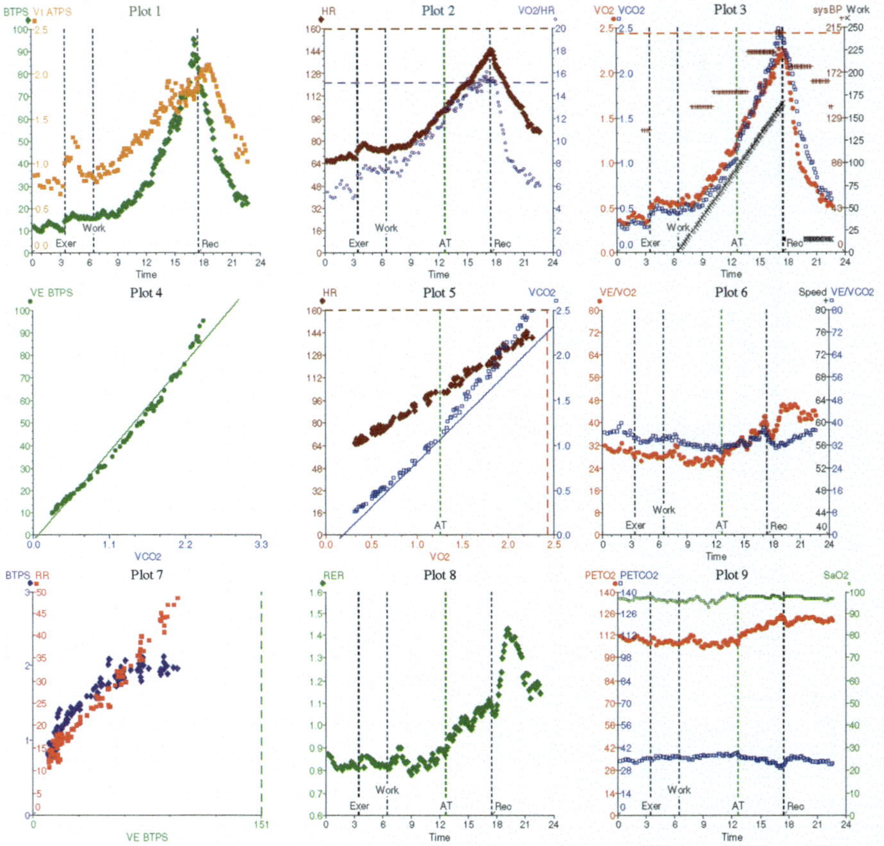

Fig. 7.9 60-year-old for liver transplant assessment. Same patient as Fig. 7.6, 2 years later following training and exercise. This is a maximal effort test, peak VO_2 23 ml/min/kg (93% of predicted) with AT of 13.2 ml/min/kg. Normal heart rate response, VO_2/WR and *O2* pulse slopes are normal, with normal ventilatory equivalents. **This illustrates an improvement in functional and aerobic capacity with training**

Liver Transplant surgery

Patients listed for liver transplant have significantly reduced exercise capacity due to a combination of cardiovascular and skeletal muscle dysfunction. This is seen in a reduced peak VO_2 and has been demonstrated in all trials relating to CPET and liver transplant patients [24–29]. Mean peak VO_2 across studies was 17.4 ml/min/kg, which is equivalent to that of a sedentary female in her seventies or eighties [11].

Authors have demonstrated a negative correlation between low peak VO_2 scores and higher MELD scores of > 17, [26, 29, 30] with lower peak VO_2 scores being a significant predictor of reduced one-year survival in those awaiting liver transplantation [29, 30]. Predictors of 1-year post-transplant mortality included severe impairment of aerobic capacity, defined as peak $VO_2 < 60\%$, [9, 24, 25] with a low AT value being more predictive than peak VO_2 [24, 26, 27]. These variables were also predictive of a significantly longer hospital stay [25–27, 29, 30]. Only one study found a low peak $VO_2 < 13.4$ ml/min/kg was associated with increased length of stay in the intensive care unit [26].

As different CEPT parameters and cut off values have been used between studies, optimal thresholds to predict pre- and post-transplant mortality are unavailable [11]. Additionally advances in surgical technique, donor characteristics, and variability of graft quality makes comparison of CPET data with mortality and survival data difficult [19].

More recently peak workload achieved as an indexed value (to body weight) has been investigated in our institution and has been found to give a better prediction of length of hospital stay compared with AT. This has been achieved by incorporating peak workload index into an analysis model of gender, MELD score and plasma sodium at time of LT [31]. Additionally, a small study investigating total work load achieved has been found to be an indepencent predictor of 1 year survival after LT [32].

Hepatic Resection surgery

In liver surgery, AT has been found to be the optimal predictor of outcome. A cut off value for AT of < 9 ml/min/kg has been predictive of short term (< 90 days) mortality and an AT of less than 11.5 ml/min/kg is predictive of long-term (3 year) mortality in hepatic resection surgery [33]. Admission to intensive care or coronary care is correlated with an AT of < 9.9 ml/min/kg and $VE/VCO_2 > 34.5$ at AT was predictive of postoperative cardiopulmonary complications in this patient group [12]. The use of peak VO_2 to predict length of stay and ICU admission is not as strong, so cut off values are not used [12, 13].

Pancreatic surgery

Studies investigating pancreatic surgery found that an AT < 10 ml/min/kg was associated with a higher risk of pancreatic fistula, formation, abdominal collections or the development of other surgical postoperative complications [33–35]. These studies found AT < 10 ml/min/kg was associated with increased length of hospital stay due to increased rate of post-operative complications [36]. In a UK cohort study of high-risk patients undergoing pancreatic cancer surgery, AT was not found to be predictive of mortality. Instead a VE/VCO_2 value at AT > 41 was associated with increased morbidity from post-operative surgical complications including pancreatic fistula, delayed gastric emptying and or haemorrhage within 30 postoperative days [37].

Pre-operative Optimisation

Poor physical fitness measured by CPET, reflects a poor physiological reserve and as discussed above can be predictive of a complicated post-operative period. Prehabilitation is defined as the "process of enhancing the functional capacity of the individual to enable him or her to withstand a stressful event" [38]. The goal of prehabilitation is to accelerate post-operative recovery and enhance physiological reserve through physical intervention.

Patients undergoing major surgery have been shown to have improvements in measures of physical fitness (VO_2 peak, AT or peak work-rate) and health related quality of life outcomes [4, 39]. A reduction in post-operative complications, specifically pulmonary complications have been observed in patients undergoing intrabdominal surgery, [36] however drawing clear conclusions on mortality has been more difficult due to heterogenicity of trial designs in terms of outcomes measured and exercise prescription [5].

The cohort of patients awaiting HPB and transplant surgery may benefit from prehabilitation, as they tend to have features associated with frailty due to liver failure or malignancy, [40, 41] including cachexia, myopenia and sarcopenia which are associated with poor long-term outcomes [41]. Sarcopenia is a decline in muscle mass and physical performance which results in a reduction in aerobic capacity (the ability for muscles to consume oxygen during exercise) [10]. Features of frailty in patients awaiting LT have been associated with increased hospital admissions/length of hospital stay, and higher rates of pre and post LT mortality [27, 42, 43]. Other measures of frailty which elicit a decline in function (hand grip strength (HGS), timed repeated chair stands and balance), have been associated with increased risk of death and delisting whilst awaiting LT [44, 45].

Recognition and screening for frailty in liver failure patients using performance-based measures such as HGS and gait speed in a 5-metre walk test, are reproducible markers of performance status. These can be easily done in an outpatient setting and identify the most vulnerable end stage liver failure patients who would benefit from the intervention of a prehabiliation programme [43]. Moreover patients with reduced physical activity status post liver transplant are at greatest risk of suffering cardiopulmonary complications, [46] which is the leading cause of non-transplant related death in this patient group [47]. A small trial consisting of a 12 week programme of aerobic and strength training in patients awaiting a liver transplant, showed this is safe and feasible in this patient group, with improvements seen in peak VO_2 following training[48]. As liver transplant centres cover large geographic areas, it may be more acceptable and feasible to carry out home based training programmes [49]. A pilot trial investigating a home based exercise programme over 12 weeks for pre LT patients, involving functional resistance exercises and daily step targets showed improvements in functional capacity and frailty measures [49]. An example of how home based exercise and increased activity can improve functional capacity is shown in Figs. 7.6 and 7.9.

Prehabilitation trials on cancer patients awaiting surgery have included a range of physical interventions including strength and or aerobic training. A four week supervised high intensity exercise programme involving patients listed for hepatic resection showed improvements in AT, peak VO_2 and peak work load achieved [6]. Other training intervention targets have included; training at intensities within 40-85% of maximal heart rate, continuous exercise at 60–65% of peak VO_2, and interval training at 100% of peak VO_2 for 30 seconds with a 60 second rest [39]. The exercise programmes ranged from 2 to 6 weeks duration, delivered using a range of modalities including cycle, jogging or step count [5]. A consensus on optimal timings and outcome measures have yet to be agreed as outcome data from clinically powered trials is awaited [5].

Post-operative Resource Allocation

Older's 1993 seminal study illustrated the utility of a low anaerobic threshold or the presence of ischaemia on CPET as being highly predictive for mortality [50]. Older and colleagues suggested that CPET variables could be used to plan peri-operative care and resource allocation in high risk patients undergoing major abdominal surgery. In 1999 Older selected 548 patients who were having major surgery and were either over 60 years or < 60 years but with evidence of cardio-pulmonary disease. Those patients who achieved an AT < 11 ml/min/kg or underwent an aortic or oesophageal surgical procedure were admitted post-operatively to ICU. Patients who demonstrated an AT > 11 ml/min/kg but showed evidence of ischemia (on CPET) or had a $VE/VCO_2 > 35$ were admitted to HDU. All other patients received ward-based care postoperatively. The 30-day mortality rates were 7.8% (ICU), 3.5% (HDU) and 0.4% (ward) [51]. This was evidence that CPET could be used to identify those patients most at risk and to aid in the correct allocation of resources.

Guidelines for the use of CPET in assessment of preoperative patients were initially based on the above findings and are now regularly updated [52] and are designed to aid clinicians in deciding on risk categories. CPET variables indicating high risk include AT < 11 ml/min/kg, VE/VCO_2 slope ≥ 35.0, peak $VO_2 < 10$ ml/min/kg, drop in systolic blood pressure during exercise and ischemia seen on ECG during the test [52].

Interpreting CPET in Patients with Liver Failure Awaiting LT

The pathological processes in liver failure and frailty often cause a greatly reduced exercise capacity due to a combination of cardiovascular and skeletal muscle dysfunction [10]. This is seen as low peak VO_2 values, a proportionate decrease in the AT value [29] and a decreased maximal workload [32]. Poor nutritional status and reduced muscle mass resulting in deconditioning means these patients will often exhibit early cessation of exercise and hyperventilation at low workloads with high ventilatory and heart rate reserves [53]. Hyperventilation is well documented in liver failure patients, this may be due to respiratory compensation from a metabolic acidosis or secondary to reduced lung compliance and basal atelectasis from large volume ascites, or pulmonary effusions [10]. At rest these patients will have a hyperdynamic circulation and may already be at or close to their compensation point, with high resting heart rates. When stressed with exercise, their stroke volume is not able to increase appropriately. From the Fick equation discussed earlier we know that O_2 pulse (VO_2/HR) can give an indication of stroke volume. The low unchanging O_2 pulse seen in some liver failure patients in response to exercise can be an indication of an inadequate stroke volume response or a lack of incrementing oxygen extraction [10].

Cirrhotic cardiomyopathy can occur in liver failure patients, the main features being a blunted contractile response to stress and impaired diastolic relaxation [10]. Most patients with this condition will stop exercise before their heart rate reaches the predicted peak [54]. However, autonomic neuropathy seen in cirrhosis [55] or beta blocker therapy [14] may be an alternative cause for a large heart rate reserve.

In patients with significant ascites, there is a higher VO_2 during unloaded exercise due to the increased work of leg movement against the abdominal weight. High values of VE/VCO_2 slope may be seen secondary to a restrictive pattern of ventilation and basal atelectasis caused by ascites or pleural effusions. Therefore, in our institution significant volume ascites will be drained 1–2 days prior to CPET testing.

Another significant cause of ventilation perfusion mismatch is seen in hepatopulmonary syndrome (HPS). When significant, HPS can cause hypoxemia at rest [56]. When less obvious, HPS can be noticed during CPET testing as raised VE/VCO_2 levels throughout the test and profoundly elevated values of VE/VCO_2 at AT. In addition, exercise may increase intrapulmonary shunting and lead to desaturation in patients with HPS [10] (Fig. 7.8).

Pulmonary hypertension, which is identified on transthoracic echo and quantified on right heart catheterisation, is routinely screened for in liver assessment work up as it is associated with high morbidity and mortality rates if untreated [57]. This can be identified on CPET with high unchanging VE/VCO_2 values, a low VO_2/WR slope, reduced VO_2 pulse, a low and decreasing end tidal CO_2 during exercise and desaturation during exercise (Fig. 7.7).

Interpreting CPET in HPB Patients

Some patients coming for HPB surgery may be deconditioned following neoadjuvant chemotherapy and have a poor nutritional status with associated muscle wasting by the time they come for their procedure. Features of deconditioning described above can also be seen in this patient group.

These patients may have evidence of neoadjuvant induced cardiomyopathy which can be seen as a cardiac limitation on CPET testing. Significant findings relating to cardiac limitation that are seen on CPET include: ECG changes on exercise, drop in systolic blood pressure > 20 mmHg or no rise in BP with exercise, a reduced VO_2/WR slope and low peak VO_2 and AT values (Fig. 7.4).

Practical Use of CPET at King's College Hospital

In our institution CPET is used along with several other investigations to help assess suitability for LT and HPB surgery. The results and assessments are collectively reviewed by the liver multidisciplinary team (MDT). Although CPET gives a useful functional assessment of a patient's exercise capacity there are several reasons why a patient may perform poorly on the test e.g.: large volume ascites, precipitous drop in Hb, concurrent infection, unfamiliarity with cycling etc. These factors are taken into consideration along with other investigations and a clinical review to give a global assessment of a patient's functional status and peri operative risk.

Summary

CPET is a dynamic objective test giving a global assessment of a patient's cardiovascular, respiratory and metabolic systems and demonstrates how the body copes with increased oxygen requirements. Quantifying a patient's oxygen uptake under physiological stress can help to predict the ability to meet the increased oxygen demands following major surgery.

Recorded and derived variables are displayed graphically on a classical Wasserman's nine panel plot, which can be grouped into graphs which display information on cardiovascular, respiratory, metabolic and ventilatory perfusion relationships. Using a systematic approach to assess the nine panels helps to interpret normal from abnormal and determine a patient's exercise capacity and cause of limitation.

CPET testing can be useful in quantifying patient risk which plays an important role in informed consent and clinical decision making. This must be done by incorporating exercise capacity into a comprehensive assessment of the patient in combination with other indicators such as cardiovascular risk factors. Liver failure patients and cancer patients awaiting hepatobiliary surgery will often show a reduced exercise capacity due to the multisystem disease process. This is illustrated in characteristic changes seen on CPET testing.

The theory that an objective test demonstrating low functional reserve can predict poor outcome following the major stressors of transplant or cancer surgery is appealing. However, it is unlikely that a single CPET derived variable can predict outcome in what is a hugely complex physiological process [58]. There is growing evidence to suggest certain CPET variables can be used to help predict length of intrahospital stay, morbidity and mortality in LT, pancreatic surgery and hepatic resection surgery. Although this can help guide MDT decisions, preoperative optimisation and post-operative resource allocation, more evidence is required from large multicentre trials evaluating CPET and surgical outcome data. From this a more effective predictor of risk might be developed incorporating CPET variables with other indicators of cardiopulmonary risk.

References

1. Prentis J, Snowden C. A role of cardiopulmonary exercise testing (CPET) in defining cardiopulmonary function before liver transplantation. Cardiovascular diseases and liver transplantation, 1st ed. edn. New York: Nova Biomedical Books; 2011.
2. Levett DZH, Jack S, Swart M, Carlisle J, Wilson J, Snowden C, Riley M, Danjoux G, Ward SA, Older P, Grocott MPW, Perioperative Exercise T, Training S. Perioperative cardiopulmonary exercise testing (CPET): consensus clinical guidelines on indications, organization, conduct, and physiological interpretation. Br J Anaesth. 2018;120(3):484–500. https://doi.org/10.1016/j.bja.2017.10.020.
3. Older P, Hall A. Cardiopulmonary exercise testing in preoperative risk assessment and patient management. BJA Br J Anaesthes. 2017;119(4):837–8. https://doi.org/10.1093/bja/aex313.
4. Levett DZ, Grocott MP. Cardiopulmonary exercise testing, prehabilitation, and enhanced recovery after surgery (ERAS). Can J Anaesthes. 2015;62(2):131–42. https://doi.org/10.1007/s12630-014-0307-6.
5. Hijazi Y, Gondal U, Aziz O. A systematic review of prehabilitation programs in abdominal cancer surgery. Int J Surg. 2017;39:156–62. https://doi.org/10.1016/j.ijsu.2017.01.111.
6. Dunne DFJ, Jack S, Jones RP, Jones L, Lythgoe DT, Malik HZ, Poston GJ, Palmer DH, Fenwick SW. Randomized clinical trial of prehabilitation before planned liver resection. BJS. 2016;103(5):504–12. https://doi.org/10.1002/bjs.10096.
7. Wasserman KH, Sue JE, Stringer DY, Sietsema WW, Sun KE, Whipp BJ. Principles of exercise testing and interpretation: including pathophysiology and clinical applications, 5th edn. Lippincott Williams & Wilkins (LWW); 2011.
8. Myers J, Arena R, Franklin B, Pina I, Kraus WE, McInnis K, Balady GJ, Cardiology CC, Nursing CC. Recommendations for clinical exercise laboratories a scientific statement from the American heart association. Circulation. 2009;119(24):3144–61. https://doi.org/10.1161/Circulationaha.109.192520.
9. Balady GJ, Arena R, Sietsema K, Myers J, Coke L, Fletcher GF, Forman D, Franklin B, Guazzi M, Gulati M, Keteyian SJ, Lavie CJ, Macko R, Mancini D, Milani RV, Cardiac AHAE, Prevention CE, Dis CPV, Quality IC. Clinician's guide to cardiopulmonary exercise testing in adults a scientific statement from the American heart association. Circulation. 2010;122(2):191–225. https://doi.org/10.1161/CIR.0b013e3181e52e69.
10. Lemyze M, Dharancy S, Wallaert B. Response to exercise in patients with liver cirrhosis: implications for liver transplantation. Dig Liver Dis. 2013;45(5):362–6. https://doi.org/10.1016/j.dld.2012.09.022.
11. Ney M, Haykowsky MJ, Vandermeer B, Shah A, Ow M, Tandon P. Systematic review: pre- and post-operative prognostic value of cardiopulmonary exercise testing in liver transplant candidates. Aliment Pharmacol Ther. 2016;44(8):796–806. https://doi.org/10.1111/apt.13771.

12. Junejo MA, Mason JM, Sheen AJ, Moore J, Foster P, Atkinson D, Parker MJ, Siriwardena AK. Cardiopulmonary exercise testing for preoperative risk assessment before hepatic resection. BJS. 2012;99(8):1097–104. https://doi.org/10.1002/bjs.8773.
13. Dunne DFJ, Jones RP, Lythgoe DT, Pilkington FJ, Palmer DH, Malik HZ, Poston GJ, Lacasia C, Jack S, Fenwick SW. Cardiopulmonary exercise testing before liver surgery. J Surg Oncol. 2014;110(4):439–44. https://doi.org/10.1002/jso.23670.
14. Wallen MP, Hall A, Dias KA, Ramos JS, Keating SE, Woodward AJ, Skinner TL, Macdonald GA, Arena R, Coombes JS. Impact of beta-blockers on cardiopulmonary exercise testing in patients with advanced liver disease. Aliment Pharmacol Ther. 2017;46(8):741–7. https://doi.org/10.1111/apt.14265.
15. Lee TH, Marcantonio ER, Mangione CM, Thomas EJ, Polanczyk CA, Cook EF, Sugarbaker DJ, Donaldson MC, Poss R, Ho KKL, Ludwig LE, Pedan A, Goldman L. Derivation and prospective validation of a simple index for prediction of cardiac risk of major noncardiac surgery. Circulation. 1999;100(10):1043–9. https://doi.org/10.1161/01.CIR.100.10.1043.
16. Moonesinghe SR, Mythen MG, Das P, Rowan KM, Grocott MPW. Risk stratification tools for predicting morbidity and mortality in adult patients undergoing major surgery: qualitative systematic review. Anesthesiol J Am Soc Anesthesiolog. 2013;119(4):959–81. https://doi.org/10.1097/aln.0b013e3182a4e94d.
17. Brown RS Jr, Lake JR. The survival impact of liver transplantation in the MELD Era, and the future for organ allocation and distribution. Am J Transplant. 2005;5(2):203–4. https://doi.org/10.1111/j.1600-6143.2005.00769.x.
18. Bambha KM, Biggins SW. Inequities of the model for end-stage liver disease: an examination of current components and future additions. Curr Opin Organ Transplant. 2008;13(3):227–33. https://doi.org/10.1097/MOT.0b013e3282ff84c7.
19. Adam R, Karam V, Cailliez VO, Grady JG, Mirza D, Cherqui D, Klempnauer J, Salizzoni M, Pratschke J, Jamieson N, Hidalgo E, Paul A, Andujar RL, Lerut J, Fisher L, Boudjema K, Fondevila C, Soubrane O, Bachellier P, Pinna AD, Berlakovich G, Bennet W, Pinzani M, Schemmer P, Zieniewicz K, Romero CJ, De Simone P, Ericzon B-G, Schneeberger S, Wigmore SJ, Prous JF, Colledan M, Porte RJ, Yilmaz S, Azoulay D, Pirenne J, Line P-D, Trunecka P, Navarro F, Lopez AV, De Carlis L, Pena SR, Kochs E, Duvoux C, centers atoc, Liver tE, Association IT. 2018 annual report of the european liver transplant registry (ELTR)—50-year evolution of liver transplantation. Transplant Int. 2018;31(12):1293–1317. https://doi.org/10.1111/tri.13358.
20. Hennis PJ, Meale PM, Grocott MPW. Cardiopulmonary exercise testing for the evaluation of perioperative risk in non-cardiopulmonary surgery. Postgrad Med J. 2011;87(1030):550–7. https://doi.org/10.1136/pgmj.2010.107185.
21. Moran J, Wilson F, Guinan E, McCormick P, Hussey J, Moriarty J. Role of cardiopulmonary exercise testing as a risk-assessment method in patients undergoing intra-abdominal surgery: a systematic review. Br J Anaesth. 2016;116(2):177–91. https://doi.org/10.1093/bja/aev454.
22. Carlisle J, Swart M. Mid-term survival after abdominal aortic aneurysm surgery predicted by cardiopulmonary exercise testing. Br J surg. 2007;94(8):966–9. https://doi.org/10.1002/bjs.5734.
23. James S, Jhanji S, Smith A, O'Brien G, Fitzgibbon M, Pearse RM. Comparison of the prognostic accuracy of scoring systems, cardiopulmonary exercise testing, and plasma biomarkers: a single-centre observational pilot study. Br J Anaesth. 2014;112(3):491–7. https://doi.org/10.1093/bja/aet346.
24. Epstein SK, Freeman RB, Khayat A, Unterborn JN, Pratt DS, Kaplan MM. Aerobic capacity is associated with 100-day outcome after hepatic transplantation. Liver Transpl. 2004;10(3):418–24. https://doi.org/10.1002/lt.20088.

25. Neviere R, Edme JL, Montaigne D, Boleslawski E, Pruvot FR, Dharancy S. Prognostic implications of preoperative aerobic capacity and exercise oscillatory ventilation after liver transplantation. Am J Transplant. 2014;14(1):88–95. https://doi.org/10.1111/ajt.12502.
26. Bernal W, Martin-Mateos R, Lipcsey M, Tallis C, Woodsford K, Mcphail MJ, Willars C, Auzinger G, Sizer E, Heneghan M, Cottam S, Heaton N, Wendon J. Aerobic capacity during cardiopulmonary exercise testing and survival with and without liver transplantation for patients with chronic liver disease. Liver Transpl. 2014;20(1):54–62. https://doi.org/10.1002/lt.23766.
27. Prentis JM, Manas DMD, Trenell MI, Hudson M, Jones DJ, Snowden CP. Submaximal cardiopulmonary exercise testing predicts 90-day survival after liver transplantation. Liver Transpl. 2012;18(2):152–9. https://doi.org/10.1002/lt.22426.
28. Ow MMG, Erasmus P, Minto G, Struthers R, Joseph M, Smith A, Warshow UM, Cramp ME, Cross TJS. Impaired functional capacity in potential liver transplant candidates predicts short-term mortality before transplantation. Liver Transpl. 2014;20(9):1081–8. https://doi.org/10.1002/lt.23907.
29. Dharancy S, Lemyze M, Boleslawski E, Neviere R, Declerck N, Canva V, Wallaert B, Mathurin P, Pruvot FR. Impact of impaired aerobic capacity on liver transplant candidates. Transplantation. 2008;86(8):1077–83. https://doi.org/10.1097/TP.0b013e318187758b.
30. Mancuzo EV, Pereira RM, Sanches MD, Mancuzo AV. Pre-transplant aerobic capacity and prolonged hospitalization after liver transplantation. GE Port J Gastroenterol. 2015;22(3):87–92. https://doi.org/10.1016/j.jpge.2015.02.001.
31. Katyayani K, Taylor YWC, Nicholson C, Rigby A, Barber S, Sarma N, Milan Z. Peak workload index during cardiopulmonary exercise testing is better predictor of length of hospitalisation than anaerobic threshold in liver transplant patients. Kings College Hospital, Abstracts from the BJA Research Forum Dundee: London, UK; 2018.
32. O'Carroll JAA, Milan Z. Peak workload during cardiopulmonary exercise testing is a predictor of one year survival following liver transplantation. 2019.
33. Kumar R, Garcea G. Cardiopulmonary exercise testing in hepato-biliary & pancreas cancer surgery—a systematic review: are we any further than walking up a flight of stairs? Int J Surg. 2018;52:201–7. https://doi.org/10.1016/j.ijsu.2018.02.019.
34. Chandrabalan VV, McMillan DC, Carter R, Kinsella J, McKay CJ, Carter CR, Dickson EJ. Pre-operative cardiopulmonary exercise testing predicts adverse post-operative events and non-progression to adjuvant therapy after major pancreatic surgery. HPB (Oxford). 2013;15(11):899–907. https://doi.org/10.1111/hpb.12060.
35. Ausania F, Vallance AE, Manas DM, Prentis JM, Snowden CP, White SA, Charnley RM, French JJ, Jaques BC. Double bypass for inoperable pancreatic malignancy at laparotomy: postoperative complications and long-term outcome. Ann R Coll Surg Engl. 2012;94(8):563–8. https://doi.org/10.1308/003588412X13373405386934.
36. Moran J, Guinan E, McCormick P, Larkin J, Mockler D, Hussey J, Moriarty J, Wilson F. The ability of prehabilitation to influence postoperative outcome after intra-abdominal operation: a systematic review and meta-analysis. Surgery. 2016;160(5):1189–201. https://doi.org/10.1016/j.surg.2016.05.014.
37. Junejo MA, Mason JM, Sheen AJ, Bryan A, Moore J, Foster P, Atkinson D, Parker MJ, Siriwardena AK. Cardiopulmonary exercise testing for preoperative risk assessment before pancreaticoduodenectomy for cancer. Ann Surg Oncol. 2014;21(6):1929–36. https://doi.org/10.1245/s10434-014-3493-0.
38. Ditmyer MM, Topp R, Pifer M. Prehabilitation in preparation for orthopaedic surgery. Orthop Nurs. 2002;21(5):43–54.
39. O'Doherty AF, West M, Jack S, Grocott MPW. Preoperative aerobic exercise training in elective intra-cavity surgery: a systematic review. Br J Anaesth. 2013;110(5):679–89. https://doi.org/10.1093/bja/aes514.
40. Lai JC, Covinsky KE, Dodge JL, Boscardin WJ, Segev DL, Roberts JP, Feng S. Development of a novel frailty index to predict mortality in patients with end-stage liver

disease. Hepatology (Baltimore, MD). 2017;66(2):564–74. https://doi.org/10.1002/hep.29219.

41. Ryan AM, Power DG, Daly L, Cushen SJ, Ní Bhuachalla Ē, Prado CM. Cancer-associated malnutrition, cachexia and sarcopenia: the skeleton in the hospital closet 40 years later. Proc Nutr Soc. 2016;75(2):199–211. https://doi.org/10.1017/S002966511500419X.
42. Lai JC, Dodge JL, Sen S, Covinsky K, Feng S. Functional decline in patients with cirrhosis awaiting liver transplantation: results from the functional assessment in liver transplantation (FrAILT) study. Hepatology (Baltimore, MD). 2016;63(2):574–80. https://doi.org/10.1002/hep.28316.
43. Kulkarni SS, Chen H, Josbeno DA, Schmotzer A, Hughes C, Humar A, Sood P, Rachakonda V, Dunn MA, Tevar AD. Gait speed and grip strength are associated with dropping out of the liver transplant waiting list. Transplant Proc. 2019;51(3):794–7. https://doi.org/10.1016/j.transproceed.2019.01.030.
44. Kotarska K, Wunsch E, Jodko L, Raszeja-Wyszomirska J, Bania I, Lawniczak M, Bogdanos D, Kornacewicz-Jach Z, Milkiewicz P. Factors affecting exercise test performance in patients after liver transplantation. Hepat Mon. 2016;16(3):e34356–e34356. https://doi.org/10.5812/hepatmon.34356.
45. Lai JC, Feng S, Terrault NA, Lizaola B, Hayssen H, Covinsky K. Frailty predicts waitlist mortality in liver transplant candidates. Am J Transpl. 2014;14(8):1870–9. https://doi.org/10.1111/ajt.12762.
46. Tanikella R, Kawut SM, Brown RS Jr, Krowka MJ, Reinen J, Dinasarapu CR, Trotter JF, Roberts KE, Mohd MA, Arnett DK, Fallon MB. Health-related quality of life and survival in liver transplant candidates. Liver Transpl. 2010;16(2):238–45. https://doi.org/10.1002/lt.21984.
47. Pruthi J, Medkiff KA, Esrason KT, Donovan JA, Yoshida EM, Erb SR, Steinbrecher UP, Fong TL. Analysis of causes of death in liver transplant recipients who survived more than 3 years. Liver Transpl. 2001;7(9):811–5. https://doi.org/10.1053/jlts.2001.27084.
48. Debette-Gratien M, Tabouret T, Antonini M-T, Dalmay F, Carrier P, Legros R, Jacques J, Vincent F, Sautereau D, Samuel D, Loustaud-Ratti V. Personalized adapted physical activity before liver transplantation: acceptability and results. Transplantation. 2015;99(1):145–50. https://doi.org/10.1097/tp.0000000000000245.
49. Williams FR, Vallance A, Faulkner T, Towey J, Durman S, Kyte D, Elsharkawy AM, Perera T, Holt A, Ferguson J, Lord JM, Armstrong MJ. Home-based exercise in patients awaiting liver transplantation: a feasibility study. Liver Transpl. 2019;25(7):995–1006. https://doi.org/10.1002/lt.25442.
50. Older P, Smith R, Courtney P, Hone R. Preoperative evaluation of cardiac-failure and ischemia in elderly patients by cardiopulmonary exercise testing. Chest. 1993;104(3):701–4. https://doi.org/10.1378/chest.104.3.701.
51. Older P, Hall A, Hader R. Cardiopulmonary exercise testing as a screening test for perioperative management of major surgery in the elderly. Chest. 1999;116(2):355–62. https://doi.org/10.1378/chest.116.2.355.
52. Guazzi M, Arena R, Halle M, Piepoli MF, Myers J, Lavie CJ. 2016 focused update: clinical recommendations for cardiopulmonary exercise testing data assessment in specific patient populations. Circulation. 2016;133(24):e694–711. https://doi.org/10.1161/CIR.0000000000000406.
53. Lemyze M, Dharancy S, Neviere R, Wallaert B. Cardiopulmonary response to exercise in patients with liver cirrhosis and impaired pulmonary gas exchange. Respir Med. 2011;105(10):1550–6. https://doi.org/10.1016/j.rmed.2011.06.011.
54. Wong F, Girgrah N, Graba J, Allidina Y, Liu P, Blendis L. The cardiac response to exercise in cirrhosis. Gut. 2001;49(2):268. https://doi.org/10.1136/gut.49.2.268.
55. Zardi EM, Zardi DM, Chin D, Sonnino C, Dobrina A, Abbate A. Cirrhotic cardiomyopathy in the pre- and post-liver transplantation phase. J Cardiol. 2016;67(2):125–30. https://doi.org/10.1016/j.jjcc.2015.04.016.

56. Krowka MJ, Cortese DA. Hepatopulmonary syndrome: current concepts in diagnostic and therapeutic considerations. Chest. 1994;105(5):1528–37. https://doi.org/10.1378/chest.105.5.1528.
57. Cosarderelioglu C, Cosar AM, Gurakar M, Pustavoitau A, Russell SD, Dagher NN, Gurakar A. Portopulmonary hypertension and liver transplant: recent review of the literature. Exp Clin Transplant. 2016;14(2):113–20.
58. Findlay JY. Exercise for all? Liver Transpl. 2012;18(2):143–5. https://doi.org/10.1002/lt.22482.

Chapter 8
Anaesthesia for Liver Transplantation

Lavinia Brezeanu, Matthew Evans and Zoka Milan

Introduction

Anaesthesia for liver transplantation (LT) is considered one of the most challenging, anaesthetic sub-speciality. There are still no binding rules that specify levels of competence or guarantee the continuity of care by anaesthetic providers [1]. It is the authors' humble opinion based on years of experience that requirements for anaesthetists involved in LT are some of the following: (1) knowledge of: (a) the pathophysiology of liver diseases and systemic manifestation of liver disease (Chap. 3), (b) cardiovascular and respiratory physiology (Chap. 3), (c) coagulation abnormalities and management (Chap. 11), (d) fluid balance, (e) blood and blood products replacement (Chap. 12), (f) pharmacology of drugs administered in patients with liver disease, (g) donor types (Chap. 4), (h) surgical aspects of LT (Chap. 5), (i) basics of immunosupression plus constant update, (2) skills of rapid blood and products transfusion, management of hypo and hypercoalugable status, maintaining haemodynamic stability based on advanced monitoring, including transoesophageal echocardiography (TOE) and (3) personality that includes (a) dedication (b) rapid decision making, (c) ability to work under stress, (d) physical and mental fitness for frequent on calls and work out of sociable hours [2], (e) good communication skills, (f) ability to work in a big team, (g) flexibility, (h) good sense for humour and probably much more that should be identified and included in the policy that should be created in the future.

L. Brezeanu (✉)
Department of Anaesthesia and Critical Care, Fundeni Clinical Institute, Bucharest, Romania
e-mail: Laviniajipa11@yahoo.com

M. Evans
Royal Surrey Hospital NHS Foundation Trust, Guilford, UK

Z. Milan
FRCA, King's College Hospital, London, UK

Z. Milan and C. Goonasekera (eds.), *Anesthesia for Hepatico-Pancreatic-Biliary Surgery and Transplantation*, https://doi.org/10.1007/978-3-030-51331-3_8

Additionally, technical skills for insertion of veno-venous bypass (VVBP) lines and understanding principle of VVBP are still desirable (Chap. 17) and recently, basic knowledge of Extra Corporeal Membrane Oxygenator (ECMO) principle of work is also required (Chap. 15).

In addition to skills related to invasive procedures required, LT anaesthesia also include the ability to fast track post LT patients (Chap. 13).

Anaesthesia for LT itself is small period of time when compared with the whole process of LT: investigations before the final diagnosis, multidisciplinary pre-assessment, waiting list time, postoperative care in Intensive Therapy Unit (ITU), recovery on medical wards and duration of life of LT patients after LT when immunosuppression is maintained and regular follow up clinics, but extremely important part of the whole process that can significantly contribute to the outcomes. There is evidence that certain anaesthetic approach can change outcomes of LT [3] and there is evidence that lack of training and experience can lead to serious complications [4].

There are three main phases of liver transplantation: dissection, anhepatic and neohepatic, while reperfusion is the main event that can cause major disturbances in haemodynamic and metabolic area.

Since the first LT operation in the UK in 1968. in Cambridge, when Dr Elisabeth Gibbs was the first anaesthetist for LT, there is a huge progress made in LT anaesthesia in last 5 decades [5].

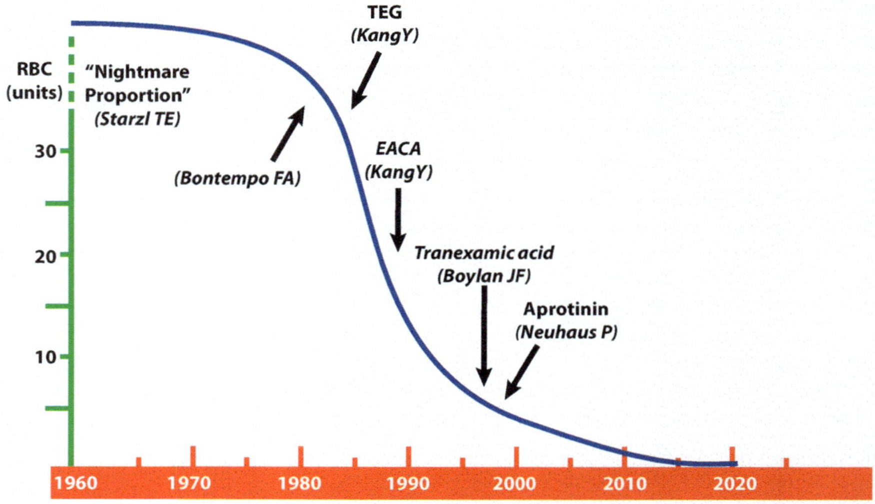

Fig. 8.1 Trends in bleeding and blood and products replacement in liver transplant programme

There is generally gradual decrease in bleeding and blood and products replacement as shown on updated Fig. 8.1. Consequently, haemodynamic instability and massive transfusion are less frequent than they have been in the past [6].

Pre assessment has also improved in last several decades (Chaps. 6 and 7). As a consequence, patients are better prepared for surgery, and anaesthetists are more in control [7].

Additional improvement in surgical techniques, postoperative care, better understanding pathophysiology and effective immunosuppression and extracorporeal organ preservation (Chap. 16) led to an important increase in the number of successful procedures and improved patients outcomes. Patients outcomes are so much better that we look less into increased survival rate, but more into shorter intensive care and hospital stay, lower number of complications and better quality of life post LT [8, 9].

Fast tracking of LT patient after surgery, and even fast tracking in ICU stay post LT are more common in recent years [7, 8].

Challenges that we meet in more recent times are: older age of LT recipients, high risk patients with advanced liver disease and impairment in cardiovascular, pulmonary, renal and coagulation systems, acute liver failure in pregnancy, severe liver trauma patients, re-do LTs, multivisceral transplants etc. [10].

Additionally, as we are trying to expand liver grafts pool, we have marginal donors that can jeopardise good results of LT programme [11].

There is no formal training for LT anaesthetists as such. Simulation training for anaesthesia for LTs is more common, particularly in large LT centres and during LT meetings [12]. Larger LT centers have fellowships that last from 6 to 12 months for external candidates and supervised on-the-job training for LT anaesthesia team members [13].

LT recipient pool is relatively small when compared with other surgeries. For example, there is approximately more than 600 operations per year in the UK, 8000 in USA and 20 000 worldwide [14, 15]. For anaesthetists, that means that there is not many anaesthetic LT jobs available. Liver transplant programs are moving towards main centres, mainly because there is an evidence that high volume centres have better outcomes [16].

There is another movement in LT programme. We are still looking for the objective parameters for the assessment of the quality of work of anaesthetics and other healthcare professionals involved in LT programme. Parameters such as length of hospital stay (LOS), length of ICU stay, the incidence of Renal replacement treatment (RRT), duration of mechanical ventilation, number and severity of complications, number of re-do procedures may become outcomes that anaesthetists and other members of LT teams should look at more closely [17, 18].

As anaesthesia for LT is complex, it is not surprise that there are numerous protocols and several articles and book chapters describing anaesthesia for LT. This chapter should be read together with all other chapters in this book and will be focused on intra-operative care during LT.

Anaesthetic Management

Liver transplantation is a high risk surgery performed under general anaesthesia and despite recent advances, it still remains a major challenge for the anaesthetist due to important multiorgan systems changes.

With advance in pre-assessment and our knowledge of different pathophysiological changes in different liver diseases (Chaps. 6 and 9), LT anaesthetists can make a plan before LT and be more in control of changes that will follow. Ethiology of liver disease, stage of liver disease measured by Child-Pough, MELD and UKELD scores, recipients co-morbidities, first of re-do LT, quality of donor's liver and experience of the surgical team can give us a rough idea whether LT will be straight forward or challenging. Despite that, we should always be ready for the different scenario.

Although massive bleeding and haemodynamic instability can be expected during LT, it is important to know that at least 1/3 of LT patients, mainly patients with primary diagnosis of PBC, PSC, autoimmune hepatitis, HCC and some metabolic diseases are not more complex than standard liver resection and that they may not require RBC transfusion [6].

Anaesthetic work starts with meeting a patient before going to operating theatre and reviewing pre-assessment form. At King's College Hospital it is two page document with the diagnosis of the primary liver disease, history and staging of liver disease, co-morbidities, cardiovascular examination (including ECG, cardiac echo, CPEX test and coronary angiography in some patients), all laboratory results, social status, reason for listing for LT and standard laboratory test results. Type of graft on the donor of surgery that can be used is also recorded on that form. It is very important to see the patient, as sometimes time before listing and LT can be long, or long enough that patient's condition can change a lot, in positive and negative way.

Depending on transplant centre, pre-medication can be used for anxiolysis, particularly if the plan is to transfer the patient sedated and ventilated to ICU at the end of surgery.

Most common causes of liver diseases and implications for LT are already presented in Chap. 9, as well as pre-assessment process and interpretation of the data extracted from there (Chap. 6).

Induction and Maintenance of Anaesthesia

The surgery is performed under general anaesthesia with the aid of invasive haemodynamic monitoring as described in Chap. 10, coagulation monitoring as described in Chap. 10 and devices for rapid fluid infusion and cell salvage [19].

LT is an emergency procedure but usually patients have enough notice time in order to be starved. Rapid sequence induction can be indicated if recipients present with ascites, recent food intake or if there is any suspicion of gastroparesis, when recipients are at risk of delayed gastric emptying. Rapid sequence induction is advised under these circumstances, despite numerous discussion currently questioning the value and the most appropriate technique [20]. LT patients should have carbohidrate solutions up to 2 hours before surgery [21].

ESLD patients have altered anaesthetic drug distribution, metabolism and elimination and all anaesthetic drugs can reduce hepatic blood flow and oxygen uptake. Cirrhotic patients have low albumin levels leading to high bioavailability of many drugs including benzodiazepines; midazolam has a longer half life, duration of action and a reduced protein binding so, in theory, judicious use is necessary for preoperative anxiolysis [22]. However, as LT is long surgical procedure during which at some point newly transplanted liver start working and majority of patients stay sedated and ventilated post surgery. Therefore longer half life of benzodiazepines and most anaesthetic drugs does not play a major role in anaesthesia for LT.

All known induction agents are used for induction of general anaesthesia for LT. Propofol is an important vasodilator and increases recipients' total hepatic blood flow during induction of anaesthesia [23]. Etomidate decreases hepatic blood flow and has an increased distribution volume leading to an unpredictable clinical recovery in short surgical procedures, effect that is not clinically relevant for anaesthesia for LT [24]. Some centres, including King's College Hospital, still use thiopentone for induction of anaesthesia for LT. There is no evidence that any induction agent is superior for induction of anaesthesia for LT. Haemodynamic stability without need for massive fluid infusion or frequent injection of vasoactive drugs is desirable during induction of anaesthesia.

Equally, despite careful consideration that muscle relaxants that do not need a liver to be metabolised are preferable for LT patients, all available muscle relaxants and analgesic agents can be used during anaesthesia for LT, particularly if we are not planning fast tracking patient at the end of LT. Neuromuscular block monitoring is advisable, and reduction of the dose of muscle relaxant either by reduction of infusion rate or by completely stopping infusion after the hepatic artery/bile duct anastomosis and using boluses if required to facilitate abdominal closure [25].

Most of patients who have Acute Liver Failure (ALF) are already intubated and ventilated patients. More time they spend in ICU before LT, more likely they are to be over sedated [26]. As most ALF patients have multiorgan failure, they are also on renal replacement therapy, which further decrease amount of anaesthetics that these patients require [27].

Prophylactic antibiotics should be administered after induction of anaesthesia and prior to skin incision and the class of antibiotic used varies according to centre protocols; redosing is necessary if massive bleeding occurs [28].

Line insertion

Apart from i.v. cannula for induction of anaesthesia, arterial and central venous catheter (CVC) are sine qua non for every LT. Ultrasound guided CVC insertion is recommended, but still not achieved in all LT centers [29]. Although less and less LT patients experience massive bleed, it is better to have big intravascular line for rapid fluid infusion ready, rather than to try to insert one when patient start to bleed. For rapid fluid infusion, some centres use Swan-Ganz sheath, some vascular catheter than can be used for RRT if required or Advanced Venous Access catheter or some use large bore peripheral vascular cannulas [29–31]. Peripheral cannulas are not reliable when rapid transfusion is required. In order to avoid large central venous cannula if not necessary, some centres use additional single lumen CVC that can be quickly replaced with larger lumen one over guidewire if needed. Veno-venous bypass line can also be used for rapid fluid administration [32]. The choice of vascular access depends on many factors, including the volume of LT centre, experience, quality of graft used, anaesthetic and surgical skills, the extent of point of care of coagulation monitoring, etc. In conclusion, large bore peripheral cannula, CVC and arterial line are compulsory for every LT anaesthesia. In more complex cases and in LT centres with different policies, additional vascular access can be provided.

Maintenance of anaesthesia

Maintenance of general anaesthesia is achieved with a balanced technique using inhalational anaesthetics, non-depolarising muscle relaxants and opioids. All volatile agents decrease mean arterial pressure (MAP) and portal blood flow [33]. Desflurane and sevoflurane have little effect on total hepatic blood flow and are preferred in fast track liver anaesthesia [34]. ESLD patients have less inhalational requirements compared to healthy subjects and this varies with the MELD score and phase of LT [35, 36].

In terms of analgesia, fentanyl is metabolised by the liver but its elimination is not altered in cirrhotic patients [37]. It can be used as continuous infusion or boluses. There is no accurate and simple method of measurement of analgesic requirement although there are some new technologies that may change it in a near future [38]. As stated in Chapter Fast track general approximately 20 ml of fentanyl is sufficient for LT for most patients. As there is not reliable assessment of intraoperative analgesia, analgesia in LT patient is more frequently overdosed than underdosed. Remifentanil can be used for LT patient, too, as alfentanil as well [39]. LT is painful because of large incision and during dissection phase. From anhepatic phase, it is less painful as liver is separated from all afferent pain stimuli and there is a general belief that pain during LT is less intense than pain during liver resection [40].

Emergency drugs such as inotropes and vasopressors should be prepared and readily available at any time during the LT in case of sudden cardiovascular (CV) instability. Noradrenaline infusion, dopamine, dobutamine, levosimendane and adrenaline are the drugs of choice. Vasopressin can also be used in case of refractory hypotension as studies showed that ESLD patients have lower vasopressin levels [41].

Cell salvage devices are routinely used during LT except when neoplasia or infection is present [19].

Intraoperative Fluids Administration Management

Amount of fluids administration

The amount of bleeding and blood products transfused have declined significantly in the last 20 years due to better surgical techniques, point of care monitoring and reduction of portal pressure [6] An individualised and thorough assessment of patients' volemic status and fluids perfused should be assessed regularly during LT. Anaesthesia for LT should follow the same principles as anaesthesia for liver resection surgery.

Excessive fluid therapy can have important adverse effects: pulmonary and graft edema, abnormal gas exchange, organ congestion, primary non function or acute kidney injury [42–45].

Present studies do not offer a clear answer regarding the ideal monitoring system and fluid therapy in LT patients. More details about haemodynamic monitoring during LT is presented in Chap. 10.

Attempts to lower the CVP by avoiding plasma transfusion during the pre-anhepatic phase have been described and have proved to reduce red blood cell transfusion [46]. After re-perfussion, when patients start worming up and vasodilatation occur, more liberal fluid replacement is advisable.

Significant blood loss during LT can sometimes occur and requires blood products and fluid transfusion in order to maintain an adequate cardiac output (CO) and organ perfusion. Massive transfusion can have major adverse effects in the postoperative period. (Chapter 12) The amount of blood products administered intraoperatively can predict patients' readmission to ICU [47].

Type of fluids

Colloids:

The use of albumin during LT reduces the amount of intraoperative fluid administration and the incidence of pulmonary oedema [48]. Albumin decreases mortality in cirrhotic patients, reduces the incidence of post reperfusion syndrome (PRS) and the use of vasopressor agents, but its use is limited by high costs.

Hetastarch is not recommended as it affects platelet aggregability and increases the risk of bleeding by decreasing the concentration of coagulation factor VIII [49].

The use of gelatines over cystalloids in liver transplant patients has not been supported by convincing evidence. Gelatines can have numerous side effects: anaphylactic reactions, decrease in thrombin generation, worsening of fibrinolysis which is specific in the anhepatic phase and can increase the risk of acute kidney injury (AKI) [50].

Cristalloids

There is no ideal crystalloid solution and all have their limitations. Isotonic crystalloids can be adequate for fluid therapy. Excessive usage of normal saline (0.9%) should be avoided as it causes hyperchloremic acidosis and increases sodium levels leading to acute central pontine myelinolysis in patients with low pre-operative Na [50]. Ringer lactate (RL) solutions are hypotonic and can increase intracellular fluid and worsen cerebral edema. Also, the lactate in RL requires liver metabolism for elimination [50]. In the first two phases of LT metabolisam of lactate is deranged, which may result in increased lactate and metabolic acidosis.

Plasmalyte has an almost normal pH and similar plasma electrolytes and osmolarity. One of the advantages is that it contains acetate which requires extrahepatic metabolism to bicarbonate. Plasmalyte does not contribute to increase lactate level in LT. However, proinflammatory and potential cardiotoxic effects have been described [51].

In conclusion, balance fluid replacement based on patients' needs is recommended. Fluid replacement should be guided by monitoring fluid input and output clinically and using haemodynamic and POC monitoring. Individualised fluid management and goal directed fluid therapy are important measures for a successful LT.

Phases of LT

Pre-anhepatic phase

This is the first surgical phase of the LT procedure. It starts with skin incision. In rare occasions patients with extensive portal hypertension, massive bleeding can start from skin incision. Octreotide infusion can reduce bleeding from the skin and varices at dissection phase of LT [52, 53]. Vasopressin may have similar effect [54]. Octreotide should start as prevention in patients with portal hypertension, rather than when patients start bleeding.

Pre-anhepatic phase continues with ascitic fluid drainage in patients with portal hypertension. Large volume drainage of ascitic fluid at the beginning of LT can decrease intraabdominal pressure (IAP), improve lung compliance and ventilation and decrease transpulmonary pressure [55]. It can also decrease central venous pressure [55]. However, in patients with large amount of ascitic fluid, fast drainage of ascitic fluid can cause significant cardiovascular strain and impaired renal function. [56] Albumin 20 or 5% and inotropic support should be ready for administration for circulating volume and blood pressure resuscitation in patients who have more than several litres of ascitic fluid [57].

Pre-anhepatic phase continues with separation of liver from surrounding structures. In some patients this phase can be bloodless. However, excessive bleeding can also occur and have a serious impact on patient's cardiovascular stability. The risk is increased and can be predicted in recipients with previous abdominal surgical interventions, previous spontaneous bacterial peritonitis (SBP), re-do LT, in the presence of portal hypertension and in patients with hypervolaemia [46]. Neutral or fluid restrictive strategy and portal vasoconstriction (i.e. with octreotide) are recommended in this phase of LT. Coagulation abnormality should not be corrected in this phase if patients are not bleeding [46]. It is important to keep all organs well perfused during dissection phase.

It continues with dissection of hilum, where hepatic portal vein, artery and bile duct are located. If liver is enlarged, i.e. polycystic liver, access to the hilum can be very difficult.

The anaesthetic goal in this first part of LT is to maintain adequate volaemic status, hemodynamic stability, electrolyte concentration, clotting profile, haemoglobin level and temperature.

Optimising patient's volaemic status is the key management during this first phase as it prepares the patient for the clamping of the IVC. Volume loading, use of vasoactive drugs, correction of hypocalcemia and maintaining K below 4 mEq/L represent important measures.

Anhepatic phase

It is the second surgical phase; It starts with clamping of the portal vein, hepatic artery (inflow) and hepatic veins (outflow). Next stage is physical removal of the liver, followed by the joining of the outflow and inflow vessels. It ends with liver graft reperfusion through portal vein in majority of cases and less frequently through the hepatic artery.

Depending on surgical technique, the anhepatic phase is characterised by cardiovascular instability as hepatic outflow is obstructed and venous blood is sequestrated in the portal system. This will lead to an important decrease in preload, CO and arterial pressures. Hemodynamic stability can be maintained with vasoactive or inotropic drugs.

Patients with good collateral venous circulation due to long standing ESLD can have minimal cardiovascular instability. Severe hemodynamic collapse can be managed by portosystemic shunting with a temporal surgical porto-systemic shunt or porto-systemic VVB. VVB has also proved extremely useful in aiding difficult liver dissections (See Chap. 17) (redo LT, adhesions, previous SBP).

The main goal in this phase is also to keep patient haemodunamicaly stable, normotermic, with normal Hb level, with K level below 4 and with low CVP.

There is no liver function in this phase. Patients can become acidotic with increased lactate level due to lack of lactate metabolism. Severity of acidosis depends on duration of anhaepatic phase, previous liver function, bleeding and blood products replacement and the amount of inotropes used. In the most extreme cases, severe acidosis may require correction with RRT [58].

Hyperkalemia is consequence of metabolic acidosis and potassium shift from intra into extracellular space or massive stored blood transfusion. Hyperkalemia should be treated before reperfussion: (1) by correcting metabolic acidosis, (2) with loop diuretics, (3) with insulin and glucose boluses or infusion that will push K into intarcellular space, (4) with bicarbonate boluses (although there is no evidence, temporary correction of low pH can reduce amount of inotropes required) (5) with hyperventilation and (6) with calcium and magnesium administration.

Worsening hyperkalemia unresponsive to previous measures can be managed with RRT. Thromethamine infusion for K control has also been described [59].

Excessive fluid resuscitation should be avoided as this can result in an important fluid overload during reperfusion which could lead to right heart failure and graft congestion. Fluid restriction is the best choice especially if standard technique is used and adequate arterial pressures are maintained with the use of vasopressors and inotropes. Noradrenaline is the vasopressor and inotrope of choice during LT and cardiac output monitoring systems can help guide the use of inotropes if necessary.

Coagulation problems are very important during this phase because blood coagulation factors synthesis does not exist. Another reason is the accumulation of tissue plasminogen activator (tPA) and other anticoagulant factors including heparinoid products which are normally metabolised by the functioning liver. Despite all these, minimal bleeding usually occurs in the anhepatic stage. No aggressive correction of coagulation abnormalities should be made since these products will be immediately metabolised after graft repefusion. Viscoelastic tests are mandatory for diagnosis and management of hyperfibrinolysis and other coagulation problems during LT.

There are studies that show the use of mannitol before IVC clamping (0.5 g/kgc) in order to avoid liver blood congestion and intraabdominal organ edema [60].

In this stage of the surgery, the anaesthetist should optimise the patient for graft reperfusion. Serum K levels should be maintained below 4 mEq/L, calcium levels should be normalised and inotropes readily available.

Neo-Hepatic Phase

The neohepatic phase begins when the donor's liver is perfused with recipient's blood, usually through the portal vein. Soon after reperfusion, the donor's liver begins working in the recipient's body.

Reperfusion is accompanied by sudden decreases in systemic vascular resistance and cardiac output, resulting in a decrease in blood pressure. Heart rate can also decrease, increase or become irregular. Reperfusion can result in worsening of pulmonary hypertension and even right heart failure and/or increase in intracranial pressure [61]. Hyperkalaemia can also develop and may be so sudden and severe that it can lead to sudden cardiac arrest.

The first definition of post-reperfusion syndrome (PRS) is a 30% decrease in the main arterial pressure for at least 1 minute that appears within the first 5 minutes after graft reperfusion [62].

Further addition includes asystole or haemodynamically significant arrhythmia, or the need to begin infusion of vasopressors during the post-reperfusion period [63].

The incidence rate of RPS varies between 10% and 50%, with most studies reporting an incidence of 30% [64, 65].

The mechanism of reperfusion syndrome PRS is complex and not fully understood. It has been suggested that the abrupt influx of cold, hyperkalaemic and acidotic blood into the circulation and release of vasoactive substances from the liver graft at the time of reperfusion contribute to PRS [66]. In addition, endothelial cell activation and non-specific immune responses at the time of reperfusion lead to overt activation of inflammation [67]. These inflammatory responses are variable among patients [67]. Some biomarkers, such as IL-6, measured after reperfusion, are useful for predicting early vascular complications and long-term survival [67].

The risk factors that contribute to reperfusion syndrome are presented in Table 8.1.

The influence of fatty liver on PRS is demonstrated by the differences in incidence of PRS when the donor liver shows moderate, mild and no steatosis (37.5% vs. 24% vs. 18.8%, respectively) [68]. This may be explained as a result of impaired hepatic micro-circulation in the steatotic liver, leading to reduced tolerance of the steatotic liver to ischaemia-reperfusion injury [70].

To prevent profound PRS, it is essential to maintain normothermia [71], normovolaemia [46] or slight hypovolaemia on inotropic support before reperfusion, with acceptable Hb level, normal to low K level, no acidosis and with vasopressors and inotropes on hand. If risk factors are present, primarily fatty liver, the surgical team should be alerted and ready to start CPR if required. Treatment when severe reperfusion syndrome occurs is mainly symptomatic.

Cardiac arrest on reperfusion is more common in patients with donor liver steatosis [65].

Table 8.1 Risk factors that contribute to reperfusion syndrome

Factors related to the donor's liver:	
	Macrosteatosis of donor's liver [66]
	Long cold ischaemic time (CIT) [66, 68]
	Age > 60 years [69]
Factors related to the recipient:	
	MELD > 30 [65]
	Fulminant hepatic failure
	Re-do LT [69]
	History of SBP [69]
	Multiple abdominal surgeries [69]
	Portal vein thrombosis [69]
	Age > 60 years [64, 69]
	BMI > 40 [69]
	Pre-operative anaemia [64]
	Pre-operative tachycardia [64]
	Pre-reperfusion hyperkalaemia [64]
Factors related to surgical technique:	
	Porto-caval shunt not performed [68]

The most common complications and consequences of PRS are:

- PAAR-persistent acidosis, the presence of a significant negative slope coefficient for base excess values measured after hepatic artery anastomosis through 72 hours post-operatively. The incidence is 10%, and it is associated with significant 30-day and in-hospital mortality rates [72].
- Flat TEG line after reperfusion, resulting from hyperfibrinolysis or heparin effect [73].
- Primary graft failure.
- Higher rates of post-operative renal failure and lower early survival rates [74].

After reperfusion, the new liver should have a good colour and should not be congested. In addition, the new liver should begin to produce bile soon after reperfusion.

The primary non-functioning liver is grey in colour, congested, does not produce bile and the patient becomes anuric. Major bleeding is the most prominent symptom of a primary non-functioning liver.

If liver function is adequate following reperfusion, arterial and bile anastomosis follow and, finally, abdominal closure can be performed.

References

1. Walia A, Mandell S, Mercaldo N, Michaels D, Robertson A, Banerjee A, et al. Anesthesia for liver transplantation in US academic centers: Institutional structure and perioperative care. Liver Transplant. 2012;18:737–43.
2. Halliday N, Martin K, Collet D, Allen E, Thorburn D. Is liver transplantation 'out-of-hours' non-inferior to 'in-hours' transplantation? A retrospective analysis of the UK transplant registry. BMJ Open. 2019;9:e024917.
3. Hevesi ZG, Lopukhin SY, Mezrich JD, Andrei AC, Lee M. Designated liver transplant anaesthesia team reduce blood transfusion, need for mechanical ventilation and duration of intensive care. Liver Transpl. 2009;15:460–5.
4. Hofer I, Spivack J, Yapont M, Zerillo J, Reich DL, Wax D. Association between anesthesiologist experience and mortality after orthotopic liver transplantation. Liver Transpl. 2015;21:89–95.
5. Gibbs E. The Cambridge first liver transplant. The history of anaesthesia society proceedings of the joint meeting of 6th March 1993 with the Section of Anaesthetics of the Royal Society of Medicine. 1993;12:20–22.
6. Findlay JY, Long TR, Joyner MJ, et al. Changes in transfusion practice over time in adult patients undergoing liver transplantation. J Cardiothorac Vasc Anesth. 2013;27:41–5.
7. Bulato IG, Heckman MG, Rawal B, Aniskevich S, Shine TS, Keaveny AP, et al. Avoiding stay in intensive care unit after liver transplantation: a score to assign location of care. Am J Transplant. 2014;14:2088–96.
8. Echeveri J, Goldaracena N, Singh AK, Sapisochin G, Selzner N, Cattral MS, et al. Avoiding ICU admission by using a fast-track protocols is safe in selected adult-to-adult live donor liver transplant recipients. Transplant Direct. 2017;3:e213. https://doi.org/10.1097/txd.0000000000000730.
9. Bonavia A, Pachunski J, Bezinover D. Perioperative anesthetic management of patients having liver transplantation for uncommon conditions. Sem Cardiovasc Vasc Anesthes. 2018;22:197–210.

10. Hessheimer AJ, Coll E, TorresF, Ruiz P, Gastaca M, Rivas JI, et al. Normothermic regional perfusion versus super-rapid recovery in controlled donation after circulatory death liver transplantation. J Hepatol 2019; 70:658–65.
11. Aggraval S, Bane BC, Boucek BC, Planinsic RM, Lutz JV, Metro DG, et al. Simulation: a teaching tool for liver transplantation anesthesiology. Clin Transplant. 2012;26:564–70.
12. https://www.cuh.nhs.uk/addenbrookes/services/clinical/anaesthesia/international_fellows_programme.html. Accessed 15 Sep 2019.
13. https://nhsbtdbe.blob.core.windows.net/umbraco-assets-corp/12250/nhsbt-liver-transplantation-annual-report-2017–2018.pdf. Accessed 21 Oct 2019.
14. https://unos.org/data/transplant-trends/. Accessed 26 Mar 2020
15. Ozhathi DK, Li Y, Smith JK, Tseng JF, Saidi RF, Bozorgzadeh A, Shah SA. Effect of centre volume and high donor risk index on liver allograft survival. HPB (Oxford). 2011;13:447–53.
16. Ooi PH, Hager A, Mazurak VC, Dajani K, Bhargava R, Gilmour SM, et al. Sarcopenia in chronic liver disease: Impact on outcomes. Liver Transpl. 2019;25:1422–38.
17. Ohnemus D, Neighbors K, Rychlik K, Venick RS, Bucuvalas JC, Sundariam SS. et al. Health-related quality of life and cognitive functioning in pediatric liver transplant recipients. Liver Transpl. 2019. https://doi.org/10.1002/lt.25634.
18. Rando K, Niemann CU, Taura P, Klinck J. Optimizing cost-effectiveness in perioperative care for liver transplantation: a model for low-to medium-income countries. Liver Transpl. 2011;17:1247–78.
19. Zdravkovic M, Berger-Estilita J, Sorbello H, Hagberg CA. An international survey about rapid sequence intubation in 10,003 anaesthetists and 16 airway experts. Anaesthesia. 2020;75:313–22.
20. Oliveira RA, Guatura GMGBDS, Peniche ACG, Costa ALS, Poveda VB. An integrative review of postoperative accelerated recovery protocols. AORN J 2017;106:324–30.
21. Rahimzadeh P, Safari S, Faiz SH, Alavian SM. Anesthesia for patients with liver disease. Hepat Mon. 2014;14:e19881.
22. Meierhenrich R, Gauss A, Muhling B, Bracht H, Radermacher P, Georgieff M, et al. The effect of propofol and desflurane anaesthesia on human hepatic blood. Anaesthesia. 2010;65:1085–93.
23. Thomson IA, Fitch W, Hughes RL, Campbell D, Watson R. Effect of certain i.v. anaesthetics on liver blood flow and hepatic oxygen consumption in the greyhound. Br J Anaesth. 1986;58:69–80.
24. Bhangui P, Bhangui P, Gupta N, Jolly AS, Bhalotra S, Sharma N, Soin AS, et al. Fast tracking in adult living donor liver transplantation: a case series of 15 patients. Indian J Anaesth. 2018;62:127–30.
25. Aragon RE, Proano A, Mongilardi N, de Ferrari A, Harrera P, Roland R, et al. Sedation practices and clinical outcomes in mechanically ventilated patients in a prospective multicentre cohort. Crit Care. 2019;23:130. https://doi.org/10.1186/s13054-019-2394-9.
26. Ostermann M, Chawla LC, Forni LG, Kane-Gill SL, Kellum JA, Koyner J et al. Drug management in acute kidney disease-Report of the acute disease quality initiative XVI meeting. Br J Clin Pharmacol. 2018;84:396–403.
27. Haidar G, Green M, American Society of Transplantation Infectious Diseases community of Practice. Intra-abdominal infections in solid organ transplant guidelines recipients: Guidelines from the American society of transplantation infectious diseases community of practice. Clin Transplant. 18:e13595.
28. Schumann R, Mandell S, Mercaldo N, Michaels D, Robertson A, Banerjee A, et al. Anesthesia for liver transplantation in United States academic centers: intraoperative practice. J Clin Anesth. 2013;25:542–50.
29. Kim SS, Ko JS, Yu JM, Kim HY. The intermittent bolus infusionsof rapid infusion system caused hypothermia during liver transplantation. Korean J Anesthesiol. 2013;65:363–4.

30. Milan Z, Agrawal S, Katyayani K, Sharma N. What happens when adequate vascular access cannot be provided for major surgery (Liver transplantation)? J Assoc Vacular Access. 2019;24:52–4.
31. Jakson P, Jankovic Z. Veno-venous bypass catheter for hepatic transplant risk unique complications. Anaesth Intens Care. 2007;35:805–6.
32. Figueira ERR, Filho JAR. Is there a place for sevoflurane to prevent liver ischemiareperfusion injury during liver transplantation? Edorium J Anesthes. 2015;1:1–5.
33. Suttner SW, Schmidt CC, Boldt J, Huttner I, Kumle B, Piper SN. Low-flow desflurane and sevoflurane anesthesia minimally affect hepatic integrity and function in elderly patients. Anesth Analg. 2000;91:206–12.
34. Hasanin AS, Mahmoud FM, Yassen KA. Entropy-guided end-tidal desflurane concentration during living donor liver transplantation. Saudi J Anaesth. 2013;7:399–403.
35. Kang JG, ko JS, Kim GS, Gwak MS, Kim YR, Lee SK. The relationship between inhalational anaesthetic requirement and the severity of liver disease in liver ransplant recipients according to three phases of liver transplantation. Transpl Proc. 2010;42:854–7.
36. Jin SJ, Jung JY, Noh MH, Lee EK, Choi BM, Song MH, et al. The population pharmacokinetics of fentanyl in patients undergoing living-donor liver transplantation. Clin Pharmacol Ther. 2011;90:423–31.
37. Sabourdin N, Diarra C, Wolk R, Piat V, Louvet N, Constant I. Pupillary pain index changes after a standardized bolus of alfentanil under sevoflurane anesthesia. First evaluation of a new pupillometric index to assess the level of analgesia during general anesthesia. Anesthetic Clin Pharmacol. 2019;128:467–79.
38. Restoux A, Grassin-Delyle S, Liu N, Paugman-Burtz C, Mantz J, Le Guen M. Pilot study of closed-loop anaesthesia for liver transplantation. Br J Anesth. 2016;117:332–40.
39. Milan Z. Analgesia after liver transplantation. World J Hepatol. 2015;7:2331–5.
40. Taneja S, Chawla YK. Perioperative use of terlipressin in adult liver transplant. Liver Transpl. 2017;23:995–6.
41. Iwaki K, Yagi S, Morita S, Hamaguchi Y, Masano Y, Yamamoto G, et al. Impact of graft quality and fluid overload on postoperative massive ascites after living donor liver transplantation. Transpl Proc. 2019;51:1779–84.
42. Jeong HW, Jung KW, Kim SO, Kwon HM, Moon YJ, Jung IG, et al. Early postoperative weight gain is associated with increased risk of graft failure in living donor liver transplant recipients. Sci Rep. 2019;9:20096.
43. Codes L, de Souza YG, D'Oliveira RAC, Bastos JLA, Bittencourt PL. Cumulative positive fluid balance is a risk factor for acute kidney injury and requirement for renal replacement therapy after liver transplantation. World J Transpl. 2018;8:44–51.
44. Feltracco P, Carollo C, Barbieri S, Pettenuzzo T, Ori C. Early respiratory complications after liver transplantation. World J Gastroenterol. 2013;19:9271–81.
45. Klink JR, Pan LTT. Lessons from liver transplantation. Anaesthesia. 2012;67:1063–75.
46. Levy MF, Greene L, Ramsay MA, Jennings LW, Ramsay KJ, et al. Readmission to the intensive care unit after liver transplantation. Crit Care Med. 2001;29:18–24.
47. Haynes G, Navickis R, Wilkes M. Albumin administration- what is the evidence of clinical benefit? A systematic review of randomized controlled trails. Eur J Anaesthesiol. 2003;20:771–93.
48. Hand WR, Whiteley JR, Epperson TI, Tam L, Crego H, et al. Hydroxyethyl starch and acute kidney injury in orthotopic liver transplantation: a single-center retrospective review. Anesth Analg. 2015;120:619–26.
49. Groeneveld AB, Navickis RJ, Wilkes MM. Update on the comparative safety of colloids: a systematic review of clinical studies. Ann Surg. 2011;253:470–83.
50. Nandhakumar A, McCluskey SA, Srinivas C, Chandy TT. Liver transplantation: advances and perioperative care. Indian J Anaesth. 2012;56:326–35.

51. Byram SV, Gupta RA, Ander M, Edelstein S, Andretta B. Effects of continuous octreotide infusion on intraoperative transfusion requirements during orthotopic liver transplantation. Transplant Proc. 2015;47:2712–4.
52. Troisi RI, Vanlander A, Giglio MC, Van Linmen J, Scudeller L, Heyse B, et al. Somatostatin as inflow modulator in liver-transplant recipients with severe portal hypertension. Ann Surg. 2019;269:1025–33.
53. Reddy MS, Kaliamoorthy I, Rajakumar A, Malleeshwaran S, Appuswamy E, Lakshmi S, et al. Double-blind randomized controlled trial of the routine perioperative use of terlipressin in adult living donor liver transplantation. Liver Transpl. 2017;23:1007–14.
54. Mayr U, Karsten E, Lahmer T, Rasch S, Thies P, Henschel B, et al. Impact of large volume paracentesis on respiratory parameters including transpulmonary pressure an on transpulmonary derived hemodynamics: a prospective study. PLoS One. 2018;13:e193654.
55. Sharma A, Fletcher A, Lipscomb GR. Pulmonary oedema after therapeutic ascitic paracentesis: a case report and literature review of the cardiac complications of cirrhosis. Eur J Gastroenterol Hepatol. 2010;22:241–5.
56. Yosry A, Soliman ZA, Eletreby R, Hamzal I, Ismail A, Elkady MA. Oral midodrine in comparable to albumin infusion in cirrhotic patients with refractory ascites undergoing large-volume paracentesis: results of a pilot study. Eur J Gastroenterol Hepatol. 2019;31:345–51.
57. Karvellas CJ, Taylor S, Bigam D, Kneteman NM, Shapiro AMJ, Romanovsky A, et al. Intraoperative continuous renal replacement therapy during liver transplantation: a pilot randomized-controlled trial (INCEPTION). Can J Anaesth. 2019;66:1151–61.
58. Adelmann D, Kronish K, Ramsay MA. Anesthesia for liver transplantation. Anesthesiol Clin. 2017;35:491–508.
59. Vater Y, Levy A, Martay K, Hunter C, Weinbroum AA. Adjuvant drugs for end-stage liver failure and transplantation. Med Sci Monit. 2004;10:RA77–88.
60. Detry O, Arkadopoulos N, Ting P, Kahaku E, Margulies J, Arnaout W, et al. Intracranial pressure during liver transplantation for fulminat hepatic failure. Transplantation. 1999;67:767–70.
61. Aggrawal S, Kang Y, Freeman JA, Fortunato FL, Pinsky MR. Postreperfusion syndrome: cardiovascular collapse following hepatic reperfusion during liver transplantation. Transpl Proc. 1987;19(Suppl 3):54–5.
62. Ramsay M. The reperfusion syndrome: have we made any progress. Liver Transpl. 2008;14:412–4.
63. Croome KP, Lee DD, Croome S, Chadha R, Livingston D, Abader P, et al. The impact of postoperative syndrome during liver transplantation using livers with significant macrosteatosis. Am J Transpl. 2019;19:2550–9.
64. Chung IS, Kim HY, Shin YH, ko JS, Gwak MS, Sim WS, et al. Incidence and predictors of post-reperfusion syndrome in living donor liver transplantation. Clin Transpl. 2012;26:539–43.
65. Zalunardo MP, Schlpfer M, Beck-Scimmer B, Seifert B, Spahn DR, et al. Impact of cytokine release on ventricular function after epatic reperfusion: a prospective observational echocardiograpy study with tissue doppler imaging. BMC Anesthesiol. 2015;15:107.
66. Faitot F, Besch C, Lebas B, Addeo P, Ellero B, Woehl-Jaegle MR, et al. Interleukin 6 at reperfusion: a predictor of hepatic and extrahepatic early complications after liver transplantation. Clin Transplant. 2018;32:e13357.
67. Paugam-Burtz C, Kavafyan J, Marckx P, Dahmani S, Sommacale D, Ramsay M, et al. Postreperfusion syndrome during liver transplantation for cirrhosis: outcomes and predictors. Liver Transpl. 2009;15:522–9.
68. Chavin KD, Taber DJ, Norcross M, et al. Safe use of highly steatotic livers by utilizinga donor/recipient clinical algorithm. Clin Transplant. 2013;27:732–41.

69. Seifelian AM, Piasecki C, Agrawal A, Davidson BR. The effect of graded steatosis on flow in the hepatic parenchymal microcirculation. Transplantation. 1999;67:195–200.
70. Lamb FJ, Rogers R. Forced-air warming maintains normothermia during orthotopic liver transplantation. Anaestesia. 1995;50:745.
71. Kim S, DeMaria S, Li J, Lin HM, Smith N, Wax D, et al. Persistent acidosis after reperfusion-A prognostic indicator of increased 30-day and in-hospital postoperative mortality in liver transplant recipients. Clin Transpl. 2019;33:e13473.
72. Kim EH, Song SH, Kim GS, Ko JS, Gwak MS, Lee SK. Evaluation of "flat-line" thromboelastography after reperfusion during liver transplantation. Transpl proc. 2015;47:457–9.
73. Lee SH, Gwak MS, Choi SJ, Shin JH, Ko JS, Lee SY, et al. Intra-operative cardiac arrests during liver transplantation-a retrospective review of the first 15 yr in Asian population. Clin Transpl. 2013;27:126–36.

Chapter 9
How Does the Aetiology of Primary Liver Disease Affect Anaesthesia for Liver Transplantation

Mussarat N. Rahim and Michael A. Heneghan

Introduction

Patients with acute liver failure (ALF) and chronic liver disease require different types of perioperative care for liver transplantation (LT). First, we describe the intensive care unit (ICU) treatment of patients with ALF and the specific considerations for the anaesthetic technique for those patients undergoing LT. The remainder of this chapter focuses specifically on the particular LT nuances for end-stage liver disease patients pertinent to the LT anaesthetist.

Acute Liver Failure

In the absence of pre-existing liver disease, acute liver failure (ALF) is characterized by the development of hepatic encephalopathy (HE) and coagulopathy (international normalized ratio (INR) $\geq$1.5) within a certain period from the exposure of a precipitant [1]. Table 9.1 shows the sub-classification of ALF [2].

Table 9.1 Classification of ALF and prognosis [2]

	Jaundice to HE time	Cerebral oedema	Coagulopathy	Prognosis
Hyperacute	0–7 days	Common	Marked	Moderate
Acute	8–28 days	Common	Marked	Poor
Subacute	1–3 months	Rare	Modest	Poor

M.N. Rahim · M.A. Heneghan (✉)
King's College Hospital, London, UK
e-mail: michael.heneghan@nhs.net

M.N. Rahim
e-mail: mussaratrahim@nhs.net

Z. Milan and C. Goonasekera (eds.), *Anesthesia for Hepatico-Pancreatic-Biliary Surgery and Transplantation*, https://doi.org/10.1007/978-3-030-51331-3_9

The most common causes of ALF include:

- Acetaminophen toxicity
- Drug-induced liver injuries, e.g. isoniazid, rifampicin and salicylates
- Viral hepatitis
- Alcoholic hepatitis
- Autoimmune hepatitis (AIH)
- Hepatic ischaemia
- Vascular occlusion, e.g. Budd Chiari syndrome
- Pregnancy associated liver failure

The pathophysiology of ALF involves cytokine release from hepatocyte necrosis and rapid loss of liver function. Severe systemic inflammation and microcirculatory alterations contribute to a clinical picture comparable to septic shock [3]. ALF can lead to multi-organ failure (MOF). Management is mainly supportive and should ideally take place in a specialist ICU with access to emergency LT [4]. Despite advances in critical care, transplant-free survival remains low. Emergency LT is the only definitive treatment for ALF in those failing supportive medical treatment and can improve survival to 75–90% [5].

Clinical Picture of ALF

Hepatic encephalopathy (HE) is a neuropsychiatric syndrome which involves changes in mental state and motor function due to accumulation of toxic products from protein breakdown and gut bacterial metabolism. HE can occur in ALF and chronic liver failure. Precipitants include infection, gastrointestinal haemorrhage, metabolic disturbances, medications, hypoglycaemia, hypoxia, uraemia and surgery. The West Haven classification describes HE as follows [6].

- Grade I = lack of awareness, shortened attention span and impaired performance
- Grade II = minimal confusion and subtle personality/behavioural changes
- Grade III = significant disorientation and confusion with somnolence
- Grade IV = coma

In addition to HE, cerebral oedema is estimated to occur in up to 80% of patients with ALF and is a poor prognostic marker. It is more prominent in patients with hyperacute ALF and ALF, potentially due to a lack of time for compensatory mechanisms to equilibrate the osmotic changes within the brain. One post-mortem series of patients with ALF showed that 25% had cerebral oedema with cerebellar tonsil and temporal lobe herniation [7]. However, cerebral oedema as a cause of death in ALF is decreasing, possibly secondary to improved early supportive care [8].

Clinical signs of elevated intracranial pressure (ICP) (e.g. hypertension, bradycardia, hypertonia, abnormal posturing and impaired pupillary reflexes) occur late and do not provide a reliable guide for early therapy. Radiological imaging is not sensitive enough to detect oedema. Direct ICP monitoring allows real-time observation and earlier detection of elevated ICP. If cerebral oedema is suspected, a retrograde jugular bulb catheter can be inserted to indirectly assess cerebral oxygenation [9].

Adaptive and non-adaptive immunity are both impaired in patients with ALF. Decreased complement synthesis, Kupffer cell dysfunction, chemotaxis, neutrophil adhesion abnormalities and superoxide production lead to impaired opsonization against bacteria/fungi and decreased endotoxin clearance [10]. Malnutrition also contributes to infective susceptibility [11].

Bacterial and fungal infections occur in 80% and a third of patients with ALF respectively [12]. Pyrexia and leucocytosis are unreliable markers of infection, as they are absent in a significant proportion of infected patients with ALF. Conversely, patients with ALF, in the absence of infection, often fulfil the criteria for systemic inflammatory response syndrome (SIRS).

Spontaneous Bacterial Peritonitis (SBP) is the presence of infection in ascitic fluid, in the absence of intra-abdominal pathology (e.g. perforation). It is caused by bacterial translocation from the gut to ascitic fluid through the lymphatics and bloodstream [13].

Metabolic acidosis is usually reflective of renal failure. Lactate metabolism to bicarbonate is dependent on hepatic function. In ALF, lactate accumulation leads to lactic acidosis [14].

Treatment of ALF

Where possible, removal of the offending agent or treatment of the underlying cause should be instituted.

N-acetylcysteine (NAC) infusion in paracetamol toxicity should be started as soon as possible. Early treatment has a positive impact on outcome. NAC administration in non-paracetamol-induced ALF has also shown clinical benefit, although the mechanism of action is unclear [15, 16].

Artificial liver support devices as a 'bridge' to LT or during recovery remain under investigation. To date, these approaches have had limited success. The molecular adsorption and recirculation system (MARS), an adaptation of haemodialysis, dialyses blood against albumin solution and removes albumin-bound toxins. Artificial support systems have shown improvement in HE, renal function and haemodynamic factors in patients with acute-on-chronic liver failure [17].

Treatment of HE involves general supportive measures, nutrition and correction of the underlying cause, e.g. SBP. Specific treatments include:

(a) Airway protection if consciousness is impaired
(b) Avoidance of long-acting sedatives/opiates which require hepatic metabolism, e.g. propofol and alfentanil are preferable to morphine and midazolam

(c) Removal of toxins with regular lactulose—also acidifies gut converting ammonia to non-absorbable ammonium
(d) Regular non-absorbable antibiotics (e.g. Rifaxamin)—modifies gut microbiome
(e) L-Ornithine-L-Aspartate (LOLA)—controversial [18].

Treatment of cerebral oedema starts when ICP remains > 25 mmHg for a substantial period. An osmotic agent can be administered at this stage. Mannitol should be avoided in patients with oliguria not on renal replacement therapy (RRT). However, if on RRT, it can be given but twice its volume should be removed [19].

Hypertonic saline is an alternative osmotic agent. Serum sodium levels should be maintained between 145–150 mmol/L. In the early stages of ALF, maintaining a high serum osmolality reduces the incidence of high ICP. If the ICP is fluctuating, it is important to ensure that the patient is adequately sedated, and interventions are minimized to prevent surges in ICP [20].

Deep sedation with thiopental is reserved for patients not responding to osmotic agents. Neuromuscular blocking (NMB) drugs are not recommended as they are associated with neuromyopathy and infection. Seizures are difficult to recognize in sedated patients but must be suspected in those with an elevated ICP and low jugular oxygen saturation (SjO2), i.e. increased cerebral oxygen consumption (Fig. 9.1). In this scenario, anti-convulsants have been shown to decrease ICP and improve SjO2. There is some evidence that moderate hypothermia (32–33 °C) can reduce ICP and improve cerebral blood flow [21]. However, further studies are required to confirm this. In practice, normothermia remains the aim.

Early enteral feeding is recommended as a supportive measure.

Complications

Complications of ALF include cerebral oedema, respiratory/renal failure, hypoglycaemia, lactic acidosis, electrolyte disturbance and sepsis [22].

Early deaths in ALF are usually secondary to cerebral oedema (raised intracranial pressure (ICP)) or cardiovascular collapse, whereas late deaths tend to be related to sepsis and MOF [18].

Broad-spectrum antibiotics (for gram-positive/negative organisms) and an anti-fungal agent should be administered early [4]. This reduces the incidence of infective episodes when compared to treating at the time of suspected infection. Unfortunately, multi-resistant organisms are increasingly prevalent. Aseptic techniques are crucial for invasive procedures.

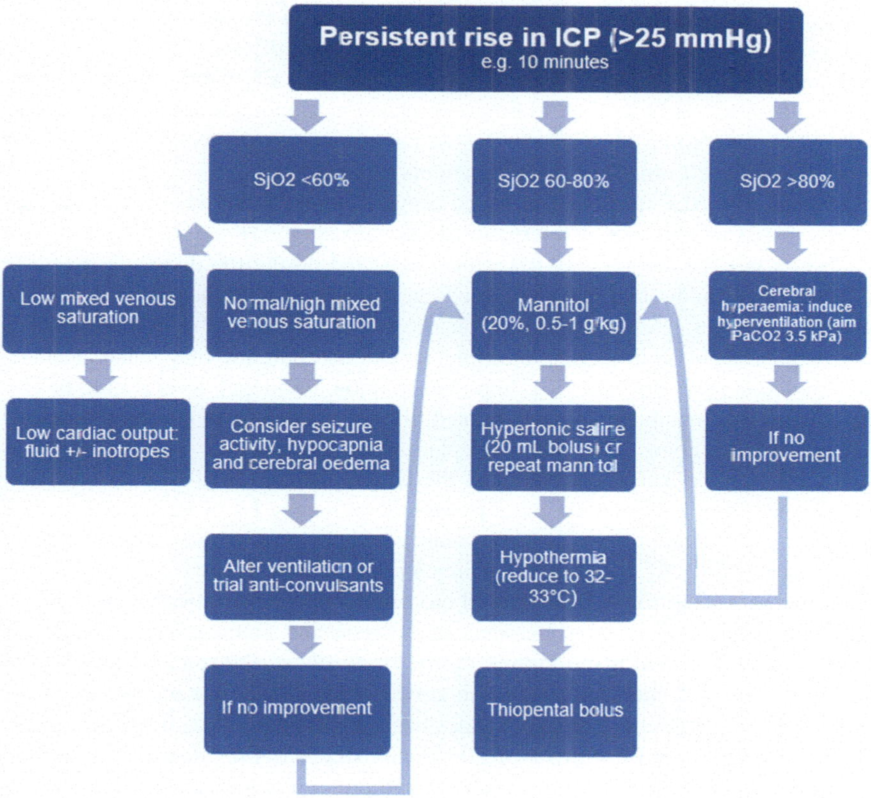

Fig. 9.1 Algorithm for the management of raised ICP

Recommendations for Anaesthesia in Patients with Acute Liver Disease

LT is still the treatment of choice for ALF patients who fulfil LT criteria [14]. The majority of patients with ALF will have grade 3 or 4 HE, multiorgan failure, a requirement for mechanical ventilation, and a need for invasive monitoring (central venous cannulation and arterial line insertion). These patients are typically receiving continuous veno-venous hemofiltration (CVVH), inotropic support, and advanced haemodynamic monitoring [8]. The use of invasive ICP monitoring has become less common over the last decade [20].

Pharmacological ICP reduction through the use of a thiopentone infusion was previously commonplace, however patients now typically receive shorter acting sedation via a combination of propofol and fenatnyl, alfentanil or remifentanil. These infusions could be used to intraoperatively maintain a lower ICP in patients with ALF undergoing LT, however, most centres opt to use volatile anaesthesia during LT, as in chronic liver disease patients receiving LT.

Patients with ALF may have deranged coagulation according to conventional laboratory tests, including a high international normalised ratio (INR). Despite this, their blood loss may be surprisingly lower than expected during the dissection phase of LT. Therefore, unless there is overt bleeding, fresh frozen plasma (FFP) should not be used to correct an elevated INR. Over use of FFP can cause hypervolaemia with a subsequent increase in surgical bleeding, an elevated ICP, and may make mechanical ventilation more difficult [23]. Importantly, a low fibrinogen level should be corrected with cryoprecipitate or concentrated fibrinogen. Thromboelastography testing is being increasingly used to guide the replacement of products.

CVVH may be instigated as part of the ICU management of ALF. It is recommended that this is continued intraoperatively as it may be of benefit during LT, by helping to maintain the acid–base balance and normo-to-hypovolaemia prior to graft reperfusion [24]. Similarly, if patients are on extracorporeal membrane oxygenation (ECMO) prior to LT, it should be continued intraoperatively.

The requirement for intraoperative anaesthesia and analgesia may be low in patients with ALF and acute kidney injury, by virtue of the reduced metabolism and elimination of anaesthetic and analgesic agents in the face of both impaired liver and renal function. Depth of anaesthesia monitoring (e.g. Bispectral Index Monitoring (BIS) or Entropy) typically demonstrates a low anaesthetic requirement prior to graft reperfusion. Additionally, the requirement for muscle relaxants can also be lower than expected. However, avoidance of an acute rise in ICP by maintaining muscle paralysis is important. Consequently some centres advocate the intraoperative use of an infusion of atracurium. Invasive ICP monitoring commonly reveals an acute rise in ICP during reperfusion.

Postoperatively, patients often have a period of sedation and ventilation on ICU prior to extubation. Those with pre-operative multiorgan failure, may require additional time to recover following LT. Younger patients undergoing LT earlier in the course of their disease, before the onset of multiorgan failure have a better chance of a more rapid recovery. Additionally, surgical approach may influence recovery. Patients receiving an auxiliary LT often have a longer recovery period, as the remaining native, damaged liver will continue to release cytokines which will have pronounced systemic effects.

Viral Hepatitis

Hepatitis B virus (HBV) infection is a global health issue. It is a virus that is transmitted through blood, bodily fluids and vertically from mother to child. It affects more than 250 million people worldwide and its prevalence varies regionally.

Transmission rates of HBV are dependent on the phase of infection and viral load. HBV infection is a concern for health care professionals particularly for those who are in contact with human blood and those who might be exposed through injuries with needle sticks and sharp instruments. Of note, the virus can survive outside the body for at least 7 days. Knowing the viral load and phase of disease (e.g. hepatitis e-antigen positivity) is useful when assessing transmission risk during surgery/anaesthesia. The full vaccination series can prevent infection in the majority of health care professionals [25].

In cases of exposure, receiving HBV vaccination and/or hepatitis B immunoglobulin within 24 hours may prevent infection. Acute infection can cause ALF in<1% of cases. In those who acquire HBV during adulthood, less than 5% of cases will develop chronic infection. Chronic HBV infection can lead to cirrhosis, hepatocellular cancer, LT and mortality. Selected patients will be on long-term indefinite therapy with nucleos(t)ide analogues (e.g. entecavir or tenofovir). These aim to suppress the virus, as opposed to cure [26].

Hepatitis delta virus (HDV) requires HBV for replication. Its prevalence is high in endemic areas such as Central/West Africa. Transmission usually occurs from mother to child during delivery, as well as through contact with blood and other bodily fluids. The clinical sequalae of HDV infection includes a spectrum of manifestations, ranging from ALF to asymptomatic carrier status. Severity of the clinical course is influenced by several factors e.g. persistent replication and genotype. HDV infection has poor virological response to interferon therapy. Novel therapeutic agents are required. Transmission can be prevented with hepatitis B immunization [27].

Similarly to HBV, Hepatitis C virus (HCV) infection can lead to both acute and chronic hepatitis. Acute HCV infection is usually self-limiting and rarely causes ALF. Conversely, chronic HCV infection develops in the majority (≈70%) of those infected. Globally, it is thought that more than 70 million people have chronic infection. HCV is primarily a blood-borne virus and transmission occurs through exposure to infected blood. Needless to say, adequate sterilization of medical equipment is essential. Unfortunately, there is no effective vaccine to prevent HCV infection. Extra-hepatic manifestations of HCV (e.g. renal disease with mixed cryoglobulinaemia and membranous glomerulonephritis) should be sought for at assessment, along with co-infection due to the routes of possible acquisition (e.g. HIV infection). Like HBV, chronic HCV infection is associated with the development of cirrhosis, hepatocellular carcinoma, LT and death [28].

Treatment is based on patient candidacy, extent of liver damage and genotype (although pan-genotypic treatment regimens are available). In the era of novel direct-acting antivirals, cure rates are excellent. In contrast to HBV, the goal of anti-viral therapy is to completely eradicate the virus. This can be predicted by the attainment of sustained virological response (i.e. undetectable HCV viral levels) at 12 weeks post-treatment. So, all newly discovered infections should be referred to the local Hepatology services for assessment of therapy. Complete eradication of HCV infection is a global aim, although access to diagnosis and treatment is the main barrier to this [29].

Alcohol Related Liver Disease

ALD can present in three ways: steatosis, alcoholic hepatitis or cirrhosis. The latter two are the most likely conditions to present to an anaesthetist.

General supportive care should be initiated in patients with ALD irrespective of presentation. Medications which provoke HE or renal dysfunction should be stopped. Patients with ALD and vitamin B1 (thiamine) deficiency are at risk of Wernicke's encephalopathy, which needs to be differentiated from HE and traumatic brain injuries. A withdrawal regimen (if required) and intravenous thiamine should be commenced. There is low threshold to commence antibiotics if an infection or variceal bleed is suspected. Malnutrition is associated with severity of liver dysfunction and outcome. Nutrition should be started early; enteral feeding preferably. Protein restriction is no longer recommended due to risks of muscle wastage. However, in severe HE, feeds containing branched-chain amino acids are an option to consider [30]. Hypotension should be aggressively managed with fluid resuscitation ± inotropes. Regular glucose monitoring is recommended. Onset of renal failure significantly worsens outcome, therefore terlipressin and HAS may be required.

Multi-organ Failure in Alcohol Related Liver Disease

Like other conditions requiring ICU admission, outcome is determined by the number of deteriorating organs. In a retrospective cohort study of patients with decompensated ALD admitted to ICU, the requirement for mechanical ventilation alone was associated with a 31% inpatient mortality. The requirement for additional organ support increased this to 85% [31]. However, these results require cautious interpretation as cause of death and previous ICU admissions were not discussed. Other studies suggest a lower mortality rate in patients with predominantly alcohol-related cirrhosis admitted to ICU (65% mortality with two organ failure) [32]. Patients with more advanced liver disease (of various aetiologies) have worse outcomes, e.g. Child-Pugh score of>12 admitted to ICU is associated with 80% mortality [33].

Non-alcoholic Fatty Liver Disease

NAFLD is one of the most common causes of CLD worldwide. It is the hepatic manifestation of metabolic syndrome (MS), which results from fat accumulation in the liver. MS is defined as the co-existence of obesity, hypertension and diabetes. Specific anaesthetic complications will be similar to those of obesity, e.g. difficult intubation. Known comorbidities associated with obesity, such as DM, cardiovascular disease, obstructive sleep apnea, metabolic syndrome, and impaired pulmonary function can impact transplant outcomes. These cardiometabolic risks are compounded by the increased incidence of hyperlipidemia, hypertension, and DM observed with immunosuppressive drugs [34, 35].

A body mass index (BMI) > 30 kg/m^2 has been considered a contraindication for LT in the past. However, patients with a high BMI and only one co-morbidity are now considered suitable for LT. We are expanding the indications for LT as we gain more experience [35].

MS, irrespective of liver disease, has negative impact on surgical outcomes and increases the risk of adverse perioperative events. In addition to death, the frequency of hypotension, hypoxaemia, hypertension and bleeding are increased in patients with MS [36]. Post-operatively, they have an increased risk of cardiac events, stroke, respiratory complications, acute kidney injury, wound complications, sepsis and prolonged length of stay [37–39]. MS has been associated with an increased incidence of atrial fibrillation, which has its own risks in the perioperative setting [40].

More specific to NAFLD, a meta-analysis on patients undergoing liver resection showed that postoperative risk was greater in those with > 30% steatosis of the liver, whilst those with < 30% steatosis did not have significantly reduced mortality [41]. Non-alcoholic steatohepatitis (NASH) is also associated with increased morbidity following hepatic resection [42].

NASH is common in patients with morbid obesity undergoing bariatric surgery (e.g. sleeve gastrectomy). Cirrhosis in these patients may be present in approximately 6%. Peri-operative mortality has been reported to be 4% in one study [43]. However, in general, bariatric surgery is well tolerated in patients with compensated cirrhosis [44, 45] and may reduce the risk of recurrent fatty liver disease post-transplantation [46].

Perioperative glycaemic control is important. Avoidance of significant hyperglycaemia can reduce perioperative morbidity/mortality. However, tight intra-operative glycaemic control may increase morbidity/mortality, due to perioperative hypoglycaemia and stroke [47].

Autoimmune Hepatitis

Autoimmune hepatitis is a chronic inflammatory condition of the liver which is characterized by circulating autoantibodies and elevated serum globulin levels [48]. It presents heterogeneously with a spectrum of clinical manifestations, such as acute hepatitis and ALF, as well as chronic liver disease and cirrhosis. Along with serological markers, liver biopsy is key in making a diagnosis. This condition can occur as an overlap syndrome with a cholestatic disorder. Once the diagnosis has been established, initial immunosuppressive therapy usually includes corticosteroids, thiopurines or mycophenolate mofetil. More potent immunosuppression may be required in severe refractory disease [48].

Some patients on long term corticosteroids may have an element of adrenal insufficiency. Perioperative "stress" doses of hydrocortisone should be given to these patients. Long-term immunosuppression makes these patients more prone to infective complications.

These candidates are relatively fit for their first LT and they are good candidates for fast tracking in centres where this is established practice. However, they can subsequently develop antibodies to the transplanted liver and consequently may require one or more re-transplantations. It is well known that a repeat LT poses a higher risk for postoperative complications and mortality.

Cholestatic Disorders

Cholestatic disorders of the liver include primary biliary cholangitis (PBC) and primary sclerosing cholangitis (PSC). PBC is a chronic autoimmune condition which slowly damages the bile ducts of the liver and, in some patients, can cause cirrhosis. Diagnosis is mainly based on cholestatic liver biochemistry and positive serology (anti-mitochondrial antibodies). Liver biopsy is not normally required. PBC can result in pruritus, metabolic bone disease, hypercholesterolaemia, cardiovascular diseases and fat malabsorption (including deficiencies of fat-soluble vitamins, e.g. vitamin K) [49]. Treatment for this condition includes ursodeoxycholic acid, obeticholic acid and the non-licenced fibrates. Responsiveness to ursodeoxycholic acid is often used to prognosticate course of disease. Severe disease often results in liver transplantation. Disease can recur post-transplantation.

PSC is another chronic progressive condition which affects the bile ducts of the liver. It results in persistent inflammation and fibrosis of the intrahepatic and extrahepatic bile ducts which leads to progressive cholestasis and eventually cirrhosis. It has an association with inflammatory bowel disease. Cholangiographic imaging may reveal characteristic multi-focal strictures and segmental dilatations. Liver biopsy is not necessary but may be useful in assessing small duct disease, overlap syndromes and excluding other conditions, e.g. IgG4-related disease. Use of ursodeoxycholic acid in these patients is controversial. Along with the other complications associated with cholestatic disorders, these patients are at increased risk of cholangiocarcinoma, gallbladder and colon cancer and require regular surveillance for these. Patients commonly develop end-stage liver disease and require LT. Once again, PSC can recur post-transplantation [50].

Patients with primary biliary cirrhosis (PBC) undergoing LT are usually well preserved and recover rapidly if they receive a good quality graft. A large proportion of patients with PBC are potential candidates for fast tracking [51].

Patients with PBC or PSC do not require any specific anaesthetic considerations. However, the presence of pulmonary hypertension is worth noting during the preoperative assessment, as this can develop before cirrhosis.

α1-Antitrysin Deficiency

α1-antitrypsin is a protease inhibitor which is encoded by the SERPINA1 gene. α1-antitrypsin deficiency is a rare inherited disorder, which causes a lack of this protective protein against proteolytic enzymes and subsequent liver and lung disease. Severity depends on the phenotype of disease, e.g. homozygosity for the Z allele conferring severe disease. Clinical manifestations of severe deficiency include early onset emphysema, liver cirrhosis and skin disease. Assessment of respiratory function is important preoperatively. Lung function tests may show an obstructive airway pattern with partial reversibility following bronchodilator inhalation. Chest imaging may reveal a pattern of emphysematous and bullous changes. Sometimes lung disease may be so severe that patients cannot undergo LT because of progression and irreversibility of lung disease [52].

Wilson's Disease

This is a rare autosomal recessive disorder of copper metabolism which leads to copper accumulation within the body. These patients have increased sensitivity to NMBs, resulting in prolonged muscle paralysis following their administration. This is related to decreased muscle function from the disease itself and long-term D-penicillamine (chelator) use. Atracurium may be a better option; due to Hofman elimination, it does not rely on hepatic or renal excretion.

Delayed intra-operative metabolism of hypnotic and sedative drugs can aggravate neuropsychiatric symptoms in patients with Wilson's disease in the post-operative phase.

D-penicillamine can impair wound healing due to inhibition of protein synthesis and collagen cross-linking [53]. Dosage should therefore be reduced perioperatively.

Haemochromatosis

Haemochromatosis is an inherited disorder of iron metabolism and results in iron overload. This can lead to iron accumulation in the heart, liver, pancreas, gonads and pituitary gland. Mainstay of treatment is with venesection with an aim of achieving a serum ferritin level <50 μg/L and transferrin saturations <50%.

These patients should be evaluated for complications such as diabetes and cardiomyopathy prior to surgery, as the presence of these influence perioperative care. Historically, these patients had poorer outcomes post-LT (likely due to underlying cardiomyopathy) compared to those with other aetiologies [54]. Outcomes have improved with better patient selection.

Vascular Conditions

Patients with Budd Chiari syndrome (characterized by hepatic venous outflow obstruction) and portal vein thrombosis are usually well established on anticoagulation prior to elective surgery. It is important that this is stopped at an appropriate time before surgery, with the arrangement of a suitable 'bridging' therapy. Pro-thrombotic agents should be avoided. Compression stockings and early post-operative mobilisation are important.

Due to the congested liver seen in patients with Budd-Chiari Syndrome, the dissection phase of LT can take longer and bleeding can be significant, despite pro-thrombotic diathesis. Administration of blood and products will further derange the hemostatic balance. Additionally, from a surgical standpoint, previous transjugular intrahepatic portosystemic shunt (TIPSS) placement can make LT technically more difficult [55].

Polycystic Liver Disease

Liver function is usually preserved in patients with polycystic liver disease. As a result, patients with a polycystic liver disease wait a long time before receiving a LT, at which point their native liver may be up to 20 kg. Consequently, surgical access to such a large liver may be difficult, and as a result blood loss during surgery may be greater. There is longstanding debate whether Veno-venous bypass should be used to make the dissection easier, shorter, and with less blood loss in this patient population.

Patients with polycystic liver disease do not usually experience hepatic failure, but rather suffer with abdominal pain due to liver distension. These patients typically have no clotting abnormalities. Careful patient selection for LT can lead to a more rapid recovery. Patients with polycystic liver disease will be in different stages of polycystic renal disease. Therefore, patients at an earlier stage of disease, without renal failure, would be expected to make a faster recovery following LT. When a combined liver and renal transplant is required, LT is commonly performed first, followed by the renal transplant. A change in the fluid replacement strategy occurs after the LT is complete. Once the new liver begins to function and clotting is stablised, fluid restriction is no longer an issue, and the aim should be to achieve normo-to-hypervolaemia with crystalloids to maintain renal perfusion. If patients were on dialysis preoperatively, CVVH may be performed intraoperatively and weaned in the postoperative period as the transplanted kidney begins to function.

Cystic Fibrosis

Although pulmonary complications remain the chief concern for patients with cystic fibrosis, their liver function can deteriorate to the point of requiring LT. In these instances, a thorough assessment of lung function is essential. In rare cases, lung transplantation and LT may be required. This should be performed at specialist centres where ECMO facilities are available [56].

Pregnancy-Related Liver Disease

The challenges posed by the physiological changes of pregnancy are well known. Although most organ functions will alter, surprisingly hepatic blood flow is unchanged during pregnancy. Nevertheless, a variety of conditions may impact liver function during pregnancy, including those described below. Importantly, the morbidity and mortality for the mother and fetus will be strongly associated with the aetiology of their liver failure.

1. **Pre-eclampsia or Pre-Eclamptic Toxaemia (PET)**: Characterized by hypertension and proteinuria. Usually presents in the 3rd trimester, but can also occur in the postpartum period. Patients should be managed in HDU as complications can develop unpredictably.
2. **HELLP syndrome**: Severe form of PET characterized by haemolysis, low platelets and elevated liver enzymes. Disseminated intravascular coagulation occurs in 20%. Acute renal failure is more common than in PET. Hepatic rupture is rare but associated with high mortality [57].
3. **Acute fatty liver of pregnancy (AFLP)**: Rare condition, debatably a variant of PET. Usually presents in the late 3rd trimester. Associated with high maternal and perinatal mortality and best managed in the ICU setting. Monitor for fulminant hepatic failure. Renal impairment, metabolic acidosis and lactataemia are also common [58].
4. **Obstetric cholestasis**: Caused by impaired bile acid excretion. Malabsorption of vitamin K is common and should be treated before central neuraxial blockade or surgery. Opioids can worsen pruritis.
5. **Viral hepatitis**: Most common cause of hepatic dysfunction in pregnancy. Higher incidence of acute hepatitis, ALF, HE and HRS during pregnancy. Risk of HBV vertical transmission is reduced with anti-viral therapy in the 3rd trimester in selected cases, and immunization of the fetus. Hepatitis E is more common in pregnancy. In these cases, the development of ALF has a mortality

rate of 30% [59]. Associated obstetric complications include premature delivery, growth restriction and perinatal mortality. Herpes simplex associated viral hepatitis in pregnancy can also cause ALF. Treatment is with acyclovir. Salvage LT is rarely required [60].

6. **Autoimmune hepatitis**: This usually improves during pregnancy. Immunosuppression should continue during pregnancy. In the absence of cirrhosis, maternal and fetal outcomes are favourable [61].
7. **Cirrhosis in pregnancy**: Pregnancy in patients with pre-existing cirrhosis is associated with high mortality. Portal Hypertension (PHTN) worsens during the 2nd trimester, thus increasing the risk of variceal bleeding. Concerns over increased risk of variceal rupture during labour often makes elective Caesarean section delivery preferable. Other complications include decompensation and maternal death. Prognosis can be predicted with pre-pregnancy MELD scores [62].

There are reports of LT during pregnancy in patients with acute or chronic or acute liver failure [63]. With an increasing number of case reports and series, we will develop a better understanding of how to manage pregnant LT patients and improve perioperative outcomes. Anaesthesia for LT in patients early in pregnancy is no different from non-pregnant patients undergoing LT. In more advanced stages of pregnancy, the physiological changes observed will represent a combination of alterations related to both liver disease and pregnancy. Due to the emotive nature of such cases, there is often a great deal of pressure on the perioperative multi-disciplinary team. Importantly, a delay in delivery, or delivery at the time of LT should be considered, as this may represent the management option with the greatest chance of success for both mother and child.

References

1. Lee WM, Stravitz RT, Larson AM. Introduction to the revised American Association for the Study of Liver Diseases Position Paper on acute liver failure 2011. Hepatology. 2012;55:965–7.
2. O'Grady JG, Schalm SW, Williams R. Acute liver failure: redefining the syndromes. Lancet. 1993;342:273–5.
3. Zoubek ME, Lucena MI, Andrade RJ, Stephens C. Systematic review: ibuprofen-induced liver injury. Aliment Pharmacol Ther. 2020 Jan 27. https://doi.org/10.1111/apt.15645. [Epub ahead of print] Review.
4. Willars C. Update in intensive care medicine: acute liver failure. Initial management, supportive treatment and who to transplant. Curr Opin Crit Care. 2014;20:202–9.
5. O'Grady J, Lake J, Howdle P, editors. Acute liver failure. Comprehensive clinical hepatology 1st ed. London: Mosby; 2000. p. 30.1–20.
6. Ferenci P, Lockwood A, Mullen K, et al. Hepatic encephalopathy—definition, nomenclature, diagnosis, and quantification: final re-port of the working party at the 11th World Congresses of Gastro-enterology, Vienna, 1998. Hepatology. 2002;35(716–21):14.
7. Ware AJ, D'Agostino AN, Combes B. Cerebral edema: a major complication of massive hepatic necrosis. Gastroenterology. 1971;61:877–84.

8. Bernal W, Hyyrylainen A, Gear A, Audimoolam VK, McPhail MJW, Auzinger G, et al. Lession from look-back in acute liver failure? A single centre experience of 3300 patients. J Hepatol. 2013;59:74–80.
9. Wright G, Shawcross D, Olde Damink SW, Jalan R. Brain cytokine flux in acute liver failure and its relationship with intracranial hypertension. Metab Brain Dis. 2007;22:375–88.
10. Barbier L, Ferhat M, Salamé E, Robin A, Herbelin A, Gombert JM, et al. Interleukin-1 family cytokines: keystones in liver inflammatory diseases. Front Immunol. 2019;10:2014.
11. Blaser A, Starkopf J, Ahazzani W, Berger MM, Casaer MP, Deane AM, et al. Early enteral nutrition in critically ill patients: ESICM clinical practice guidelines. Intensive Care Med. 2017;43:380–98.
12. Rosenblatt R, Shen N, Tafesh Z, Cohen-Mekelburg S, Crawford CV, Kumar S, et al. The North American Consortium for the study of end-stage liver disease-acute-on-chronic liver failure score accurately predicts survival: an external validation using a National Cohort. Liver Transpl. 2020;26:187–95.
13. Wieser A, Li H, Zhang J, Liss I, Markwardt D, Hornung R, et al. Evaluating the best empirical antibiotic therapy in patients with acute-on-chronic liver failure and spontaneous bacterial peritonitis. Dig Liver Dis. 2019;51:1300–7.
14. Bernal W, Wang Y, Maggs J, Willars C, Sizer E, Auzinger G, Wendon J et al. Development and validation of a dynamic outcome prediction model for paracetamol-induced acute liver failure: a cohort study. Lancet Gastroenterol Hepatol. 2016;1:217–225.
15. Lee WM, Hynan LS, Rossaro L, Fontana RJ, Stravitz RT, Larson AM et al. Acute Liver Failure Study Group. Intravenous N-acetylcysteine improves transplant-free survival in early stage non-acetaminophen acute liver failure. Gastroenterology. 2009;137:856–64.
16. Darweesh SK, Ibrahim MF, El-Tahawy MA. Effect of N-acetylcysteine on mortality and liver transplantation rate in non-acetaminophen-induced acute liver failure: a multicenter study. Clin Drug Investig. 2017;37:473–82.
17. Kjaergard LL, Liu J, Als-Nielsen B, Gluud C. Artificial and bioartificial support systems for acute and acute-on-chronic liver failure: a systematic review. JAMA. 2003;289:217–22.
18. Bernal W, Lee WM, Wendon J, Larsen FS, Williams R. Acute liver failure. A curable disease by 2024? J Hepatol. 2015;62:S112–S120.
19. de-Lima-Oliveira M, Salinet ASM, Nogueira RC, de Azevedo DS, Paiva WS, Teixeira MJ et al. Intracranial hypertension and cerebral autoregulation: a systematic review and meta-analysis. World Neurosurg. 2018;113:110–124.
20. Rajajeje V, Fontana RJ, Courey AJ, Patil PG. Protocol based invasive intracranial pressure monitoring in acute liver failure: feasibility, safety and impact on management. Crit Care. 2017;21:178.
21. Jalan L, Damink S, Deutz N, Lee A, Hayes P. Moderate hypothermia for uncontrolled intracranial hypertension in acute liver failure. Lancet. 1999;354:1164–8.
22. Guerra JF, Quezada JL, Cancino A, Arrese M, Wolff R, Benítez C, et al. Liver transplantation: development, learning curve and results after the first 300 cases. Rev Med Chil. 2019;147:955–64.
23. Bernal W, Caldwell SH, Lisman T. Nails in the coffin of fresh frozen plasma to prevent or treat bleeding in cirrhosis? J Hepatol. 2020;72:12–13.
24. Coelho S, Fonseca JN, Gameiro J, Jorge S, Velosa J, Lopes JA. Transient and persistent acute kidney injury in acute liver failure. J Nephrol. 2019;32:289–96.
25. Turton KL, Meier-Stephenson V, Badmalia MD, Coffin CS, Patel TR. Host Transcription factors in Hepatitis B virus RNA synthesis. Viruses. 2020; 30 12(2).
26. Kim SU, Seo YS, Lee HA, Kim MN, Lee EJ, Shin HJ et al. Cancer Epidemiol Biomarkers Prev. 2020 Jan 27. pii: Cebp.0614.2019. https://doi.org/10.1158/1055-9965.epi-19-0614. [Epub ahead of print].
27. Hefele L, Vannachone S, Khounvisith V, Phonethipsavanh N, Sayasone S, Kounnavong S et al. Lasting benefit of infant Hepatitis B vaccination in adolescents in the Lao People's

Democratic Republic. Int J Infect Dis. 2020 Jan 31. pii: S1201-9712(20)30058-8. https://doi.org/10.1016/j.ijid.2020.01.055. [Epub ahead of print].
28. Rial-Crestelo D, Sepúlveda MA, González-Gasca FJ, Geijo-Martínez P, Martínez-Alfaro E, Barberá JR, et al. Does fibrosis really regress in HIV/hepatitis C virus co-infected patients after treatment with direct antiviral agents? AIDS. 2020;34:427–32.
29. Soria A, Fava M, Bernasconi DP, Lapadula G, Colella E, Valsecchi MG et al. Comparison of three therapeutic regimens for genotype-3 Hepatitis C virus infection in a large real-life multicentre cohort. Liver Int. 2020 Jan 22. https://doi.org/10.1111/liv.14386. [Epub ahead of print].
30. Palma E, Riva A, Moreno C, Odena G, Mudan S, Manyakin N et al. Perturbations in mitochondrial dynamics are closely involved in the progression of alcoholic liver disease. Alcohol Clin Exp Res. 2020 Feb 4. https://doi.org/10.1111/acer.14299. [Epub ahead of print].
31. Mackle IJ, Swann DG, Cook B. One year outcome of intensive care patients with decompensated alcoholic liver disease. Br J Anaesth. 2006;97:496–8.
32. Cholongitas E, Senzolo M, Patch D, et al. Risk factors, sequential organ failure assessment and model for end-stage liver disease scores for predicting short term mortality in cirrhotic patients admitted to intensive care unit. Aliment Pharmacol Ther. 2006;23:883–93.
33. Rabe C, Schmitz V, Paashaus M, et al. Does intubation really equal death in cirrhotic patients? Factors influencing outcome in patients with liver cirrhosis requiring mechanical ventilation. Intensive Care Med. 2004;30:1564–71.
34. Spinosa M, Stine JG. Nonalcoholic fatty liver disease- evidence for a thrombophilic state? Curr Pharm Des. 2020 Jan 30. https://doi.org/10.2174/1381612826666200131101553. [Epub ahead of print].
35. Diwan TS, Lee TC, Nagai S, Benedetti E, Posselt A, Bumgardner G et al. Obesity, transplantation, and bariatric surgery: an evolving solution for a growing epidemic. Am J Transpl. 2020 Jan 21. https://doi.org/10.1111/ajt.15784. [Epub ahead of print].
36. Pomares J, Palomino R, Gómez CJ, Gómez-Camargo D. Metabolic syndrome and perioperative complications during elective surgery using general anesthesia. Rev Colomb Anestesiol. 2012;40:106–12.
37. Bhayani NH, Hyder O, Frederick W, et al. Effect of metabolic syndrome on perioperative outcomes after liver surgery: a National Surgical Quality Improvement Program (NSQIP) analysis. Surgery. 2012;152:218–26.
38. Lohsiriwat V, Pongsanguansuk W, Lertakyamanee N, Lohsiriwat D. Impact of metabolic syndrome on the shortterm outcomes of colorectal cancer surgery. Dis Colon Rectum. 2010;53:186–91.
39. Glance LG, Wissler R, Mukamel DB, et al. Perioperative outcomes among patients with the modified metabolic syndrome who are undergoing noncardiac surgery. Anesthesiology. 2010;113:859–72.
40. Tanner RM, Baber U, Carson AP, et al. Association of the metabolic syndrome with atrial fibrillation among United States adults (from the REasons for Geographic and Racial Differences in Stroke [REGARDS] Study). Am J Cardiol. 2011;108:227–32.
41. de Meijer VE, Kalish BT, Puder M, Ijzermans JN. Systematic review and meta-analysis of steatosis as a risk factor in major hepatic resection. Br J Surg. 2010;97(9):1331–9.
42. Reddy SK, Marsh JW, Varley PR, Mock BK, Chopra KB, Geller DA, Tsung A. Underlying steatohepatitis, but not simple hepatic steatosis, increases morbidity after liver resection: a case-control study. Hepatology. 2012;56:2221–30.
43. Brolin RE, Bradley LJ, Taliwal RV. Unsuspected cirrhosis discovered during elective obesity operations. Arch Surg. 1998;133(1):84.
44. Pestana L, Swain J, Dierkhising R, Kendrick ML, Kamath PS, Watt KD. Bariatric surgery in patients with cirrhosis with and without portal hypertension: a single-center experience. Mayo Clin Proc. 2015;90:209–15.

45. Sharpton SR, Terrault NA, Posselt AM. Outcomes of Sleeve gastrectomy in obese liver transplant candidates. Liver Transpl. 2019;25:538.
46. Diwan TS, Rice TC, Heimbach JK, Schauer DP. Liver transplantation and bariatric surgery: timing and outcomes. Liver Transpl. 2018;24:1280.
47. Wiener RS, Wiener DC, Larson RJ. Benefits and risks of tight glucose control in critically ill adults: a meta-analysis. JAMA. 2008;300:933–44.
48. Sciveres M, Nastasio S, Maggiore G. Novel Diagnostic and Therapeutic Strategies in Juvenile Autoimmune Hepatitis. Front Pediatr. 2019;7:382. 10.3389/fped.2019.00382. eCollection 2019. Review.
49. Harms MH, de Veer RC, Lammers WJ, Corpechot C, Thorburn D, Janssen HLA et al. Number needed to treat with ursodeoxycholic acid therapy to prevent liver transplantation or death in primary biliary cholangitis. Gut. 2019 Dec 16. pii: gutjnl-2019-319057. https://doi.org/10.1136/gutjnl-2019-319057. [Epub ahead of print].
50. Tibdewal P, Bhatt P, Jain A, Gupta D, Bhatia S, Shukla A. Clinical profile and outcome of primary sclerosing cholangitis: a single-centre experience from western India. Indian J Gastroenterol. 2019;38:295–302.
51. Bulatao IG, Heckman MG, Rawal B, Aniskevich S, Shine TS, Keaveny AP, et al. Avoiding stay in the intensive care unit after liver transplantation: a score to assign location of care. Am J Transplant. 2014;14:2088–96.
52. Zamora M. Surgery for patients with Alpha 1 Antitrypsin Deficiency: a review. Am J Surg. 2019;218:639–47.
53. Yarze JC, Martin P, Muñoz SJ, Friedman LS. Wilson's disease: current status. Am J Med. 1992;92(6):643.
54. Farrell FJ, Nguyen M, Woodley S, Imperial JC, Garcia-Kennedy R, Man K, Esquivel CO, Keeffe EB. Outcome of liver transplantation in patients with hemochromatosis. Hepatology. 1994;20(2):404.
55. Liu ZX, Zhu JQ, Ma J, Kou JT, Li XL, He Q. Deceased donor liver transplantation for Budd-Chiari syndrome: long-segmental thrombosis of the inferior vena cava with extensive collateral circulation. Hepatobiliary Pancreat Dis Int. 2019 Dec 4. pii: S1499-3872(19)30249-8. https://doi.org/10.1016/j.hbpd.2019.11.008. [Epub ahead of print] .
56. Morrell MR, Kiel SC, Pilewski JM. Organ Transplantation for cystic fibrosis. Semin Respir Crit Care Med. 2019;40:842–56.
57. Brady CW. Liver disease in pregnancy: what's new. Hepatol Commun. 2020;4:145–56.
58. de Vasconcelos Gaspar A, Ascensão TC, Santos Silva I. Acute fatty liver of pregnancy: rare, but potentially fatal. Am J Case Rep. 2020 Jan 29;21:e921122 10.12659/AJCR.921122.
59. Khuroo MS, Kamili S. Aetiology, clinical course and outcome of sporadic acute viral hepatitis in pregnancy. J Viral Hepatol. 2003;10:61–9.
60. Thurman RH, König K, Watkins A, Weerasiri T, Permezel M. Fulminant herpes simplex virus hepatic failure in pregnancy requiring liver transplantation. Aust N Z J Obstet Gynaecol. 2010;50(5):492–4.
61. Westbrook RH, Yeoman AD, Kriese S, Heneghan MA. Outcomes of pregnancy in women with autoimmune hepatitis. J Autoimmun. 2012;38:239–44.
62. Westbrook RH, Yeoman AD, O'Grady JG, Harrison PM, Devlin J, Heneghan MA. Model for end-stage liver disease score predicts outcome in cirrhotic patients during pregnancy. Clin Gastroenterol Hepatol. 2011;9:694–9.
63. Jankovic Z, Stamenkovic D, Duncan B, Prasad R, Davies M. Successful outcome after a technically challenging liver transplant during pregnancy. Transplant Proc. 2007;39:1704–6.

Chapter 10
Haemodynamic Monitoring During Liver Transplant Surgery

Annabel Blasi, Gianni Biancofiore and David Green

Introduction

Haemodynamic monitoring (HM) is fundamental under anaesthesia for liver transplantation (LT) given the previously described haemodynamic profiles of patients with end-stage liver disease (ESLD) or acute liver failure, potential rapid and significant blood loss, fluid shifts, vascular clamping and unclamping, the long anhepatic phase of LT, reperfusion syndrome, and primary liver nonfunction. Significant haemodynamic changes can affect graft reperfusion, myocardial performance, and the functions of all other organs [1]. There is no standard for HM during LT. The fact that there is such a variety of options for HM shows that each has advantages and disadvantages in terms of accuracy, validity, and reproducibility. Our impression is that the type of HM used may depend on LT centre volume, the experience of the anaesthetists, the economic status of the country, legislation, preoperative assessment and optimisation, surgical technique, and many other factors. Although different mechanical, electronic, and optical systems provide HM data, the human brain must understand and interpret these data and use them to better understand haemodynamic changes (which are just part of a much more complex process) and the choice of treatment. Knowledge of the value of monitor-derived data and the most frequent complications during anaesthesia for LT specifically is essential in the decision-making process. In this chapter we present the most common HM used during LT, with a summary of recent knowledge on this topic.

A. Blasi (✉)
Anaesthetic Department, Hospital Clinic Barcelona, IDIBAPS, Barcelona, Spain
e-mail: ablasi@clinic.cat

G. Biancofiore
Transplant Anaesthesia and Critical Care, University Hospital of Pisa, Pisa, Italy

D. Green
King's College Hospital, London, UK

Z. Milan and C. Goonasekera (eds.), *Anesthesia for Hepatico-Pancreatic-Biliary Surgery and Transplantation*, https://doi.org/10.1007/978-3-030-51331-3_10

Invasive Blood Pressure (IBP) Measurement

As the noninvasive blood pressure (NIBP) monitoring that is mandatory for all surgical procedures is not accurate enough for LT surgery, invasive blood pressure (IBP) monitoring is used for all LT patients worldwide. There is ongoing debate as to whether to use radial artery blood pressure (RABP), which reflects peripheral IBP, or femoral artery blood pressure (FABP), which reflects central IBP, or both at the same time [2]. RABP is widely accepted as the only method of measuring IBP and as part of beat-to-beat arterial pressure-based cardiac output (CO) monitoring, such as PiCCO, LiDCO, and FloTrac/Vigileo® [3]. However, PiCCO monitoring requires a central IBP signal via the femoral artery (FABP) and also for TP thermodilution for calibration. Flotrac has gone through 4 major software upgrades and is still unreliable as a SV monitor in conditions such as vasodilation often found in liver patients. LiDCO is the only monitor that has been validated as accurate using the radial artery as it is looks at the power of the overall waveform not the contour. It is also calibrated via the injection of a peripheral indicator.

The main argument against using RABP is more pronounced hypotension immediately after reperfusion compared to FABP [4]. The only reasonable explanation for this is that extreme peripheral vasodilation at the time of reperfusion decreases distal pressure disproportionately more compared to central pressure [4]. There are several disadvantages of measuring FABP: ischaemia is a rare but very serious complication [6]; when VV bypass is used, one groin has to be saved for the bypass; a haematoma may form during insertion of the FABP cannula; and if or when the aorta is clamped for arterial conduit, FABP cannot be assessed for at least 30 min at a time, although haemodynamic changes can be profound.

One study suggested that NIBP in addition to RABP may be an alternative to FABP for evaluating haemodynamic instability during reperfusion [5].

Central Venous Pressure

Measuring central venous pressure (CVP) is routine for all LT patients. The preload of the right atrium and ventricle is traditionally measured using CVP [3]. However, right ventricular preload is the volume of venous return to the heart, which determines CO according to the Frank–Starling law. Filling pressure is an indirect and inaccurate indicator of filing volume. In addition, frequent changes in the position of the liver also affect the CVP reading during LT surgery [7].

Although CVP is not an accurate assessment of volume status, many units use direct RABP and CVP measurements as the only HM during LT, partly because they cannot afford more sophisticated HM. However, there is no evidence that more advanced HM contributes to better outcomes following LT [8].

Pulmonary Artery Catheter (PAC)

A PAC directly measures right pulmonary systolic and diastolic artery pressure (PAP), pulmonary artery wedge pressure (PAWP), can assess mixed venous oxygen saturation (SvO_2) and can be used for the assessment of the cardiac output (CO), the cardiac index (CI) and systemic and pulmonary vascular resistance (SVR and PVR),

Although patients with ESLD have hyperdynamic circulation with a high CO and low SVR, CO is the haemodynamic variable most frequently used to monitor the cardiovascular state when circulatory instability occurs during LT [9].; PAC CO remains the clinical gold standard for assessing CO [10]. However, given the rapid haemodynamic changes during LT, the ability of a PAC to guide haemodynamic management during LT is limited [11].

This is because pressure measured using a PAC depend not only on the volume of the chamber (Frank–Starling law) but also on several mechanical factors that can affect intrathoracic pressure, such as positive end expiratory pressure (PEEP) or surgical retraction on the diaphragm.

There is less cardiac performance for a given preload compared to the normal curve during decreased left ventricular contractility/systolic heart failure (rarely seen in cirrhotic myocardiopathy). This is represented by a downward shift in the normal Frank–Starling curve [12].

However, a decrease in afterload will cause an upward shift in the ventricular performance curve in a similar fashion, leading to an increase in inotropy.

Conversely, an increase in afterload will cause a downward shift in the normal Frank–Starling curve, leading to a decrease in inotropism.

Changes in compliance of the myocardium, such as diastolic dysfunction and valvular pathologies (which can be present in patients with cirrhosis), also explain the poor correlation between pulmonary pressure (CVP/PAWP) and cardiac performance (SV/CO) [3].

Standard measurement of CO with a PAC involves injecting 5–10 mL cold 5% dextrose into the right atrium, which decreases the temperature in the pulmonary artery. The rate of blood flow is inversely proportional to the change in temperature over time [13]. The accuracy of PAC-derived CO depends on several factors, such as the respiratory cycle and temperature, and the volume and speed of the injectate, so the determination needs to be performed carefully at least three times giving the median value. The accuracy of thermodilution also decreases because of tricuspid pathology and/or intracardiac shunt [3]. Graft reperfusion is the most critical phase of LT, and a PAC can underestimate the actual CO because of the sudden release of blood and cold preservation storage fluids from the new liver, creating fluctuations in temperature. The CO reading is also affected if the anaesthetist administers a large volume of fluid during reperfusion to treat hypotension [3].

Semi-continuous measurement of CO can be achieved by a PAC-modified device that contains a filament to generate a hot instead of a cold water injection.

The correlation between the two techniques is good, which means it does not overcome the limitation of intermittent thermodilution during reperfusion [14, 15].

Modified PAC catheters provide continuous measurement of CO (CCO) and measurement of the right ventricle end-diastolic volume (RVEDV) and SVO_2. Della Rocca et al. conducted a multicentre study assessing the correlation between stroke volume index (SVI), RVEDVI, and filling pressure (CVP and PAOP) at four predefined phases of LT in 244 patients. SVI was strongly associated with cRVEDVI, although the correlations between SVI and CVP and PAOP were less strong [16]. The limitations of measuring cRVEDV originate from the thermodilution technique. In addition, the thermal filament of the catheter must be placed correctly in the right ventricle, as changes in the R wave of the electrocardiogram (arrhythmia or any other beat-to-beat variation in myocardial pacing) can affect the value [17].

Continuous monitoring of mixed venous saturation (SVO_2) requires insertion of a PAC. This parameter integrates data on CO, haemoglobin (Hb), and arterial oxygen saturation into a composite parameter; it is the percentage of oxygen bound to Hb in the blood returning to the right side of the heart. SVO_2 reflects the amount of oxygen remaining after the tissues remove oxygen. SVO_2 helps determine when a patient's body is extracting more oxygen than normal. Increasing extraction is the body's way of meeting the oxygen needs of tissue [18]. SVO_2 informs whether CO and oxygen delivery is sufficient to meet the patient's needs. Normal values are 65–75%; this denotes tissue oxygen extraction of 25%–35% and a normal PVO_2 of 35–45 mmHg [18].

Central venous saturation ($ScVO_2$): $ScVO_2$ can be measured directly from blood drawn from the superior venous system via a central venous catheter. Central venous saturation has been proposed as a less invasive alternative to SVO_2 for intraoperative HM. However, a study performed during LT showed that $ScVO_2$ cannot be considered equivalent to SVO_2 because of a lack of agreement between parameters during hepatectomy and after reperfusion. By contrast, in one study, good agreement between parameters was observed during the first stage of LT (hepatectomy). In that study, $ScVO_2$ overestimated SVO_2: 87 ± 7 versus 82.8 ± 7.3. The lack of a correlation can be explained by the increase in oxygen consumption by the graft after hours of ischaemia [19].

Unfortunately, SVO_2 and $ScVO_2$ have not been validated in patients with cirrhosis [20]. Although the normal ranges are not well defined in this population, the intraoperative trend in values during LT is very helpful as a guide for managing these patients clinically.

With all of the modifications of PACs, the only strong indication for standard PAC use during LT is pulmonary hypertension. Mean PA pressure>50 mmHg is a contraindication to LT because of high mortality (70–100%) [21].

With advances in preassessment, pulmonary hypertension can be detected by echocardiography. Transthoracic echocardiography (TTE) overestimates pulmonary artery pressure in patients with ESLD. When PAP measured using TTE indicates severe pulmonary hypertension, a PAC should be placed to directly monitor pulmonary artery pressure and calculate pulmonary vascular resistance [22]. Patients with severe pulmonary hypertension should be removed from the transplant waiting list and should undergo treatment for pulmonary hypertension. They should be relisted if PAP reaches values that permit LT. Patients with mild (mean PA pressure = 25–35 mmHg) and moderate (mean PA pressure = 35–45 mmHg) pulmonary hypertension need close monitoring and follow-up. Repeated measurement of PAP is indicated if patients are on the waiting list for more than 6 months. As a result of using this protocol, we rarely have patients with severe pulmonary hypertension. Thus, the need for a PAC during LT is reduced to almost 0 when adequate preassessment and optimisation are performed. On the rare occasions when patients end up in the operating theatre with severe pulmonary hypertension, transoesophageal echocardiography (TOE) is a good diagnostic tool for assessing pulmonary hypertension and guiding intraoperative treatment of PH [23].

Potential complications during PAC positioning are neither frequent nor negligible. In a review of the placement of 3,730 PACs for cardiac surgery, the incidence of serious mechanical complications related to PAC catheterisation was 0.1%: a right ventricular free-wall perforation, one knotting of the catheter, and two ruptures of the pulmonary artery [24]. The incidence of thrombotic complications may be as high as 53% [25]. Serious infection leading to a fatal outcome resulted when a catheter was left in situ after LT. Less serious complications include transient arrhythmia while inserting the catheter [24]. Complications due to vascular puncture may be reduced dramatically but not eradicated completely by inserting an ultrasound-guided catheter. We are aware of sporadic severe complications, sometimes with fatal outcomes, that have not been reported.

Transoesophageal Echocardiography

Recent surveys have reported the frequency of TOE use during LT at 87–94% in centres in the United States. About 38% of respondents reported using TOE routinely, and the rest used TOE in special circumstances. There is no uniformity across institutions with regard to the required certification needed to perform TOE in these settings, with up to 88% of users lacking certification in echocardiography [26].

The greatest strength of intraoperative TOE is its ability to directly visualise the right and left sides of the heart in real time. TOE can be used to assess right ventricle (RV) and left ventricle (LV) performance (systolic/diastolic dysfunction and wall abnormalities); volume preload; and intraoperative, but often devastating, rare conditions that cannot be otherwise easily detected, such as intracardiac air/thrombosis and Takosubo cardiomyopathy [27–31]. At the very least, the use of TOE in emergency situations, such as during unrelenting hypotension and/or unexplained hypoxia, is crucial [32–34].

A standard TOE examination of the most clinically relevant parameters is recommended immediately after inducing anaesthesia to assess baseline cardiac structure, ventricular function, and volume status.

Assessment of Ventricular Function

Left ventricular global systolic function can be assessed by simply visualising the size of the left ventricular chamber and its homogeneous contractile function in patients with coronary artery disease (32% of LT candidates with moderate to severe cirrhosis > 50 years display severe coronary artery disease on coronary angiography) [35].

Ischaemia can be detected in real time by regional wall motion abnormality. In fact, in one study TOE was more sensitive than EKG at detecting myocardial ischaemia [36].

Right ventricular function can be assessed by visualising the right ventricular area, the right–left area ratio, the shape of the right ventricle, its contractility, and the tricuspid annular plane systolic excursion (TAPSE). The normal range for TAPSE is not established in patients with cirrhosis.

The incidence of diastolic dysfunction ranges from 30 to 50% in LT candidates [37, 38]. It can be diagnosed by measuring the E/A ratio. The E/A ratio represents the ratio of peak velocity blood flow from gravity during early diastole (the E wave) to peak velocity flow during late diastole caused by atrial contraction (the A wave); it is a marker of left ventricular function. The E/A ratio in normal individuals is < 0.8. Values > 1.5 are highly suggestive of diastolic dysfunction [39].

Assessment of Volume

TOE has an important role in assessing hyper- and hypovolemia during LT by directly measuring left and right end-diastolic volume (area) or simply visualising the size and wall motion of the right and left ventricles. TOE findings are more accurate than CVP and PAOP [40, 41].

Respiratory variation in the superior vena cava can be used to define a positive response to a fluid challenge during mechanical ventilation. The threshold superior vena cava collapsibility of 36%, calculated as (maximum diameter on expiration—minimum diameter on inspiration)/maximum diameter on expiration), allows discrimination between fluid responsiveness (defined as an increase in CI of at least 11% induced by volume expansion) and no fluid responsiveness in patients with sepsis [42].

Patients with upper septal left ventricular hypertrophy may be at high risk for left ventricular outflow tract obstruction, which is severe hypotension caused by occluded left ventricular outflow with the anterior leaflet of the mitral valve [43, 44].

TOE can also be used to assess characteristics of major vessels, such as volume status, based on size and flow in the SVC, the suprahepatic anastomosis structure of the SVC, or the presence of a thrombus in the IVC and hepatic veins, assessing the reasons for allograft congestion and haemodynamic instability [45, 46].

TOE has the following significant limitations:

(a) It is operator dependent and requires significant training. The American Society of Echocardiography recommends a training program involving 300 TTEs and 50 TOEs and performing 50–75 TOE examinations a year to maintain proficiency [47], which is not achievable for most LT anaesthetists. Performing TEEs without formal qualifications has been questioned in the past.
(b) PAP is difficult to assess in the absence of tricuspid regurgitation.
(c) The transgastric view (mid-short axis) is the best view for visualising left end-diastolic volume; however, it is largely unavailable during LT because of posterior retraction of the stomach [3].
(d) Positioning of the retractors during the operation can affect the quality of the TOE and the images that can be obtained.
(e) There is a potential for serious misinterpretation, and inexperienced anaesthesiologists may mistake unfamiliar but normal anatomy as abnormal.
(f) Complications related to placement of the TOE, such as oesophageal perforation and variceal bleeding, are rare (<0.8%) but can be serious [48–50]. The most likely cause of variceal haemorrhage is increased variceal wall tension, which is exacerbated by intraoperative clamping of the hepatic vein. For this reason, limited manipulation of the probe during the anhepatic phase is needed.

As with any procedure involving intubation of the oesophagus, there is a small but not nonexistent risk for dental injury, oropharyngeal injury, oesophageal perforation, Mallory–Weiss tear, endotracheal tube displacement, or laryngeal palsy. Signs of oesophageal injury, such as a persistently sore throat, dysphagia, or haematemesis, should be monitored postoperatively [51].

Unfortunately, measurements of CO from a PAC and TOE are not interchangeable, and the degree of correlation varies with the MELD score. Overall, CO is underestimated by TOE compared to a PAC [52–54].

With the exception of pulmonary hypertension, which requires placement of a PAC, TOE is a suitable tool for monitoring LT as a standard of care in trained hands. The use of TOE in addition to a PAC may be a useful diagnostic option for the most serious cases.

Pulse Contour Continuous Cardiac Output Devices

PiCCO System Monitoring During LT

CO can be derived from arterial pulse pressure [55].

The Pulse Contour Cardiac Output (PiCCO; Pulsion Medical System, Munich, Germany) system requires placement of a thermodilution catheter into the femoral artery. It measures the blood temperature changes induced by a bolus of saline, derives a thermodilution curve, and calculates CO using an arterial waveform analysis algorithm. The PiCCO system provides continuous data on CO changes using pulse contour analysis [56].

Initial Transaortic (Transpulmonary) Thermodilution Bolus

This method of haemodynamic monitoring is less invasive than a PAC but still requires access to the femoral artery. It measures global end-diastolic volume and is used to calculate intrathoracic blood volume, a preload index, and extravascular lung water as a parameter of lung function. Thus, this method is used more frequently in the intensive care unit with complex post-LT patients.

This device allows the computation of stroke volume (SV) from an arterial pressure waveform. The arterial pressure waveform can be altered with significant changes in vascular tone (i.e., vasoconstriction as a consequence of the use of vasopressors).

When vasodilators are used, PiCCO underestimates CO by 40%. Recalibration is required when any major change occurs (i.e., rapid blood loss) but at that time we usually have no time for re-calibration.

Dynamic indices of fluid responsiveness, such as variation in stroke volume, pulse pressure, or systolic pressure, are the best indicators of responsiveness to fluid therapy, but they do not indicate the need for fluids.

This method has not been fully validated on ESLD patients, and many clinicians refrain from fully replacing fluids based on dynamic indices.

LiDCO Haemodynamic Monitoring During LT

The LiDCO device uses a lithium indicator as a diluent rather than thermodilution to calibrate the pulse waveform to CO [9]. The main difference between LiDCO and the other methods is that LiDCO relies on the arterial signal sampled (radial vs. femoral), the dilutional curve to obtain transpulmonary CO (lithium vs. cold saline), and the algorithm used to compute continuous CO.

LiDCO Plus Ltd., Cambridge, UK

This noninvasive device allows clinicians to measure CO based on the peripheral arterial pulse.

Because LiDCO measurements are derived from the radial artery pressure waveform, a peripheral artery site may not accurately reflect aortic pressure under conditions of extreme splanhnic vasodilation and systemic hypotension, often with concomitant vasopressor administration [3].

It is less precise than a PAC, in particular in haemodynamically unstable patients.

Available evidence suggests that the agreement between the two technologies is not always consistent, as the validity of LiDCO Plus during LT following abrupt haemodynamic changes needs further elucidation [3].

Positive side of LiDCO Plus monitor is that data recorded beat to beat can be stored and used for medicolegal or research purpose [9].

FloTrac/Vigileo Haemodynamic Monitoring During LT

FloTrac/Vigileo haemodynamic monitoring (Edwards Lifesciences, Irvine, CA, USA) uses a noninvasive device that allows CO measurements based on the peripheral arterial pulse system and does not require intermittent CO bolus calibration.

Its results correlate poorly with standard thermodilution CI measurements, in particular when SVR is low and haemodynamic changes are rapid, leading to pharmacological interventions.

The features of cirrhotic patients with a high CO and a low SVR are causative factors that limit all three methods during LT.

Several studies have found a poor correlation between waveform analysis CO calculations and PAC thermodilution during LT, in Child–Pugh class B and C patients for both the FloTrac and LiDCO devices [57].

This can be attributed to the haemodynamic profile of patients with cirrhosis (hyperdynamic circulation and low cardiac performance) and the sudden changes inherent in LT. In these patients, the degree of inaccuracy of FloTrac is proportional to the patient's systemic vascular resistance, with lower resistance being less correlated with reference thermodilution values [58, 59].

By contrast, FloTrac underestimates CO in LT patients whose CO exceeds 8 L/min [60]. Moreover, the algorithm used by these systems to calculate CO from the arterial waveform is based on factors that reflect the compliance and resistance of the arterial tree at the moment of calibration, and recalibration is needed when these parameters change. Biancofiore et al. determined CI with a PAC and by FloTrac/Vigileo (software version 01.10) simultaneously in 31 cirrhotic patients undergoing LTx. They reported that the FloTrac/Vigileo system underestimated CI and showed poor agreement with standard thermodilution CI measurements. The FloTrac/Vigileo system failed to reliably trend CI data below an acceptable level. A significant offset or bias was detected between the CI readings at a low SVR that was related to the degree of peripheral vasodilation [59]. Another study by the same investigators assessed the accuracy and reliability of a third-generation (version 3.02) FloTrac/Vigileo algorithm software by measuring pulse contour analysis–derived CI and PAC thermodilution–derived CI in the same setting. The version 3.02 FloTrac/Vigileo software significantly reduced the adverse effects of pulse contour CO reading bias in low peripheral resistance states and improved the overall precision of the system. However, although the trending ability of the new software improved, it remained well below current benchmarks for monitoring cirrhotic patients undergoing LT [58].

Continuous analyses of the arterial waveform introduced the so-called dynamic indices (variation in systolic volume, systolic pressure, and pulse pressure), which are the best indicators of response to fluid therapy in other settings [61]. This parameter fails to predict fluid responsiveness in cirrhotic patients during LT [62]. Nevertheless, the variation in systolic volume measured using FloTrac versus the variation in systolic volume measured using Doppler transthoracic echocardiography (calculated as the velocity time integral of aortic blood flow) showed acceptable bias, limits of agreement, and similar performance in terms of fluid responsiveness [63].

All peripheral arterial waveform analyses become less reliable for LT intraoperative monitoring as disease progresses from Child–Pugh class A to Child–Pugh class B and class C [15, 53].

References

1. Fukazawa K, Yamada Y, Gologorsky E, Arheart KL, Pretto EA. Hemodynamic recovery following postreperfusion syndrome in liver transplantation. J Cardiothorac Vasc Anesth. 2014;28:994–1002.
2. Arnal D, Garutti I, Perez-Peña J, Olmedilla L, Tzenkov IG. Radial to femoral arterial blood pressure differences during liver transplantation. Anaesthesia. 2005;60:766–71.
3. Feltracco P, Biancofuore G, Ori C, Saner FH, Della Rocca G. Limits and pitfalls of haemodynamic monitoring systems in liver transplantation surgery. Minerva Anesthesiologica. 2012;78:1372–84.
4. Krenn CG, De Wolf AM. Current approach to intraoperative monitoring in liver transplantation. Curr Opin Organ Transpl. 2008;13:285–90.
5. Lee M, Weinberg L, Pearce B, Scurrah N, Story DA, Pillai P, et al. Agreement between radial and femoral arterial blood pressure measurements during orthotopic liver transplantation. Crit Care Resusc. 2015;17:101–7.
6. Al-Talabani BG, Kareem T, Hassan T, Rasheed J. Limb amputation of an infant with transposition of great arteries using spinal anaesthesia. Edorium J Anesth. 2018;4:100016A05BA2018.
7. Lichtenegger P, Schiefer J, Graf A, Berlakovich G, Faybik P, Baron DM et al. The association of pre-operative anaemia with survival after orthotopic liver transplantation. Anaesthesia. 2019 Nov 7. https://doi.org/10.1111/anae.14918. [Epub ahead of print].
8. Rando K, Niemann CU, Taura P, Klinck J. Optomizing cost-effectiveness in perioperative care for liver transplantation: a model for low-to medium income countries. Liver Transpl. 2011; 17: 1247–78.
9. Milan Z, Taylor C, Armstrong D, Davies P, Roberts S, Rupnik B, et al. Does preoperative beta-blocker use influence intraoperative hemodynamic profile and post-operative course of liver transplsntation? Transpl Proc. 2016;48:11–5.
10. Lee M, Weinberg L, Pearce B, Scurrah N, Story DA, Pillai P, et al. Agreement in hemodynamic monitoring during orthotopic liver transplantation: a comparison of Flo Trac/

Vigileo at two monitoring sites with Pulmonary artery catheter thermodilution. J Clin Monit Comput. 2017;31:343–51.
11. Vetrung L, Bignmi E, Barbariol F, Langiano N, De Lorenzo F, Matellon C, et al. Cardiac output measurement in liver transplantation patients using pulmonary artery and transpulmonary thermodilution: a comparative study. J Clin Monit Comput. 2019;33:223–31.
12. Sequeira V, van der Velden J. The Frank-Starling Law: a jigsaw of titin proportions. Biophys Rev. 2017;9:259–67.
13. https://www.edwards.com/gb/devices/Hemodynamic-Monitoring/swan-ganz-catheters. Accessed 21 November 2019.
14. Bottiger BW, Sinner B, Motsch J, Bach A, Bauer H, Martin E. Continuous versus intermittent thermodilution cardiac output measurement during orthotopic liver transplantation. Anaesthesia. 1997;52:207–14.
15. Naik BI, Durieux ME. Hemodynamic monitoring devices: putting it all together. Best Pract Res Clin Anaesthesiol. 2014;28:477–88.
16. Di Marco P, Della Rocca G, Costa MG, Feltracco P, Biancofiore G, Begliomini B, et al. Continuous right ventricular end diastolic volume and right ventricular ejection fraction during liver transplantation: a multicenter stud. Liver Transpl. 2007;13:767–8.
17. Wagner JG, Leatherman JW. Right ventricular end-diastolic volume as a predictor of the hemodynamic response to a fluid challenge. Chest. 1998;113:1048–54.
18. Kim KM, Ko JS, Gwak MS, Kim GS, Cho HS. Comparison of mixed venous oxygen saturation after in vitro calibration of pulmonary artery catheter with that of pulmonary artery blood in patients undergoing donor liver transplantation. Transpl Proc. 2013;45:1961–9.
19. Dahmani S, Paugam-Burtz C, Gauss T, Alves M, Le Bihan E, Necib S, et al. Comparison of central and mixed venous saturation during liver transplantation in cirrhotic patients: a pilot study. Eur J Anaesthesiol. 2010;27:714–9.
20. el-Masry A, Mukhtar AM, el-Sherbeny AM, Fathy M, el-Meteini M. Comparison of central venous oxygen saturation and mixed venous oxygen saturation during liver transplantation. Anaesthesia. 2009;64:372–82.
21. Ramsay MA, Simpson BR, Nguyen AT, Ramsay KJ, East C, Klintmalm GB. Severe pulmonary hypertension in liver transplant candidates. Liver Transpl Surg. 1997;3:494–500.
22. Krowka MJ, Fallon MB, Kawut SM, Fuhrmann V, Heimbach JK, Ramsay MAE, et al. International Liver Transplant Society practice guidelines. Transplantation. 2016;100:1440–52.
23. DuBroock HM, Salgia RJ, Sussman NL, Bartolome SD, Kadry Z, Mulligan DC, et al. Portopulmonary hypertension: a survey of practice patterns and provider attitudes. Transpl Direct. 2019;5:e456.
24. Bossert T, Gummert JF, Bittner HB, Barten M, Walther T, Falk V, et al. Swan-Ganz catheter-induced severe complications in cardiac surgery: right ventricular perforation, knotting, and rupture of a pulmonary artery. J Card Surg. 2006;21:292–5.
25. Connors AF, Castele RJ, Farhat NZ, Tomashefski JF. Complications of right heart catheterization. Chest. 1985;88:567–72.
26. Wax DB, Torres A, Scher C, Leibowitz AB. Transesophageal echocardiography utilization in high-volume liver transplantation centers in the United States. J Cardiothorac Vasc Anesth. 2008;22:811–3.
27. Suriani RJ. Transesophageal echocardiography during organ transplantation. J Cardiothorac Vasc Anesth. 1998;12:686–94.
28. Fahy BG, Hasnain JU, Flowers JL, Plotkin JS, Odonkor P, Ferguson MK. Transesophageal echocardiographic detection of gas embolism and cardiac valvular dysfunction during laparoscopic nephrectomy. Anesth Analg. 1999;88:500–4.
29. Sharma A, Pagel PS, Bhatia A. Intraoperative iatrogenic acute pericardial tamponade: use of rescue transesophageal echocardiography in a patient undergoing orthotopic liver transplantation. J Cardiothorac Vasc Anesth. 2005;19:364–6.

30. Eagle SS, Thompson A, Fong PP, Pretorius M, Deegan RJ, Hairr JW, et al. Takotsubo cardiomyopathy and coronary vasospasm during orthotopic liver transplantation: separate entities or common mechanism? J Cardiothorac Vasc Anesth. 2010;24:629–32.
31. Tiwari AK, D'Attellis N. Intraoperative left ventricular apical ballooning: transient Takotsubo cardiomyopathy during orthotopic liver transplantation. J Cardiothorac Vasc Anesth. 2008;22:442–5.
32. Shanewise JS, Cheung AT, Aronson S, Stewart WJ, Weiss RL, Mark JB, et al. ASE/SCA guidelines for performing a comprehensive intraoperative multiplane transesophageal echocardiography examination: recommendations of the American Society of Echocardiography Council for Intraoperative Echocardiography and the Society of Cardiovascular Anesthesiologists Task Force for Certification in Perioperative Transesophageal Echocardiography. J Am Soc Echocardiogr. 1999;12:884–900.
33. Soong W, Sherwani SS, Ault ML, Baudo AM, Herborn JC, De Wolf AM. United States practice patterns in the use of transesophageal echocardiography during adult liver transplantation. J Cardiothorac Vasc Anesth. 2014;28:635–9.
34. Vetrugno L, Barbariol F, Baccarani U, Forfori F, Volpicelli G, Della Rocca G. Transesophageal echocardiography in orthotopic liver transplantation: a comprehensive intraoperative monitoring tool. Crit Ultrasound J. 2017;9:15.
35. Carey WD, Dumot JA, Pimentel RR, Barnes DS, Hobbs RE, Henderson JM, et al. The prevalence of coronary artery disease in liver transplant candidates over age 50. Transplantation. 1995;59:859–64.
36. Smith JS, Cahalan MK, Benefiel DJ, Byrd BF, Lurz FW, Shapiro WA, et al. Intraoperative detection of myocardial ischemia in high-risk patients: electrocardiography versus two-dimensional transesophageal echocardiography. Circulation. 1985;72:1015–21.
37. Carvalheiro F, Rodrigues C, Adrego T, Viana J, Vieira H, Seco C, et al. Diastolic dysfunction in liver cirrhosis: prognostic predictor in liver transplantation? Transplant Proc. 2016;48:128–31.
38. Nagueh SF, Smiseth OA, Appleton CP, Byrd BF, Dokainish H, Edvardsen T, et al. Recommendations for the evaluation of left ventricular diastolic function by echocardiography: an update from the American Society of Echocardiography and the European Association of Cardiovascular Imaging. Eur Hear J Cardiovasc Imaging. 2016;17:1321–60.
39. Falletta C, Filì D, Nugara C, Di Gesaro G, Minà C, Baravoglia CMH, et al. Diastolic dysfunction diagnosed by tissue Doppler imaging in cirrhotic patients: Prevalence and its possible relationship with clinical outcome. Eur J Intern Med. 2015;26:830–4.
40. Cheung AT, Savino JS, Weiss SJ, Aukburg SJ, Berlin JA. Echocardiographic and hemodynamic indexes of left ventricular preload in patients with normal and abnormal ventricular function. Anesthesiology. 1994;81:376–87.
41. Burtenshaw AJ, Isaac JL. The role of trans-oesophageal echocardiography for perioperative cardiovascular monitoring during orthotopic liver transplantation. Liver Transpl. 2006;12:1577–83.
42. Vieillard-Baron A, Chergui K, Rabiller A, Peyrouset O, Page B, Beauchet A, et al. Superior vena caval collapsibility as a gauge of volume status in ventilated septic patients. Intensive Care Med. 2004;26(30):1734–9.
43. Essandoh M, Otey AJ, Dalia A, Dewhirst E, Springer A, Henry M. Refractory hypotension after liver allograft reperfusion: a case of dynamic left ventricular outflow tract obstruction. Front Med. 2016;16:3.
44. Maraj S, Jacobs LE, Maraj R, Contreras R, Rerkpattanapipat P, Malik TA, et al. Inducible left ventricular outflow tract gradient during dobutamine stress echocardiography: an association with intraoperative hypotension but not a contraindication to liver transplantation. Echocardiography. 2004;21:681–5.

45. De Marchi L, Lee J, Rawtani N, Nguyen V. Intraoperative transesophageal echocardiogram during orthotopic liver transplantation: TEE to the rescue! Semin Cardiothorac Vasc Anesth. 2018;22:146–9.
46. Khurmi N, Seman M, Gaitan B, Young S, Rosenfeld D, Giorgakis E, et al. Nontraditional use of TEE to evaluate hepatic vasculature and guide surgical management in orthotopic liver transplantation. Case Rep Transpl. 2019;19:1–6.
47. Douglas PS, Khandheria B, Stainback RF, Weissman NJ, Brindis RG, Patel MR, et al. ACCF/ASE/ACEP/ASNC/SCAI/SCCT/SCMR 2007 Appropriateness Criteria for Transthoracic and Transesophageal Echocardiography Developed in accordance with the principles and methodology outlined by ACCF: Patel MR, Spertus JA, Brindis RG, Hendel RC, Douglas PS, Peterson E, Wolk MJ, Allen JM, Raskin IE. ACCF proposed method for evaluating the appropriateness of cardiovascular imaging. J Am Coll Cardiol. 2005;46:1606–13.
48. Markin NW, Sharma A, Grant W, Shillcutt SK. The safety of transesophageal echocardiography in patients undergoing orthotopic liver transplantation. J Cardiothorac Vasc Anesth. 2015;29:588–93.
49. Burger-Klepp U, Karatosic R, Thum M, Schwarzer R, Fuhrmann V, Hetz H, et al. Transesophageal echocardiography during orthotopic liver transplantation in patients with esophagoastric varices. Transpl J. 2012;94:192–6.
50. Dalia AA, Flores A, Chitilian H, Fitzsimons MG. A comprehensive review of transesophageal echocardiography during orthotopic liver transplantation. J Cardiothorac Vasc Anesth. 2018;32:1815–24.
51. Mazilescu LI, Bezinover D, Paul A, Saner FH. Unrecognized esophageal perforation after liver transplantation. J Cardiothorac Vasc Anesth. 2018;32:1407–10.
52. Perilli V, Avolio AW, Sacco T, Modesti C, Gaspari R, Caserta R, et al. Use of an Esophageal echo-doppler device during liver transplantation: preliminary report. Transpl Proc. 2009;41:198–200.
53. Perilli V, Aceto P, Modesti C, Ciocchetti P, Sacco T, Vitale F, et al. Low values of left ventricular ejection time in the post-anhepatic phase may be associated with occurrence of primary graft dysfunction after orthotopic liver transplantation: results of a single-centre case-control study. Eur Rev Med Pharmacol Sci. 2012;16:1433–40.
54. Boucaud C, Bouffard Y, Dumortier J, Gaillac N, Sagnard P, Graber MC, et al. Transoesophageal echo-Doppler vs. thermodilution cardiac output measurement during hepatic vascular exclusion in liver transplantation. Eur J Anaesthesiol. 2008;25:485–9.
55. Hamilton WF, Remington JW. The measurement of the stroke volume from the pressure pulse. Am J Physiol Content. 1947;148:14–24.
56. https://www.aci.health.nsw.gov.au/__data/assets/pdf_file/0005/306590/Pulse_Contour_Cardiac_Output_Learning_Package.pdf. Accessed 21 November 2019.
57. Krejci V, Vannucci A, Abbas A, Chapman W, Kangrga IM. Comparison of calibrated versus uncalibrated arterial pressure—based cardiac output monitors during orthotopic liver transplantation. Liver Transpl. 2010;16:773–82.
58. Biais M, Nouette-Gaulain K, Cottenceau V, Vallet A, Cochard JF, Revel P, et al. Cardiac output measurement in patients undergoing liver transplantation: pulmonary artery catheter versus uncalibrated arterial pressure waveform analysis. Anesth Analg. 2008;106:1480–6.
59. Biancofiore G, Critchley LAH, Lee A, Yang X, Bindi LM, Esposito M et al. Evaluation of a new software version of the FloTrac/Vigileo (version 3.02) and a comparison with previous data in cirrhotic patients undergoing liver transplant surgery. Anesth Analg. 2011;113:515–22.
60. Della Rocca G, Costa MG, Chiarandini P, Bertossi G, Lugano M, Pompei L, et al. Arterial pulse cardiac output agreement with thermodilution in patients in hyperdynamic conditions. J Cardiothorac Vasc Anesth. 2008;22:681–7.

61. Pinsky MR, Teboul J-L. Assessment of indices of preload and volume responsiveness. Curr Opin Crit Care. 2005;11:235–9.
62. Gouvêa G, Diaz R, Auler L, Toledo R, Martinho JM. Evaluation of the pulse pressure variation index as a predictor of fluid responsiveness during orthotopic liver transplantation. Br J Anaesth. 2009;103:238–43.
63. Biais M, Nouette-Gaulain K, Roullet S, Quinart A, Revel P, Sztark F. A comparison of stroke volume variation measured by VigileoTM/FloTracTM system and aortic doppler echocardiography. Anesth Analg. 2009;109:466–9.

Chapter 11
Point of Care Viscoelastic Haemostasis Monitoring During Liver Transplant Surgery

Antonio Leon-Justel and Joe Macmillan

Introduction

Liver transplantation (LT) is regarded as a surgical intervention with potential for massive blood loss and replacement. Although the volumes of blood loss and replacement during LT have decreased over the past few decades [1], there remains potential for improvement.

Research into the complex nature of liver disease coagulopathy has led to the concept that the haemostatic profile in these patients is 're-balanced'; moreover, stable patients exhibit a reduced reserve, rather than an inherent bleeding diathesis, and can be readily tipped towards a bleeding or thrombotic tendency [2]. The various phases of LT along with fluid and blood product administration may contribute to additional disturbances in coagulation [3].

Monitoring haemostatic changes is a key aspect of timely and adequate intervention to prevent massive bleeding and thromboembolic events. Perioperative monitoring includes clinical observation of the operating field, traditional coagulation laboratory tests, point of care (POC) haemostatic monitoring, and monitoring of other parameters. In this chapter, we will discuss monitoring methods with a focus on current POC monitoring techniques, data interpretation, and recent evidence related to the benefit of POC haemostatic monitoring during LT.

A. Leon-Justel (✉)
Macarena University Hospital, Seville, Spain
e-mail: antonio.leonj.sspa@juntadeandalucia.es

J. Macmillan
King's College Hospital, London, UK

Z. Milan and C. Goonasekera (eds.), *Anesthesia for Hepatico-Pancreatic-Biliary Surgery and Transplantation*, https://doi.org/10.1007/978-3-030-51331-3_11

'What Laboratory Tests Should We Use to Guide Coagulation and Transfusion Management During Liver Transplantation?'

Patients with liver failure have reduced levels of both pro- and anticoagulant proteins (Table 11.1); thus, all components of coagulation are considerably altered, such that pro- and anticoagulant systems are maintained in equilibrium. Disruption during the perioperative period can tip this balance toward either bleeding or thrombosis.

Conventional coagulation tests, including the international normalised ratio (INR), prothrombin time (PT), activated prothrombin time (APTT), platelet count (Plt), fibrinogen level, and haemoglobin (Hb) level do not reflect the coagulation system in the blood, because of the following factors:

- They are based on plasma alone and do not reflect interactions among platelets, vascular endothelium, and fibrinolytic factors.
- Activated prothrombin time and prothrombin time/international normalised ratio are sensitive to deficiencies in clotting factors, but not to the reduction of anti-coagulant factors present in patients with liver disease.
- An elevated INR does not predict bleeding complications [4].

Table 11.1 Alterations in anti- and pro-hemostatic factors in patients with liver disease

Anti-hemostatic	Pro-hemostatic
Platelets ↓Platelet count ↓Platelet activation ↑Nitric oxide ↑Prostacyclin	**Platelets** ↑vWF ↓ADAMTS 13 ↑Platelet hyperreactivity
Coagulation factors Reduced production of thrombopoetin ↓Factors II, V, VII, IX, X, XI, XIII ↓Fibrinogen	**Coagulation factors** ↓Protein C ↓Protein S ↓AT III ↓α2 macroglobulin
Fibrinolysis ↑Fibrinolysis ↓TAFI ↑tPA	↓Heparin co-factor II ↓ADAMTS-13 ↓Plasminogen
↓Vitamin K ↓α2 anti-plasmin ↓Production of thrombopoetin	↑Factor VIII ↑PAI ↑Procoagulant changes in fibrin structure

tTAFI thrombin activatable fibrinolysis inhibitor; *tPA* tissue plasminogen activator; *vWF* Von Willebrand factor; *ADAMTS 13* A disintegrin and metalloproteinase with a thrombospendin type 1 motif member 13; *AT* antithrombin; *PAI* plasminogen activator inhibitor

- Platelet count does not reflect the functional status of platelets [5]. Patients with end-stage liver disease are known to have a low platelet count and an elevated level of Von Willebrand factor, which may result in normal platelet function despite the low platelet count.
- Conventional coagulation tests are limited by the length of time from sampling to results.
- Conventional coagulation tests are generally unable to detect fibrinolysis, clot quality, or hypercoagulability [6–8].
- Fibrinogen level is the only conventional coagulation test that can indicate bleeding diathesis during LT [9].
- A low starting haemoglobin level is significantly associated with red blood cell transfusion rates; a low starting fibrinogen level is significantly associated with the platelet transfusion rate [10].

Many authors have suggested using a viscoelastic test (VT) as an alternative or complement to conventional coagulation tests to assess haemostasis during LT [11]. They assert that coagulation is a dynamic process and may be better studied using a global haemostasis assay, such as a VT.

Viscoelastic Tests

VTs measure the interactions among coagulation factors, inhibitors, and cellular components during clot formation and lysis phases over time. VTs provide valuable information regarding balance in the haemostatic system by examining the rate and total thrombin generated, individual haemostatic capacity, whole blood clot formation, and/or fibrin polymerisation, clot structure, and stability in artificially created conditions. VTs can be performed rapidly, thus providing immediate information useful for assessment of haemostatic status and its management in the majority of LT patients.

Thromboelastography (TEG; Haemonetics Corp., Rosemont, IL, USA) and thromboelastometry (TEM; ROTEM®, TEM International GmbH, Munich, Germany) are methods for assessment of changes in viscosity and elasticity, respectively, during the clotting process using whole blood. Both technologies are similar and provide similar information, with some differences in the parameters used.

Thromboelastography

TEG was developed in 1948 by Hartert [12]. When Kim introduced TEG to the LT programme, perioperative blood replacement decreased by 10 units per LT [13].

TEG uses a small instrument that can be easily implemented in the anaesthesia room. The instrument consists of two mechanical parts: a heated (37 °C) cuvette or cup, which oscillates, and a pin suspended freely from a torsion wire (Fig. 11.1). Freshly drawn blood is placed in the cuvette; the motion of the cuvette does not affect the pin while the sample remains liquid. However, when a clot begins to form, the fibrin strand 'couples' the motion of the cup to the pin; the shear modulus and elasticity of the clot is then transmitted through the pin and amplified to yield the TEG trace, which is recorded on heat-sensitive paper moving at a rate of 2 mm/min. The quantitative TEG variables are presented in Fig. 11.2 [14].

Normal values for TEG parameters and interpretation of TEG in terms of transfusion requirements are presented in Tables 11.2 and 11.3.

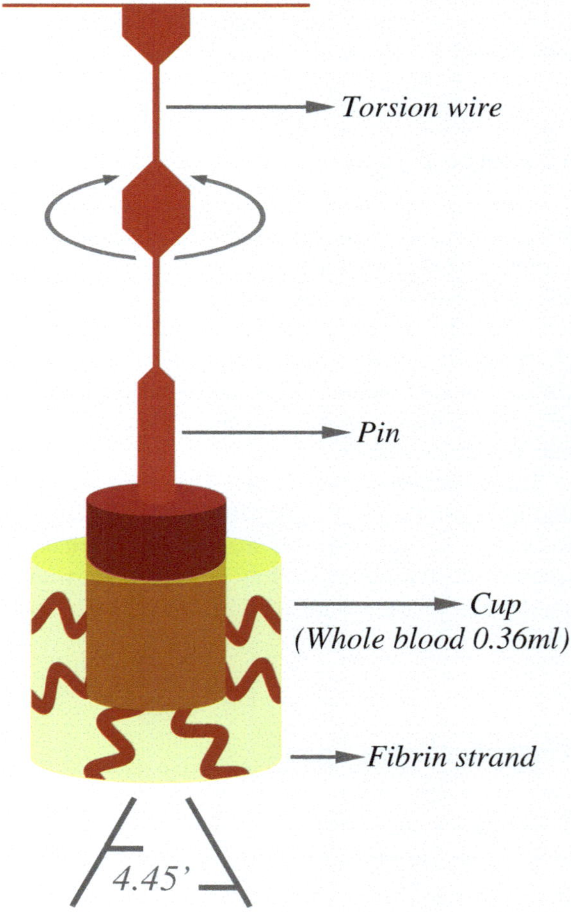

Fig. 11.1 Principles of thromboelastography

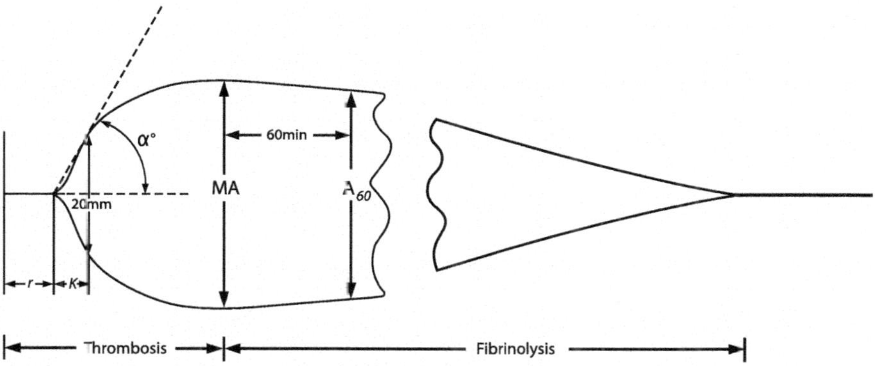

Fig. 11.2 Quantification of thromboelastography (TEG) variables. R = Reaction time, K = Clot formation time, Alpha angle = angle formed by the slope of the TEG, MA = maximum amplitude, A_{60} = amplitude of the tracing 60 min after MA is achieved

Table 11.2 Interpretation of Tromboelastography (TEG)

Parameter	Range	Description	Measures
R-time	5–10 min	Time to initial clot formation	Clotting factors
K-time	1–3 min	Time for fibrin to reach 20 mm	Fibrinogen/platelet number
α angle	53–72°	Slope between R and K	Fibrinogen/platelet number
MA	5–7.7 cm	Max amplitude	Platelet number and function
G value	5.3–12 dynes/s	Clot strength	Entire coagulation system
LY30	0–3%	Clot lysis at 30 min following	MA Fibrinolysis

Table 11.3 Interpretation for Tromboelastography (TEG) in terms of transfusion management

Value	Interpretation	Action
R time > 10 min	Low clotting factors	FFP
K-time > 3 min	Low fibrinogen or platelet number/function	Cryoprecipitate/platelets
α angle < 40°	Low fibrinogen or platelet number/function	Cryoprecipitate/platelets
MA < 45 mm	Low platelet function	Platelets
LY30 > 3%	Increased fibrinolysis	Tranaxemic acid or EACA

EACA Epsilon amincaproic acid

Thromboelastometry

TEM uses a principle very similar to that of TEG. The quantitative TEM variables are presented in Figs. 11.3, 11.4 and 11.5 and Table 11.4.

Clotting time (CT) is the point at which clots begin to form. It corresponds to the activation of thromboplastin with the formation of the first fibrin clots, and

Table 11.4 Interpretation of TEM

Parameter	Range	Description	Measures
CT		Time to initial clot formation	Low fibrinogen
CFT		Thrombin formation (kinetics)	Low fibrinogen and platelets
α angle		State of coagulability	
MCF		Max amplitude	Platelet and fibrinogen number/ function Platelet and fibrinogen
A10	<35 mm	Fibrinogen to clot strength	↓Fibrinogen of fib polimerisation
LI30			
ML	<15%	Maximal lysis	

CT clotting time; *CFT* clot formation time; *MCF* Maximum clot formation; *Fib* fibrinogen

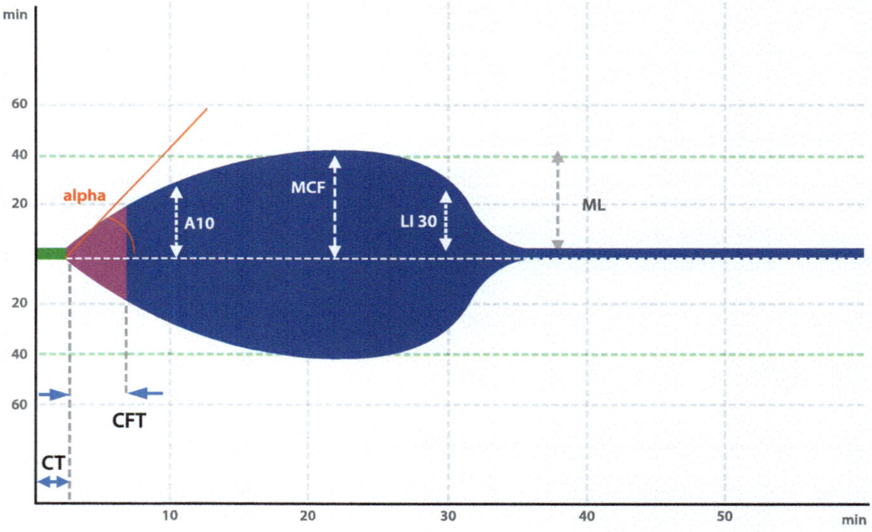

Fig. 11.3 Typical thromboleastometry tracings

reaches an amplitude of 2-mm. This is the point at which thrombin initially forms and the clot is polymerised. During this phase, coagulation factors and the effects of inhibitors can be assessed. Prolonged CT is not unusual during LT. It is rarely associated with a clotting factor deficit, as in liver disease. Pro- and anticoagulant pathways are both altered and are maintained in equilibrium. Prolonged CT is more frequently associated with low fibrinogen (FIBTEM, maximum clot firmness [MCF] <7).

Clot formation time (CFT) represents the kinetics of thrombin formation, fibrin polymerisation, and clot stabilisation through interactions among platelets, fibrinogen, and factor XIII. Prolonged CFT is associated with low levels of fibrinogen and/or a low platelet count.

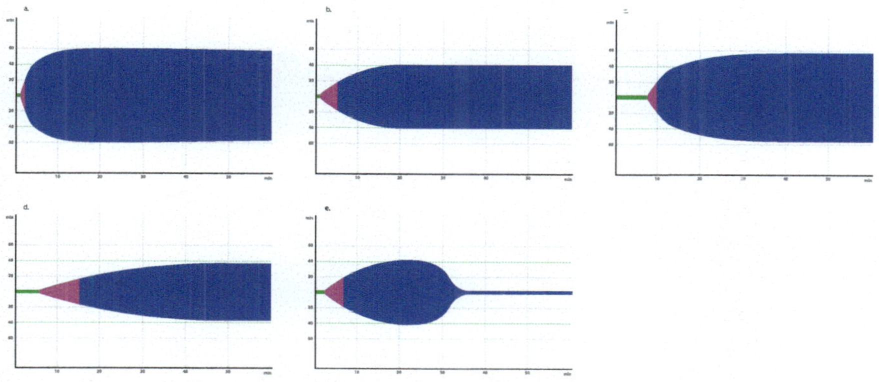

Fig. 11.4 Examples of TEM results: **a** normal TEM **b** CFT reduction due abnormal contribution to clot strength of platelets or fibrinogen **c** Long CT due an Insufficient generation of thrombin (deficit of coagulations factors or inhibitor presence) **d** Mix alteration, long CT with low MCF due abnormal contribution to clot strength of platelets or fibrinogen **e** Hyperfibrinolysis

Alpha angle indicates the patient's state of coagulability. A more acute angle indicates a greater tendency toward hypocoagulability. Conversely, a more obtuse angle indicates a greater tendency toward hypercoagulability.

MCF is the maximal amplitude of the graph. It represents peak clot stability, which is the result of fibrin polymerisation and interactions among platelets, fibrinogen, and factor XIII. MCF is an indicator of clot consistency and quality. The key determinants of whole blood clot strength are factor XIII, platelets, and fibrin/fibrinogen. The relative contributions of platelets and fibrin to clot amplitude (strength) are approximately 80% and 20%, respectively [15, 16]. Low MCF is associated with platelet dysfunction or a low platelet count, and/or fibrinogen dysfunction or low fibrinogen levels.

A05 to A30 is an assessment of clot firmness that is reflected by the graph amplitude between the 5- and 30-min time points. A10 is an earlier indicator of the contribution of platelets and fibrinogen to clot strength. Low graph amplitude at A10 (<35–40-mm) is normally associated with abnormal platelet and/or fibrinogen levels or function (an additional FIBTEM test should be completed to assess the final diagnostic).

Maximum lysis (ML) is the reduction in clot firmness after MCF. The clot is stable if ML is<15%. Hyperfibrinolysis occurs when ML is>15%.

Coagulation can be further assessed by utilising ROTEM®: INTEM, EXTEM, FIBTEM, HEPTEM, and APTEM. These tests have different reagents and their names are related to their roles or reagents that they use.

EXTEM: The EXTEM reagent is a tissue factor that activates the extrinsic coagulation pathway. It is a good screening test to assess the general status of coagulation during LT. Onset of clot formation is 70 sec. This test provides an assessment of the extrinsic pathway and evaluates the contributions of vitamin K-dependent factors II, VII, IX, and X.

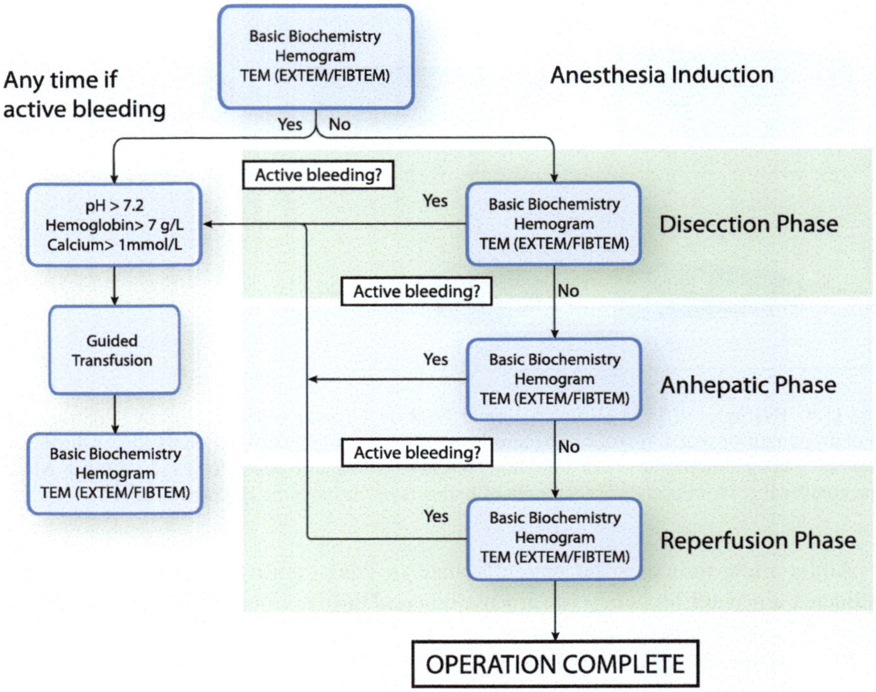

Fig. 11.5 Dynamic hemostasis monitoring based on POC laboratory test. During the anesthesia induction phase, should be performed a basal study including: basic biochemistry panel (acid-basic test, ionized calcium, lactic acid and hemoglobin), Blood Cell count (three population analysis) and ROTEM®. EXTEM is a good screening test to assess the general status of the coagulation and additional FIBTEM could be used as needed. Preventively correct abnormal results are not recommended

INTEM: The INTEM reagents are phospholipids and ellagic acid. This test constitutes an assessment of the intrinsic pathway (activation is triggered in the contact phase by ellagic acid). INTEM evaluates the contributions of factors XII, XI, IX, VIII, X, V, II, I, and von Willebrand. INTEM is a complementary test to EXTEM, which provides a general measure of coagulation during LT.

FIBTEM: The FIBTEM reagent is cytochalasin, which is a fungus-produced alkaloid that inhibits platelet activity. FIBTEM is used when there is an abnormal reduction in clot strength, as demonstrated by EXTEM or INTEM. FIBTEM helps to distinguish whether the reduction in clot strength is due to abnormal platelet or fibrinogen function and/or concentration. Therefore, FIBTEM can be used to guide administration of fibrinogen concentrate or cryoprecipitate and may reduce the administration of fresh frozen plasma (FFP), platelets, and red blood cell transfusions.

A10 and MCF show the contribution of fibrinogen to clot strength. Low A10 or MCF are related to low levels of fibrinogen (<1 mmol/L) or poor fibrinogen polymerisation, which are not uncommon in patients with cirrhosis.

HEPTEM: The reagents for HEPTEM are phospholipids, ellagic acid, and heparinase. Heparinase degrades any heparin that may be present in the sample. Activation is similar to that of the INTEM test. If HEPTEM corrects the change in CT relative to INTEM, then the cause of prolonged CT is due to heparinised blood; otherwise, prolonged CT represents a coagulation factor deficiency.

APTEM: The reagent for APTEM is aprotinin, a tissue factor. Aprotinin is a bovine pancreatic trypsin inhibitor that also inhibits plasmin. It serves as an adjunct to EXTEM to predict the clinical effect of fibrinolysis inhibitors in patients with hyperfibrinolysis. The effects of APTEM mimic treatment with tranexamic acid.

'How Do We Use POC Laboratory Tests to Support Coagulation and Transfusion Management During Liver Transplantation?'

Blood transfusions are associated with increases in infectious and respiratory complications, longer intensive care unit (ICU) length of stay, and higher rates of reoperation and mortality among affected patients [17]. In addition, transfusion of packed red blood cells is associated with an increased incidence of hepatic artery thrombosis [18, 19]. Uses of cryoprecipitate, platelets, and FFP are associated with reduced graft survival at 1 and 5 years [18, 19].

With the increased understanding of POC testing, there have been considerable developments regarding the management of bleeding patients. Recent recommendations have been developed using guided transfusion models based on dynamic monitoring of patient coagulation status.

In 2017, the European Society of Anaesthesiology recommended application of interventional algorithms incorporating pre-defined triggers and targets based on intraoperative VTs. These guidelines provided individualised haemostatic intervention in patients with perioperative bleeding (level of evidence 1C) [20]. In a similar approach, the American Society of Anaesthesiologists Task Force on Perioperative Blood Management suggested the use of VTs for intraoperative patient monitoring [21].

According to published data, the best approach to reduce the transfusion requirement and improve patient outcome after LT involves dynamic coagulation monitoring and guided therapy using POC laboratory testing. Dynamic coagulation monitoring and guided therapy involve the performance of different POC tests during the procedure to detect coagulopathy early, as well as to perform targeted early therapy. Figure 11.6 describes a proposal for dynamic monitoring during LT.

Baseline tests should be performed at the induction of anaesthesia, including a basic biochemistry panel (acid-basic test, ionised calcium, lactic acid, and haemoglobin), blood cell count (three population analysis), and TEG or ROTEM®. EXTEM is a good screening test to assess the general status of coagulation. FIBTEM can also be used if necessary.

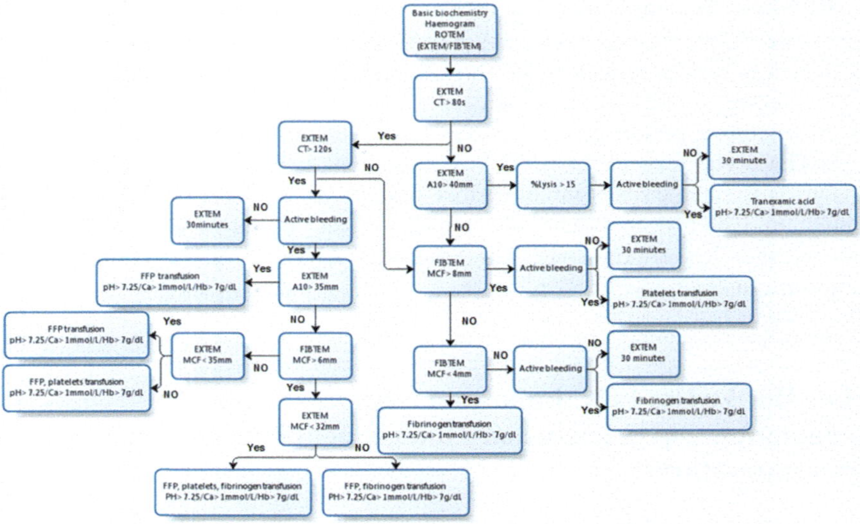

Fig. 11.6 POC guided therapy in LT. Flowchart showing details of the steps, assessment performed, and treatments administered. All the samples were analyzed for basic biochemistry, hemogram, and TEM (EXTEM and FIBTEM assay). CT: coagulation time (s); A10: clot amplitude 10 min (mm); MCF: maximum clot firm (mm); ionized calcium (mmol/L); Hb, hemoglobin (g/dL), FFP: fresh frozen plasma

The same testing protocol should be used during the dissection and anhepatic phase. Blood loss during liver resection is a major determinant of perioperative outcome. During the dissection and anhepatic phase, it is typical to find abnormal results, long CT, or low A10 and MCF because of the reduced levels of clotting factors due to surgical bleeding and the use of a high volume of crystalloids. Careful attention to fibrinogen levels is essential and use of FIBTEM is necessary if a long EXTEM-CT (CT > 80 sg) and low EXTEM-A10 (A10 < 35–40 mm) are observed. Hypofibrinogenemia (fibrinogen < 1 mmol/L) due to reduced synthesis, as well as dysfibrinogenemia, are commonly detected in LT candidates. In addition, fluid administration and bleeding during LT may result in extensive haemodilution and coagulopathy, with a reduction of plasma fibrinogen that is inversely proportional to the degree of bleeding and haemodilution [22].

Acidosis, hypocalcaemia, and hypothermia should be considered; they affect platelets, clotting factors, and fibrinolytic enzymes released from damaged cells, all of which can lead to increased fibrinolysis of previously formed blood clots.

Graft reperfusion is a critical step during LT. Haemodynamic disturbances are typical and can contribute further to disturbances in coagulation status, which is characterised by hyperfibrinolysis and global reduction of all factors. Coagulation disorders are strongly related to the abnormal contributions of platelets and fibrinogen. EXTEM A10/MCF and FIBTEM A10/MCF are useful for assessment of coagulation status and guidance of targeted therapy [23]. Hyperfibrinolysis is detected by EXTEM-ML > 15%, which is normalised by adding aprotinin

(APTEM) or tranexamic acid. Tranexamic acid is recommended to minimise bleeding during major surgery and/or to treat bleeding due to hyperfibrinolysis [24] (e.g., dose of 20–25 mg/kg) (level of evidence 1B).

The surgical field should be visually assessed for the presence of excessive microvascular or surgical bleeding. If active bleeding is detected, a basic study panel to detect early coagulopathy should be performed.

Hypothermia and acidosis induce coagulopathy. A core temperature < 34 °C inhibits thrombin generation, fibrinogen synthesis, and platelet function; it also increases fibrinolysis. Therefore, maintenance of a patient's body temperature within normal limits using different warming devices can reduce coagulopathy and bleeding during LT.

Acidosis (pH < 7.1) inhibits thrombin generation and platelet function, but accelerates fibrinogen degradation. Reversal of acidosis with a pharmacological agent does not correct acidosis-induced coagulopathy. However, prevention of acidosis using CVVH can avoid coagulopathy. As blood pH decreases from 7.4 to 7.0, FVII activity in vitro decreases by > 90% and FVII/TF activity decreases by > 60%.

The combination of hypothermia and acidosis, rarely present during LT, is more likely to cause coagulopathy, than each of these factors separately. In thromboelastometric studies of healthy volunteers, hypothermia-induced coagulopathy was reportedly exacerbated by acidosis, whereas acidosis without hypothermia had no significant effect on coagulation [25].

It is important to recognise that thromboelastometry performed at 37 °C may overestimate the integrity of coagulation in patients experiencing hypothermia and acidosis.

Hypocalcaemia can also increase coagulopathy during LT. The positively charged ionised calcium enhances fibrin polymerisation, coagulation factor activity, and platelet activity. The calcium level should be monitored hourly during LT. Some centres administer a calcium infusion during LT. If the ionised calcium concentration is low during a massive transfusion, boluses should be administered to maintain normocalcaemia (>1 mmol/L).

There are more complex guidelines for POC test-guided therapy in LT patients. The key points of the proposed POC test-guided therapy (Fig. 11.7) approach are as follows:

- Do not use a prophylactic transfusion based on an abnormal coagulation test.
- Coagulation disorders should not be corrected before or at the time of the transplantation, in the absence of uncontrolled bleeding [23].
- Fluid restriction reduces bleeding during LT [24] (level of evidence 1B).
- No FFP or platelets should be administered if the patient is not actively bleeding; rescue therapy should be used, rather than prophylactic or preventive therapy.
- After POC laboratory testing has been performed, a fibrinogen concentrate should be administered as first-line therapy in patients with clinically relevant diffuse bleeding and reduced clot firmness detected by the TEG, ROTEM®, or FIBTEM assays [25].

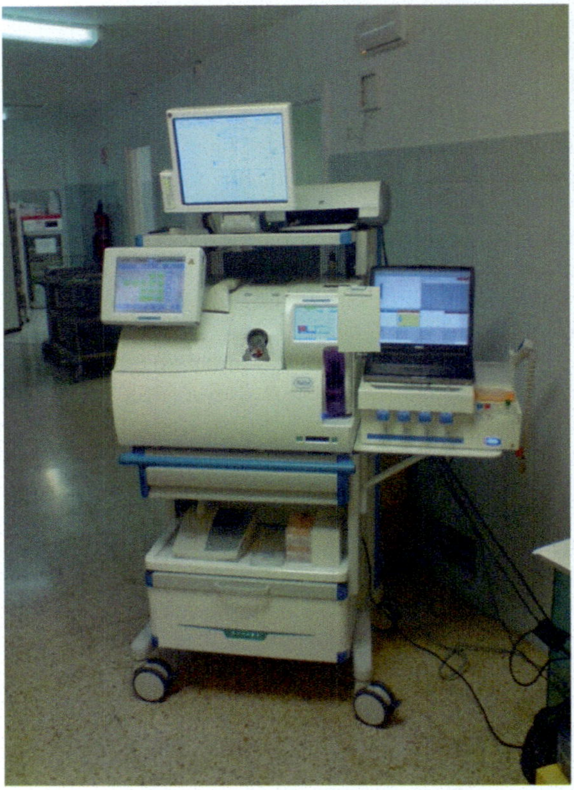

Fig. 11.7 Mov1Lab placed into the clean aisle next to the operation room. Virgen del Rocio University Hospital (Spain)

- FFP transfusion alone is insufficient to correct hypofibrinogenemia [24] (level of evidence 1C).
- An increased risk of thrombotic complications has been reported in association with fibrinogen transfusion [26].

An important concern is the personnel who should be running and interpreting the tests. The tests can be run by the operating room staff (nurse or anaesthesiologist) or by laboratory staff who are present in the operating room to complete and interpret the tests, in conjunction with the anaesthesiologist.

Various manufacturers provide the POC laboratory tests needed to support dynamic coagulation monitoring and goal-guided transfusion. Figure 11.7 shows an example unit (Mov1Lab® from Roche Diagnostic). It is mobile and can be placed in the operating room. It is used at the Virgen del Rocio University Hospital (Spain) and has been adapted to support haemostasis during high-risk surgeries, such as LT. Mov1Lab provides blood gas, acid-base, metabolic (including, glucose, sodium, potassium, ionised calcium and lactate) and blood cell (three-population analysis) analyses in a ROTEM® supported integrated system.

'Can POC Laboratory Testing Improve Patient Outcomes and Reduces Costs During LT?'

The benefits of using POC test-based haemostasis and transfusion management during LT surgery have been controversial [27]. However, POC test-based haemostasis and transfusion management are increasingly used in this setting and have gained recognition in terms of successful outcomes [28]. There is increasing evidence that using POC testing within a haemostasis management strategy is associated with reduced FFP usage and increased use of fibrinogen-containing products in LT patients [3].

Leon-Justel et al. reported a significant reduction in transfusion requirement when they compared a new approach, based on POC laboratory testing, with a previous practice based on conventional coagulation testing performed at the main lab: red blood cell transfusions dropped from 5 to 3 units, FFP dropped from 2 to 0 units, and platelets dropped from 1 to 0 units. In addition, total avoidance of transfusion was greater in the POC group, such that 24% of patients completely avoided allogeneic blood transfusion, compared with only 5% in the conventional group ($p<0.001$). Massive intraoperative transfusions were reduced from 13 to 2% [28]. Leon-Justel et al. also reported that the rate of re-exploration due to bleeding was>50% lower for patients treated using the POC testing approach [28]. Only 2% of patients under POC monitoring developed acute kidney injury [28]. Hendriks et al. [29] reported that 24% of patients underwent surgical re-intervention due to bleeding during the initial hospitalisation period.

A Cochrane review [32] regarding the effectiveness of transfusion strategies guided by POC devices in patients with severe bleeding found no evidence that POC monitoring improves mortality. A cost-effectiveness analysis suggested that the POC testing approach is cost-saving and more effective than standard laboratory monitoring during LT. Leon-Justel et al. and Craig et al. reported a cost-savings when using the POC testing approach [28].

Conclusion

POC testing was introduced many years ago and continues to improve. Training and consistent interpretation of data are important for effective POC testing. Notably, POC testing has reduced the use of blood, FFP, and platelets, whereas it has increased the use of fibrinogen-containing products. As the use of blood and blood products has decreased, the cost of treatment and the number of complications have both decreased. POC testing has not shown an effect on mortality; however, there is evidence for an increased frequency of thrombo-embolic complications.

References

1. Findlay JY, Long TR, Joyner MJ, Heimbach JK, Wass CT. Changes in transfusion practice over time in liver transplantation. J Cardiothorac Vasc Anesth. 2013;27:41–5.
2. Milan Z, Katyayani K, Cubas G, Unic-Stojanovic D, Cooper M, Bras P, et al. Trends in transfusion practice over 20 years in paediatric liver transplantation. Vox Sang. 2019;114:355–62.
3. Clevenger B, Mallet SV. Transfusion and coagulation management in liver transplantation. World J Gastroenterol. 2014;20:6146–58.
4. Yoon JK, Cheon JH, Choi YJ, Byoen GJ, Ahn JH, Choi EJ, et al. The correlation between conventional coagulation tests and thromboelastography in each phase of liver transplantation. Clin Transpl. 2019;33:e13478.
5. Bernal W, Caldwell S, Lisman T. Nails in the coffin of fresh frozen plasma to prevent or treat bleeding in cirrhosis. J Hepatol. 2010;72:12–3.
6. Werner MJM, de Meijer VE, Adelmeijer J, de Kleine RHJ, Scheenstra R, Bontemps STH et al. Evidence for a rebalanced haemostatic system in paediatric liver transplantation: a prospective cohort study. Am J Transpl. 2019 Dec 16. https://doi.org/10.1111/ajt.15748. [Epub ahead of print].
7. De Pietri L, Montalti R, Nicolini D, Troisi RI, Moccheggiani F, Vivarelli M. Perioperative thromboprophylaxis in liver transplant patients. World J Gastroenterol. 2018;24:2931–48.
8. Moore HB, D'Alessandro A, Moore EE, Wither M, Lawson PJ, Huebner BR, et al. Increase in post-reperfusion sensitivity to tissue plasminogen activator-mediated fibrinolysis during liver transplantation is associated with abnormal metabolic changes and increased blood product utilisation. Blood Transfus. 2019;17:312–20.
9. Craig J, Aguiar-Ibanez R, Bhattacharya S, Downie S, Duffy S, Kohli H, et al. The clinical and cost effectiveness of thromboelastography/thromboelastometry. HTA Programme: Health Technology Assessment Report 11 June 2008.
10. Massicotte L, Carrier FM, Denault AY, Karakiewicz P, Hevesi Z, McCormack M, et al. Development of a predictive model for blood transfusions and bleeding during liver transplantation: an observational cohort study. J Cardiothorac Vasc Anesth. 2018;32:1722–30.
11. Lichtenegger P, Schiefer J, Graf A, Berlakovich G, Faybik P, Baron DM et al. The association of pre-operative anaemia with survival after orthotopic liver transplantation. Anaesthesia. 2019 Nov 7. https://doi.org/10.1111/anae.14918. [Epub ahead of print].
12. Hartert H. [Blutgerinnungstudien mit der Thrombelastographic einen neven Untersuchungsverfahren.]. Klin Wochenschr. 1948; 26:577–83.
13. Kang Y. Liver Transplantation: historical perspedtive. In: Subramaniam K, Sakai T, editors. Anesthesia and perioperative care for organ transplantation. Springer, p. 319–33.
14. Mallet SV, Cox DJ. Thromboelastography. BJA. 1992;69:307–13.
15. Harr JN, Moore EE, Chin TL, Ghasabyan A, Gonzalez E, Wohlauer MV, et al. Platelets are dominant contributors to hypercoagulability after injury. J Trauma Acute Care Surg. 2013;74:756–62.
16. Harr JN, Moore EE, Ghasabyan A, Chin TL, Sauaia A, Banerjee A, et al. Functional fibrinogen assay indicates that fibrinogen is critical in correcting ab normal clot strength following trauma. Shock. 2013;39:45–9.
17. Maegele M, Brockamp T, Nienaber U, Probst C, Schoechl H, Görlinger K, et al. Predictive models and algorithms for the need of transfusion including massive transfusion in severely injured patients. Transfus Med Hemother. 2012;39:85–97.
18. Kozek-Langenecker SA1, Ahmed AB, Afshari A, Albaladejo P, Aldecoa C, et al. Management of severe perioperative bleeding: guidelines from the European Society of Anaesthesiology: first update 2016. Eur J Anaesthesiol. 2017;34:332–95.
19. Practice Guidelines for Perioperative Blood Management. An updated report by the American Society of Anesthesiologists Task Force on Perioperative Blood Management. Anesthesiology. 2015;122:241–75.

20. Sabate A, Dalmau A. Fibrinogen: a clinical update on liver transplantation. Transpl Proc. 2015;47:2925–8.
21. Blasi A, Beltran J, Pereira A, Martinez-Palli G, Torrents A, Balust J et al. An assessment of thromboelastometry to monitor blood coagulation and guide transfusion support in liver transplantation. Transfusion. 2012;52: 1989e98.
22. Sun Y, Jia LL, Yu WL, Yu HL, Sheng MW, Du HY. The changes of intraoperative body temperature in adult liver transplantation: a retrospective study. Hepatobiliary Pancreat Dis Int. 2018;17:496–501.
23. Lisman T1, Stravitz RT. Rebalanced hemostasis in patients with acute liver failure. Semin Thromb Hemost. 2015;41:468–73.
24. Villarreal JA, Yoeli D, Ackah RL, Sigireddi RR, Yoeli JK, Kueht ML et al. Intraoperative blood loss and transfusion during primary pediatric liver transplantation: a single-center experience. Pediatr Transpl. 2019 Jun;23:e13449.
25. Nielsen VG, Levy JH. Fibrinogen and bleeding: old molecule—new ideas. Anesth Analg. 2007;105:902–3.
26. Dickneite G, Pragst I, Joch C, Bergman GE. Animal model and clinical evidence indicating low thrombogenic potential of fibrinogen concentrate (Haemocomplettan P). Blood Coagul Fibrinolysis. 2009; 20:535e40.
27. Feltracco P, Brezzi M, Barbieri S, Galligioni H, Milevoj M, Carollo C, et al. Blood loss, predictors of bleeding, transfusion practice and strategies of blood cell salvaging during liver transplantation. World J Hepatol. 2013; 5:1–15.
28. Leon-Justel A, Noval-Padillo JA, Alvarez-Rios AI, Mellado P, Gomez-Bravo MA, Álamo JM, et al. Point-of-care haemostasis monitoring during liver transplantation reduces transfusion requirements and improves patient outcome. Clin Chim Acta. 2015;446:277–83.
29. Hendriks HG, van der Meer J, de Wolf JT, Peeters PM, Porte RJ, de Jong K, et al. Intraoperative blood transfusion requirement is the main determinant of early surgical re-intervention after orthotopic liver transplantation. Transpl Int. 2005; 17:673–9.

Chapter 12
How to Reduce Bleeding and Blood Transfusion During Liver Transplantation

Luc Massicotte and Zoltan Hevesi

Historically, orthotopic liver transplantation (OLT) has been associated with major blood loss and the need for massive blood product transfusions [1]. However, a significant decrease in blood loss and blood product requirements has been observed during OLT over the last 2 decades [2]. This development can be explained by increasing experience, improvements in surgical and anesthetic techniques, and a better understanding of the various hemostatic abnormalities encountered during OLT. Nonetheless, there is a wide range of blood product transfusion rates between various organ transplantation centers—and between different clinicians at the same centers as well—and this is true even for patients who do not have significant coagulation defects at baseline [3, 4].

Transfusion of blood products is associated with mortality and morbidity (infection, sepsis, reduced graft function, renal injury, immunosuppressive effects, transfusion related acute lung injury and transfusion associated cardiac overload) [5–10]. To reduce bleeding and transfusion of blood products, one must understand the physiology and coagulation abnormalities associated with cirrhosis. Patients with cirrhosis and portal hypertension have an altered blood volume distribution [11, 12]. The cirrhotic liver causes a blood flow obstruction in the portal vein and the compensatory increased secretion of vasoactive substances leads to an increased splanchnic pooling.

Before exploring the best approach for treating the coagulopathic derangements in liver failure, it is essential to understand normal hemostasis. The liver produces all coagulation factors with an extra-hepatic contribution of factor VIII by the endothelial cells which is increased during periods of stress. So, factor VIII—bound to von Willebrand factor (vWF)—is increased in cirrhotic patients.

L. Massicotte (✉)
CHUM (Centre Universitaire de l'Université de Montréal), 1051 Sanguinet, Montreal, QC H2X0C1, Canada
e-mail: Luc.massicotte@umontreal.ca

Z. Hevesi
University of Wisconsin, Madison, USA

Z. Milan and C. Goonasekera (eds.), *Anesthesia for Hepatico-Pancreatic-Biliary Surgery and Transplantation*, https://doi.org/10.1007/978-3-030-51331-3_12

In addition, the liver synthesizes the most important antithrombotic modulating factors (protein S, protein C, and antithrombin III) and key components of the fibrinolytic system (plasminogen and alpha 2-antiplasmin) as well. The liver is also essential for the clearance of activated coagulation factors from the circulation, which function is often impaired in hepatic failure.

In the pathologic state of end-stage liver disease (ESLD), numerous disturbances in this delicate balance arise. The coagulation system is adversely affected by low levels of prothrombotic factors and antithrombotic modulators at the same time. Deficient coagulation factors prolong the prothrombin time (PT), the INR (International normalized ratio) and the activated partial thromboplastin time (PTT); on the other hand, low levels of antithrombotic compounds may result in hyper-coagulable tendencies. Coincidentally, the fibrinogen level is normal or increased typically, but an excessive sialic acid content in the fibrinogen molecules results in a functionally abnormal fibrinogen [13, 14]. A combination of dysfibrinogenemia and a low level of factor XIII compromise fibrin polymerisation. Furthermore, the fibrinolytic system is also affected by liver disease because the concentrations of plasminogen and alpha 2-antiplasmin are often low, whereas an enlarged endothelial area may increase the concentration of the tissue plasminogen activator. Additionally, despite normal or even increased platelet production, the number of circulating platelets is reduced in the presence of portal hypertension with splenic sequestration. In patients with liver cirrhosis, the effect of thrombocytopenia is balanced by an increase in vWF multimers (platelet adhesive protein) and a low plasma level of the cleaving protease, a disintegrin and metalloproteinase with a thrombospondin type 1 motif, member 13 (ADAMST 13). It is well known that fibrinolysis during OLT is a contributor to nonsurgical bleeding; but, conventional tests of coagulation were found to be poor predictors of fibrinolysis. An increased concentration of tissue-type plasminogen activator concentration results in an accelerated fibrinolysis during the pre-anhepatic and anhepatic phases of surgery, and it frequently worsens immediately after graft reperfusion. In summary, hepatic dysfunction brings forth exceedingly complex changes in the natural balance of the normal state of hemostasis. The imbalance between coagulation and its inhibition, as well as the impaired regulation between fibrin polymerisation and fibrinolysis results in all forms of coagulopathy. Treating this global hemostatic imbalance is the sine qua non of managing patients for OLT.

The cause of bleeding during OLT is multifactorial [15]. Obviously, the extensive surgical trauma plays a major role in the origin of bleeding. This bleeding can be augmented in patients who had multiple prior abdominal surgeries, peritonitis, chemo-embolization and portal hypertension with varicose veins. Defects in the hemostatic system contribute to the bleeding. Hemostatic disturbances can be divided into those present before the OLT and those originating during surgery. The later can be classified according to the three main systems of hemostasis: coagulation, platelet function, and fibrinolysis. Hyper-fibrinolysis is an important cause of nonsurgical bleeding during OLT.

How to Decrease Bleeding and the Need for Transfusion

Management of Coagulopathy

New concepts affecting our understanding of conventional tests of coagulation in end-stage liver disease were discussed above and should be considered during the intraoperative management of these patients. Despite these new concepts, many liver transplantation centers follow the American Society of Anesthesiologists' (ASA) generic guidelines for the transfusion of blood products; threshold for red blood cell (RBC) transfusion: hemoglobin (Hb) of 60–100 g/L, threshold for plasma transfusion: INR higher than 1.5 (10–15 ml/kg), threshold for platelet transfusion: platelet count of less than 50×10^9 /L, cryoprecipitate trigger: a fibrinogen lower than 2 g/L [16]. For more than two decades now, various studies have shown that it is not necessary to correct coagulation defects before the anhepatic phase [17, 18]. A more recent study found that the transfusion of plasma for the purpose of correcting coagulation defects was not associated with a reduction in RBC transfusion. In fact, the opposite occurred [4]. Transfusion of plasma (10–15 ml/kg) at the beginning of the surgery increased central venous pressure (CVP), and the abnormally high intravascular volume resulted in portal venous congestion and increased bleeding. Furthermore, transfusion of plasma does not correct perfectly the coagulopathy reflected in an abnormal INR value. A series of 200 consecutive OLTs without any transfusion of plasma corroborates theses concepts [19]. Lately, many liver transplantation centers have adopted the "wait-and-se" approach of rescue therapy instead of prophylactic interventions.

Can bleeding be reduced by administering some pro-coagulant factor or medication? Recombinant factor VIIa was found to control bleeding in patients with complex acquired coagulation defect but two randomized trials failed to show efficacy when the drug was given prophylactically [20, 21]. On the other hand, anti-fibrinolytic agents are commonly used because fibrinolysis plays an important role in bleeding. Aprotinin—an inhibitor of plasmin with antiinflammatory properties—has been shown to decrease the need for transfusion during OLTs [22]; however, its use is no longer recommended because of recent evidence suggesting a dose-dependent increase in mortality, renal failure and other cardiovascular events [23]. Epsilon-aminocaproic acid (EACA) and tranexamic acid are the remaining frequently used anti-fibrinolytic agents, with the former being the more common. Neither drug has been studied as extensively as aprotinin was and there are fewer randomized controlled trials confirming their efficacy. Both are lysine analogs that inhibit plasminogen-to-plasmin conversion by adhering to lysine-binding sites on plasminogen. A study in 2011, comparing aprotinin to tranexamic acid in OLT, did not find any difference in bleeding, transfusion requirement and mortality. Tranexamic acid was as efficient as aprotinin [24].

Prothrombin complex concentrate (PCC) contains factors II, VII, IX, X and proteins C and S; and, it offers an attractive alternative for the treatment of coagulation factor deficits. Additionally, fibrinogen concentrate is also available to correct low fibrinogen concentrations.

Monitoring

The ability to predict intraoperative blood loss and transfusion requirements would be of great help to ensure optimal blood product use and to enable data-driven therapy for patients at high risk for bleeding. TEG (thromboelastography) and ROTEM (rotation thromboelastometry) are point-of-care tests to monitor coagulation and to provide clinical decision support. TEG and ROTEM analyzers work based on thromboelastographic principles. Both measure the viscoelastic properties of whole blood, coagulation generation and lysis. The instruments provide important global hemostatic information about the plasma-platelet-leucocyte interaction and clot tensile strength. ROTEM results are available more rapidly than those from laboratory-based conventional coagulation testing and provide more detailed information regarding coagulation speed, platelet function, clot strength and fibrinolysis. Kang et al. [25] used thromboelastogram (TEG) to achieve a decrease in red blood cell (RBC) use during OLT in the 1980's. ROTEM analysis includes plasmatic coagulation and fibrinolytic factors and inhibitors, as well as all circulating blood cells. Additionally, it provides important information about the quality of the final blood clot. The ROTEM provides four independent measuring channels; and, assays with different activators and additives are commercially available to detect and differentiate specific hemostatic defects such as hyperfibrinolysis, heparin and protamine effects, hypofibrinogenemia, fibrin polymerization disorders, coagulation factor deficiencies and thrombocytopenia. ROTEM has been mostly studied in cardiac surgery: two large observational and retrospective studies from Dr. Gorlinger et al. [26] and Karkouti et al. [27] found significantly reduced blood loss and decreased need for RBC and platelet transfusions. Unfortunately, at this time, only nine prospective randomized trials are available on 224 patients. Moreover, there is no prospective randomized study that compares TEG or ROTEM to conventional coagulation tests in OLT; however, some observational studies support the usefulness of both technologies. Most frequently, it is the guidance of antifibrinolytic therapy that TEG and ROTEM are used for [28]. Many centers adopted the use of TEG and ROTEM for OLTs.

Transfusion Threshold

It seems intuitively obvious that the skills of the surgeons would make a great difference in outcome but this complex issue is very difficult to objectively assess. For example, a team of two senior surgeons does not perform the same way as a team consisting of a junior surgeon and a trainee—fellow or resident—does.

It has been shown that the level of experience of the anesthesia team is also a major determinant of reduced blood loss, transfusion of blood products, need for post-operative mechanical ventilation and the duration of intensive care [29]. Furthermore, collaborative anesthesia-surgery interactions result in a more relaxed work environment and considerably increased academic productivity for members of the transplant team. As we described previously, there is a major variability of clinical care in the field of transplantation which includes major differences in transfusion practices [3, 4]. Generally speaking, more junior anesthesiologists tend to be more aggressive when correcting a low Hgb concentration or a coagulation defect [30]. Different thresholds for transfusion of RBCs or pro-coagulant products will result in different transfusion rates. Prophylactic transfusion of plasma increases the CVP, increases the congestion of the splanchnic bed and increases the bleeding and transfusions of RBCs. Consequently, adopting a threshold of 80 g/L instead of 70 or 60 for transfusing RBCs will increase the volume of RBCs transfused. Differences in institutional practices are likely to influence the use of all blood components. Inconsistent coagulation management methods with varying transfusion thresholds and algorithms for blood component intervention result in differences in the use of blood products with no clear effect on perioperative blood loss. The variable use of anti-fibrinolytics, which have been found effective in decreasing blood loss and transfusion in OLT, may be an additional factor in this area. Standardized, published evidence-based care is a more desirable and economical approach but, unfortunately, it is not the universal norm at this time.

Physical Measures

The conventional strategy for optimizing cardiac output was limited to generous intravenous fluid administration—to maintain arterial pressure and a renal perfusion—during periods of caval compression and clamping. This approach has been increasingly questioned and replaced on the basis of our improved understanding of the physiology of ESLD. During liver transplantation, bleeding is not usually caused by problems with major vessels but by transections in the complex mesh of portosystemic collateral veins; therefore, a causal connection was proposed between portal hyperemia, blood loss and overall fluid management. Patients with cirrhosis show alterations in the arterial and venous pressure-volume relationships, with a blunted cardiac output response to acute intravenous volume expansion [31]. Moreover, in severe cirrhosis, the regional blood volume distribution is altered. There is hardly any increase in central and arterial blood volume, while the non-central blood volume—mostly the splanchnic blood volume—increases. Consequently, blood volume expansion results in splanchnic venous pooling and congestion. In addition, the indiscriminate administration of blood products or crystalloid and colloid solutions may worsen coagulopathy by diluting or changing the balance between clotting factors. This hypothesis may partly explain the decreased need for blood transfusion when a low CVP was maintained [2]. In this study, the low CVP was achieved by utilizing phlebotomy and adhering to a restrictive fluid management before the anhepatic phase. The phlebotomy consisted of withdrawing blood from the introducer of the pulmonary artery catheter without any crystalloid or colloid volume replacement at the beginning of the case while CVP was monitored from the proximal port of the pulmonary artery catheter. Avoiding hemodilution led to a preservation of the coagulation factors level. Criteria for a phlebotomy were a hemoglobin concentration above 85 g/L and a normal renal function [2]. A drop of more than 20% of the arterial pressure from the induction of anesthesia was considered a contraindication for using phlebotomy; and, the phlebotomy was interrupted if the blood pressure dropped by more than 20% in spite of intravenous vasopressor administrations. The typical quantity of blood withdrawn was proportional to the patients' body mass, about 7–10 ml/kg. The normal CVP was restored only after the unclamping of the inferior vena cava. The intraoperatively withdrawn blood was returned to the patient at the end of the surgery unless indicated earlier. Norepinephrine, phenylephrine and/or vasopressin infusions were added to maintain an adequate blood pressure as necessary per the judgment of the clinicians. Because, portal venous pressure cannot be measured reliably intraoperatively, CVP is often used as a surrogate measure; however, one must use discretion and critical thinking when using CVP to guide intravenous fluid therapy because CVP is not an accurate and sensitive indicator of the overall intravascular volume status [32]. Fluid restriction to reduce portal perfusion requires liberal use of vasopressors and risks systemic and especially renal hypoperfusion: there is a limited amount of data available related to this concern and the published evidence is contradictory [4, 30].

Phlebotomy is an effective tool for decreasing portal venous pressure [33] but it is not an end by itself or a miracle treatment. From a series of 800 consecutive OLTs, phlebotomy decreased blood loss by a mean of 500 ml per case [30]. In a transplant center where the mean blood loss is 10 liters, phlebotomy will not make a significant difference; but, for a center where the typical blood loss is about 1500 ml, the median RBC transfusion rate may decrease to zero [34].

Some centers use diuretics to lower the CVP with good results in reducing transfusion of RBCs [35]. However, the use of furosemide is controversial because ESLD patients are often total body volume overloaded and are also generally intravascular volume depleted at the same time. Mannitol, however, has several characteristics that make its use advantageous during OLT. Patients with end-stage liver disease may have edema of the abdominal organs because of the congested blood flow through the fibrosed liver and the very prevalent hypoalbuminemia. The hyper-osmolar mannitol solution may facilitate the removal of free water from these organs, particularly in the setting of hepatorenal syndrome. It may also provide renal protection during the anhepatic stage. Furthermore, mannitol has potential free radical scavenging and antioxidant properties which may offer additional benefits such as a decreased incidence of post-reperfusion hypotension. Optimal dosing of mannitol is 0.5–1 g/kg during the anhepatic phase or just before cross-clamping. Nitroglycerin may be helpful in achieving a lower CVP as well in patients whose blood pressure tolerates it. In addition, using lower tidal volumes

6–8 ml/kg) for mechanical ventilation and avoiding positive end-expiratory pressure may help in minimizing CVP and, therefore, decrease the risk of bleeding.

An additional pharmacological strategy is intravenous vasopressin administration which has been shown to significantly reduce portal venous pressure and flow in the native liver without decreasing the cardiac output during OLT [12, 36, 37]. Patients with liver disease are known to have low endogenous levels of vasopressin and the use of exogenous intravenous vasopressin results in an increase in systemic vascular resistance and perfusion pressure. Using small bolus doses of vasopressin to treat episodes of hypotension is another method to circumvent the need for transfusion.

There is general agreement in the surgical community that conservation of the vena cava (piggyback technique) decreases blood use [38]; however, there are transplantation centers with exceptionally low transfusion rates despite practicing the classical cross clamping of the vena cava and using an interposition graft [2].

Intraoperative blood salvage has gained acceptance for OLT as another means of reducing banked RBC transfusion. In a study on 150 OLTs, the blood salvage resulted in a decrease of 2 RBC units per patient. The use of blood salvage is economical not only because RBC is expensive but a limited resource as well. The presence of a hepatocellular carcinoma (HCC) is not a contraindication to cell salvage as long as a leuko-reduction filter is used in the transfusion set.

Conclusion

Patients with cirrhosis or end-stage liver disease have a coagulation abnormality that is difficult to evaluate with conventional coagulation tests. There is a simultaneous decrease in pro-coagulant and anti-coagulant factors with a fragile and often poorly rebalanced hemostasis. At this time, a "wait and see" approach of rescue therapy is superior to the available prophylactic methods for correcting coagulation defects. TEG or ROTEM use is advisable for coagulation monitoring during liver transplantation. A combination of various published evidence-based physical and pharmacological strategies are available for the clinician to reduce bleeding and the need for blood transfusion.

References

1. Butler P, Israel L, Nusbacher J, et al. Blood transfusion in liver transplantation. Transfusion. 1985;25:120.
2. Massicotte L, Lenis S, Thibeault L, et al. Effect of low central venous pressure and phlebotomy on blood product transfusion requirements during liver transplantation. Liver Transpl. 2006;12:117.
3. Ozier Y, Pessione F, Samain E, et al. Institutional variability in transfusion practice for liver transplantation. Anesth Analg. 2003;97:671.

4. Massicotte L, Sassine MP, Lenis S, et al. Transfusion predictors in liver transplant. Anesth Analg. 2004;98:1245.
5. Brand A. Immunological aspects of blood transfusions. Transpl Immunol. 2002;10:183.
6. Hensler T, Heinemann B, Sauerland S, et al. Immunologic alterations associated with high blood transfusion volume after multiple injury: effects on plasmatic cytokine and cytokine receptor concentrations. Shock. 2003;20:497.
7. Massicotte L, Sassine MP, Lenis S, et al. Survival rate changes with transfusion of blood products during liver transplantation. Can J Anesth. 2005;52:148.
8. Ramos E, Dalmau A, Sabate A, et al. Intraoperative red blood cell transfusion in liver transplantation: influence on patient outcome, prediction of requirements, and measures to reduce them. Liver Transpl. 2003;9:1320.
9. Pereboom IT, de Boer MT, Haagsma EB, et al. Platelet transfusion during liver transplantation is associated with increased postoperative mortality due to acute lung injury. Anesth Analg. 2009;108:1083.
10. de Boer MT, Christensen MC, Asmussen M, et al. The impact of intraoperative transfusion of platelets and red blood cells on survival after liver transplantation. Anesth Analg. 2008;106:32.
11. Kiszka-Kanowith M, Henriksen JH, Moller S, et al. Blood volume distribution in patients with cirrhosis: aspects of the dual-head gamma-camera technique. J Hepatol. 2001;35:605.
12. : Mukhtar A, Salah M, Aboulfetouh F, et al. The use of terlipressin during living donor liver transplantation: effects on systemic and splanchnic hemodynamic and renal function. Crit Care Med. 2011;39:1329.
13. Tripodi A, Mannucci PM. The coagulopathy of chronic liver disease. N Engl J Med. 2011;365:147.
14. Lisman T, Porte RJ. Value of preoperative hemostatic testing in patients with liver disease for preoperative hemostatic management. Anesthesiology. 2017;126:338.
15. Porte RJ. Coagulation and fibrinolysis in orthotopic liver transplantation: current views and insights. Semin Hemost. 1993;19:191.
16. ASA guidelines. http://www.asahq.org/publicationandservices/transfusion.pdf.
17. Reyle-Hahn M, Rossaint R. Coagulation techniques are not important in directing blood product transfusion during liver transplantation. Liver Transpl. 1997;6:659.
18. Dupont J, Messiant F, Declerck N, et al. Liver transplantation without the use of fresh frozen plasma. Anesth Analg. 1996;83:681.
19. Massicotte L, Beaulieu D, Thibeault L, et al. Coagulation defects do not predict blood product requirements during liver transplantation. Transplantation. 2008;85:956.
20. Planinsic RM, van des Merr J, Testa G, et al. Safety and efficacy of a single bolus administration of recombinant factor VIIa in liver transplantation due to chronic liver disease. Liver Transpl. 2005;11:895.
21. Lodge JP, Jonas S, Jones RM, et al. Efficacy and safety of repeated perioperative doses of recombinant factor VIIa in liver transplantation. Liver Transpl. 2005;11:973.
22. Porte RJ, Molenaar IQ, Begliomini B, et al. Aprotinin and transfusion requirements in liver transplantation: a multicenter randomised double-blind study. Lancet. 2000;355:1301.
23. Mangano DT, Tudor IC, Dietzel C. The risk associated with aprotinin in cardiac surgery. N Engl J Med. 2006;354:353.
24. Massicotte l, Denault AY, Beaulieu, et al. Aprotinin versus tranexamic acid during liver transplantation: impact on blood product requirements and survival. Transplantation. 2011;91:1273–8.
25. Kang YG, Martin DJ, Marquez J. Intraoperative changes in blood coagulation and thromboelastography monitoring in liver transplantation. Anesth Analg. 1985;64:888.
26. Gorlinger K, Dirkman D, Hanke AA, et al. First line therapy with coagulation factor concentrates combined with point-of care coagulation testing is associated with decreased allogenic blood transfusion in cardiac surgery: a retrospective, single-center cohort study. Anesthesiology. 2001;115:1179.

27. Karkouti K, Callum J, Wijeysundera DN, et al. Point-of-care hemostatic testing in cardiac surgery: a stepped-wedge clustered randomized controlled trial. Circulation. 2016;134:1152.
28. Roullet S, Pillot J, Freyburger G, et al. Rotation thromboelastometry detects thrombocytopenia and hypofibrinogenaemia during orthotopic liver transplantation. Br J Anaesth. 2010;104:422.
29. Hevesi ZG, Lopukhin SY, Mezrich JD, et al. Designated liver transplant anesthesia team reduces blood transfusion, need for mechanical ventilation, and duration of intensive care. Liver tranpl. 2009;15:460.
30. Massicotte L, Carrier FM, Karakiewicz P, et al. Impact of MELD score-based organ allocation on mortality, bleeding, and transfusion in liver transplantaqtion: a before-after observational cohort study. JCardiothoracic Vasc Anesth. 2019, Mar 8. pii: S1053-0770(19)30268-X. https://doi.org/10.1053/j.jvca.2019.03.008. [Epub ahead of print].
31. Hadegue A, Moreau R, Gaudin C, et al. Total effective vascular compliance in patients with cirrhosis: a study of the response to acute blood volume expansion. Hepatology. 1992;18:809.
32. Gelman S. Venous function and central venous pressure: a physiology story. Anesthesiology. 2008;108:735.
33. Massicotte L, Perreault MA, Denault AY, et al. Effects of phlebotomy and phenylephrine infusion on portal venous pressure and systemic hemodynamics during liver transplantation. Transplantation. 2010;89:920.
34. Massicotte L, Carrier FM, Denault AY, et al. Development of a predictive model for blood transfusion, and bleeding during liver transplantation: an observational cohort study. J Cardiothorac Vasc. 2018;32:1722.
35. Shan WLP, Barkun J, Metrakos P, et al. Blood product use during orthotopic liver transplantation. Can J Anesth. 2004;51:1045.
36. Vater Y, Levy A, Martay K, et al. Adjuvant drugs for end-stage liver failure and transplantation. Med Sci Monit. 2004;10:77.
37. Wagener G, Gubitosa G, Renz J, et al. Vasopressin decreases portal vein pressure and flow in the native liver during liver transplantation. Liver Transpl. 2008;14:1664.
38. Groenland TH, porte RJ, Metselaar HJ. Liver transplantation and risk of bleeding. Curr Opin Organ Transpl. 2007;12:287.

Chapter 13
Fast Tracking in a Liver Transplant Programme

Stephen Aniskevich, Ryan Chadha and Sher Lu Pai

Introduction

As the practice of transplant medicine evolves, physicians have been able to manage these increasingly complex patients in ways previously thought impossible. These improvements have advanced the acceptable criteria for listing recipients, allowing for older and sicker patients to receive organs, and increased the donor pool by utilizing extended criteria organs, and have improved postoperative care. Concurrent with this, the field of transplant anesthesiology has also evolved and developed methods to improve outcomes in these patient populations. With the routine use of invasive monitoring and intraoperative transesophageal echocardiography and a better understanding of transfusion physiology, there has been enhanced recognition and management of intraoperative complications.

Physicians are now challenging the next "impossible" doctrine and applying the principles of fast track anesthesia to liver transplant recipients. Fast track anesthesia is the practice of extubating patients immediately at the end of surgery, recovering the patient briefly in the post-anesthesia care unit (PACU), and admitting the patient directly to the surgical ward, bypassing the intensive care unit entirely. In this chapter, we will review the history of early extubation and its evolution toward fast track anesthesia and describe its application in the care of transplant recipients.

S. Aniskevich (✉) · R. Chadha · S. L. Pai
Division of Hepatobiliary and Abdominal Transplant Anesthesiology, Department of Anesthesiology and Perioperative Medicine, Mayo Clinic Florida, 4500 San Pablo Rd, Jacksonville, FL 32224, USA
e-mail: aniskevich.stephen2@mayo.edu

Z. Milan and C. Goonasekera (eds.), *Anesthesia for Hepatico-Pancreatic-Biliary Surgery and Transplantation*, https://doi.org/10.1007/978-3-030-51331-3_13

History

Prior to the 1970s, clinicians felt that prolonged postoperative ventilation following major surgery was beneficial because it decreased the work of breathing and ensured adequate oxygenation while allowing patients to recover from the stress of surgery. This was especially true in the cardiac surgical literature where the recommendations of the time were to leave the patient intubated for up to 24 hours after surgery [1–3]. Some even advocated preemptive tracheostomy for management of potential pulmonary complications [4]. Starting in the early to mid-1970s, a trend to shorten this time emerged as clinicians realized that prolonged artificial respiration carried significant morbidity and mortality risks. In 1974, Midell first described early extubation following cardiac valve surgery [5]. In this study, 90 of the 100 patients were able to be extubated immediately in the postoperative period with 62 patients having no respiratory complications and 28 patients requiring only up to 2 hours of postoperative ventilation prior to extubation. In 1977, two more authors published articles evaluating early extubation in the immediate postoperative period. Klineberg and colleagues developed criteria based on specific surgical and physiological parameters to be suitable for early extubation at their facility. They reported that 62.5% of patients could be extubated within 5 hours of surgery and up to 91% with 20 hours using these guidelines [6]. Furthermore, when properly performed, early extubation resulted in significantly shorter length of stay in the ICU and hospital. Prakash, et al., also challenged the idea of prolonged ventilation following complex cardiac surgery [7]. Using a nitrous/narcotic anesthetic and specific respiratory criteria measured on mechanical and spontaneous ventilation modes, Prakash was able to extubate 123 of 142 patients within 3 hours of surgery. The majority of these extubations occurred within 1 hour from surgery's end. Only 5 patients who initially passed the criteria required reintubation. Taken together, these three early studies revealed that with proper clinical evaluation, the majority of the patients could be safely extubated in the immediate postoperative period following major cardiac surgery.

As evidence accumulated that early extubation was feasible and potentially beneficial following complex cardiac surgery, transplant anesthesiologists began applying the same principles to patients undergoing liver transplantation. As with cardiac surgery, detractors argued that a period of assisted ventilation allowed for intensivists to optimize physiologic and hemodynamic parameters. In 1989, a team from Mayo Clinic Rochester reported an average of 26 hours of ventilator support in their first 100 liver transplant patients, mainly due to poor nutritional status, ongoing hepatic dysfunction, neurologic conditions, or primary lung disease [8]. Carton suggested that routine transplant cases needed up to 36 hours on a ventilator and a six day ICU stay [9]. In support of early extubation, several animal studies at the time began reporting on the detrimental effects of mechanical ventilation on liver function. Multiple mechanisms including decreased venous return resulting in a reduction in cardiac output, transmission of venous backpressure via the inferior vena cava to the liver sinusoids, and an increase in intrahepatic tissue pressure from inspiratory diaphragmatic descent were theorized. Brendenberg and Paskanik evaluated the effects of positive end expiratory pressure (PEEP) in dogs. They found that increasing PEEP resulted in a decreased cardiac output and subsequently a reduction in hepatic arterial flow [10]. In this study, a dextran infusion to maintain cardiac output countered the decrease in portal blood flow when administered during application of 15 cm H_2O of PEEP. Brienza, in a pig model, showed PEEP decreased both hepatic artery and portal venous flow related to venous back-pressure and an increase in surrounding tissue pressure [11]. However, these initial animal studies have been recently challenged by research showing PEEP may actually have little to no effect on graft hemodynamics. Saner et al., examined the effects of PEEP on patients receiving living donor liver transplant [12]. They showed that a PEEP of 10 mbar (approx. 10 cm H_2O) significantly increased central venous and pulmonary capillary pressures, but had no effect on hepatic vein, portal vein, or hepatic artery pressures. Keifer et al., examined the effects of PEEP in six patients with acute lung injury and found inconsistent changes in splanchnic blood flow, with no changes in hepatosplanchnic metabolism and liver function with PEEPs up to 14 cm H_2O [13]. Holland et al., evaluated liver function in a small cohort of patients undergoing elective cardiac surgery using indocyanine green, a dye eliminated exclusively by the liver [14]. They reported that a PEEP of 10 mbar (10 cm H_2O) over 2 hours did not compromise either liver function or gastric perfusion. Krenn et al., reported that short term application of pressure controlled ventilation with PEEP levels up to 10 cmH_2O did not influence indocyanine green metabolism in postoperative orthotopic liver transplant recipients [15].

Despite the conflicting data regarding positive pressure ventilation on liver function and blood flow, there is a robust amount of evidence showing that early extubation is beneficial. Prolonged mechanical ventilation has been associated with ventilator associated pneumonia, tracheal injury, and deconditioning; the risks of which can be lessened with early extubation [16–18]. Early extubation following liver transplantation is not without risk, however. Transplant recipients present with multiple comorbidities, have undergone a complex surgery associated with bilateral rectus muscle transection, and have the potential for injury to the chest wall and diaphragm from retraction [19]. It is therefore of paramount importance to identify candidates who have the highest likelihood of success for early extubation. In 1990, Rossaint et al., reported the first application of early extubation following liver transplantation in a small cohort of patients [20]. They suggested that fluid restriction may improve the ability to extubate liver recipients immediately following surgery. By administering crystalloids, packed red blood cells, and fresh frozen plasma only when there was a drop in the cardiac index, the team was able to extubate 5 patients immediately after surgery and 34 of 37 patients within six hours of transplant. Building on this, Mandell et al., studied patients who were successfully extubated within eight hours following liver transplantation at two centers and identified several criteria that predicted the ability to safely extubate patients [21]. Her team also found that patients capable of early extubation had significantly shorter ICU stays, lower nursing acuity, and fewer laboratory tests performed, which translated to over a 50% reduction in cost to the patient. Neelakanta also described the safe extubation of 18 patients in the operating room, but did not find a benefit with regard to ICU or hospital stay [22]. More importantly, Neelakanta found no difference in outcomes when the early extubation group was compared to matched controls. Plevak, et al., showed that by forming an interdisciplinary care team and developing an integrated care plan for the first 48 hours postoperatively, the time to extubation and ICU stay could be safely reduced [23].

As experience with early extubation grew, clinicians attempted to define specific criteria that would predict successful extubation and limit the likelihood of reintubation. Glanemann et al., retrospectively analyzed 546 patients following orthotopic liver transplantation. His group found that patients presenting with deteriorating clinical conditions such as acute liver failure, re-transplantation, massive transfusion, prolonged reperfusion syndrome, and preoperative mechanical ventilation predicted those who would need prolonged postoperative ventilatory support [24]. In 2002, Mandell's group at the University of Colorado published the first paper on fast track liver transplantation. This three year study evaluated early extubation and transfer to the surgical ward, bypassing the ICU entirely. Of the 147 patients enrolled, all but 36 were able to transfer directly to the surgical ward following a stay in the PACU [25]. Only 3 patients initially admitted to the ward were subsequently transferred to the ICU and there was no impact on long term graft function in the study group. Even though the researchers used a defined anesthetic protocol that limited the amount of respiratory depression, the decision to extubate was based on clinical judgement and the team found a pronounced learning curve. As the study progressed and the clinicians gained experience and confidence with the fast track concept, there was an increase in the number of attempts and improvement in the success rates [25]. Cammu et al., described using a total intravenous technique utilizing propofol, remifentanil, and cisatracurium to facilitate early extubation following living donor transplantation. In this extremely small study, patients without pre-existing encephalopathy or acute liver failure who received less than 10 units of red cells, were hemodynamically stable with good donor function, and had an alveolar-arterial gradient <200 mmHg were successfully extubated at the end of the procedure [26]. That same year, Ulukaya reported the first application of early extubation following pediatric liver transplantation [27]. Multiple studies followed evaluating factors to predict the success of early extubation [28–32]. It quickly became obvious that a wide range of variables play a role in predicting candidates for successful extubation and regional variances in donor selection, perioperative management, physician experience, and institutional biases all can affect outcomes [17, 33]. In an attempt to give guidance, Skurzak et al., compared 52 non-extubated patients with 545 extubated patients and devised the "safe operating room extubation after liver transplantation (SORELT) score". Composed of both major and minor criteria, the authors found that patients who fulfilled the SORELT score derived criteria were considered safe for extubation in the operating room [34] (Table 13.1). As experience in early extubation improved and was shown to not affect long-term patient outcomes, attention returned to the idea set forth by Mandell in 2002 and

Table 13.1 SORELT score criteria

Major criteria	Minor criteria
Intraoperative administration of ≥7 units of packed red blood cells	Inpatient
Lactate level ≥3.4 mmol/L at the completion of surgery	Surgery lasting ≥5 hours
	Administration of vasoactive medication infusions at the end of surgery

Consider extubation if patient has less than 2 major; 1 major and 2 minor; or 3 minor criteria
Adapted from Skurzak et al. [34]

Table 13.2 Variables used to devise Fast tracking probability score

Preoperative	Intraoperative
Age at transplant	PRBC transfused
Body mass index	Operative time
Gender	Vasopressor requirement in last hour of surgery
MELD	
Inpatient versus outpatient	
Primary versus redo transplant	

From Bulatao et al. [36]

clinicians began evaluating the ability to bypass the ICU completely, a process coined "fast tracking". Taner et al., evaluated 1045 transplant recipients over a 5-year period and found that approximately 60% were able to bypass the ICU and be admitted directly to the floor [35]. Their study had a 1.9% failure rate after fast tracking to the surgical ward. The reasons for failed fast tracking were surgical complications, cardiac arrhythmias, myocardial infarction, renal failure, and respiratory distress. Bulatao et al., at the same institution developed a scoring system to predict the ability to bypass ICU admission. Using nine readily available pre- and intraoperative clinical variables, the authors were able to validate a scoring system that predicts the likelihood of successful fast tracking [36] (Table 13.2). Echeverri et al., were able to show that fast tracking was feasible following living donor liver transplantation [37]. Both the studies by Taner and Echeverri utilized an elevated level of postoperative care that falls in the spectrum between ICU and the standard surgical ward. Taner described 1:1 nursing for up to 24 hours following transplant, continuous telemetry, and an integrated team approach, whereas Echeverri utilized a step-down unit with similar characteristics as described by Taner but not to the level of a full ICU admission [35, 37].

Aside from the medical benefits, early extubation and direct admission to the surgical ward without ICU admission is cost effective [21, 28, 35, 38]. In a time where hospitals are looking to efficiently manage care and resources, avoiding unnecessary time in the ICU can translate to better cost containment and availability of these high acuity beds for patients more in need. The savings associated with early extubation and fast tracking appears to be related to both a reduction in room charges and testing associated with mechanical ventilation. Mandell and Taner showed savings related to a reduction in the length of hospitalization following transplantation, the number of chest radiographs performed, and the frequency of arterial blood gas sampling [21, 35]. Loh et al., found that fast tracking likely resulted in an average reduction in post-transplant length of stay of 2.5–3.2 days [38]. This would translate to a conservative cost savings of approximately $39–50 million per year in the United States alone. This benefit may be especially important in developing countries with limited high acuity care resources [39, 40].

Anesthesia for Fast Track

Most studies have employed a balanced anesthetic technique with a goal to limit respiratory depression and facilitate early extubation [20, 22–27, 29, 31, 34, 35, 37, 40–43]. The majority of studies utilize either thiopental or propofol combined with a narcotic for induction, followed by inhalational agents, neuromuscular blockade, and intermittent narcotics for maintenance of anesthesia.

Isoflurane, sevoflurance, and desflurane have all been used in studies examining early extubation. Maintenance has also been performed utilizing propofol infusions [40]. Dosing of these agents may be difficult due to alterations in drug metabolism that occur during the anhepatic phase of the transplant, as well as, concomitant comorbidities [44–47]. For instance, propofol concentrations may increase during the anhepatic phase and could potentially interfere with the ability to extubate following a successful surgery [46, 48]. Some authors have advocated for the use of bispectral index (BIS) monitoring to help with titration and prevent a relative over dosage [44, 45]. Restoux described a successful closed loop anesthetic model utilizing propofol and remifentanil combined with BIS monitoring in 13 patients undergoing orthotopic liver transplantation [49]. All the patients were transferred to the ICU still intubated so the utility of this methodology with relation to immediate early extubation has not been evaluated.

Nearly every modern neuromuscular blocking agent has been utilized in studies evaluating early extubation [40]. Most often the benzoisoquinolones, atracurium and cis-atracurium, are utilized due to their metabolism that is independent of hepatic function. Vecuronium, rocuronium, and pancuronium have also been explored; however, these agents rely on hepatic metabolism to varying degrees and may result in prolonged neuromuscular blockade in the setting of delayed or primary graft non-function. The introduction of sugammadex into the anesthesiologist's armamentarium may lessen this risk and ensure rapid return of neuromuscular function following rocuronium or vecuronium [50]. Prospective studies evaluating sugammadex in liver transplant recipients are lacking, however. To ensure a return of normal muscle strength, neuromuscular monitoring should be performed on all patients prior to extubation.

Adequate pain control without significant respiratory depression is paramount in patients selected for early extubation. Typically, the majority of patients have a decreased need for postoperative pain control compared to patients without end-stage liver disease [51–53]. The mechanism for this is multifactorial and may relate to decreased metabolism of endogenous opioid neuropeptides, preexisting encephalopathy, and decreased hepatic clearance of administered opioids [54]. Supporting this, researchers in Korea found that as model for end-stage liver disease scores increased, patients had lower postoperative pain scores and required less postoperative pain medication [52]. Remifentanil may be advantageous in this regard as it is rapidly metabolized by nonspecific tissue and plasma esterases independent of liver function allowing for easy titration. Fentanyl is frequently utilized in studies examining early extubation, presumably due to its rapid metabolism compared to morphine or hydromorphone. In contrast to remifentanil, all other opioids undergo varying degrees of hepatic metabolism and should be carefully titrated to prevent over sedation.

Implementing a Fast Track Program—The Mayo Clinic Florida Model

On average, Mayo Clinic Florida performs 160 orthotopic deceased donor liver transplants annually with 30% having a biological MELD between 21–30 and 20% having a biological MELD of 31–40 [43]. The institution implemented a fast track anesthesia practice in 2002 and has successfully fast tracked approximately 60% of the 3000 livers performed since that time. Our failure rate of patients transferring to the ICU after admission to the post anesthesia care unit or surgical ward is approximately 2% and typically relates to the experience level of the attending anesthesiologist [35]. Implementation of this program involved a coordinated plan involving all levels of providers to ensure buy-in and resolve concerns related to changing the status quo from postoperative ICU care. Hospital administration was also involved early and often in the decision making process as significant capital investment is needed at the outset to ensure adequate staffing and monitoring. The surgical ward was modified to function similar to a standard step-down unit allowing for continuous telemetry and 1:1 nursing coverage for up to the first 24 hours after surgery. Additionally, the program has 24 hour in-house midlevel practitioners covering the service with dedicated hepatologist and surgical oversight. Transplant critical care physicians are available at all times to assist the floor service with emergencies. A small, yet highly specialized team of consultants in transplant anesthesiology was developed to allow for consistency of care and experience in dealing with conditions and complications in this patient population.

A protocolized approach to intraoperative management is followed by the anesthesiologists at the institution. A rapid sequence induction using propofol,

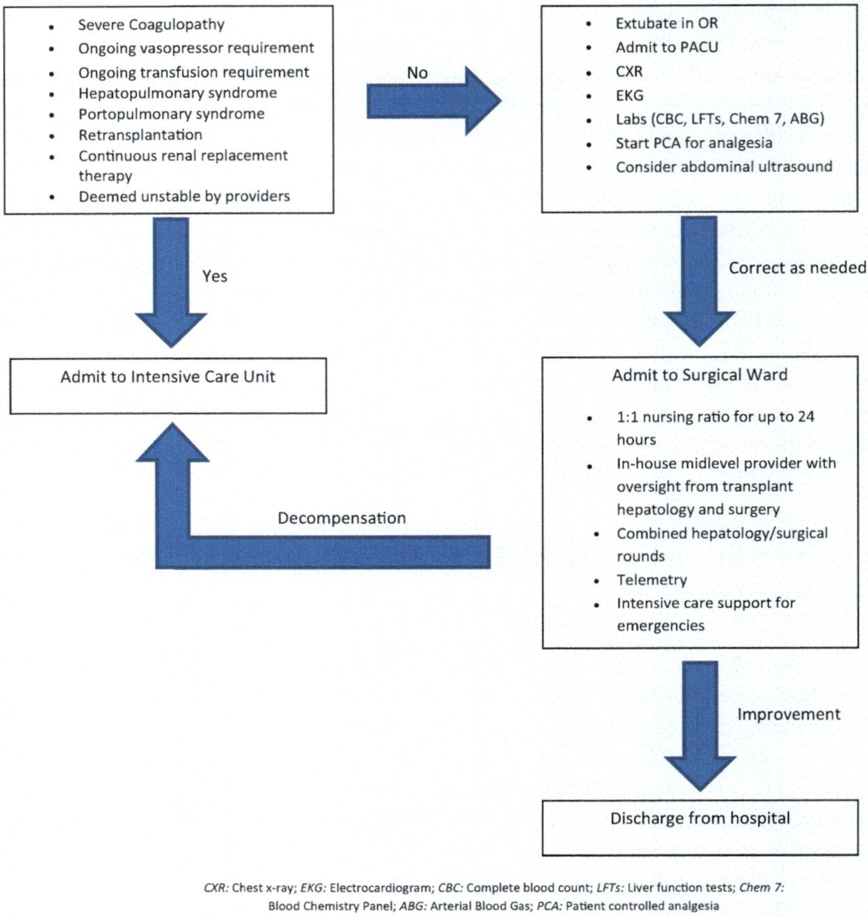

Fig. 13.1 Generalized postoperative liver transplant flowchart at Mayo Clinic Florida

fentanyl, and succinylcholine is performed followed by maintenance with sevoflurane and intermittent fentanyl dosing. The total fentanyl dose administered intraoperatively is limited to 1000 micrograms in opioid naïve patients and long acting narcotics are generally avoided until the patient is extubated. In the absence of renal failure, rocuronium is used for neuromuscular blockade and reversed with sugammadex at the end of surgery. If the patient is anuric, cisatracurium is substituted for rocuronium and titrated to maintain a train-of-four of 1 or less. The decision to extubate is based on the clinical judgement of the attending anesthesiologist in consultation with the transplant surgeon. In general, patients with severe hepato-pulmonary or porto-pulmonary syndrome, re-transplantation, requiring ongoing transfusions and/or vasopressor support, or needing continuous renal replacement therapy are admitted to the ICU (Fig. 13.1). Intraoperative high-volume transfusion is not considered a requirement for ICU admission unless there is airway edema or persistent coagulopathy with a high likelihood of needing more than 2 units of blood products over the first several hours postoperatively. Similarly, MELD score itself is not used to determine postoperative care but may alert the provider to significant comorbidities than may preclude fast tracking. After admission to the PACU, patients are evaluated for adequate pain control and undergo an electrocardiogram and chest x-ray. Blood electrolytes, complete blood count, thromboelastrogram, and coagulation profiles are obtained and corrected, if necessary. Pain control is achieved with patient controlled analgesia. After an average of 2 hours of observations, patients are discharged to the surgical ward when they meet standard PACU discharge criteria.

References

1. Dammann JF Jr, Thung N, Christ L 2nd, Littlefield JB, Muller WH Jr. The management of the severely ill patient after open-heart surgery. J Thorac Cardiovasc Surg. 1963;45:80–90.
2. Lefemine AA, Harken DE. Postoperative care following open-heart operations: routine use of controlled ventilation. J Thorac Cardiovasc Surg. 1966;52(2):207–16.
3. Macrae WR, Masson AH. Assisted ventilation in the post-bypass period. Br J Anaesth. 1964;36:711–7.
4. Robertson DS. Tracheostomy and open heart surgery. Proc R Soc Med. 1964;57:855–64.
5. Midell AI, Skinner DB, DeBoer A, Bermudez G. A review of pulmonary problems following valve replacement in 100 consecutive patients: the case against routine use of assisted ventilation. Ann Thorac Surg. 1974;18(3):219–27.
6. Klineberg PL, Geer RT, Hirsh RA, Aukburg SJ. Early extubation after coronary artery bypass graft surgery. Crit Care Med. 1977;5(6):272–4.
7. Prakash O, Jonson B, Meij S, et al. Criteria for early extubation after intracardiac surgery in adults. Anesth Analg. 1977;56(5):703–8.
8. Plevak DJ, Southorn PA, Narr BJ, Peters SG. Intensive-care unit experience in the Mayo liver transplantation program: the first 100 cases. Mayo Clin Proc. 1989;64(4):433–45.
9. Carton EG, Plevak DJ, Kranner PW, Rettke SR, Geiger HJ, Coursin DB. Perioperative care of the liver transplant patient: part 2. Anesth Analg. 1994;78(2):382–99.
10. Bredenberg CE, Paskanik AM. Relation of portal hemodynamics to cardiac output during mechanical ventilation with PEEP. Ann Surg. 1983;198(2):218–22.
11. Brienza N, Revelly JP, Ayuse T, Robotham JL. Effects of PEEP on liver arterial and venous blood flows. Am J Respir Crit Care Med. 1995;152(2):504–10.
12. Saner FH, Olde Damink SW, Pavlakovic G, et al. Positive end-expiratory pressure induces liver congestion in living donor liver transplant patients: myth or fact. Transplantation. 2008;85(12):1863–6.
13. Kiefer P, Nunes S, Kosonen P, Takala J. Effect of positive end-expiratory pressure on splanchnic perfusion in acute lung injury. Intensive Care Med. 2000;26(4):376–83.
14. Holland A, Thuemer O, Schelenz C, van Hout N, Sakka SG. Positive end-expiratory pressure does not affect indocyanine green plasma disappearance rate or gastric mucosal perfusion after cardiac surgery. Eur J Anaesthesiol. 2007;24(2):141–7.
15. Krenn CG, Krafft P, Schaefer B, et al. Effects of positive end-expiratory pressure on hemodynamics and indocyanine green kinetics in patients after orthotopic liver transplantation. Crit Care Med. 2000;28(6):1760–5.

16. Papadimos TJ, Hensley SJ, Duggan JM, et al. Implementation of the "FASTHUG" concept decreases the incidence of ventilator-associated pneumonia in a surgical intensive care unit. Patient Saf Surg. 2008;2:3.
17. Mandell MS, Campsen J, Zimmerman M, Biancofiore G, Tsou MY. The clinical value of early extubation. Curr Opin Organ Transplant. 2009;14(3):297–302.
18. Razonable RR, Findlay JY, O'Riordan A, et al. Critical care issues in patients after liver transplantation. Liver Transplant Off Publ Am Assoc Study Liver Dis Int Liver Transplant Soc. 2011;17(5):511–27.
19. Avolio AW, Gaspari R, Teofili L, et al. Postoperative respiratory failure in liver transplantation: risk factors and effect on prognosis. PLoS One. 2019;14(2):e0211678.
20. Rossaint R, Slama K, Jaeger M, et al. Fluid restriction and early extubation for successful liver transplantation. Transplant Proc. 1990;22(4):1533–4.
21. Mandell MS, Lockrem J, Kelley SD. Immediate tracheal extubation after liver transplantation: experience of two transplant centers. Anesth Analg. 1997;84(2):249–53.
22. Neelakanta G, Sopher M, Chan S, et al. Early tracheal extubation after liver transplantation. J Cardiothorac Vasc Anesth. 1997;11(2):165–7.
23. Plevak DJ, Torsher LC. Fast tracking in liver transplantation. Liver Transplant Surg: Off Publ Am Assoc Study Liver Dis Int Liver Transplant Soc. 1997;3(4):447–8.
24. Glanemann M, Langrehr J, Kaisers U, et al. Postoperative tracheal extubation after orthotopic liver transplantation. Acta Anaesthesiol Scand. 2001;45(3):333–9.
25. Mandell MS, Lezotte D, Kam I, Zamudio S. Reduced use of intensive care after liver transplantation: patient attributes that determine early transfer to surgical wards. Liver Transplant: Off Publ Am Assoc Study Liver Dis Int Liver Transplant Soc. 2002;8(8):682–7.
26. Cammu G, Decruyenaere J, Troisi R, de Hemptinne B, Colardyn F, Mortier E. Criteria for immediate postoperative extubation in adult recipients following living-related liver transplantation with total intravenous anesthesia. J Clin Anesth. 2003;15(7):515–9.
27. Ulukaya S, Arikan C, Aydogdu S, Ayanoglu HO, Tokat Y. Immediate tracheal extubation of pediatric liver transplant recipients in the operating room. Pediatr Transplant. 2003;7(5):381–4.
28. Quiroga M, Rodriguez MG, Montalvan C, et al. Trends in mechanical ventilation and immediate extubation after liver transplantation in a single center in Chile. Transplant Proc. 2004;36(6):1683–4.
29. Biancofiore G, Bindi ML, Romanelli AM, et al. Fast track in liver transplantation: 5 years' experience. Eur J Anaesthesiol. 2005;22(8):584–90.
30. Glanemann M, Busch T, Neuhaus P, Kaisers U. Fast tracking in liver transplantation. Immediate postoperative tracheal extubation: feasibility and clinical impact. Swiss Med Wkly. 2007;137(13–14):187–91.
31. Zeyneloglu P, Pirat A, Guner M, Torgay A, Karakayali H, Arslan G. Predictors of immediate tracheal extubation in the operating room after liver transplantation. Transplant Proc. 2007;39(4):1187–9.
32. Lee S, Sa GJ, Kim SY, Park CS. Intraoperative predictors of early tracheal extubation after living-donor liver transplantation. Korean J Anesthesiol. 2014;67(2):103–9.
33. Biancofiore G, Tomescu DR, Mandell MS. Rapid recovery of liver transplantation recipients by implementation of fast-track care steps: what is holding us back? Semin Cardiothorac Vasc Anesth. 2018;22(2):191–6.
34. Skurzak S, Stratta C, Schellino MM, et al. Extubation score in the operating room after liver transplantation. Acta Anaesthesiol Scand. 2010;54(8):970–8.
35. Taner CB, Willingham DL, Bulatao IG, et al. Is a mandatory intensive care unit stay needed after liver transplantation? Feasibility of fast-tracking to the surgical ward after liver transplantation. Liver Transplant: Off Publ Am Assoc Study Liver Dis Int Liver Transplant Soc. 2012;18(3):361–9.
36. Bulatao IG, Heckman MG, Rawal B, et al. Avoiding stay in the intensive care unit after liver transplantation: a score to assign location of care. Am J Transplant: Off J Am Soc Transplant Am Soc Transpl Surg. 2014;14(9):2088–96.

37. Echeverri J, Goldaracena N, Singh AK, et al. Avoiding ICU admission by using a fast-track protocol is safe in selected adult-to-adult live donor liver transplant recipients. Transplant Direct. 2017;3(10):e213.
38. Loh CA, Croome KP, Taner CB, Keaveny AP. Bias-corrected estimates of reduction of post-surgery length of stay and corresponding cost savings through the widespread national implementation of fast-tracking after liver transplantation: a quasi-experimental study. J Med Econ. 2019;1.
39. Rando K, Niemann CU, Taura P, Klinck J. Optimizing cost-effectiveness in perioperative care for liver transplantation: a model for low- to medium-income countries. Liver Transplant: Off Publ Am Assoc Study Liver Dis Int Liver Transplant Soc. 2011;17(11):1247–78.
40. Wu J, Rastogi V, Zheng SS. Clinical practice of early extubation after liver transplantation. Hepatobiliary Pancreat Dis Int: HBPD INT. 2012;11(6):577–85.
41. Biancofiore G, Romanelli AM, Bindi ML, et al. Very early tracheal extubation without predetermined criteria in a liver transplant recipient population. Liver Transplant: Off Publ Am Assoc Study Liver Dis Int Liver Transplant Soc. 2001;7(9):777–82.
42. Mandell MS, Stoner TJ, Barnett R, et al. A multicenter evaluation of safety of early extubation in liver transplant recipients. Liver Transplant: Off Publ Am Assoc Study Liver Dis Int Liver Transplant Soc. 2007;13(11):1557–63.
43. Aniskevich S, Pai SL. Fast track anesthesia for liver transplantation: review of the current practice. World J Hepatol. 2015;7(20):2303–8.
44. Kang JG, Ko JS, Kim GS, Gwak MS, Kim YR, Lee SK. The relationship between inhalational anesthetic requirements and the severity of liver disease in liver transplant recipients according to three phases of liver transplantation. Transplant Proc. 2010;42(3):854–7.
45. Toprak HI, Sener A, Gedik E, et al. Bispectral index monitoring to guide end-tidal isoflurane concentration at three phases of operation in patients with end-stage liver disease undergoing orthotopic liver transplantation. Transplant Proc. 2011;43(3):892–5.
46. Takizawa D, Hiraoka H, Nakamura K, Yamamoto K, Horiuchi R. Propofol concentrations during the anhepatic phase of living-related donor liver transplantation. Clin Pharmacol Ther. 2004;76(6):648–9.
47. Baron-Stefaniak J, Gotz V, Allhutter A, et al. Patients undergoing orthotopic liver transplantation require lower concentrations of the volatile anesthetic sevoflurane. Anesth Analg. 2017;125(3):783–9.
48. Wu J, Zhu SM, He HL, Weng XC, Huang SQ, Chen YZ. Plasma propofol concentrations during orthotopic liver transplantation. Acta Anaesthesiol Scand. 2005;49(6):804–10.
49. Restoux A, Grassin-Delyle S, Liu N, Paugam-Burtz C, Mantz J, Le Guen M. Pilot study of closed-loop anaesthesia for liver transplantation. Br J Anaesth. 2016;117(3):332–40.
50. Aniskevich S, Leone BJ, Brull SJ. Sugammadex: a novel approach to reversal of neuromuscular blockade. Expert Rev Neurother. 2011;11(2):185–98.
51. Donovan KL, Janicki PK, Striepe VI, Stoica C, Franks WT, Pinson CW. Decreased patient analgesic requirements after liver transplantation and associated neuropeptide levels. Transplantation. 1997;63(10):1423–9.
52. Ko JS, Shin YH, Gwak MS, Jang CH, Kim GS, Lee SK. The relationship between postoperative intravenous patient-controlled fentanyl analgesic requirements and severity of liver disease. Transplant Proc. 2012;44(2):445–7.
53. Moretti EW, Robertson KM, Tuttle-Newhall JE, Clavien PA, Gan TJ. Orthotopic liver transplant patients require less postoperative morphine than do patients undergoing hepatic resection. J Clin Anesth. 2002;14(6):416–20.
54. Pai SL, Aniskevich S, Rodrigues ES, Shine TS. Analgesic considerations for liver transplantation patients. Curr Clin Pharmacol. 2015;10(1):54–65.

Chapter 14
Acute Kidney Injury in Hepatico-Pancreatic-Biliary Surgery and Liver Transplantation

Won Ho Kim

Abbreviations

ACR	acute cellular rejection
AKI	acute kidney injury
AKIN	acute kidney injury network
CKD	chronic kidney disease
GFR	glomerular filtration rate
HPB	hepatico-pancreatic-biliary
HRS	hepatorenal syndrome
IGFBP-7	insulin-like growth factor-binding protein-7
KDIGO	Kidney Disease Improving Global Outcomes
mTOR	mammalian target of rapamycin
LDLT	living-donor liver transplantation
MELD	model for end-stage liver disease
NGAL	neutrophil gelatinase-associated lipocalin
RIFLE	risk, injury, failure, loss of function, end-stage renal disease
RRT	renal replacement therapy
SBP	spontaneous bacterial peritonitis
TIMP-2	tissue inhibitor of metalloprotease-2

W. H. Kim (✉)
Department of Anesthesiology and Pain Medicine, Seoul National University College of Medicine, 101, Daehak-no, Jongno-gu, Seoul, Republic of Korea
e-mail: wonhokim@snu.ac.kr

Z. Milan and C. Goonasekera (eds.), *Anesthesia for Hepatico-Pancreatic-Biliary Surgery and Transplantation*, https://doi.org/10.1007/978-3-030-51331-3_14

Introduction

Acute kidney injury (AKI) has been recognized as a clinically relevant complication after cardiac and non-cardiac surgery due to its association with long-term mortality and chronic kidney disease (CKD) [1–4]. Even small increases in serum creatinine after surgery are of substantial prognostic relevance [1, 2]. AKI has also been recognized as a clinically relevant complication after hepatico-pancreatic-biliary (HPB) surgery as well as liver transplantation due to its association with hospital length of stay, mortality and poor graft survival [5–15]. Although its incidence has been reported to be as high as 68% after liver transplantation [6, 7, 16–22] and 20% after liver resection [12, 15], effective preventive or therapeutic strategies have not yet been established. Therefore, it is important to identify a modifiable risk factor such as perioperative medications or intraoperative hemodynamic parameters and to prevent its occurrence. However, although numerous studies and literature reported risk factors of AKI, the causal relationship has rarely been demonstrated by randomized trials with adequate power. Furthermore, well-designed randomized trials with a sufficient number of participants which demonstrated a significant reduction in the incidence of AKI were rare. AKI after HPB surgery has not been investigated as thoroughly as AKI after liver transplantation. However, its clinical implication in HBP surgery was also consistently reported.

Definitions

Three criteria have been developed to define AKI including risk, injury, failure, loss of function, end-stage renal disease (RIFLE) criteria, acute kidney injury network (AKIN) criteria, and Kidney Disease: Improving Global Outcomes (KDIGO) criteria [9]. Details of the three criteria are shown in Table 14.1. AKIN and KDIGO criteria abandoned glomerular filtration rate (GFR) criteria and urine output criteria are applied to all three criteria. All criteria have been used in previous studies of HPB surgery and liver transplantation [2, 12–14, 16, 23, 24]. Serum creatinine criteria of KDIGO defines AKI based on the postoperative increase in serum creatinine (Stage 1: 1.5–1.9 within 7 days or ≥0.3 mg/dL increase within 48 hours; stage 2: 2–2.9; stage 3: more than 3-fold increase of baseline, respectively within the first 7 days after transplantation. The most recent preoperative serum creatinine is used as a baseline. For surgical patients, the routine preoperative measurement of baseline serum creatinine and daily follow-up of serum creatinine made the serum creatinine criteria of AKI widely available.

A recent study suggested that an increase in creatinine of ≥0.3 mg/dL within 48 hours may have a different clinical implication from the 1.5 fold increase from baseline. However, it has not been evaluated in HPB surgery patients [25]. There were studies which reported optimal cutoff for urine output criteria could

Table 14.1 Diagnostic criteria of acute kidney disease

	RIFLE		AKIN		KDIGO	
Criteria	Creatinine definition	Criteria	Creatinine definition	Criteria	Creatinine definition	Urine Output[a]
Risk	≥1.5-fold increase from baseline SCr OR decrease in GFR ≥25%	Stage 1	≥0.3 mg/dL increase OR ≥1.5 fold increase from baseline SCr within 48 hours	Stage 1	≥0.3 mg/dL increase within 48 hours OR 1.5–1.9 times baseline within 7 days	<0.5 ml/kg/h for >6 hours
Injury	≥2 fold increase from baseline SCr OR decrease in GFR ≥50%	Stage 2	≥2 fold increase from baseline SCr within 48 hours	Stage 2	2.0–2.9 times baseline within 7 days	<0.5 ml/kg/h for 12 hours
Failure	≥3 fold increase from baseline SCr OR increase to ≥4 mg/dL or decrease in GFR ≥75%	Stage 3	≥3 fold increase from baseline SCr within 48 hours OR increase to ≥4.0 mg/dL with an acute increase of >0.5 mg/dl within 48 hours OR initiation of RRT	Stage 3	≥ 3 times baseline within 7 days OR increase to ≥4.0 mg/dL with an acute increase of >0.5 mg/dL OR initiation of RRT	<0.3 ml/kg/h for 24 hours OR Anuria for >12 hours

RIFLE = risk, injury, failure, loss, end-stage kidney disease; AKIN = acute kidney injury network; KDIGO = Kidney Disease: Improving Global Outcomes; sCr = serum creatinine; GFR = glomerular filtration rate; RRT = renal replacement therapy
[a]Urine output criteria are applied to all three criteria

be different in surgical setting [26–28]. The optimal urine output criteria of AKI in patients undergoing major abdominal surgery was suggested as 0.3 mL/kg/min [27]. For patients with decompensated liver cirrhosis, the urine output is frequently reduced due to their high renal sodium and water retention [29]. In addition, patients with refractory ascites who are not responsive to diuretic therapy can have stable serum creatinine levels but oliguria criteria of AKI could be met. As these patients surely do not have AKI, oliguria criteria could not be applied to for these patients with stable creatinine levels.

Diagnosis of AKI in patients with liver cirrhosis is currently a matter under discussion [30]. Serum creatinine level is a poor marker of renal dysfunction in patients with muscle wasting and ascites [31]. In 2010, the International Club of Ascites and Acute Dialysis Quality Initiative reported the criteria for the diagnosis of AKI in a patient with cirrhosis [32]. Serum creatinine criteria consist of a rise by $\geq$0.3 mg/dl within 48 hours or elevation of $\geq$50% from baseline. However, the urine output criteria were eliminated. Hepatorenal syndrome (HRS) type 1 was regarded as a special form of AKI and HRS type 2 is a specific form of chronic kidney disease in patients with cirrhosis. Acute worsening of renal function in patients with chronic kidney disease was defined as having acute-on-chronic kidney disease.

Biomarker for Early Detection and Guidance for Management

Traditionally, clearance of endogenous markers of creatinine has been used to measure renal function. As an endogenous marker, cystatin C is an alternative measurement of GFR [33, 34]. Serum cystatin C itself or as part of the equation of GFR independently predicted patient mortality [35, 36]. In patients with liver cirrhosis, conventional tools used to differentially diagnose AKI including fractional excretion of sodium have poor correlation with biopsy finding [37, 38].

During liver transplantation, a large amount of crystalloid administration and transfusion may result in hemodilution of serum creatinine further delaying the diagnosis of AKI. Biomarkers of renal damage and stress response were investigated due to this limitation of creatinine [39]. Marker of acute tubular injury including neutrophil gelatinase-associated lipocalin (NGAL), kidney injury molecule-1, and interleukin-18 have been extensively studied in patients with liver cirrhosis and waiting for liver transplantation [40–43]. Urinary NGAL was reported to predict AKI preoperatively, during surgery and immediate postoperatively [44–46], and also identify patients at risk of chronic kidney disease [47]. Recently, the insulin-like growth factor-binding protein 7 (IGFBP7) and the tissue inhibitor of metalloprotease-2 (TIMP-2) are introduced as urinary cell cycle arrest biomarkers [48]. TIMP-2 was reported to be helpful to differentiate between reversible and irreversible AKI after liver transplantation [49].

However, in general, the performance of urinary and plasma biomarkers was inconsistent and variable [50–53] partly due to the nonrenal cause of biomarker elevation [54]. Further large prospective trials are required to validate biomarkers for prediction and early detection of AKI after liver transplantation.

Risk Factors of Acute Kidney Injury After HPB Surgery

AKI after HPB surgery has been understudied compared to AKI after liver transplantation. This may be because the incidence of AKI after HPB surgery was reported to be relatively low and the clinical implication has not been well recognized. However, studies of liver resection reported 8-20% of AKI incidence and AKI is associated with longer hospital length of stay, higher postoperative morbidity rates and mortality [11–15, 55–58].

Prior studies reported the risk factor of AKI after liver resection surgery for hepatocellular carcinoma [11–15, 55–58]. Surgical technique of laparoscopic approach was reported to reduce the occurrence of AKI compared to open approach [59]. Significant predictors reported included older age [12, 55–57], female [55], body-mass index [55], model for end-stage liver disease (MELD) score [11, 57], preoperative alanine transaminase level [15, 56], preoperative hypertension [14, 15, 55], diabetes mellitus [15, 55, 58], baseline renal function [14, 15], preoperative hematocrit value [55], major hepatectomy [11, 12], duration of surgery [11, 13, 55], open surgical approach [55], intraoperative amount of surgical bleeding [12], and Pringle maneuver [55].

Pringle maneuver is a hepatic inflow occlusion technique to reduce intraoperative bleeding and has been a subject of debate due to the concern of ischemic liver injury. Pringle maneuver was also significantly associated with AKI possibly due to hypotension and ischemia-reperfusion injury [55]. However, other retrospective study reported that continuous Pringle maneuver has no influence on overall survival regardless of occlusion time [60]. A recent retrospective study reported that the effect of infrahepatic inferior vena cava semi-clamping could reduce blood loss during hepatic resection but the risk of AKI could be increased depending on the duration and mean blood pressure after clamping [61].

Several studies have evaluated the association between anesthesia-related parameters and AKI after hepatectomy. A small retrospective study examined the association of intraoperative hydroxyethyl starch with AKI after living donor hepatectomy [62]. There was no significant difference in the incidence of AKI after propensity score matching. A recent study evaluated the prognostic value of AKI determined by AKIN criteria of serum creatinine and urine output and reported that urine output criteria could result in overestimation of AKI and undermined the prognostic value of AKIN criteria [12]. Epidural analgesia for major hepatectomy was associated with a higher risk of AKI, while no difference in minor hepatectomy [63]. In another study, postoperative renal function was compared between epidural and intravenous patient-controlled analgesia after living-donor hepatectomy and reported no significant difference [56].

Regarding pancreatic resection, the influence of surgical approach type was evaluated in a previous retrospective study [64]. Laparoscopic surgery was associated with a reduced incidence of AKI after propensity score matching. The left renal vein could be used for venous reconstruction of the portal vein or superior mesenteric vein during HPB surgery. Left renal vein harvest was an independent risk factor for AKI but did not affect the long-term renal function during three years after surgery [65].

Preoperative baseline poor renal function was consistently reported to be associated with postoperative AKI [66, 67]. A previous large retrospective cohort study of more than 1,000 pancreatic resections revealed the association between preoperative CKD and postoperative morbidity including acute renal failure requiring new-onset hemodialysis [66]. Preoperative serum creatinine $\geq$1.8 mg/dL was suggested as a useful marker of renal insufficiency and was associated with an increased risk of morbidity and respiratory failure [66]. Analysis of a retrospective cohort of more than 16,000 patients undergoing pancreatectomy revealed that preoperative CKD of any stage was associated with morbidity including AKI and this association was consistent over all age groups [67]. AKI after pancreatic resection was more frequent in patients with diabetes mellitus but diabetes mellitus was not significantly associated with major complication rate except the post-resection fistula formation.

Risk Factors of AKI After Liver Transplantation

Recipient and Donor Characteristics

Previously-reported risk factor of AKI after liver transplantations are summarized in Table 14.2. Baseline characteristics of the recipient have been reported to be associated with AKI after liver transplantation—such as high MELD score [6, 17, 68]. Among the components of MELD score, preoperative PT-INR was strongly associated with AKI, suggesting the importance of severity of the underlying liver disease. HRS prior to liver transplantation is a significant predictor of worse renal function after liver transplantation [69]. A substantial proportion of patients with end-stage liver disease and AKI is considered to have underlying chronic kidney disease [70]. Non-alcoholic steatohepatitis is a growing indication for liver transplantation and is associated with increased risk of AKI [16].

The incidence of AKI is lower after living donor liver transplantation (LDLT) compared to deceased donor liver transplantation [16]. This is because LDLT is usually performed as an elective procedure when the recipient is optimized with minimal cold ischemic time and relatively healthy donor graft. Extended criteria donors are associated with AKI requiring hemodialysis and chronic kidney disease after liver transplantation [73]. Donation after circulatory death is associated

Table 14.2 Risk factors of acute kidney injury according to the stages relative to liver transplantation surgery

Stages relative to surgery	Risk factors
Preoperative	Baseline severity of liver cirrhosis (MELD score) [6, 17, 68]
	Intrinsic medical renal disease [70]
	Baseline renal function [70]
	Hepatorenal syndrome [69]
	Non-alcoholic steatohepatitis [16]
	Preoperative low hematocrit [17, 71]
	Donor
	Deceased donor versus living donor [22]
	Circulatory death versus brain death [72]
	Extended criteria donor [73]
	ABO-incompatible transplantation [21]
Intraoperative	Baseline systemic congestion (elevated central venous pressure, right ventricular end-diastolic volume) [71, 74]
	Hemodynamic derangement (arterial blood pressure, low cardiac output, low mixed venous oxygen saturation, low oxygen delivery) [71, 74, 75]
	Transfusion of red blood cells [17, 71]
	Postreperfusion syndrome [17, 20]
	Severe portal hypertension [71, 76]
	Portal vein thrombosis [71, 76]
	Previous abdominal surgery [71, 76]
	Small for size graft syndrome (living-donor) [6, 17, 77]
Postoperative	Calcineurin inhibitor (cyclosporine, tacrolimus) exposure [17, 18]
	Hypoalbuminemia [78]
	Postoperative bleeding and reoperation [79, 80]
	Retransplantation [79, 80]
	Early allograft dysfunction [79, 80]
	Heart failure after transplantation

MELD score = Model for end-stage liver disease score

with a higher risk of posttransplant AKI than brain death [72]. Normothermic or hypothermic liver graft machine perfusion is a promising technique to mitigate ischemic reperfusion injury [81].

Although the feasible mechanism was not revealed, the incidence of AKI was reported to be higher in ABO-incompatible liver transplantation [21]. Risk factors of AKI after LDLT are generally similar to those after deceased donor liver transplantation [6, 17]. Notably for LDLT, small for graft size syndrome was reported to be significantly associated with postoperative renal dysfunction [6, 17, 77].

Surgical and Intraoperative Factors

Intraoperative hemodynamic variables have been investigated as modifiable risk factors in patients undergoing liver transplantation [71, 74, 75]. Intraoperative arterial blood pressure, baseline central venous pressure, baseline right ventricular end-diastolic pressure and mixed venous oxygen saturation during anhepatic phase were reported to be associated with the development of posttransplant AKI [71, 74]. All these hemodynamic variables are related to cardiac output and arterial oxygen content, which are components of intraoperative oxygen delivery [82]. Poor oxygen delivery due to renal hypoperfusion is one of the potential mechanisms of the posttransplant AKI. During liver transplantation, frequent decrease in hemoglobin concentration and cardiac output occurs by clamping inferior vena cava and significant surgical bleeding [83]. These fluctuations may result in poor oxygen delivery to major organs including kidney which is vulnerable to ischemic injury, leading to AKI. Adequacy of major organ oxygenation could be estimated by DO_2I adapted to oxygen demand [84]. However, the optimal strategies for maintaining DO_2I during liver transplantation surgery adapted to meet oxygen needs is still unknown [85]. The prognostic implication of intraoperative hemodynamic management on postoperative AKI and mortality as well as the optimal target of intraoperative hemodynamic management has not yet been investigated.

Prolonged hypotension and hemodynamic instability following unclamping of portal vein, i.e. postreperfusion syndrome was recognized as a risk factor for AKI though ischemic reperfusion injury [17, 20]. Ischemic reperfusion injury also triggers inflammation and cellular damage in renal tubule, contributing to the development of AKI [86]. To mitigate hemodynamic instability during surgery, piggyback technique avoiding complete vena cava clamping is adopted in many institutions. Additionally, temporary portocaval shunt [87] or extracorporeal venovenous bypass could be considered to prevent hemodynamic instability and congestions in the kidney [88]. However, it has not been evaluated whether decreasing the incidence of postreperfusion syndrome could reduce the risk of AKI.

Propofol is reported to have a protective effect against ischemia-reperfusion injury in liver transplantation [89, 90]. A recent study compared the propofol intravenous anesthesia with desflurane versus desflurane alone regarding postoperative complications in pairs of adult donor and recipients of liver transplantation [91]. However, complication and AKI rates were not significantly different between groups.

Since severe portal hypertension, portal vein thrombosis and previous abdominal surgery can result in blood loss and renal hypoperfusion, these variables can be considered as predictors of posttransplant AKI [71, 76]. Preoperative anemia and intraoperative transfusion amounts are also reported as risk factors of AKI [17, 71].

Postoperative Factors

Administration of CNI is a risk factor of posttransplant AKI [17, 18]. The risk of AKI could be relieved with a combination of CNI with mycophenolate [17]. Postoperative hypoalbuminemia was considered to be associated with an increased free fraction of CNI, increasing the risk of AKI [78]. Reoperation, bleeding, heart failure, retransplantation, early allograft dysfunction were suggested as a postoperative risk factor of AKI [79, 80].

Although a considerable number of risk factors have been identified in previous studies, a risk prediction model for AKI has rarely been developed possibly due to the difficulty in gathering a sufficient number of cases of liver transplantation. A recent study reported better performance of a machine-learning approach—gradient boosting machine to predict AKI after liver transplantation [92].

Strategies to Prevent AKI After HPB Surgery

There have been few studies to investigate any specific strategy to prevent AKI after this specific subset of surgeries. As mentioned above, as an open surgical approach was significantly associated with a higher risk of AKI [55, 59], the laparoscopic approach should be considered.

A recent study evaluated the effect of a closed-loop system for continuous monitoring and control of intraoperative blood glucose during hepatectomy on the incidence of postoperative AKI [93]. The target range of blood glucose of 100-150 mg/dL was maintained by the programmed infusion of insulin in an artificial endocrine pancreas group. Strict blood glucose control by artificial pancreas yielded suppressing elevations in serum creatinine concentrations.

Strategies to Prevent AKI After Liver Transplantation

Although plenty of risk factors were identified to predict AKI after liver transplantation, prospective trials which showed a significant reduction in the risk of AKI by modifying any risk factor have rarely been reported.

Preoperative Preventions

Nephrotoxic agent including diuretics, nonsteroidal anti-inflammatory agents, radiocontrast agent and aminoglycoside should be avoided [94]. Spontaneous bacterial peritonitis (SBP) should be controlled with early administration of antibiotics and albumin [95]. Prophylaxis of SBP with norfloxacin delays the development of HRS [96]. Type-1 HRS is considered as a form of AKI and its mainstay treatment consists of vasopressor of terlipressin in a combination of albumin [97]. Since recurrence of HRS is common even in responders of terlipressin and albumin, terlipressin should be considered a bridge to transplantation. When terlipressin is not available, norepinephrine could be an effective alternative [98].

However, in a recent randomized trial, terlipressin was reported to be superior to norepinephrine for AKI in acute on chronic liver failure [73]. Although terlipressin and albumin could also reverse type 2 HRS, recurrence is common and a large proportion of patients eventually develop CKD [72, 99].

In patients with high stages of AKI are managed with renal replacement therapy (RRT). However, the timing of initiation of RRT remains a topic of debate. Previous meta-analyses suggested that earlier initiation of RRT in critically ill patients with AKI may decrease mortality [81]. However, the ideal timing of initiation of RRT has not been established in patients with cirrhosis or patients undergoing liver transplantation. Initiation of RRT in patients with positive fluid balance before the onset of severe AKI may prevent underestimation of AKI [100] and mitigate renal injury [76].

Intraoperative Prevention and Management

A recent trial of major abdominal surgery including transplantation demonstrated that urinary biomarker (TIMP-2 and IGFBP7)-guided KDIGO bundle care significantly reduce the incidence of AKI [101]. The KDIGO bundle included optimization of fluid status and perfusion pressure along with discontinuation of a nephrotoxic agent. Although the effect of hemodynamic optimization is promising, randomized trials are required to establish specific hemodynamic goals and algorithm of hemodynamic management.

Pharmacologic interventions have rarely been evaluated for their effect on the risk of AKI after liver transplantation, although randomized trials of drugs to prevent ischemia-reperfusion injury have been performed [102]. The drugs evaluated in another surgical setting such as cardiovascular surgeries showed largely no significant effects [103]. Further studies are required to find effective pharmacologic agents to mitigate the risk of AKI.

Remote ischemic conditioning has been introduced as a promising non-pharmacologic strategy to mitigate ischemia-reperfusion injury and protect major organs. A previous small randomized trial reported that remote ischemic postconditioning in cycles of intermittent clamping performed in the upper limb after graft reperfusion was reported to reduce the stage 1 posttransplant AKI [104]. However, this finding should be validated in further studies with sufficient power.

Postoperative Management of Immunosuppressive Agent

Calcineurin inhibitors (CNI) including cyclosporine and tacrolimus markedly improved liver graft survival rate and are still the mainstay of immunosuppressive agents after liver transplantation. However, their long-term use is associated with CNI nephrotoxicity which may result in AKI and CKD. Possible mechanisms of

CNI nephrotoxicity included renal artery vasoconstriction and thrombotic microangiopathy [105]. Minimizing CNI use could preserve or even improve renal function in patients undergoing liver transplantation without increasing rejection rate or mortality [106].

Reducing CNI dosage can be achieved by combination therapy with a mammalian target of rapamycin (mTOR) inhibitors including everolimus and sirolimus. Previous studies have demonstrated that the use of mTOR inhibitors led to an improvement in renal function. However, the effect of the sirolimus on the renal function within the first month of the immediate postoperative phase showed conflicting results [107–109]. A previous multicenter randomized phase II study compared standard dose tacrolimus versus reduced dose tacrolimus with sirolimus reporting an increased risk of graft loss and mortality in the sirolimus group [108]. Although other studies of sirolimus reported a renal protective effect of the regimen with reduced or without CNI beyond the first month, the incidence of acute cellular rejection (ACR) and adverse events was high [107, 109]. Studies with everolimus with minimized CNI use was associated with improved renal function without an increase in ACR or mortality [110]. However, everolimus was associated with an increased risk of overall infection. Furthermore, CNI reduction with mTOR inhibitors was not shown to be beneficial beyond the first year of transplantation [53, 111].

Delayed administration of CNI with short-term induction of monoclonal or polyclonal antibodies of daclizumab or belatacept has been used to protect renal function with conflicting results [112–115]. Failure to improve renal function [112] or higher rates of ACR [115] still requires further trials for an adequate conclusion. A recent trial tested the use of induction therapy with basiliximab, a monoclonal antibody, along with mycophenolic acid could eliminate CNI administration with improved renal function without an increased rate of ACR [116].

CNI dose reduction with continuous use of mycophenolate mofetil was reported to be beneficial regarding renal protection with no increased rates of ACR [17, 117]. However, the use of mycophenolate mofetil alone without CNI is associated with an increased incidence of ACR.

Summary

AKI is common after liver transplantation or HPB surgery and influences postoperative mortality. AKI develops from multifactorial etiology including hemodynamic and inflammatory factors as well as ischemia-reperfusion injury. AKI can be triggered by perioperative infection, nephrotoxic medication, poor renal perfusion, decreased oxygen delivery and transfusion. Pretransplant AKI and HRS increase the risk of posttransplant AKI and long-term renal dysfunction. Effective strategies optimizing preoperative renal function and preventing the development of posttransplant AKI are required to avoid poor postoperative patient outcomes after liver transplantation or HBP surgery. Biomarkers were investigated with diagnostic values yet to be defined. A novel biomarker may assist in early identification of acute tubular injury for early diagnosis of AKI and guiding patient management to prevent further deterioration of renal function. Further clinical trials are required to find an optimal regimen of immunosuppressive agents to minimize the nephrotoxicity of CNI. Randomized trials are required to find the modifiable perioperative risk factors of AKI and their causal relationship should be proven to mitigate the risk of AKI. Given the multifactorial etiology and numerous risk factors, a multimodal approach should be required to prevent AKI and improve the outcomes of liver transplantation.

References

1. Paramesh AS, Roayaie S, Doan Y, Schwartz ME, Emre S, Fishbein T, et al. Post-liver transplant acute renal failure: factors predicting development of end-stage renal disease. Clin Transplant. 2004;18:94–9.
2. Trinh E, Alam A, Tchervenkov J, Cantarovich M. Impact of acute kidney injury following liver transplantation on long-term outcomes. Clin Transplant. 2017;31.
3. Hobson CE, Yavas S, Segal MS, Schold JD, Tribble CG, Layon AJ, et al. Acute kidney injury is associated with increased long-term mortality after cardiothoracic surgery. Circulation. 2009;119:2444–53.
4. Bell S, Dekker FW, Vadiveloo T, Marwick C, Deshmukh H, Donnan PT, et al. Risk of postoperative acute kidney injury in patients undergoing orthopaedic surgery–development and validation of a risk score and effect of acute kidney injury on survival: observational cohort study. BMJ. 2015;351:h5639.
5. O'Riordan A, Wong V, McQuillan R, McCormick PA, Hegarty JE, Watson AJ. Acute renal disease, as defined by the RIFLE criteria, post-liver transplantation. Am J Transplant. 2007;7:168–76.
6. Utsumi M, Umeda Y, Sadamori H, Nagasaka T, Takaki A, Matsuda H, et al. Risk factors for acute renal injury in living donor liver transplantation: evaluation of the RIFLE criteria. Transpl Int. 2013;26:842–52.
7. Lebron Gallardo M, Herrera Gutierrez ME, Seller Perez G, Curiel Balsera E, Fernandez Ortega JF, Quesada GG. Risk factors for renal dysfunction in the postoperative course of liver transplant. Liver Transpl. 2004;10:1379–85.
8. Barri YM, Sanchez EQ, Jennings LW, Melton LB, Hays S, Levy MF, et al. Acute kidney injury following liver transplantation: definition and outcome. Liver Transpl. 2009;15:475–83.
9. Thomas ME, Blaine C, Dawnay A, Devonald MA, Ftouh S, Laing C, et al. The definition of acute kidney injury and its use in practice. Kidney Int. 2015;87:62–73.
10. Wyatt CM, Arons RR. The burden of acute renal failure in nonrenal solid organ transplantation. Transplantation. 2004;78:1351–5.
11. Lim C, Audureau E, Salloum C, Levesque E, Lahat E, Merle JC, et al. Acute kidney injury following hepatectomy for hepatocellular carcinoma: incidence, risk factors and prognostic value. HPB (Oxford). 2016;18:540–8.
12. Bressan AK, James MT, Dixon E, Bathe OF, Sutherland FR, Ball CG. Acute kidney injury following resection of hepatocellular carcinoma: prognostic value of the acute kidney injury network criteria. Can J Surg. 2018;61:E11–6.
13. Garnier J, Faucher M, Marchese U, Meillat H, Mokart D, Ewald J, et al. Severe acute kidney injury following major liver resection without portal clamping: incidence, risk factors, and impact on short-term outcomes. HPB (Oxford). 2018;20:865–71.

14. Tomozawa A, Ishikawa S, Shiota N, Cholvisudhi P, Makita K. Perioperative risk factors for acute kidney injury after liver resection surgery: an historical cohort study. Can J Anaesth. 2015;62:753–61.
15. Slankamenac K, Breitenstein S, Held U, Beck-Schimmer B, Puhan MA, Clavien PA. Development and validation of a prediction score for postoperative acute renal failure following liver resection. Ann Surg. 2009;250:720–8.
16. Hilmi IA, Damian D, Al-Khafaji A, Planinsic R, Boucek C, Sakai T, et al. Acute kidney injury following orthotopic liver transplantation: incidence, risk factors, and effects on patient and graft outcomes. Br J Anaesth. 2015;114:919–26.
17. Park MH, Shim HS, Kim WH, Kim HJ, Kim DJ, Lee SH, et al. Clinical risk scoring models for prediction of acute kidney injury after living donor liver transplantation: a retrospective observational study. PLoS One. 2015;10:e0136230.
18. Inoue Y, Soyama A, Takatsuki M, Hidaka M, Muraoka I, Kanematsu T, et al. Acute kidney injury following living donor liver transplantation. Clin Transplant. 2012;26:E530–5.
19. Chen J, Singhapricha T, Hu KQ, Hong JC, Steadman RH, Busuttil RW, et al. Postliver transplant acute renal injury and failure by the RIFLE criteria in patients with normal pretransplant serum creatinine concentrations: a matched study. Transplantation. 2011;91:348–53.
20. Jun IG, Kwon HM, Jung KW, Moon YJ, Shin WJ, Song JG, et al. The impact of postreperfusion syndrome on acute kidney injury in living donor liver transplantation: a propensity score analysis. Anesth Analg. 2018;127:369–78.
21. Jun IG, Lee B, Kim SO, Shin WJ, Bang JY, Song JG, et al. Comparison of acute kidney injury between ABO-compatible and ABO-incompatible living donor liver transplantation: a propensity matching analysis. Liver Transpl. 2016;22:1656–65.
22. Hilmi IA, Damian D, Al-Khafaji A, Sakai T, Donaldson J, Winger DG, et al. Acute kidney injury after orthotopic liver transplantation using living donor versus deceased donor grafts: a propensity score-matched analysis. Liver Transpl. 2015;21:1179–85.
23. Karapanagiotou A, Dimitriadis C, Papadopoulos S, Kydona C, Kefsenidis S, Papanikolaou V, et al. Comparison of RIFLE and AKIN criteria in the evaluation of the frequency of acute kidney injury in post-liver transplantation patients. Transplant Proc. 2014;46:3222–7.
24. Kundakci A, Pirat A, Komurcu O, Torgay A, Karakayali H, Arslan G, et al. Rifle criteria for acute kidney dysfunction following liver transplantation: incidence and risk factors. Transplant Proc. 2010;42:4171–4.
25. Sparrow HG, Swan JT, Moore LW, Gaber AO, Suki WN. Disparate outcomes observed within Kidney Disease: Improving Global Outcomes (KDIGO) acute kidney injury stage 1. Kidney Int. 2019;95:905–13.
26. Hori D, Katz NM, Fine DM, Ono M, Barodka VM, Lester LC, et al. Defining oliguria during cardiopulmonary bypass and its relationship with cardiac surgery-associated acute kidney injury. Br J Anaesth. 2016;117:733–40.
27. Mizota T, Yamamoto Y, Hamada M, Matsukawa S, Shimizu S, Kai S. Intraoperative oliguria predicts acute kidney injury after major abdominal surgery. Br J Anaesth. 2017;119:1127–34.
28. Kunst G, Ostermann M. Intraoperative permissive oliguria—how much is too much? Br J Anaesth. 2017;119:1075–7.
29. Wong F. Management of ascites in cirrhosis. J Gastroenterol Hepatol. 2012;27:11–20.
30. Wong F. The evolving concept of acute kidney injury in patients with cirrhosis. Nat Rev Gastroenterol Hepatol. 2015;12:711–9.
31. Sherman DS, Fish DN, Teitelbaum I. Assessing renal function in cirrhotic patients: problems and pitfalls. Am J Kidney Dis. 2003;41:269–78.
32. Wong F, Nadim MK, Kellum JA, Salerno F, Bellomo R, Gerbes A, et al. Working Party proposal for a revised classification system of renal dysfunction in patients with cirrhosis. Gut. 2011;60:702–9.
33. Levitsky J, Baker T, Ahya SN, Levin ML, Friedewald J, Gallon L, et al. Outcomes and native renal recovery following simultaneous liver-kidney transplantation. Am J Transplant. 2012;12:2949–57.

34. Vagefi PA, Qian JJ, Carlson DM, Aparici CM, Hirose R, Vincenti F, et al. Native renal function after combined liver-kidney transplant for type 1 hepatorenal syndrome: initial report on the use of postoperative Technetium-99 m-mercaptoacetyltriglycine scans. Transpl Int. 2013;26:471–6.
35. Gowrishankar M, VanderPluym C, Robert C, Bamforth F, Gilmour S, Senthilselvan A. Value of serum cystatin C in estimating renal function in children with non-renal solid organ transplantation. Pediatr Transplant. 2015;19:27–34.
36. Shlipak MG, Matsushita K, Arnlov J, Inker LA, Katz R, Polkinghorne KR, et al. Cystatin C versus creatinine in determining risk based on kidney function. N Engl J Med. 2013;369:932–43.
37. Trawale JM, Paradis V, Rautou PE, Francoz C, Escolano S, Sallee M, et al. The spectrum of renal lesions in patients with cirrhosis: a clinicopathological study. Liver Int. 2010;30:725–32.
38. Wadei HM, Geiger XJ, Cortese C, Mai ML, Kramer DJ, Rosser BG, et al. Kidney allocation to liver transplant candidates with renal failure of undetermined etiology: role of percutaneous renal biopsy. Am J Transplant. 2008;8:2618–26.
39. Chawla LS, Bellomo R, Bihorac A, Goldstein SL, Siew ED, Bagshaw SM, et al. Acute kidney disease and renal recovery: consensus report of the Acute Disease Quality Initiative (ADQI) 16 Workgroup. Nat Rev Nephrol. 2017;13:241–57.
40. Fagundes C, Pepin MN, Guevara M, Barreto R, Casals G, Sola E, et al. Urinary neutrophil gelatinase-associated lipocalin as biomarker in the differential diagnosis of impairment of kidney function in cirrhosis. J Hepatol. 2012;57:267–73.
41. Barreto R, Elia C, Sola E, Moreira R, Ariza X, Rodriguez E, et al. Urinary neutrophil gelatinase-associated lipocalin predicts kidney outcome and death in patients with cirrhosis and bacterial infections. J Hepatol. 2014;61:35–42.
42. Belcher JM, Sanyal AJ, Peixoto AJ, Perazella MA, Lim J, Thiessen-Philbrook H, et al. Kidney biomarkers and differential diagnosis of patients with cirrhosis and acute kidney injury. Hepatology. 2014;60:622–32.
43. Belcher JM, Garcia-Tsao G, Sanyal AJ, Thiessen-Philbrook H, Peixoto AJ, Perazella MA, et al. Urinary biomarkers and progression of AKI in patients with cirrhosis. Clin J Am Soc Nephrol. 2014;9:1857–67.
44. Niemann CU, Walia A, Waldman J, Davio M, Roberts JP, Hirose R, et al. Acute kidney injury during liver transplantation as determined by neutrophil gelatinase-associated lipocalin. Liver Transpl. 2009;15:1852–60.
45. Portal AJ, McPhail MJ, Bruce M, Coltart I, Slack A, Sherwood R, et al. Neutrophil gelatinase–associated lipocalin predicts acute kidney injury in patients undergoing liver transplantation. Liver Transpl. 2010;16:1257–66.
46. Wagener G, Minhaz M, Mattis FA, Kim M, Emond JC, Lee HT. Urinary neutrophil gelatinase-associated lipocalin as a marker of acute kidney injury after orthotopic liver transplantation. Nephrol Dial Transplant. 2011;26:1717–23.
47. Cullaro G, Pisa JF, Brown RS Jr, Wagener G, Verna EC. Early postoperative neutrophil gelatinase-associated lipocalin predicts the development of chronic kidney disease after liver transplantation. Transplantation. 2018;102:809–15.
48. Gocze I, Koch M, Renner P, Zeman F, Graf BM, Dahlke MH, et al. Urinary biomarkers TIMP-2 and IGFBP7 early predict acute kidney injury after major surgery. PLoS One. 2015;10:e0120863.
49. Levitsky J, Baker TB, Jie C, Ahya S, Levin M, Friedewald J, et al. Plasma protein biomarkers enhance the clinical prediction of kidney injury recovery in patients undergoing liver transplantation. Hepatology. 2014;60:2017–26.
50. Singal AK, Jackson B, Pereira GB, Russ KB, Fitzmorris PS, Kakati D, et al. Biomarkers of renal injury in cirrhosis: association with acute kidney injury and recovery after liver transplantation. Nephron. 2018;138:1–12.

51. Aberg F, Lempinen M, Hollmen M, Nordin A, Makisalo H, Isoniemi H. Neutrophil gelatinase-associated lipocalin associated with irreversibility of pre-liver transplant kidney dysfunction. Clin Transplant. 2014;28:869–76.
52. Jeong TD, Kim S, Lee W, Song GW, Kim YK, Chun S, et al. Neutrophil gelatinase-associated lipocalin as an early biomarker of acute kidney injury in liver transplantation. Clin Transplant. 2012;26:775–81.
53. Abdelmalek MF, Humar A, Stickel F, Andreone P, Pascher A, Barroso E, et al. Sirolimus conversion regimen versus continued calcineurin inhibitors in liver allograft recipients: a randomized trial. Am J Transplant. 2012;12:694–705.
54. Hryniewiecka E, Gala K, Krawczyk M, Paczek L. Is neutrophil gelatinase-associated lipocalin an optimal marker of renal function and injury in liver transplant recipients? Transplant Proc. 2014;46:2782–5.
55. Kim M, Kiran RP, Li G. Acute kidney injury after hepatectomy can be reasonably predicted after surgery. J Hepatobiliary Pancreat Sci. 2019;26:144–53.
56. Ham SY, Kim EJ, Kim TH, Koo BN. Comparison of perioperative renal function between epidural and intravenous patient-controlled analgesia after living-donor hepatectomy: a retrospective study. Transplant Proc. 2018;50:1365–71.
57. Cho E, Kim SC, Kim MG, Jo SK, Cho WY, Kim HK. The incidence and risk factors of acute kidney injury after hepatobiliary surgery: a prospective observational study. BMC Nephrol. 2014;15:169.
58. Tsai MS, Lin CL, Chang SN, Lee PH, Kao CH. Diabetes mellitus and increased postoperative risk of acute renal failure after hepatectomy for hepatocellular carcinoma: a nationwide population-based study. Ann Surg Oncol. 2014;21:3810–6.
59. Moon YJ, Jun IG, Kim KH, Kim SO, Song JG, Hwang GS. Comparison of acute kidney injury between open and laparoscopic liver resection: propensity score analysis. PLoS One. 2017;12:e0186336.
60. Xu W, Xu H, Yang H, Liao W, Ge P, Ren J, et al. Continuous Pringle maneuver does not affect outcomes of patients with hepatocellular carcinoma after curative resection. Asia Pac J Clin Oncol. 2017;13:e321–30.
61. Imamura T, Yamamoto Y, Sugiura T, Okamura Y, Ito T, Ashida R, et al. Infrahepatic inferior vena cava semi-clamping can reduce blood loss during hepatic resection but still requires monitoring to avoid acute kidney injury. World J Surg. 2019;43:2038-47.
62. Kim SK, Choi SS, Sim JH, Baik J, Hwang S, Lee SG, et al. Effect of hydroxyethyl starch on acute kidney injury after living donor hepatectomy. Transplant Proc. 2016;48:102–6.
63. Kambakamba P, Slankamenac K, Tschuor C, Kron P, Wirsching A, Maurer K, et al. Epidural analgesia and perioperative kidney function after major liver resection. Br J Surg. 2015;102:805–12.
64. Park YS, Jun IG, Go Y, Song JG, Hwang GS. Comparison of acute kidney injury between open and laparoscopic pylorus-preserving pancreaticoduodenectomy: propensity score analysis. PLoS One. 2018;13:e0202980.
65. Loveday BPT, Dib MJ, Sequeira S, Alotaiby N, Visser R, Barbas AS, et al. Renal outcomes following left renal vein harvest for venous reconstruction during pancreas and liver surgery. HPB (Oxford). 2019;21:114–20.
66. Squires MH 3rd, Mehta VV, Fisher SB, Lad NL, Kooby DA, Sarmiento JM, et al. Effect of preoperative renal insufficiency on postoperative outcomes after pancreatic resection: a single institution experience of 1,061 consecutive patients. J Am Coll Surg. 2014;218:92–101.
67. Antoniak D, Are C, Vokoun C, Samson K, Smith L, Shiffermiller J. The relationship between age and chronic kidney disease in patients undergoing pancreatic resection. J Gastrointest Surg. 2018;22:1376–84.
68. Durand F, Francoz C, Asrani SK, Khemichian S, Pham TA, Sung RS, et al. Acute kidney injury after liver transplantation. Transplantation. 2018;102:1636–49.
69. MacDonald AJ, Nadim MK, Durand F, Karvellas CJ. Acute kidney injury in cirrhosis: implications for liver transplantation. Curr Opin Crit Care. 2019;25:171–8.

70. Francoz C, Nadim MK, Durand F. Kidney biomarkers in cirrhosis. J Hepatol. 2016;65:809–24.
71. Kim WH, Oh HW, Yang SM, Yu JH, Lee HC, Jung CW, et al. Intraoperative hemodynamic parameters and acute kidney injury after living donor liver transplantation. Transplantation. 2019;103:1877-86.
72. Angeli P, Gines P, Wong F, Bernardi M, Boyer TD, Gerbes A, et al. Diagnosis and management of acute kidney injury in patients with cirrhosis: revised consensus recommendations of the International Club of Ascites. J Hepatol. 2015;62:968–74.
73. Arora V, Maiwall R, Rajan V, Jindal A, Muralikrishna Shasthry S, Kumar G, et al. Terlipressin is superior to noradrenaline in the management of acute kidney injury in acute on chronic liver failure. Hepatology. 2018;71:600-10.
74. Kim WH, Lee HC, Lim L, Ryu HG, Jung CW. Intraoperative oliguria with decreased SvO(2) predicts acute kidney injury after living donor liver transplantation. J Clin Med. 2018;8.
75. Goren O, Matot I. Update on perioperative acute kidney injury. Curr Opin Crit Care. 2016;22:370–8.
76. Durand F, Francoz C, Asrani SK, Khemichian S, Pham TA, Sung RS, et al. Acute Kidney Injury after Liver Transplantation. Transplantation. 2018;102:1636-49.
77. Lee SK, Park JB, Kim SJ, Choi GS, Kim DJ, Kwon CH, et al. Early postoperative renal dysfunction in the adult living donor liver transplantation. Transplant Proc. 2007;39:1517–9.
78. Chow FS, Piekoszewski W, Jusko WJ. Effect of hematocrit and albumin concentration on hepatic clearance of tacrolimus (FK506) during rabbit liver perfusion. Drug Metab Dispos. 1997;25:610–6.
79. Wadei HM, Lee DD, Croome KP, Mai ML, Golan E, Brotman R, et al. Early allograft dysfunction after liver transplantation is associated with short- and long-term kidney function impairment. Am J Transplant. 2016;16:850–9.
80. Cabezuelo JB, Ramirez P, Rios A, Acosta F, Torres D, Sansano T, et al. Risk factors of acute renal failure after liver transplantation. Kidney Int. 2006;69:1073–80.
81. Karvellas CJ, Farhat MR, Sajjad I, Mogensen SS, Leung AA, Wald R, et al. A comparison of early versus late initiation of renal replacement therapy in critically ill patients with acute kidney injury: a systematic review and meta-analysis. Crit Care. 2011;15:R72.
82. McLellan S, Walsh T. Oxygen delivery and haemoglobin. Contin Educ Anaesth Crit Care Pain. 2004;4:123–6.
83. Rudnick MR, Marchi LD, Plotkin JS. Hemodynamic monitoring during liver transplantation: a state of the art review. World J Hepatol. 2015;7:1302–11.
84. Vallet B, Futier E. Perioperative oxygen therapy and oxygen utilization. Curr Opin Crit Care. 2010;16:359–64.
85. Lees N, Hamilton M, Rhodes A. Clinical review: goal-directed therapy in high risk surgical patients. Crit Care. 2009;13:231.
86. Paugam-Burtz C, Kavafyan J, Merckx P, Dahmani S, Sommacale D, Ramsay M, et al. Postreperfusion syndrome during liver transplantation for cirrhosis: outcome and predictors. Liver Transpl. 2009;15:522–9.
87. Belghiti J, Noun R, Sauvanet A. Temporary portocaval anastomosis with preservation of caval flow during orthotopic liver transplantation. Am J Surg. 1995;169:277–9.
88. Pratschke S, Meimarakis G, Bruns CJ, Kaspar M, Prix N, Zachoval R, et al. Temporary intraoperative porto-caval shunt: useless or beneficial in piggy back liver transplantation? Transpl Int. 2013;26:90–8.
89. Tsai YF, Lin CC, Lee WC, Yu HP. Propofol attenuates ischemic reperfusion-induced formation of lipid peroxides in liver transplant recipients. Transplant Proc. 2012;44:376–9.
90. Gajate Martin L, Gonzalez C, Ruiz Torres I, Fernandez Martin C, Martin Grande A, Elias Martin E, et al. Effects of the hypnotic agent on primary graft dysfunction after liver transplantation. Transplant Proc. 2016;48:3307–11.

91. Shin S, Joo DJ, Kim MS, Bae MI, Heo E, Lee JS, et al. Propofol intravenous anaesthesia with desflurane compared with desflurane alone on postoperative liver function after living-donor liver transplantation: a randomised controlled trial. Eur J Anaesthesiol. 2019;36:656-66.
92. Lee HC, Yoon SB, Yang SM, Kim WH, Ryu HG, Jung CW, et al. Prediction of acute kidney injury after liver transplantation: machine learning approaches vs. logistic regression model. J Clin Med. 2018;7.
93. Mita N, Kawahito S, Soga T, Takaishi K, Kitahata H, Matsuhisa M, et al. Strict blood glucose control by an artificial endocrine pancreas during hepatectomy may prevent postoperative acute kidney injury. J Artif Organs. 2017;20:76–83.
94. Elia C, Graupera I, Barreto R, Sola E, Moreira R, Huelin P, et al. Severe acute kidney injury associated with non-steroidal anti-inflammatory drugs in cirrhosis: a case-control study. J Hepatol. 2015;63:593–600.
95. Sort P, Navasa M, Arroyo V, Aldeguer X, Planas R, Ruiz-del-Arbol L, et al. Effect of intravenous albumin on renal impairment and mortality in patients with cirrhosis and spontaneous bacterial peritonitis. N Engl J Med. 1999;341:403–9.
96. Fernandez J, Navasa M, Planas R, Montoliu S, Monfort D, Soriano G, et al. Primary prophylaxis of spontaneous bacterial peritonitis delays hepatorenal syndrome and improves survival in cirrhosis. Gastroenterology. 2007;133:818–24.
97. Nadim MK, Durand F, Kellum JA, Levitsky J, O'Leary JG, Karvellas CJ, et al. Management of the critically ill patient with cirrhosis: a multidisciplinary perspective. J Hepatol. 2016;64:717–35.
98. Israelsen M, Krag A, Allegretti AS, Jovani M, Goldin AH, Winter RW, et al. Terlipressin versus other vasoactive drugs for hepatorenal syndrome. Cochrane Database Syst Rev. 2017;9:Cd011532.
99. Rodriguez E, Henrique Pereira G, Sola E, Elia C, Barreto R, Pose E, et al. Treatment of type 2 hepatorenal syndrome in patients awaiting transplantation: effects on kidney function and transplantation outcomes. Liver Transpl. 2015;21:1347–54.
100. Liu KD, Thompson BT, Ancukiewicz M, Steingrub JS, Douglas IS, Matthay MA, et al. Acute kidney injury in patients with acute lung injury: impact of fluid accumulation on classification of acute kidney injury and associated outcomes. Crit Care Med. 2011;39:2665–71.
101. Gocze I, Jauch D, Gotz M, Kennedy P, Jung B, Zeman F, et al. Biomarker-guided intervention to prevent acute kidney injury after major surgery: the prospective randomized BigpAK study. Ann Surg. 2018;267:1013–20.
102. Ryu HG, Jung CW, Lee CS, Lee J. Nafamostat mesilate attenuates Postreperfusion Syndrome during liver transplantation. Am J Transplant. 2011;11:977–83.
103. Kim WH, Hur M, Park SK, Jung DE, Kang P, Yoo S, et al. Pharmacological interventions for protecting renal function after cardiac surgery: a Bayesian network meta-analysis of comparative effectiveness. Anaesthesia. 2018;73:1019–31.
104. Kim WH, Lee JH, Ko JS, Min JJ, Gwak MS, Kim GS, et al. Effect of remote ischemic postconditioning on patients undergoing living donor liver transplantation. Liver Transpl. 2014;20:1383–92.
105. Remuzzi G, Bertani T. Renal vascular and thrombotic effects of cyclosporine. Am J Kidney Dis. 1989;13:261–72.
106. Kong Y, Wang D, Shang Y, Liang W, Ling X, Guo Z, et al. Calcineurin-inhibitor minimization in liver transplant patients with calcineurin-inhibitor-related renal dysfunction: a meta-analysis. PLoS One. 2011;6:e24387.
107. Teperman L, Moonka D, Sebastian A, Sher L, Marotta P, Marsh C, et al. Calcineurin inhibitor-free mycophenolate mofetil/sirolimus maintenance in liver transplantation: the randomized spare-the-nephron trial. Liver Transpl. 2013;19:675–89.
108. Asrani SK, Wiesner RH, Trotter JF, Klintmalm G, Katz E, Maller E, et al. De novo sirolimus and reduced-dose tacrolimus versus standard-dose tacrolimus after liver transplantation: the 2000-2003 phase II prospective randomized trial. Am J Transplant. 2014;14:356–66.

109. Weir MR, Pearson TC, Patel A, Peddi VR, Kalil R, Scandling J, et al. Long-term follow-up of kidney transplant recipients in the spare-the-nephron-trial. Transplantation. 2017;101:157–65.
110. Lin M, Mittal S, Sahebjam F, Rana A, Sood GK. Everolimus with early withdrawal or reduced-dose calcineurin inhibitors improves renal function in liver transplant recipients: a systematic review and meta-analysis. Clin Transplant. 2017;31.
111. Levitsky J, O'Leary JG, Asrani S, Sharma P, Fung J, Wiseman A, et al. Protecting the kidney in liver transplant recipients: practice-based recommendations from the American Society of Transplantation Liver and Intestine Community of Practice. Am J Transplant. 2016;16:2532–44.
112. Calmus Y, Kamar N, Gugenheim J, Duvoux C, Ducerf C, Wolf P, et al. Assessing renal function with daclizumab induction and delayed tacrolimus introduction in liver transplant recipients. Transplantation. 2010;89:1504–10.
113. Neuberger JM, Mamelok RD, Neuhaus P, Pirenne J, Samuel D, Isoniemi H, et al. Delayed introduction of reduced-dose tacrolimus, and renal function in liver transplantation: the 'ReSpECT' study. Am J Transplant. 2009;9:327–36.
114. Yoshida EM, Marotta PJ, Greig PD, Kneteman NM, Marleau D, Cantarovich M, et al. Evaluation of renal function in liver transplant recipients receiving daclizumab (Zenapax), mycophenolate mofetil, and a delayed, low-dose tacrolimus regimen vs. a standard-dose tacrolimus and mycophenolate mofetil regimen: a multicenter randomized clinical trial. Liver Transpl. 2005;11:1064–72.
115. Klintmalm GB, Feng S, Lake JR, Vargas HE, Wekerle T, Agnes S, et al. Belatacept-based immunosuppression in de novo liver transplant recipients: 1-year experience from a phase II randomized study. Am J Transplant. 2014;14:1817–27.
116. Saliba F, Duvoux C, Gugenheim J, Kamar N, Dharancy S, Salame E, et al. Efficacy and safety of everolimus and mycophenolic acid with early tacrolimus withdrawal after liver transplantation: a multicenter randomized trial. Am J Transplant. 2017;17:1843–52.
117. Goralczyk AD, Bari N, Abu-Ajaj W, Lorf T, Ramadori G, Friede T, et al. Calcineurin inhibitor sparing with mycophenolate mofetil in liver transplantion: a systematic review of randomized controlled trials. Am J Transplant. 2012;12:2601–7.

Chapter 15
Use of Extracorporeal Membrane Oxygenation During Liver Transplantation

Marc Giménez-Milà, Antoni Sabaté and Pádraig Ó. Scanaill

Introduction

Patients with end-stage liver disease (ESLD are candidates for liver transplantation (LT). Those presenting for LT have a high risk of respiratory and cardiovascular events perioperatively. LT patients with cardiorespiratory failure refractory to maximal conventional therapy may be considered for extracorporeal life support [1]. Recent advances in technology and clinical experience with this technology have lead to the increased use of Extracorporeal Membrane Oxygenation ECMO in this patient group.

ECMO is an established rescue therapy for refractory cardiorespiratory failure [2]. It can be classified into two types depending on the organ failure it supports: veno-venous ECMO (VV-ECMO) for severe respiratory failure and veno-arterial ECMO (VA-ECMO) for refractory cardiogenic shock. The utility of extracorporeal membrane oxygenation in treating ESLD perioperatively has been well described [3]. ECMO may be used as a rescue therapy, both preoperatively to facilitate LT and postoperatively to provide continued supportive therapy in the critical care unit.

In this chapter, we discuss the principles of ECMO, the current evidence on its use in LT and some points to consider when using it in ESLD patients.

M. Giménez-Milà (✉) · A. Sabaté
Department of Anaesthesia and Critical Care, Biomedical Research Institute of Bellvitge (IDIBELL), Bellvitge University Hospital, Barcelona, Spain
e-mail: gimimarc@gmail.com

P. Ó. Scanaill
Department of Anaesthesia, Kings College Hospital, London SE5 9RS, UK

Z. Milan and C. Goonasekera (eds.), *Anesthesia for Hepatico-Pancreatic-Biliary Surgery and Transplantation*, https://doi.org/10.1007/978-3-030-51331-3_15

Principles of ECMO

Generally, VA-ECMO supports both cardiac and respiratory function, where as VV-ECMO predominantly supports respiratory function. An ECMO circuit is essentially a modification of the cardiopulmonary bypass circuit [4]. The principles of ECMO involve venous blood being removed from the patient, oxygenated, having carbon dioxide removed and returned to the arterial system. A membrane oxygenator is incorporated into the extracorporeal circuit to allow for oxygenation, and a 'sweep gas' to control carbon dioxide. A centrifugal pump is incorporated to allow for continuous flow. Similar to the cardiopulmonary bypass circuit, a heat exchanger and pressure detectors are incorporated for safety. Recent modifications have allowed the ECMO circuit to be smaller and more portable than previous versions [4]. ECMO has traditionally been used as a short-term supportive therapy, however, with advancement in modern circuit technology, its use may be extended to several months as clinically indicated [5]. Once established, ECMO can significantly improve patient haemodynamics and provide time for recovery of organ function or be used as a bridge to definitive therapy.

Circuit Configuration

In adults, the most common configurations for VV-ECMO are: (1) femoral-jugular or (2) placement of an internal jugular dual lumen cannula. The first configuration consists of an access cannula in the femoral vein (with the tip in the inferior vena cava), while the return cannula sits in the internal jugular vein (with the tip in the superior vena cava). It is important to ensure adequate distance between cannula tips in order to minimise the risk of recirculation. In the dual-lumen cannula configuration, a single-vessel cannulation is made via the internal jugular vein, with the return cannula tip proximal to the heart (Fig. 15.1).

VV-ECMO was first established in 1972, with its first description of successful use in acute respiratory distress syndrome (ARDS) that developed in a patient after polytrauma [7]. The use of ECMO was paramount globally in the treatment of severe respiratory failure secondary to H1N1 in 2009 [8]. In the same year, the CESAR trial explored the benefits of ECMO versus conventional care in patients with severe respiratory failure [9]. Patients were randomised according to their Murray score to receive conventional ventilation or referral to an ECMO centre. Those randomised to the ECMO group were transferred to a specialised ECMO centre, where a 12-hour period of ARDS standard management was performed. The Murray scoring system includes four criteria for the development of ARDS [10]. It accounts for the PaO2/FiO2 (P/F) ratio, quadrants affected on chest x-ray, lung compliance and PEEP level on ventilator. ECMO was indicated when the Murray score was more than 3 or uncompensated hypercapnia with respiratory acidosis. If there was an improvement after the 12 hours, ECMO was not

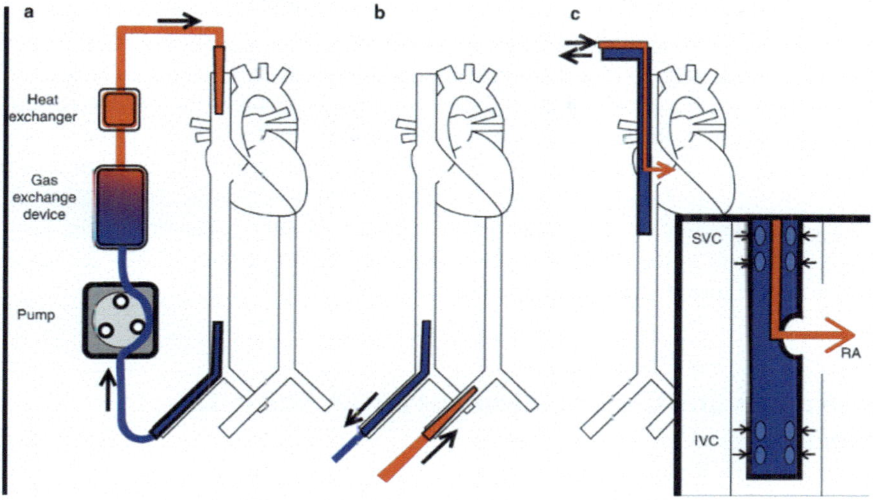

Fig. 15.1 **a** Femoral-jugular VV-ECMO configuration used in cases of severe respiratory failure. **b** Peripheral VA-ECMO where blood is drained from femoral vein and returned into the femoral artery. **c** VV-ECMO with dual lumen cannula configuration. Reproduced with permission of Springer Link [6]

commenced. This happened in 22 out of 90 patients. Although treatment group exhibited survival benefit at 6 months compared with the conventionally treated group (63% vs. 47%; relative risk 0.69 (95% confidence interval 0.5–0.97), conclusions should be drawn cautiously. This is because in 24% of patients in the intervention arm, ECMO was not deemed necessary. Therefore, what the CESAR trial tells us is that survival from severe respiratory failure improves when the patient is transferred to an ECMO centre. This highlights the importance of involving specialist units when considering extracorporeal life support.

In 2018, the EOLIA study tried to elucidate doubts generated after the CESAR trial publication around the use of VV-ECMO in ARDS (11). The 60-day mortality in the VV-ECMO group (35%) was lower than in control group (46%) but did not reach statistical significance ($p=0.09$). 35 patients in the control group (28%) were crossed-over to treatment group due to refractory hypoxaemia with a mortality of 57%. The study was stopped early based due to futility. A post hoc analysis of the EOLIA results revealed decreased mortality at 60-days in the ECMO group. A signal from the data suggests that ECMO provides a survival benefit in patients with severe respiratory failure however this benefit is less than the 20% which was the estimated absolute risk reduction initially proposed by Combes et al. [11].

In parallel, an Australian group published the first score to predict survival once ECMO is commenced [12]. The RESP score integrates age, suspected diagnosis, duration of mechanical ventilation and other comorbidities prior to starting ECMO. Survival is estimated by using a logistic regression and helps clinicians with decision to institute the therapy.

The indications for VA-ECMO are refractory cardiogenic shock or witnessed cardiac arrest in which there is no return of spontaneous circulation. VA-ECMO is used as a bridge to recovery, or definitive therapy. VA-ECMO can also be used in patients with primary respiratory failure with associated heart failure due to septic cardiomyopathy. In adults, circuit configuration is similar to the one previously described with the difference of the return cannula; inserted in the femoral artery for peripheral configuration or in the ascending aorta for central configuration. In cases of peripheral cannulation, another perfusion catheter is inserted in the femoral artery distal to the outflow cannula infusing blood from the ECMO circuit in order to avoid ipsilateral limb ischaemia.

Indications and Contraindications for ECMO in LT Patients

Indications for ECMO in LT are no different from that of the general population. Potential reversibility of organ dysfunction and severity of respiratory and or circulatory dysfunction are used as indications for ECMO. Similar to the general population, contraindications to ECMO in the LT population include: high patient frailty, uncontrolled coagulopathy, disseminated malignancy and patient or relatives refusal of treatment. Prior to considering ECMO for a LT patient, a full multi-disciplinary discussion involving intensivists, anaesthetists, transplant physicians, surgeons and haematologists should occur to tailor to individual patients.

In the preoperative period, VV-ECMO could be used as "bridge" in patients with acute liver failure or chronic liver failure and reversible cardiovascular instability awaiting LT [13].

Intraoperatively, ECMO has been used in extremely haemodynamically unstable patients [14, 15].

In the postoperative period VV-ECMO has been used in ARDS [3, 16], pneumonia [17] and HPS [18–20]. VA-ECMO has been used in cases with fulminant pulmonary embolism and portopulmonary hypertension (Fig. 15.2).

ECMO and Liver Transplant

In the last decade, reports on the use of ECMO on adult and paediatric patients undergoing LT have consolidated this therapy in selected cases. Park and colleagues [17] published a retrospective study recruiting 18 patients that required VV-ECMO due to ARDS and severe pneumonia refractory to conventional ICU management. Eight patients (44%) were successfully weaned from ECMO after a mean of 10.4 days (±6.8 days) with a survival of 100% at 13 months. No factors of failure of therapy amongst their population could be found possibly due

Configura-tion	Indication	pa-tients	Popula-tion	timing	Outcome	Reference
VV-ECMO	ARDS/pneu-monia	18	Adult	Post-OLT	44% survival	Park et al
VV-ECMO	HPS	1	Paediatric	Post-OLT	Survival	Fleming et al
VV-ECMO	HPS	1	Adult	Post-OLT	Survival	Sharma et al
VV-ECMO	HPS	1	Adult	Pre-OLT	Survival	Monsel et al
Unknown	ARDS	1	Adult	Post-OLT	Death (massive intracranial bleed)	Jeng et al
VV-ECMO	ARDS	9	Adult	Post-OLT	45% survival	Choi et al
VV-ECMO	Pulm Haem-orrhage	1	Paediatric	Pre- OLT	Survival	Fujita et al
VA-ECMO	Pulm Haem-orrhage	1	Paediatric	Pre-OLT	Survival	Son et al
VV-ECMO	ARDS	3	Paediatric	Pre-OLT	66% survival	Nandhabalan et al
VV-ECMO	HPS	1	Adult	Post-OLT	Survival	Auzinger et al
VA-ECMO	Cardiogenic shock	1	Adult	Intra-OLT	Survival	Sun et al
VA-ECMO	Pulmonary embolism	1	Adult	Intra-OLT	Death (9 weeks after OTH)	Szocik et al
VA-ECMO	Porto-pulmo-nary Hyper-tension	1	Adult	Intra-OLT	Died (septic shock)	Martucci et al
VV&VA-ECMO	Acute pulmo-nary& car-diac failure	8	Adult	Post-OLT	38% survival	Braun at al

Fig. 15.2 Published uses of ECMO in liver transplantation

to limited sample size. Choi and colleagues (5), in a 9 patient cohort, reported a survival rate of 45% that is in line with outcomes in general non-transplant population.

Hepatopulmonary syndrome (HPS) is a potential cause of hypoxaemia in ESLD patients that arises due to ventilation/perfusion mismatch with intrapulmonary vasodilation and intra-pulmonary shunting. It was previously considered to be a contraindication but transplantation has shown to improve oxygenation better than maximal conventional medical therapy. In a few patients, refractory hypoxaemia due to HPS can evolve into graft dysfunction and multi-organ failure unless extracorporeal support is instituted. There are case reports of successful use of VV-ECMO after LT in the paediatric [18] and adult population [19, 20]. In one patient, ECMO was instituted prior to transplantation, which was weaned off in the operating theatre at the end of LT. In the other two, ECMO was continued in the postoperative period for a period of time.

In the paediatric population, Fujita et al. [21] reports pre-transplant VV-ECMO usage in a 10-week old child with pulmonary haemorrhage for four days while awaiting a second LT. Although the patient required further subsequent re-do LT, the authors report a 15-month survival benefit. VA-ECMO has been successfully used in a five-year old patient with fulminant Wilson disease before transplantation to treat life-threatening pulmonary haemorrhage [22]. In this case, cannulation was performed accessing right carotid artery and right internal jugular vein. A case series of three paediatric ARDS patients treated with VV-ECMO prior to LT offered a 66% survival [23].

Pulmonary embolism is a potentially fatal complication during LT. Szocik et al. report a case of sudden haemodynamic compromise during the anhepatic phase of a LT [24]. An immediate transoesophageal echocardiography revealed a large thrombus in the right atrium and right ventricle. Peripheral VA-ECMO was instituted without complications and the patient was discharged home on day 12 but one week later he was re-admitted with a large thrombus in inferior vena cava, which was sadly fatal.

Severe cardiovascular compromise with portopulmonary hypertension or valve disease are also relative contraindications for liver transplantation. However, there are descriptions of successful use of VA-ECMO to treat severe mitral and tricuspid regurgitation during LT [15]. VA-ECMO has been used to treat portopulmonary hypertension which resulted in intra-transplant cardiac arrest [25]. Unfortunately, the postoperative period was complicated with septic shock and the patient passed away on the 8th postoperative day.

In comparison with the general intensive care population, there are a few issues to bear in mind when instituting ECMO before or after LT. Such issues include coagulopathy and vascular anastomosis performed during the procedure.

Coagulopathy

Complex homeostasis in patients with ESLD is disrupted once extracorporeal support is commenced. A balance needs to be met between the risk of bleeding and thrombosis.

Bleeding remains a concern, especially in those patients with evidence of pulmonary haemorrhage or previous intracranial haematoma [16]. Improvements in circuit design, with heparin-bonded tubing, and less thrombogenic oxygenators, has allowed reduction or even avoidance of systemic anticoagulation for VV- ECMO support [24, 26]. In cases of ECMO treatments without heparin and simultaneous use of continuous veno-venous hemofiltration, regional citrate has been used successfully to prolong filter life and minimise clot formation and embolisation [27]. In cases of VA-ECMO, avoidance of unfractionated heparin (UFH) may lead to significant morbidity due to arterial clot formation and embolic events.

Dosing of UFH, in most ECMO centres, is based on activated clotting time (ACT) and aPTT ratio (APR) aiming for a target of 180–220 seconds and 1.5–2.5 respectively. The aPTT is affected by some conditions that may be present in some patients with ESLD like the presence of lupus anticoagulant or changes in factor VIII, IX, XI and XII levels. In these cases, the measurement of anti-Xa levels may be of help to guide anticoagulation therapy because it only reflects UFH effect. Normal range of anti-Xa levels while on ECMO are considered to be between 0.3 and 0.5 IU/ml.

Heparin induced thrombocytopenia (HIT) is an immune-mediated complication seen after exposure to heparin [28]. It is suspected clinically in arterial and/or venous thrombosis, associated with decreased platelet count after 5–10 episodes of heparin exposure and having excluded other causes of thrombocytopenia. The diagnosis is based on clinical and laboratory criteria. The 4T score is a clinical probability scoring system and a score of>4 indicates an intermediate or high probability of HIT. If HIT is suspected, heparin should be discontinued and alternative anticoagulants started while waiting for confirmatory laboratory tests. Danaparoids and thrombin inhibitors (such as argatroban) are the most frequent alternative anticoagulants used.

Patients with ESLD may exhibit more difficulties on diagnosing HIT because of chronic thrombocytopenia [29]. With this in mind, precautions should be taken when approaching patients with suspected HIT, notwithstanding the use of non-heparin anticoagulation which may be difficult to monitor, making the affected LT population prone to bleeding events.

Vascular Anastomosis

The surgical technique during liver transplantation (piggyback versus classic technique) will have an impact on vascular access for ECMO cannulation due to risk of injury to the venous anastomosis. In order to minimise this risk, fluoroscopic guidance is mandatory during guidewire insertion and cannula positioning. When a dual lumen cannula is chosen, the use of transoesophageal echocardiography can help minimise the risk of tamponade by providing direct vision during cannula placement. There have been case reports describing malposition of the dual cannula, entering into the blind end of the donor vena cava impairing venous drainage of the liver [23, 26] resulting in venous congestion of the graft. The dual lumen cannula in adults can be 27 or 31 Fr in both cases measuring 29 cm in length. In femoral-jugular configuration, the tip of femoral cannula should be checked with fluoroscopy or ultrasound to ensure venous drainage of liver graft is not compromised.

Conclusions

The applicability of extracorporeal respiratory and circulatory support is expanding in the perioperative care of patients undergoing LT. The most frequent reported indications are hepatopulmonary syndrome and ARDS in the context of ESLD. Vascular access, haemorrhagic diathesis and immunosuppression are factors to consider when proceeding with ECMO in this population. The use of echocardiography is recommended to confirm cannula position.

Although it may relieve refractory cardiorespiratory failure, a clear multidisciplinary plan with transplant physicians, surgeons and intensivists should be made before instituting ECMO to confirm reversibility of dysfunction and options of re-listing should the graft fail. While waiting for further robust evidence, a multidisciplinary approach should be used to guarantee a balance between expectations and futility.

References

1. Auzinger G, Willars C, Loveridge R, Vercueil A, Best T, Wendon J. Extracorporeal membrane oxygenation before and after adult liver transplantation: worth the effort? Crit Care. 2014;18(Suppl 1):p203.
2. Marasco S, Lukas G, McDonald M, McMillan J, Ihle B. Review of ECMO (Extra Corporeal Membrane Oxygenation) support in critically ill adult patients. Heart Lung Circ. 2008;17:41–7.
3. Choi NK, Hwang S, Kim KW, Park GC, Yu YD, Jung SH, et al. Intensive pulmonary support using extracorporeal membrane oxygenation in adult patients undergoing liver transplantation. Hepatogastroenterology. 2012;59:1189–93.
4. Lequier L, Horton S, McMullan M, Bartlett R. Extracorporeal membrane oxygenation circuitry. Pediatr Crit Care Med. 2013;14:S7–12.
5. Wiktor A, Haft J, Bartlett R, Park P, Raghavendran K, Napolitano L. Prolonged VV ECMO (265 days) for ARDS without technical complications. 2015;61:205–6.
6. Werner NL, Park PK. Extracorporeal Membrane Oxygenation (ECMO)/Extracorporeal Carbon Dioxide Removal ($ECCO_2R$). In: Martin N, Kaplan L, editors. Principles of adult surgical critical care. Cham: Springer; 2016.
7. Hill J, O'Brien T, Murray J, Dontigny L, Bramson M, Osborn J, et al. Prolonged extracorporeal oxygenation for acute post-traumatic respiratory failure (shock-lung syndrome)—use of the bramson membrane lung. N Engl J Med. 1972;286:629–34.
8. Zangrillo A, Biondi-Zoccai G, Landoni G, Frati G, Patroniti N, Pesenti A, et al. Extracorporeal membrane oxygenation (ECMO) in patients with H1N1 influenza infection: a systematic review and meta-analysis including 8 studies and 266 patients receiving ECMO. Crit Care. 2013;17:R30.
9. Peek GJ, Mugford M, Tiruvoipati R, et al. Efficacy and economic assessment of conventional ventilatory support versus extracorporeal membrane oxygenation for severe adult respiratory failure (CESAR): a multicentre randomized controlled trial. Lancet. 2009;374:1351–63.
10. Murray JF, Matthay MA, Luce JM, Flick MR. An expanded definition of the adult respiratory distress syndrome. Am Rev Respir Dis. 1988;138:720–3.
11. Combes A, Hajage D, Capellier G, et al. Extracorporeal membrane oxygenation for severe acute respiratory distress syndrome. N Engl J Med. 2018;24(378):1965–75.

12. Schmidt M, Bailey M, Sheldrake J, et al. Predicting survival after ECMO for severe acute respiratory failure: the Respiratory ECMO Survival Prediction (RESP)-score. Am J Respir Crit Care Med. 2014;1(189):1374–82.
13. Dell'Amore A, Botta L, Gallieri S, Arpesella G. Extracorporeal membrane oxygenator assistanceas "bridge" to combined heart and liver transplantation. Transplant Proc. 2006;38:3004–5.
14. Braun HJ, Pulcrano ME, Weber DJ, Padilla BE, Ascher NL. The utility of ECMO after liver transplantation: experience at a high-volume transplant center and review of the literature. Transplantation. 2019;103:1568–73.
15. Sun X, Qiu W, Chen Y, et al. Utilization of extracorporeal membrane oxygenation for a severe cardiocirculatory dysfunction recipient in liver transplantation a case report. Medicine (Baltimore). 2018;97:e12407.
16. Jeng LB, Cheng MH, Lee WC, et al. Extracorporeal membrane oxygenation therapy for adult respiratory distress syndrome developing post liver transplantion. Transplant Proc. 1994;26:2237–8.
17. Park YH, Hwang S, Park HW, et al. Effect of pulmonary support using extracorporeal membrane oxygenation for adult liver transplant recipients with respiratory failure. Transplant Proc. 2012;44:757–61.
18. Fleming G, Cornell T, Welling T, et al. Hepatopulmonary syndrome: use of extracorporeal life support for life-threatening hypoxia following liver transplantation. Liver Transpl. 2008;14(7):966–70.
19. Sharma NS, Wille KM, Guzman ED. Extracorporeal membrane oxygenation after liver transplantation in a patient with hepatopulmonary syndrome and an atrial septal defect. Int J Ar f Organs 2015;38:170–2.
20. Monsel A, Mal H, Brisson H, et al. Extracorporeal membrane oxygenation as a bridge to liver transplantation for acute respiratory distress syndrome-induced life-threatening hypoxaemia aggravated by hepatopulmonary syndrome. Crit Care. 2011;15:R234.
21. Fujita S, Hemming AW, Fujikawa T, et al. Expanded efficacy and indication of extracorporeal membrane oxygenation for preoperative pulmonary bleeding on pediatric cadaveric orthotopic liver transplantation. Transplantation. 2005;79(11):1637. Erratum in: Transplantation. 2014;98(9):e86.
22. Son SK, Oh SH, Kim KM, et al. Successful liver transplantation following veno-arterial extracorporeal membrane oxygenation in a child with fulminant Wilson disease and severe pulmonary hemorrhage: a case report. Pediatr Transplant. 2012;16(7):E281–5.
23. Nandhabalan P, Loveridge R, Patel S, et al. Extracorporeal membrane oxygenation and pediatric liver transplantation, "a step too far?": results of a single-center experience. Liver Transpl. 2016;22:1727–33.
24. Szocik J, Rudich S, Csete M. ECMO resuscitation after massive pulmonary embolism during liver transplantation. Anesthesiology. 2002;97:763–4.
25. Martucci G, Burgio G, Lullo F, et al. Veno-arterial extracorporeal membrane oxygenation as an intraoperative rescue option in case of portopulmonary hypertension recognized during liver transplantation. Minerva Anestesiol. 2017;83:1336–7.
26. Auzinger G, Willars C, Loveridge R, Best T, Vercueil A, Prachalias A, et al. Extracorporeal membrane oxygenation for refractory hypoxemia after liver transplantation in severe hepato-pulmonary syndrome: a solution with pitfalls. Liver Transpl. 2014;20:1141–4.
27. Shum HP, Kwan AM, Chan KC, et al. The use of regional citrate anticoagulation continuous venovenous hemofiltration in extracorporeal membrane oxygenation. ASAIO J. 2014;60:413–8.
28. Cuker A, Arepally GM, Chong BH, et al. American Society of Hematology 2018 guidelines for management of venous thromboembolism: heparin-induced thrombocytopenia. Blood Adv. 2018;2:3360–92.
29. Assfalg V, Hüser N. Heparin-induced thrombocytopenia in solid organ transplant recipients: the current scientific knowledge. World J Transplant. 2016;24(6):165–73.

Chapter 16
Liver Preservation with Extracorporeal Perfusion

Miriam Cortes-Cerisuelo

Abbreviations

ALT	alanine transaminase
AST	aspartate aminotransferase
ATP	adenosine triphosphate
CIT	cold ischaemia time
cDCD	controlled DCD
DCD	donors after circulatory death
COR	controlled oxygenated rewarming
DBD	donors after brain death
EAD	early allograft dysfunction
ECD	extended criteria donors
HAT	hepatic artery thrombosis
HBOC	hemoglobin-based oxygen carrier
HTK	histidine tryptophan ketoglutarate
IC	Ischaemic cholangiopathy
IGL-1	Institute George Lopez-1
IRI	ischaemia reperfusion injury
LT	liver transplantation
MP	machine perfusion
NECMO	normothermic extra-corporeal membrane oxygenation
NMP	normothermic machine perfusion
NRP	normothermic regional perfusion
PBG	peribiliary glands
PNF	primary non-function

M. Cortes-Cerisuelo (✉)
Liver Transplant Surgeon, Institute of Liver Studies, King's College Hospital, London, UK
e-mail: m.cortescerisuelo@nhs.net

Z. Milan and C. Goonasekera (eds.), *Anesthesia for Hepatico-Pancreatic-Biliary Surgery and Transplantation*, https://doi.org/10.1007/978-3-030-51331-3_16

pSCS-NMP	post–static cold storage normothermic machine perfusion
RCT	randomized controlled trial
SCS	static cold storage
UW	University of Wisconsin
WIT	warm ischaemia time

Donor Liver Preservation Injury

Liver transplantation (LT) involves a sequence of events starting with donor organ procurement, storage and transportation, finishing with the implantation of the donor liver in the recipient; this has been possible thanks to the development of organ preservation techniques which allow not only the reduction of damage to the donor liver during the procurement but also the safe storage and transport of organs from the donor hospital to the transplant centre until it is implanted into the recipient.

The most common modality of organ preservation has been static cold storage (SCS) with special preservation solutions such as University of Wisconsin (UW), Celsior, histidine tryptophan ketoglutarate (HTK) and Institute George Lopez-1 (IGL-1). From these, UW solution has been the most commonly used since it was developed by Belzer and Southard and introduced in the clinical practice in 1987 [1]. The rationale behind SCS is the suppression of the metabolism during the period in which the donor liver doesn't receive oxygen and nutrients. According to Van't Hoff's rule, at 4 °C, the metabolic rate is 10% compared to normothermic conditions, allowing preservation times for more than 15 hours. However, there is an associated cold preservation injury that happens during SCS such as cell swelling, anaerobic metabolism with depletion of ATP and reactive oxygen species (ROS) production which are highly toxic, producing cell membrane damage. There is also increased intracellular calcium concentration which is a signal of ischemic mechanisms leading to cell death, mitochondrial dysfunction and ATP-dependant cytoskeletal dysfunction, resulting in sinusoidal endothelial cell damage, causing platelet and leukocyte adhesion, and consequently microcirculatory disturbances and an inflammatory immune response after reperfusion [2–4].

The composition of the preservation solutions mentioned above have been designed to address preservation injury and minimise the effect of SCS. Once the liver is taken out of the ice to initiate the vascular anastomosis in the recipient, it will progressively rewarm in anoxic conditions as it hasn't been reperfused, resulting in increasing energetic demand and further depletion of ATP. This period, since the liver is out of ice until it is reperfused, is called warm ischaemia time (WIT) and should be less than 50 minutes as it has been described as an independent predictor of post-transplant survival [5].

On reperfusion of the donor liver in the recipient there will be a cascade of events which will happen as a consequence of pre-existing preservation and re-warming injury during the vascular anastomosis, characterised by mitochondrial injury, cell death, microcirculatory disturbances and intravascular thrombosis as a consequence of platelet and leukocyte adhesion. These events will activate an inflammatory immune response that will result in amplified local tissue destruction, which will trigger the activation of cell death program. This additional damaged is called ischaemia reperfusion injury (IRI), and it has been directly related to the length of the SCS (also called cold ischaemia time (CIT)) and to the risk of post-transplant complications [6].

Organ Preservation Modalities

The success of LT has led to an increasing demand for donor livers, and a significant number of patients on the waiting list for transplant. In order to expand the donor pool, there is an increasing utilization of extended criteria donors (ECD) such as the elderly, elevated body mass index, livers with steatosis and donors after circulatory death (DCD) among other [7, 8]. While these options may decrease the time on the waiting list, these livers are more susceptible to cold preservation injury and to prolonged CIT, therefore they can present with higher degree of IRI, affecting short and long-term outcomes [9]; For this reason, the transplant community has been focused on alternative preservation techniques to minimise IRI, improve or minimise the liver damage during the procurement and storage, to assess liver quality and to increase organ utilization (Table 16.1).

These new alternative preservation techniques have emerged in the last 10 years with numerous experimental and clinical research being undertaken, involving mainly ex situ but also in situ machine perfusion (MP) techniques. It is predicted that it may become the standard of care in the near future [10].

Ex Situ Machine Perfusion

The term ex situ MP implies that the donor liver will be placed on MP once it has been procured from the donor. The first ex situ organ perfusion of donor livers was

Table 16.1 Advantages of the different modalities of machine perfusion

Characteristics	SCS	NMP	HOPE	NRP
Extend preservation times	–	+++	++	++
Viability assessment to extend donor pool	–	++	+	++
Bile duct regeneration	–	?	+	?
Logistic advantages	+++	+	+++	++
Simplicity	+++	+	++	+
Affordability	+++	+	+	+
Portability	+++	+	+	++
Target therapies	–	++	+	?

[a]*SCS* static cold storage; *HOPE* hypothermic oxygenated machine perfusion; *NMP* normothermic machine perfusion; *NRP* normothermic regional perfusion

Table 16.2 In-situ and ex situ machine perfusion modalities

Procurement	Transport	Pre-implantation	
Cold flush	Cold	Cold	Static cold storage
Cold flush	Normothermia	Normothermia	Preservation MP
Cold flush	Cold	Normothermia	pSCS-NMP
Cold flush	Cold	Hypothermia	HOPE
Normothermia	Cold	Cold	NRP
Cold	Cold	Hypotermia + normothermia	COR

[a]*MP* machine perfusion; *NMP* normothermic machine perfusion; *NRP* normothermic regional perfusion; *pSCS-NMP* post–static cold storage normothermic machine perfusion

successfully performed by Brettschneider and Starzl et al. in 1967 using a series of canine liver grafts [11]. Since then, MP techniques have been widely explored in animal models and also in the clinical practice establishing the following significant advantages when compared to SCS [12]:

1. Preservation of donor livers providing oxygen and nutrients.
2. Reconditioning and improvement of the donor organs quality, especially those livers from ECD, minimising the risk of IRI.
3. Functional assessment and viability of the donor livers with MP under physiological conditions (37° C) to help surgeons in the decision making of whether to utilize that liver.
4. Improve transplant logistics.
5. Utilization of therapeutic strategies during the perfusion time to improve donor quality.
6. Decrease organ immunogenicity.

Different methods of ex situ machine perfusion have been explored and developed by different authors over the years, and can be mainly classified according to the temperature settings, portal ± arterial perfusion, oxygenation, whether the MP is flow or pressure controlled and also the timing of when the organ is placed in the machine and for how long.

For instance, with respect to the temperature settings, the liver can be preserved in hypothermia (0–12 °C), midthermia (13–24 °C), subnormothermia (25–34 °C) and normothermia (35–38 °C). From these, hypothermic and normothermic modalities have currently gained popularity in the clinical practice. Regarding the timing of when the liver is placed in the machine, MP can be initiated immediately after organ procurement, before the organ is stored on ice for transportation (pre-static cold storage), or once the liver has been retrieved and transported to the transplant center in the ice box and then placed in the MP before implantation (Post-static cold storage). If the liver is place on MP after a very brief period of SCS in the donor hospital, while the liver is prepared, and after being procured with minimal SCS, until the implantation in the recipient, this is called "Preservation Machine Perfusion" (Table 16.2).

Normothermic Oxygenated Machine Perfusion

Normothermic machine perfusion (NMP) is a modality of ex situ machine perfusion and replicates physiological conditions once the donor liver is procured. Using blood as a perfusate allows real-time assessment of the donor liver viability, measuring oxygen consumption, bile production and lactate clearance among others. Another significant advantage is that it may allow ex situ perfusion of donor livers for extended period of time [13–17]. In a porcine LT model, NMP preserved the graft viability up to 72 h of perfusion [13]. The first human randomized controlled trial (RCT) using NMP in donor livers was performed in 2013 which successfully demonstrated the safety and feasibility of this technique [18]. Subsequently, in 2018, the same team, led by Peter Friend, performed the first RCT comparing the efficacy of NMP against conventional SCS in the adult population. In the NMP arm, the donor liver was attached to the NMP device following procurement, and it was then perfused throughout the duration of preservation. The authors demonstrated a significant reduction in the peak of aspartate aminotransferase (AST) level and the incidence of early allograft dysfunction (EAD) in NMP livers after transplantation, both biomarkers of early and late graft and patient survival [19]. However, this study failed to show a survival benefit due to the limited number of patients, although they did show improved organ utilization and longer preservation times [20].

The same group subsequently published the results of a multicentre, prospective study using post–static cold storage normothermic machine perfusion (pSCS-NMP) in 31 donor livers to facilitate organ procurement, logistics and reduce costs. Essentially the donor liver is placed in the machine on arrival to the transplant centre, after a period of SCS during transport from the donor centre. They demonstrated that pSCS-NMP is feasible and safe, which may facilitate the clinical adoption of the technique [21].

A recent study published by Jassem et al. analysed the underlying mechanisms of NMP on reducing IRI [22]. They showed that NMP can alter the gene-expression profile from proinflammation to prohealing and regeneration within the liver, reducing the number of pro-inflammatory cytokines such as interferon gamma (IFN-γ) and interleukin (IL)-17, together with a reduction in neutrophil infiltration on histological examinations post-reperfusion, when compared to SCS.

Other benefits of normothermic machine perfusion

The Birmingham group demonstrated other potential advantages when using NMP. They compared intraoperative thromboelastography characteristics (R time, K time, α-angle, maximum amplitude, G value, and LY30) in liver transplants recipients who received NMP liver grafts, to a propensity score-matched control group where the grafts were preserved by traditional SCS. They showed that NMP liver grafts showed better coagulation profiles intraoperatively, in terms of shorter K and R + K times, a significantly larger α-angle, MA and G values and less hyperfibrinolysis than SCS, translating into less platelet and coagulation factor correction during surgery [23].

NMP also offers the possibility of a pharmacological intervention before implantation. The group from Birmingham showed a decrease of fat content of steatotic donor livers discarded for transplantation after providing a pharmacological enhancement of the donor livers during ex situ normothermic MP. After 6 hours of treatment they showed a reduction of tissue triglycerides by 38% and macrovesicular steatosis by 40%. These livers also showed an increased performance in terms of urea production and lower vascular resistance [24, 25].

Viability assessment

In order to increase organ utilization when using NMP, some authors have proposed different parameters to assess donor liver viability to aid surgical decision making when deciding to use these organs. These criteria include not only a healthy and homogeneous appearance of the graft during perfusion but also the liver's ability to clear lactate, produce bile, maintain pH, perfusate AST and stable pressure and flow dynamics. Additionally, Watson et al. suggested biliary pH as a potential biomarker to predict post-transplant cholangiopathy [10, 26, 27].

Different studies assessing donor livers have been carried out to develop clinical criteria for functional assessment during MP to predict complications such as primary non-function (PNF) and ischaemic cholangiopathy (IC). These livers have previously been discarded by other teams for different reasons including steatosis, poor perfusion, prolonged withdrawal phase in cases of DCD, prolonged CIT; and have had a prolonged period of SCS before being paced in NMP. Mergental et recently proposed a combination of viability criteria to predict graft function after using NMP for 6 hours, in 12 livers discarded for transplantation in the UK by all transplant centres, 8 of these being DCD [28]. They proposed lactate clearance and/or bile production as major criteria, in combination with additional minor criteria such as stable arterial and portal flows, perfusate pH, and favorable macroscopic assessment by the transplant surgeon.

Porte et al. analysed the bile production in 12 livers discarded by other centres, after placing them in NMP [26]. They observed that a cumulative bile production of ≥30 g during 6 hours of NMP was associated with significantly lower release of transaminases and potassium into the perfusion fluid and better hepatobiliary function, as reflected by a normalization of glucose and lactate levels in the perfusate, and higher biliary secretion of bilirubin in the bile. In order to make these techniques more clinically applicable, they suggested that the minimum duration of NMP needed to discriminate viable and potentially transplantable livers from non-viable livers is 2.5 hours.

The Cambridge group lead by Watson et al., published their experience transplanting 12 discarded livers in the UK placed in NMP after a median cold storage time of 427 minutes, being 9 of these livers from DCD donors [27]. Their assessment was based on perfusate transaminases and bile pH, as well as glucose concentration and the ability of the liver to maintain pH without supplemental bicarbonate. The authors observed a significant correlation between the alanine transaminase (ALT) in the perfusate measured after 2 hours of NMP and the peak ALT post-transplant levels within the first week of transplantation. The transplanted cohort presented a high incidence of IC which let them to hypothesise that the liver's capacity to produce an alkaline bile (pH>7.4) might be a good marker of cholangiocyte function, instead of the absolute amount of bile production, which may possibly help to select of organs with a low risk of developing IC.

Interestingly, they also postulate that avoidance of hyperoxia during perfusion may prevent postreperfusion syndrome and vasoplegia. High concentrations of oxygen in tissues can result in the formation of ROS and reactive nitrogen species, that can mediate reperfusion injury and cause difficult to manage vasoplegia, as well as damaging the endothelial glycocalyx [29, 30].

Additional research is needed to validate these viability markers, therefore their interpretation needs to be cautious until further randomised clinical trials are completed.

Hypothermic Oxygenated Machine Perfusion

Hypothermic oxygenated perfusion (HOPE) is another modality of ex situ liver perfusion in hypothermic conditions where perfusion flow is pressure controlled. The first report using HOPE in patients undergoing LT was in 2010 by Guarrera et al. [31]. They included 20 patients that received donor livers treated by HOPE for 3–7 hours and compared the results to a matched SCS group revealing significantly lower rates of biliary complications and shorter hospital stay in the HOPE group.

Subsequently, the group from Dutkowski, Zurich, published the first results in humans HOPE in DCD livers receiving 1–2 hours of MP before implantation with functional WIT up to 36 minutes. When compared to DBD liver grafts preserved in static cold storage only, LT with DCD livers treated with HOPE failed to present increased coagulopathy during liver transplantation, reperfusion syndrome, increased blood loss, as well as a lower incidence of early allograft dysfunction (EAD) and acute kidney injury [32]. No cases of PNF, hepatic artery thrombosis (HAT) or IC were observed. The same group is leading a multicenter RCT using HOPE versus SCS in DBD LT, which aims to study the efficacy of HOPE of liver grafts before transplantation in reducing postoperative morbidity and mortality. In this study livers are perfused for 1–2 hours before implantation.

Mechanistic behind oxygenated hypothermia

Post-static cold storage end-ischemic HOPE (1–2 hours) results in a reduction of hepatocyte apoptosis and necrosis, mitochondrial and nuclear injury, endothelial injury, activation of Kupffer cells and the host immune response. It also replenishes ATP storage and reduces vascular resistance within the graft [33]. All these contribute to reduced IRI and biliary complications [34]. In addition, the lower incidence of biliary complications found in livers treated with HOPE reported by Porte et al., has been related to the reduced severity of mural stroma necrosis and injury of the deep peribiliary glands (PBG) after reperfusion, when compared to livers preserved in SCS only, as the severity of this damage has been associated to the development of IC [35, 36].

LT with DCD livers are known to have 3-fold higher risk of developing IC after transplantation compared with DBD liver grafts, with a reported incidence between 16 and 31% in DCD versus 3–13% in DBD liver grafts [37–39]. This type of biliary complication often requires multiple endoscopic interventions, hospital re-admissions and can lead to re-transplantation in 16% of patients and death in 6% [40, 41]. Porte et al. published their results after using dual perfusion HOPE (DHOPE), involving both arterial and portal perfusion, in DCD LT for 2 hours after conventional SCS, at a temperature of 10–12 °C, examining the effect on reperfusion injury of the bile ducts. In contrast to a control group of DCD LT without HOPE, they found no increase in the severity of histological biliary injury after reperfusion in the DHOPE group [36].

Currently, the recruitment phase of a prospective randomised trial to further demonstrate the protective effect of HOPE in the development of biliary complications in livers from DCD donors has just finalised and the results will be published within the next year (ClinicalTrials.gov, NCT02584283).

Viability assessment

The viability assessment during hypothermia differs from normothermia as the liver is not fully metabolically active. It's been described that the transaminase levels in the perfusate may reflect the degree of hepatocellular injury, which may correlate with post-transplant levels in the recipient [42, 43]. The group from Dutkowski has recently proposed measuring the released mithocondrial flavin in the machine perfusate as a marker of mithocondrial complex I injury, as it strongly correlated with lactate clearance and coagulation factors during the first 48 hours after LT [44].

Other benefits of hypothermic oxygenated perfusion

It is known that IRI is accompanied by acute hyperkalemia in the recipient which can lead to life threatening arrhythmia and cardiac arrest. In a recent publication, Porte et al. showed an additional benefit of HOPE, as he demonstrated that reperfusion of hypothermic machine perfusion livers was associated with lower serum potassium levels in the patients receiving HOPE preserved livers when compared to the transplantation of conventional SCS preserved livers [45].

In an allogeneic animal liver and kidney transplant models, HOPE has also shown the potential to protect livers from acute rejection by reducing T-cell and macrophage activation, and cytokine release within the transplanted graft. Further research is required to explore the potential of HOPE in reducing the intensity of the immunosuppression regimen in transplanted patients in order to decrease the medication side effects, possibly becoming a part of tolerogenic strategies [46, 47].

In Situ Machine Perfusion

In contrast to the techniques explained above, in vivo or in situ MP implies that the liver is connected to a MP circuit while it is still in the donor, in normothermic conditions using blood, before perfusing it with cold preservation solution and finishing the procurement. The main in vivo MP technique is called normothermic regional perfusion (NRP), previously termed normothermic extra-corporeal membrane oxygenation (NECMO) and it has mainly been developed in Spain for uncontrolled DCD donors (Maastricht II) [48]. In recent years, in situ NRP is becoming more popular and it is mainly being used in controlled DCD (cDCD) procurements as it minimizes the ischemic injury to the abdominal organs, reducing the complication rates following transplantation, with similar outcomes when compared to DBD livers. This technique has also been associated with increased recovery rates of DCD livers in UK, Spain and in the United States [49–51].

The Spanish group recently published their results of the largest propensity-matched nationwide observational cohort study of LT using livers recovered from cDCD. Half of the livers were recovered after a period of in situ NRP followed by a period of SCS and the remaining were preserved with SCS after rapid recovery with cold solution [52]. They showed a significant reduction in the rates of overall biliary complications and IC, re-transplantation and graft loss.

Watson et al. describe their experience in two UK centers with LT from cDCD using in situ NRP and compared their results with a contemporaneous cohort of LT with cDCD and SCS alone [53]. They showed that NRP is an independent factor in reducing the incidence of IC in DCD livers following transplantation, as no liver from a donor undergoing NRP prior to recovery developed cholangiopathy. They also showed that a lower recipient sodium at the time of surgery, older donor age, and a donor outside the local hospital was independently associated with the development of IC. They speculate that this finding may be related to early reperfusion in the donor that may benefit the biliary tree, which is more sensitive to ischaemia than hepatocytes, or to bile composition which can be affected by the organ hypoperfusion and the acidotic state during DCD procurement. In this series, livers treated with NRP also showed significantly lower rates of PNF and an increased utilisation rate when compared to UK data, as NRP offers the possibility of doing a viability test during NRP as opposed to SCS or HOPE.

Further steps

Recently Porte et al. advocated that HOPE and NMP can have a complementary effect if applied sequentially [54]. While DHOPE resuscitates the mitochondria and increases hepatic ATP storage, NMP enables viability assessment of the donor organ prior to transplantation. Therefore, they used sequence of DHOPE for 1 hour at 10 °C, followed by controlled oxygenated rewarming (COR) for another hour (gradually increasing temperature by about 1 °C per 2 minutes) and finally NMP at 37 °C using a new hemoglobin-based oxygen carrier (HBOC) perfusion fluid in 7 DCD livers declined for transplantation. Their viability criteria were based on the normalisation of pH and lactate in the perfusate, bile production and biliary pH within 150 minutes of NMP. Five of the 7 livers tested fulfilled the criteria and were subsequently transplanted. They observed a 100% patient and graft survival, in addition to no clinical evidence of non-anastomotic strictures of the biliary tree during the median follow-up of 6.5 months.

Conclusions

Novel ex situ and in situ perfusion technologies are rapidly gaining popularity in the transplant community worldwide, with increasing evidence of better outcomes in LT. Additionally, strategies to prevent IRI and the development of IC in ECD are vital to increase the utilisation of donor organs worldwide. Current research is being undertaken using these different perfusion techniques alone or in combination to minimize the ischemic damaged suffered during cold preservation of donor livers and to increase the donor pool to satisfy the current demand for organs.

Definitions:

- **CIT**: time from cross-clamping and cold perfusion of the donor liver to removal of the organ from cold storage solution before implantation in the recipient.

- **PNF**: it is the most severe presentation of graft dysfunction characterized by liver necrosis, rapid increase in serum transaminase, coagulopathy, increased lactate levels, hemodynamic instability, hypoglycemia, respiratory and renal failure. It happens during the first 72 h from implantation excluding other causes of liver failure, and the only treatment is emergency retransplantation, othrewise it leads to death.
- **IC**: also called non-anastomotic strictures (NAS) or ischaemic type biliary lesions (ITBL) are defined as ischemic biliary lesions after LT with irreversible damaged to the bile ducts, with a spectrum of disease characterized from single to diffuse intrahepatic strictures in the absence of HAT. They are diagnosed with MRCP or direct cholangiography of the bile ducts. The clinical manifestations of NAS usually develop within the first 3 months after LT but not all cases will require retransplantation depending on the severity and geographic spectrum.
- **Functional WIT**: is defined as the period from sustained fall of systolic blood pressure (i.e. at least 2 minutes) below 50 mmHg or non-invasive oxygen saturation below 70% until the onset of in situ cold perfusion during DCD procurement.

References

1. Belzer F, Southard J. Organ preservation and transplantation. Prog Clin Biol Res. 1986;224:291–303.
2. Taylor M. Biology of cell survival in the cold: the basis for bio-preservation of tissue and organs. In: Baust JC, Baust JM, editors. Advances in biopreservation. Boca Raton, Fla: CRC/Taylor & Francis; 2007. p. 15–62.
3. Villa R, Fondevila C, Erill I. Real-time direct measurement of human liver allograft temperature from recovery to transplantation. Transplantation. 2006;81:483–6.
4. Ikeda T, Yanaga K, Kishikawa K, Kakizoe S, Shimada M, Sugimachi K. Ischemic injury in liver transplantation: difference in injury sites between warm and cold ischemia in rats. Hepatology. 1992;16:454–61.
5. Cameron A, Ghobrial R, Yersiz H, Farmer D, Lipshutz G, Gordon S, et al. Optimal utilization of donor grafts with extended criteria: a single-center experience in over 1000 liver transplants. Ann Surg. 2006;243:748–53.
6. Turrens J. Mitochondrial formation of reactive oxygen species. J Physiol. 2003;552:335–44.
7. Abt P, Crawford M, Desai N, Markmann J, Olthoff K, Shaked A. Liver transplantation from controlled non-heart-beating donors: an increased incidence of biliary complications. Transplantation. 2003;75:1659–63.
8. Detry O, Deroover A, Meurisse N, Hans M, Delwaide J, Lauwick S, et al. Donor age as a risk factor in donation after circulatory death liver transplantation in a controlled withdrawal protocol programme. Br J Surg. 2014;101:784–92.
9. Barshes N, Horwitz I, Franzini L, Vierling J, Goss J. Waitlist mortality decreases with increased use of extended criteria donor liver grafts at adult liver trans-plant centers. Am J Transplant. 2007;7:1265–70.
10. Mergental H, Stepheson B, Laing R, Kirkham A, Neil D, LL W, et al. Development of clinical criteria for functional assessment to predict primary nonfunction of high-risk livers using normothermic machine perfusion. Liver Transpl. 2018;24:1453–69.

11. Yanaga K, Makowka L, Lebeau G, Hwang R, Shimada M, Kakizoe S, et al. A new liver perfusion and preservation system for transplantation research in large animals. J Invest Surg. 1990;3:65–75.
12. Karangwa S, Dutkowski P, Fontes P, Friend P, Guarrera J, Markmann J, et al. Machine perfusion of donor livers for transplantation: a proposal for standardized nomenclature and reporting guidelines. Am J Transplant. 2016;16:2932–42.
13. Butler A, Rees M, Wight D, Casey N, Alexander G, White D, et al. Successful extracorporeal porcine liver perfusion for 72 hr. Transplantation. 2002;73:1212–8.
14. Imber C, St Peter S, Lopez de Cenarruzabeitia I, Pigott D, James T, Taylor R, et al. Advantages of normothermic perfusion over cold storage in liver preservation. Transplantation. 2002;73:701–9.
15. Schon M, Kollmar O, Wolf S, Schrem H, Matthes M, Akkoc N, et al. Liver transplantation after organ preservation with normothermic extracorporeal perfusion. Ann Surg. 2001;233:114–23.
16. St Peter S, Imber C, Lopez I, Hughes D, Friend P. Extended preservation of non-heart-beating donor livers with normothermic machine perfusion. Br J Surg. 2002;89:609–16.
17. Fondevila C, Hessheimer A, MH M, Munoz J, Taura P, Calatayud D, et al. Superior preservation of DCD livers with continuous normothermic perfusion Ann Surg 2011;254:1000–7.
18. Ravikumar R, Jassem W, Mergental H, Heaton N, Mirza D, Perera M, et al. Liver transplantation after ex vivo normothermic machine preservation: a phase 1 (first-in-man) clinical trial. Am J Transplant. 2016;16:1779–87.
19. Olthoff K, Kulik L, Samstein B, Kaminski M, Abecassis M, Emond J, et al. Validation of a current definition of early allograft dysfunction in liver transplant recipients and analysis of risk factors. Liver Transpl. 2010;16:943–9.
20. Nasralla D, Coussios C, Mergental H, Akhtar M, Butler A, Ceresa C, et al. A randomized trial of normothermic preservation in liver transplantation. Nature. 2018;557:50–6.
21. Ceresa C, Nasralla D, Watson C, AJ B, Coussios C, Crick K, et al. Transient cold storage prior to normothermic liver perfusion may facilitate adoption of a novel technology. Liver Transpl. 2019;25:1503–13.
22. Jassem W, Xystrakis E, Ghnewa Y, Yuksel M, Pop O, Martinez-Llordella M, et al. Normothermic Machine Perfusion (NMP) inhibits proinflammatory responses in the liver and promotes regeneration. Hepatology. 2019;70:682–95.
23. Ionescu M, Tillakaratne S, Hodson J, Gunson B, Nasralla D, Pinter Carvalheiro da Silva Boteon A, et al. Normothermic machine perfusion enhances intraoperative hepatocellular synthetic capacity: a propensity score-matched analysis. Transplantation. 2019;103:198–207.
24. Nativ N, Maguire T, Yarmush G, Brasaemle D, Henry S, Guarrera J, et al. Liver defatting: an alternative approach to enable steatotic liver transplantation. Am J Transplant. 2012;12:3176–83.
25. Boteon Y, Attard J, Boteon P, Wallace L, Reynolds G, Hubscher S, et al. Manipulation of lipid metabolism during normothermic machine perfusion: effect of defatting therapies on donor liver functional recovery. Liver Transpl. 2019;25:1007–22.
26. Sutton M, op den Dries S, Karimian N, Weeder P, de Boer M, Wiersema-Buist J, et al. Criteria for viability assessment of discarded human donor livers during ex vivo normothermic machine perfusion. PLoS One. 2014;9:e110642.
27. Watson C, Kosmoliaptsis V, Randle L, Gimson A, Brais R, Klinck J, et al. Normothermic perfusion in the assessment and preservation of declined livers before transplantation: hyperoxia and vasoplegia-important lessons from the first 12 cases. Transplantation. 2017;101:1084–98.
28. Mergental H, Perera M, Laing R, Muiesan P, Isaac J, Smith A, et al. Transplantation of declined liver allografts following Normothermic ex-situ evaluation. Am J Transplant. 2016;16:3235–45.

29. Murphy M. How mitochondria produce reactive oxygen species. Biochem J. 2009;417:1–13.
30. van Golen R, Reiniers M, Vrisekoop N, Zuurbier C, Olthoff P, Van Rheenen J, et al. The mechanisms and physiological relevance of glycocalyx degradation in hepatic ischemia/reperfusion injury. Antioxid Redox Signal. 2014;21:1098–118.
31. Guarrera J, Henry S, Samstein B, Odeh-Ramadan R, Kinkhabwala M, Goldstein M, et al. Hypothermic machine preservation in human liver transplantation: the first clinical series. Am J Transplant. 2010;10:372–81.
32. Dutkowski P, Schlegel A, de Oliveira M, B M, Neff F, Clavien P. HOPE for human liver grafts obtained from donors after cardiac death. J Hepatol. 2014;60:765–77.
33. Dutkowski P, Graf R, Clavien P. Rescue of the cold preserved rat liver by hypothermic oxygenated machine perfusion. Am J Transplant. 2006;6:903–12.
34. Dutkowski P, Polak W, Muiesan P, Schlegel A, Verhoeven C, Scalera I, et al. First comparison of hypothermic oxygenated perfusion versus static cold storage of human donation after cardiac death liver transplants: an international-matched case analysis. Ann Surg. 2015;262:764–70.
35. Op den Dries S, Sutton M, Karimian N, de Boer M, Wiersema-Buist J, Gouw A, et al. Hypothermic oxygenated machine perfusion prevents arteriolonecrosis of the peribiliary plexus in pig livers donated after circulatory death. PLoS One. 2014;9:e88521.
36. van Rijn R, van Leeuwen O, Matton A, Burlage L, Wiersema-Buist J, van den Heuvel M, et al. Hypothermic oxygenated machine perfusion reduces bile duct reperfusion injury after transplantation of donation after circulatory death livers. Liver Transpl. 2018;24:655–64.
37. den Dulk A, Sebib K, K, de Rooij B, Sutton M, Braat A, Inderson A, et al. High peak alanine aminotransferase determines extra risk for nonanastomotic biliary strictures after liver transplantation with donation after circulatory death. Transpl Int. 2015;28:492–501.
38. Dubbeld J, Hoekstra H, Farid W, Ringers J, Porte R, Metselaar H, et al. Similar liver transplantation survival with selected cardiac death donors and brain death donors. Br J Surg. 2010;97:744–53.
39. O'Neill S, Roebuck A, Khoo E, Wigmore S, Harrison E. A meta-analysis and meta-regression of outcomes including biliary complications in donation after cardiac death liver transplantation. Transpl Int. 2014;27:1159–74.
40. Blok J, Detry O, Putter H, Rogiers X, Porte R, van Hoek B, et al. Long-term results of liver transplantation from donation after circulatory death. Liver Transpl. 2016;22:107–1114.
41. Verdonk R, Buis C, Porte R, van der Jagt E, Limburg A, van den Berg A, et al. Anastomotic biliary strictures after liver transplantation: causes and consequences. Liver Transpl. 2006;12:726–35.
42. Liu Q, Vekemans K, Iania L, Konuta M, Parkkinen J, Heedfeld V, et al. Assesssing warm ischemic injury of pig livers at hypothermic machine perfusion. J Surg Res. 2014;186:379–89.
43. Pacheco E, Silva OJ, Sankarankutty A, Ribeiro MJ. Analysis of the liver effluent as a marker of preservation injury and early graft performance. Transplant Proc. 2010;42:435–9.
44. Muller X, Schlegel A, Kron P, Eshmuminov D, Wurdinger M, Meierhofer D, et al. Novel real-time prediction of liver graft function during hypothermic oxygenated machine perfusion before liver transplantation. Ann Surg. 2019;270:783–90.
45. Burlage L, Hessels L, Rijn R, Matton A, Fujiyoshi M, Van de Berg A, et al. Opposite acute potassium and sodium shifts during transplantation of hypothermic machine perfusion donor livers. Am J Transplant. 2019;19:1061–71.
46. Schlegel A, Kron P, Graf R, Clavien P, Dutkowski P. Hypothermic Oxygenated Perfusion (HOPE) downregulates the immune response in a rat model of liver transplantation. Ann Surg. 2014;260:931–7.
47. Kron P, Schlegel A, Muller X, Gaspert A, Clavien P, Dutkowski P. Hypothermic oxygenated perfusion: a simple and effective method to modulate the immune response in kidney transplantation. Transplantation. 2019;103:e128–36.

48. Fondevila C, Hessheimer A, Ruiz A, Calatayud D, Ferrer J, Charco R, et al. Liver transplant using donors after unexpected cardiac death: novel preservation protocol and acceptance criteria. Am J Transplant. 2007;7:1849–55.
49. Magliocca J, Magee J, Rowe S, et al. Extracorporeal support for organ donation after cardiac death effectively expands the donor pool. J Trauma. 2005;58:1095–101.
50. Ruiz P, Gastaca M, Bustamante F, Ventoso A, Palomares I, Prieto M, et al. Transplantation. 2018;Ahead of print.
51. Oniscu G, Randle L, Muiesan P, Butler A, Currie I, Perera M, et al. In situ normothermic regional perfusion for controlled donation after circulatory death—the United Kingdom experience. Am J Transplant. 2014;14:2846–54.
52. Hessheimer A, Coll E, Torres F, Ruíz P, Gastaca PR, JI, MG, et al. Normothermic regional perfusion vs. super-rapid recovery in controlled donation after circulatory death liver transplantation J Hepatol. 2019;70:658–65.
53. Watson C, Hunt F, Messer S, Currie I, Large S, Sutherland A, et al. In situ normothermic perfusion of livers in controlled circulatory death donation may prevent ischemic cholangiopathy and improve graft survival. Am J Transplant. 2019;19:1745–58.
54. de Vries Y, Matton A, Nijsten M, Werner M, Van Den Berg A, De Boer M, et al. Pretransplant sequential hypo- and normothermic machine perfusion of suboptimal livers donated after circulatory death using a hemoglobin-based oxygen carrier perfusion solution. Am J Transplant. 2019;19:1202–11.

Chapter 17
Veno-Venous Bypass in Liver Transplantation

Krishna Prasad Rao and Zoka Milan

Introduction and Brief History

Thomas Starzl performed the first successful liver transplant in 1963 [1]. His approach included explant of the entire liver and resection of the recipient retrohepatic inferior vena cava (IVC) with interposition and anastomosis of the donor IVC in an end-to-end fashion [1]. This required complete caval cross-clamping for a long period of time, resulting in decreased venous return from abdominal organs and the lower extremities, and hemodynamic instability [2]. Initially, mortality rates following liver transplantation (LT) were high, owing to massive haemorrhage and cardiovascular instability during the long anhepatic phase [3–5]. Veno-venous bypass (VVB) system was introduced two decades after the first OLT to ameliorate this hemodynamic instability by diverting blood from the IVC and splanchnic circulation to the right heart, through axillary, subclavian or internal jugular vein, thus increasing haemodynamic stability during the anhepatic phase of OLT [4].

In 1979, Calne et al. described the use of a partial cardiopulmonary bypass technique (femoro-axillary bypass with a pump-oxygenator) for collecting blood from the IVC and returning it to the axillary vein in a clinical setting [6]. Although hemodynamic stability was achieved, systemic heparinization resulted in major bleeding [6]. Subsequently, Griffith described a VVB technique in clinical LT with no requirement for systemic anticoagulation, via use of heparin-coated VVB tubing [5].

K. P. Rao (✉)
Consultant Anaesthetist, Leeds Teaching Hospitals, Leeds, UK
e-mail: Krishna-prasad.rao@nhs.net

Z. Milan
King's College Hospital, London, UK

Z. Milan and C. Goonasekera (eds.), *Anesthesia for Hepatico-Pancreatic-Biliary Surgery and Transplantation*, https://doi.org/10.1007/978-3-030-51331-3_17

Principle of VVB in LT Surgery

The VVB system is composed of heparin-coated tubes connected to a centrifugal pump (Fig. 17.1). Femoral and internal jugular bypass cannulae are frequently inserted after induction of anaesthesia. The tip of the jugular cannula should be in the distal end of the superior vena cava, and that of the femoral cannula should be in the external iliac vein [7–12].

VVB is often initiated prior to extensive retrohepatic dissection. Tubes are primed with normal saline, debubbled and, when appropriate, connected to outflow (femoral) and inflow (axillar, internal jugular) vessels. The third cannula is inserted by surgeons in portal vein and connected to the same outflow tube as the femoral cannula using a y-connector tube. The flow from the portal vein can reach half of the total outflow.

Pump flow ranges from 1.5 to 6 l/min [13]. Reduced flow or high pressure in the tubes requires checking of the cannulae for kinking, dislocation or disconnection. In rare cases, porto-jugular VVB can be carried out without femoral involvement. The average duration of VVB is 100 min (range: 70–158 min) [6, 13]. VVB terminates after reperfusion of the liver. Some units return blood from the circuit

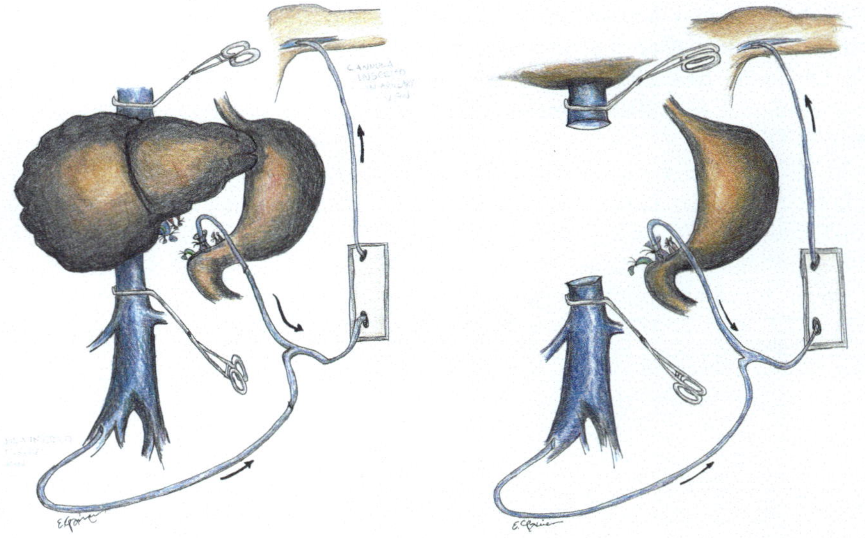

Fig. 17.1 **a** Veno-venous by pass; A cannula is inserted in right femoral vein and another into proximal portal vein. Both circulation systems are connected redirecting both systemic and portal circulation to an extracorporeal pump. The venous return is achieved via a third cannula previously inserted in the left axillary vein. Once satisfactory flows within the extracorporeal circulation are achieved, clamps are applied to supra- and infra-hepatic IVC. The cirrhotic liver is ready to be explanted. **b** Anhepatic phase of caval replacement type liver transplantation. Recipient on veno-venous by pass. The cirrhotic liver has been explanted along with native IVC

through the internal jugular vein (IJV) to LT patients. This manoeuvre can save one unit of transfused blood after the termination of VVB [14].

Femoral and jugular cannulae is removed short after graft reperfusion; rarely does it remain in place until the end of the case, and the insertion site of the skin is closed with a suture [15]. Manual compression of the suture site for five minutes should be maintained to complete haemostasis [15]. Even with the recipient in a hypocoagulable state, this maneuver is adequate for haemostasis [15]. Minimal subcutaneous haematoma formation at the right internal jugular vein site may be seen after the LT, but it is usually not clinically significant [15].

The main complications of VVB are air embolism caused by trapped air in the circuit or circuit disconnection, bleeding when the VVB cannula is disconnected from the circuit or when the jugular cannula is outside of the blood vessel (blood drained under pressure into the thoracic cavity), and thromboembolic complications [16–22]. Hypothermia is another very common complication of VVB [23].

Cannulation Technique

Most VVB cannulae vary in size from 18–21 Fr. Most centres use a kink-resistant 21 Fr catheter with 17 cm effective length and 7 mm internal diameter and a 60 cm radiopaque dilator (Figs. 17.2 and 17.3). Both the cannulae and dilators are made of soft polyurethane. Each cannula has a large distal end hole and smaller holes on four sides up to 6 cm from the tapered tip, which facilitates easy insertion (Fig. 17.2).

The first insertion techniques involved cannulation of the femoral and axillary vein via a surgical cutdown process at the beginning of the operation, followed by portal cannulation after dissection of the hepato-duodenal ligament [7]. Numerous complications were reported with use of open techniques, including nerve injuries (brachial and femoral), seromas, lymphoceles and painful neuromas [17]. The incidence of axillary lymphoceles has been reported to be 12–20%, with operative repair required in up 70% of cases according to one retrospective study [17, 24]. Many complications likely go unreported.

A percutaneous Seldinger technique of VVB cannula insertion was first described in 1994 by Ozaki et al. [8]. In this technique, an inflow cannula is inserted via the internal jugular vein (IJV), and an outflow cannula is inserted via the femoral vein. When this technique was developed, large-bore cannulae were inserted without ultrasound (US) guidance or X-ray determination of cannula positioning before VVB. Since then, numerous studies have shown that percutaneous cannula placement is safer, quicker and has a reduced incidence of major complications compared with surgical dissection technique [1–12]. However, it does not eliminate the risk of complications related to line insertion [22]. VVB cannulae can be inserted into the same IJV as central venous catheters (CVCs), and even larger cannulae, such as Swan-Ganz catheter sheaths or vascular catheters, for dialysis. Jugular VVB cannulae have side ports for infusion. Infusions can be administered through the VVB cannula port only if they exceed the VVB circuit pressure (approximately 150 mmHg).

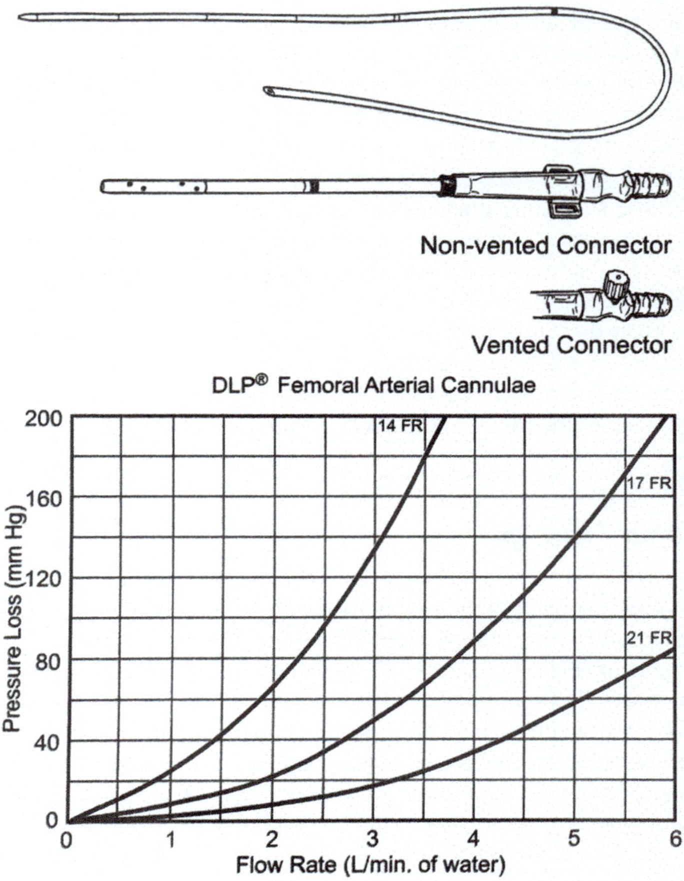

Fig. 17.2 Venovenous bypass (VVB) cannula sizes and flow rates. A large skin and subcutaneous tissue incision must be made before the VVB cannula and introducer can be advanced

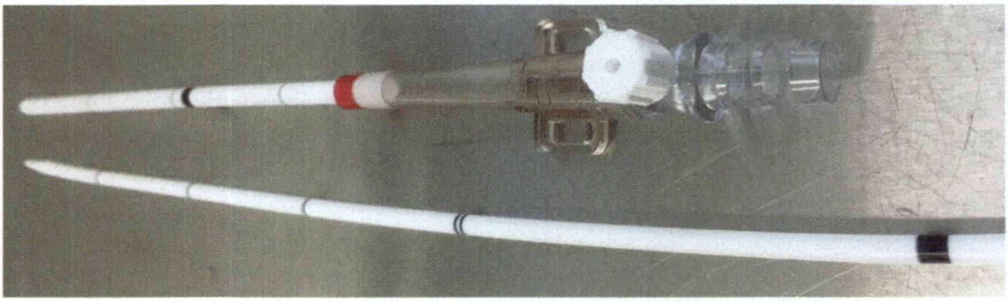

Fig. 17.3 VVB cannula and dilator

All current indications for VVB are relative, and may include severe portal hypertension and bleeding, anticipated difficult explant (e.g. enlarged caudate lobe, previous abdominal surgery and adhesions, IVC thrombus, large polycystic liver, etc.], fulminant hepatic failure, renal and cardiac dysfunction and Budd-Chiary syndrome [25–31]

Haemodynamic Effects of IVC and Portal Vein Clamp, and Role of VVB

In the anhepatic phase, the IVC and portal vein are clamped. This results in sudden loss of venous return, a decrease in cardiac output (CO), mean arterial pressure (MAP) and central venous pressure (CVP), an increase in pulmonary capillary wedge pressure (PCWP), and a subsequent decrease in cerebral blood flow, renal perfusion pressure, intestinal congestion and gut oedema [4].

VVB, by diverting blood from abdomen and lower extremities into right heart, allows more time for surgery during the anhepatic phase, while also allowing a relatively stable CO to be maintained and, consequently, adequate MAP for renal and abdominal perfusion [24]. VVB also decreases portal hypertension, intestinal congestion and oedema, such that surgical blood loss is reduced [11].

Veroli et al. reported increased perioperative morbidity and mortality when there was a >50% reduction in CO during the anhepatic phase [26]. They proposed that VVB be used in patients with a >30% drop in MAP and/or >50% drop in the cardiac index (CI) after test clamping for 5 minutes [26]. Several LT units use clamp testing to decide whether or not to proceed with VVB. To avoid unnecessary insertion of a large bypass cannula at induction of general anaesthesia, an additional single-lumen CVC can be used as a guide for bypass cannula insertion, if the patient requires bypass.

Several factors modulate hemodynamic stability during the anhepatic phase, including the extent of cardiac dysfunction, the presence of good collateral circulation in patients with long-standing liver disease, pre-load status prior to clamping of the IVC, cardiac reserve, the use of vasopressors, and various compensatory mechanisms [14]. Various factors in combination appear to determine the overall hemodynamic status of the patient. As all of these factors are known before the start of LT, informed preoperative decisions about the usage of VVB can be made for the majority of patients.

Effects of VVB on Renal Function

The anatomical position of renal veins, which are situated below hepatic veins, suggests that the IVC clamp should have a negative effect on renal vein flow, and that VVB should facilitate renal vein outflow [27–31]. Historically, VVB was considered to preserve renal function and reduce the incidence of renal failure following LT [32]. However, clinical findings do not universally support this. For example, Shaw et al. [7] demonstrated lower post-operative creatinine levels in their VVB group, while in their retrospective study Johnson et al. [9] found no significant difference in either renal function or the need for renal replacement therapy (RRT) following LT. In a randomized controlled trial (RCT), Grande et al. [25] demonstrated that the proposed reno-protective effects of VVB were of little clinical significance, with low MAP being the single most important factor in renal dysfunction. In a Korean study, Kim et al. reported that VVB had no effect on renal function in patients with previously normal renal parameters [33]. Published data from numerous studies comparing various surgical techniques with VVB remain controversial regarding the preservation of renal function [27, 28]. Sun et al. demonstrated a reduction in acute kidney injury associated with the use of VVB in patients with previously impaired renal function (37.2% vs. 50.8%) [31]. It appears that other factors, such as liver graft quality, perioperative volume status, use of nephrotoxic medication, perioperative perfusion pressure and blood loss and replacement, influence renal function following LT [21].

Reasons for the Gradual Decrease in the Use of VVB

After the piggyback surgical technique and temporary porto-caval shunting were introduced, the use of VVB gradually decreased. The costs of carrying out VVB, and the need for a technician to be present at all times, also contributed to the declining usage of VVB [34]. A number of other factors led to the virtual abandonment of this technique, including the 10–30% morbidity associated with line insertion and the VVB procedure, hypothermia, and the increased operative time and warm ischemia time [21, 26, 32, 35].

Complications

Percutaneous insertion of large-bore cannulae for venous access for VVB is associated with certain risks, and there are also complications related to the use of VVB circuits. Although the overall complication rate of VVB is 10–30%, according to a large retrospective survey, serious morbidity and mortality is rare [16–19].

A case series of 312 patients investigating large-bore percutaneous access during OLT found that the incidence of serious morbidity was 1.28%, and that of mortality was 0.32% [17]. Another study analysed 1,206 consecutive OLT complications directly related to invasive monitoring, and found that VVB cannulae contributed to <1% of them [36]. These reported complication rates are from a period before US was routinely used for bypass cannula placement. It is important to note that there are numerous serious unreported complications of VVB cannula insertion.

Hypothermia is the most commonly encountered deleterious effect of routine VVB, but its incidence can be reduced by using heparin-bonded heat exchangers, which are not available in the majority of LT centers [37, 38]. The use of the subclavian vein for VVB is associated with increased risk of vascular injury, as well as the potential for uncontrolled bleeding upon cannula removal [16]. The use of VVB can result in PRS, which is characterized by a profound decrease in MAP and CO following reperfusion due to systemic vasodilation and myocardial depression. It is postulated that exposure to extracorporeal circuits leads to activation of pro-inflammatory cytokines, and hence exacerbates hypotension due to vasodilation [39]. One study reported that the incidence of PRS with use of VVB was up to 30%, while other studies have shown a lower incidence [40].

The introduction of US-guided VVB cannulae, and the use of TOE guidance, certainly reduced the rate of complications. TOE can be useful even when the tip of the cannula is outside of the field of the TOE, if the catheter tip is in the right atrium (which can be determined using the "bubble test.") [41]. However, cannula insertion is inherently time-sensitive because of the need to minimize the warm ischemia time (WIT). Additionally, as VVB is rarely used, the new generation of LT anaesthetists are less familiar with the techniques of large-bore cannula insertion and VVB, and with the potential complications of the latter. However, with regular US-guided percutaneous catheter placement and the use of TOE, we can confidently assume that complication rates will generally decrease.

Clinical Outcomes

Shaw et al. found that, compared to when it was not used, VVB improved the 30-day survival of patients after OLT (73% vs. 91.5%), but no significant difference was reported at 6 months [7]. A major retrospective analysis from Toronto University Hospital compared the outcomes between two different periods, 1986–1992 (corresponding to routine VVB use) and 1994–1996 (corresponding to selective VVB use). The 1-year survival rate among 332 patients in the selective group was 89.7%, compared with 71.9% in the routine use group [26]. Lerut et al. published a prospective feasibility study of 202 consecutive grafts, and concluded that OLT with IVC preservation, without the use of VVB or portocaval shunting, is possible in nearly all primary transplants, and in the majority of re-transplants, with graft survival of 92–94% [42].

A Cochrane review examined the published literature up until 2010 to assess the risks and benefits of VVB for OLT [32]. Only three RCTs with a high risk of bias were eligible and, although none reported graft survival, there were no significant differences in renal failure or blood transfusion requirement rates. A VVB-related complication rate of 28.6% was also reported [32].

Does the Surgical Approach Influence VVB Use?

The piggyback technique (PBT) was first described by Calne and Williams in 1968 and subsequently popularized by Tzakis in 1989 [5, 43]. A modification of this technique by Belghiti et al. [44] which included partial side-clamping of the IVC as well as establishing a temporary porto-caval shunt, was increasingly adopted thereafter.

Since then, numerous studies have been published comparing different IVC preservation techniques with or without selective use of VVB. The advantages of such techniques are summarized below [45–52].

1. Reduced warm ischaemic time (WIT) and surgical time
2. Improved hemodynamic stability
3. No need for VVB, and hence reduced morbidity
4. Lower transfusion requirements
5. Shorter intensive care unit and hospital stay
6. Reduced operating costs.

Preservation of renal function, and graft and patient survival, were largely comparable among the techniques.

Therefore, the hemodynamic profiles of liver transplantation with IVC preservation techniques appear similar with versus without VVB, with minimal impact on renal function and negligible differences in overall long-term mortality. Nearly all primary transplants can be safely be performed without the use of bypass.

Is Routine VVB Use Still Necessary?

According to a national survey carried out in the USA in 2003, half of all adult LT centres, and 37% of all programs, routinely used VBP [35]. Conversely, a UK-wide survey conducted in 2018 revealed wide variation among centres, two of which lacked the infrastructure to support a VVB service [34].

A survey of major American centres published by Chari et al. [26] in the late 1990s showed that use of VVB was decreasing, which was attributed to the immense progress made in newer surgical techniques, including the PBT. The survey also pointed out differences among surgical approaches to liver transplantation among centres (IVC preservation, porto caval shunt, etc). However, a newly established LT program in Germany revived the use of VVB, with a lower incidence of renal failure and low morbidity reported in a series of 163 patients [36]. Therefore, VVB is likely being used selectively rather than routinely in that program.

Current indications for VVBP are summarised in Table 17.1.

In conclusion, major advances in both surgical and anaesthetic approaches towards the management of LT have been made since 1963. There are some theoretical benefits to the routine use of VVB, but these have not been consistently

Table 17.1 Relative indications for veno-venous bypass

1. Severe portal hypertension
2. Extensive blood loss during hepatectomy
3. Hemodynamic instability during portal occlusion or cross clamping
4. Acute liver failure
5. Budd Chiarri syndrome
6. Pre-existing Cardiac disease a. Ischemic heart disease b. Cirrhotic cardiomyopathy c. Severe Pulmonary hypertension
7. Polycystic liver
8. Some re-do liver transplants

demonstrated in the literature. With routine use of IVC-preserving techniques, all primary transplants, and most re-transplants, can be safely performed without VVB, with no major differences in clinical outcome. The use of VVB is also associated with higher costs, and greater staff and training requirements. A few established centres continue to use VVB as their standard approach to OLT, which probably reflects the experience and preferences of their surgical teams.

Finally, there is a paucity of high-quality RCTs on the diverse surgical techniques for OLT, with or without VVB, and this topic therefore remains controversial.

References

1. Starzl TE, Marchioro TL, Vonkaulla KN, Hermann G, Brittain RS, Wadell WR. Homotransplantation of the liver in humans. Surg Gynecol Obstet. 1963;117:659–76.
2. Moore FD, Wheele HB, Demissianos HV, Smith LL, Balankura O, Abel K, et al. Experimental whole-organ transplantation of the liver and of the spleen. Ann Surg. 1960;152:374–87.
3. Gibbs E. The Cambridge first liver transplant. The history of anaesthesia society Proceedings of the joint meeting of 6th March 1993 with the section of anaesthetics of the royal society of medicine. 1993;12, p. 20–2.
4. Estrin JA, Belani KG, Ascher NL, Lura D, Payne W, Najarian JS. Hemodynamic changes on clamping and unclamping of major vessels during liver transplantation. Transpl Proc. 1989;21:3500–5.
5. Griffith BP, Shaw BW Jr, Hardesty RL, Iwatsuki S, Bahnson HT, Starzl TE. Veno-venous bypass without systemic anticoagulation for transplantation of the human liver. Surg Gynecol Obstet. 1985;160:270–2.
6. Calne RY, Smith DP, McMaster P, Craddock GN, Rolles K, Farman JV, et al. Use of partial cardiopulmonary bypass during the anhepatic phase of orthotopic liver grafting. Lancet. 1979;2:612–4.
7. Shaw BW Jr, Martin DJ, Marquez JM, Kang YG, Bugbee AC Jr, Iwatsuki S, et al. Venous bypass in clinical liver transplantation. Ann Surg. 1984;200:524–34.
8. Ozaki CF, Langnas AN, Bynon JS, Pillen TJ, Kangas J, Vogel, et al. A percutaneous method for venovenous bypass in liver transplantation. Transplantation. 1994;57:472–3.

9. Johnson SR, Marterre WF, Alonso MH, Hanto DW. A percutaneous technique for venovenous bypass in cadaver liver transplantation and comparison with the open technique. Liver Transpl Surg. 1996;2:354–61.
10. Tisone G, Mercadante E, Dauri M, Colella D, Anselmo A, Romagnoli J, et al. Surgical versus percutaneous technique for veno-venous bypass during orthotopic liver transplantation: a prospective randomised study. Transplant Proc. 1999;31:3162–3.
11. Frenette L, Cox J, Singer D, Ronderos J, Steele S, Eckhoff D, et al. Five years of experience with percutaneous cannula for establishing venous bypass access in orthotopic liver transplantation. Transplant Proc. 1996;28:2974–7.
12. Bendetti E, Pirenne J, Troppmann C, Hakim N, Greussner R, Cochrane R, et al. A percutaneous technique for venous return cannula insertion for veno-venous bypass in hepatic transplantation. Transplantation. 1995;59:789–91.
13. Scherer RU, Giebler RM, Schmutzler MJ, Gunnicker FM, Kox WJ. Shunt flow and caval pressure gradient during veno-venous bypass in human orthotopic liver transplantation. Br J Anaesth. 1993;70:689–90.
14. Cheema SP, Hughes A, Webster NR, Bellamy MC. Cardiac function during orthotopic liver transplantation with veno-venous bypass. Anaesthesia. 1995;50:776–8.
15. Sakai T, Gligor S, Diulus J, McAffee R, Marsh JW, Planinsic RM. Insertion and management of percutaneous veno-venous bypass cannula for liver transplantation: a reference for transplant anesthesiologists. Clin Transplant. 2010;24:585–91.
16. Jakson P, Jankovic Z. Veno-venous bypass catheter for hepatic transplant risk unique complications. Anaesth Intensive Care. 2007;35:805–6.
17. Budd JM, Isaac JL, Bennet J, Freeman JW. Morbidity and mortality associated with large-bore percutaneous venovenous bypass cannulation for 312 orthotopic liver transplantations. Liver Transpl. 2001;7:359–62.
18. Jankovic Z, Boon A, Prasad R. Fatal haemothorax following large-bore percutaneous cannulation before liver transplantation. Br J Anaesth. 2005;95:472–6.
19. Khoury GF, Mann ME, Porot MJ, Abdul-Rasool IH, Busuttil RW. Air embolism associated with venovenous bypass during orthotopic liver transplantation. Anaesthesiology. 1987;67:848–51.
20. Paulsen AW, Whitten CW, Ramsay MA, Klintmalm GB. Considerations for anesthetic management during veno-venous bypass in adult hepatic transplantation. Anesth Analg. 1989;68:489–96.
21. Reddy K, Mallett S, Peachey T. Venovenous bypass in orthotopic liver transplantation: time for a rethink? Liver Transpl. 2005;11:741–9.
22. Johnson MW, Powelson JA, Auchincloss H Jr, Delmonico FL, Cosimi AB. Selective use of veno-venous bypass in orthotopic liver transplantation. Clin Transplant. 1996;10:181–5.
23. Khoury GF, Kaufman RD, Musich JA. Hypothermia related to the use of venovenous bypass during liver trasnplantation. Eur J Anesthesiol. 1990;7:501–3.
24. Belghiti J, Noun R, Sauvanet A, Durand F, Aschehoug J, Erlinger S, et al. Transplantation for fulminant and subfulminant hepatic failure with preservation of portal and caval flow. Br J Surg. 1995;82:986–9.
25. Grande L, Rimola A, Cugat E, Alvarez L, Garcia-Valdecasas JC, Taura P, et al. Effect of venovenous bypass on perioperative renal function in liver transplantation: results of a randomized, controlled trial. Hepatology. 1996; 23:1418–28.
26. Chari RS, Gan TJ, Robertson KM, Bass K, Camargo CA Jr, Greig PD, et al. Venovenous bypass in adult orthotopic liver transplantation: routine or selective use? J Am Coll Surg. 1998;186:683–90.
27. Corti A, Degasperi A, Colussi S, Mazza E, Amici O, Cristalli A, et al. Evaluation of renal function during orthotopic liver transplantation. Minerva Anestesiol. 1997;63:221–8.
28. Kuo PC, Alfrey EJ, Garcia G, Haddow G, Dafoe DC. Orthotopic liver transplantation with selective use of veno-venous bypass. Am J Surg. 1995;170:671–5.

29. Strachan A, Hannon V, Melikian CN. Do we still need a bypass service in liver transplantation? A survey of UK practice. Transplantation. 2018;102:S861.
30. Sun K. Venovenous bypass is associated with a lower incidence of acute kidney injury after liver transplantation in patients with compromised pretransplant renal function. Anesth Analg. 2017;125:1463–70.
31. Mossdorf A, Ulmer F, Junge K, Heidenhain C, Hein M, Temizel I. Bypass during liver transplantation: anachronism or revival? Gastroenterol Res Pract. 2015; Article ID 967951.
32. Gurusamy KS, Koti R, Pamecha V, Davidson BR. Veno-venous bypass versus none for liver transplantation. Cochrane Database Syst Rev. 2011;3. Article ID CD007712.
33. Kim DY, Huh IY, Cho YW, Park ES, Park SE, Nah YW, et al. Experience without using venoveno bypass in adult orthotopic liver transplantation. Korean J Anesthesiol. 2011;60:19–24.
34. Lerut J, Ciccarelli O, Roggen F, Laterre PF, Danse E, Goffette P, et al. Cavocaval adult liver transplantation and retransplantation without venovenous bypass and without portocaval shunting: a prospective study in adult liver transplantation. Transplantation. 2003;75:1740–5.
35. Shumann R. Intraoperative resource utilization in anaesthesia for liver transplantation in the United States: a survey. Anaesth Analg. 2003;97:21–8.
36. Lu S, Matsusaki T, Abuelkasem E. Complications related to invasive hemodynamic monitors during adult liver transplantation. Clin Transplant. 2013;27:823–8.
37. Scholz T, Solberg R, Okkenhaug C, Videm V, Gallimore MJ, Mathisen O, et al. Veno-venous bypass in liver transplantation: heparin-coated perfusion circuits reduce the activation of humoral defense systems in an vitro model. Perfusion. 2001;16 285–92.
38. Khoury GF, Kaufman RD, Musich JA, Mogard M. Neurotensin and vasoactive intestinal peptide levels during orthotopic liver transplantation in man. Transplantation. 1988;46:601–2.
39. Aggarwal S, Kang Y, Freeman JA, Fortunato FL, Pinsky MR. Postreperfusion syndrome: cardiovascular collapse following hepatic reperfusion during liver transplantation. Transplant Proc. 1987;19:54–5.
40. Nanashima A, Pillay P, Crawford M, Nakasuji M, Verran DJ, Painter D. Analysis of postrevascularization syndrome after orthotopic liver transplantation: the experience of an Australian liver transplantation centre. J Hepatobiliary Pancreat Surg. 2001;8:557–63.
41. Burtenshaw AJ, Issac JL. Role of trans-oesophageal echo for perioperative cardiovascular monitoring during orthoptic liver transplantation. Liver Transpl 2005;11:741–2.
42. Lerut JP, Molle G, Donataccio M. Cavocaval liver transplantation without venovenous bypass and without temporary portocaval shunting: the ideal technique for adult liver grafting? Transplant Int. 1997;10:171–2.
43. Tzakis A, Todo S, Starzl TE. Orthotopic liver transplantation with preservation of the inferior vena cava. Ann Surg. 1989;210:649–52.
44. Belghiti J, Panis Y, Sauvanet A, Gayet B, Fekete´ F. A new technique of side to side caval anastomosis during orthotopic hepatic transplantation without inferior vena caval occlusion. Surg Gynecol Obstet. 1992;175:270–2.
45. Iserr MR, Massarollo PC, de Carvalho EM, Baia CE, Kavakama J, de Andrade Lima P, et al. Randomized trial comparing pulmonary alterations after conventional with venovenous bypass versus piggy back liver transplantation. Liver Transpl. 2004;10:425–33.
46. Jones R, Hardy KJ, Fletcher DR, Michell I, McNicol PL, Angus PW. Preservation of the inferior vena cava in orthotopic liver transplantation with selective use of veno-venous bypass: the piggy back operation. Transplant Proc. 1992;24:189–91.
47. Margarit C, Lazaro JL, Balsells J, Charco R, Murio E, Edo A, et al. Recipient hepatectomy with preservation of inferior vena cava reduces the need for veno-venous bypass in liver trans- plantation. Transpl Int. 1994;7(Suppl. 1):S152–4.

48. Shokouh-Amiri MH, Osama GA, Bagous WA, Grewal HP, Hathway DK, Vera SR, et al. Choice of surgical technique influences perioperative outcomes in liver transplantation. Ann Surg. 2000;231:814–23.
49. Jovine E, Mazziotti A, Grazi GL, Ercolani G, Masetti M, Morganti M, et al. Piggy-back versus conventional technique in liver transplantation: report of a randomized trial. Transpl Int. 1997;10:109–12.
50. Hesse UJ, Berrevoet F, Troisi R, Pattyn P, Mortier E, Decruyenaere J, et al. Hepato-venous reconstruction in orthotopic liver transplantation with preservation of the recipients' inferior vena cava and veno-venous bypass. Langenbecks Arch Surg. 2000;385:350–6.
51. Stieber AC. One surgeons experience with piggy-back versus the standard technique in orthotopic liver trans- plantation: is one better than the other? Hepatogastroenterology. 1995;42:403–5.
52. Khan S, Silva MA, Tan YM, John A, Gunson B, Buckels JA, et al. Conventional versus piggyback technique of caval implantation; without extra- corporeal veno-venous bypass. A comparative study. Transpl Int. 2006;19:795–801.

Part III
Liver Resection

Chapter 18
Biology of Liver Tumors and Outcomes of Liver Surgery

Elissaios A. Kontis

Introduction

Surgical resection of malignant liver tumours offers the best long-term survival outcomes. Traditionally, liver resection was considered a major undertaking associated with increased perioperative risks. Advances in surgical technique and anaesthesia have made liver resection a safer procedure, currently performed around the world, with morbidity and mortality similar to that of other major intrabdominal procedures. Hepatico-pancreatic-billiary (HPB) surgeons have the responsibility of selecting those patients who are both fit to undergo a major procedure, but also who will benefit most from tumour resection. The latter part entails understanding the biology of liver tumours.

Cancer treatment comprises of two "pillars"; those are chemotherapy which aims to achieve systemic control and surgery which aims to achieve locoregional control of the disease. Patient selection is imperative and there are comprehensive guidelines based upon the natural history of each disease to help clinicians on their decision making [1]. The natural history of the disease reflects the biology of the tumour itself. Hereafter we aim to present the indications and current outcomes of liver resection in the treatment of the most common liver malignancies.

E.A. Kontis (✉)
Institute of Liver Studies, King's College Hospital, NHS Foundation Trust, London, UK
e-mail: e.kontis@nhs.net

Z. Milan and C. Goonasekera (eds.), *Anesthesia for Hepatico-Pancreatic-Biliary Surgery and Transplantation*, https://doi.org/10.1007/978-3-030-51331-3_18

Liver Malignancies

The liver is a common site of both primary and secondary malignancies. Primary liver cancer is the 6th most common cancer worldwide of which Hepatocellular Carcinoma (HCC) and Cholangiocarcinoma (CCA) are the most frequent [2]. The liver is also a common site for secondary malignancies; the main mechanisms to account for the high incidence of liver metastases are: (i) the dual blood supply of the liver (portal and systemic circulation) and (ii) the fenestrated sinusoidal epithelium [2, 3]. An overview of all primary and secondary malignancies of the liver appears in Table 18.1. There was an estimate of more than 42,000 new cases in 2019, accounting for 2.4% of all new cancer diagnoses and there were an estimated 31,780 deaths, accounting for 5.2% of all cancer deaths [4]. Hereafter we will summarize current evidence for the commonest liver malignancies for which adults undergo liver resection: Colorectal liver metastases, hepatocellular carcinoma (HCC), cholangiocarcinoma (CCA) and Neuroendocrine Tumours (NET), before discussing their oncological outcomes.

Primary Liver Tumors

Hepatocellular Carcinoma (HCC)

HCC is the most common primary liver malignancy arising from hepatocytes and represents a complex disease with a dismal prognosis. The most important risk factor among HCC patients is the presence of concomitant liver cirrhosis which has a major impact on both their treatment and long-term survival. Cirrhosis is both an independent risk factor for mortality and a risk factor for the development of HCC. A number of grading systems have been developed over the years to assess the severity of cirrhosis (Child-Turcotte-Pugh (CTP), Model for End Stage Liver Disease (MELD), MELD-Na, United Kingdom Model for End-Stage Liver Disease (UKELD) etc.). For one to comprehend the profound impact of liver cirrhosis upon overall health, the 3 month mortality for a patient with intermediate stage of cirrhosis such as CTP stage B (10–12 points) is 11.2% while for a patient with a MELD score of 20–29 the 3 month mortality is 19.6% [5]. Consequently, the functional status of the remaining liver parenchyma is of paramount importance when considering liver resection for HCC with concomitant cirrhosis.

HCC has a wide spectrum of available treatments, with both curative and non-curative intent. In Europe the most comprehensive and widely implemented system to offer guidance among the available treatment options is the Barcelona Clinic Liver Cancer (BCLC) staging, classification and treatment algorithm [6]. The BCLC system, by taking into account the performance status of the patient, the burden of disease (HCC) and liver function, offers guidance on the available

Table 18.1 List of all malignant tumors of the liver (primary and secondaries) as well as pediatric malignancies

Primary (cell origin)	Secondary (primary tumor)	Pediatric
Hepatocellular carcinoma (hepatocytes)	**Colorectal**	**Hepatoblastoma**
Cholangiocarcinoma (biliary epithelium) – Intrahepatic – Hilar – Extrahepatic (Common Bile Duct, Gallbladder cancer)	**Neuroendocrine** – Foregut (Lung, thymus, stomach, *duodenum*, *pancreas*, bile duct, gallbladder) –**Midgut** (*small intestine*, appendix, *proximal colon*) – Hindgut (distal colon, rectum)	Rhabdomyosarcoma of the extrahepatic bile ducts
	Breast	**Hepatocellular carcinoma**
Epitheloid hemangioendothelioma (Mesenchymal)	Gastric cancer	Embryonal sarcoma
Hepatic angiosarcoma	Pancreas	Leiomyosarcoma
Undifferentiated (embryonal) sarcoma (Mesenchymal)	Melanoma	Angiosarcoma
Other sarcomas (Kaposi's, hepatobiliary rhabdomyosarcoma, etc) (Mesenchymal)	Sarcoma	Primary hepatic rhabdoid tumor
Primary hepatic lymphoma (hematopoietic)	Renal caner	Primary hepatic non-Hodgkin's lymphoma
	Reproductive tract – Testicular – *Ovarian* – Endometrial	Malignant germ cell tumors
	Lung	Wilm's tumor
	Oesophagus	Osteogenic sarcoma
	Head and Neck	Desmoplastic small round cell tumor
	Unknown primary	Rhabdomyosarcoma
	Secondaries from hematopoietic neoplasms (Hodgkin's, non-Hodgkin's, leukemia, langerhan's histiocytosis)	Metastatic – Adrenocortical – Malignant peripheral nerve cell tumor – Colon cancer
	Gastrointestinal Stromal Tumors—GIST's	Rhabdoid tumor
	Other	

Underlined are the most common primary tumors in each category known to metastasize to the liver in adults

treatments which include radiofrequency, resection, liver transplantation (LT), transarterial chemoembolization (TACE), systemic chemotherapy and supportive care. The key discrimination among the above available treatments is that patients with Very Early (0) or Early stage (A) disease can be offered potentially curative treatment options based on the degree of preserved liver function (i.e. ablation, resection or LT), while patients with Intermediate stage (B) or Advanced stage (C) disease are offered with non-curative treatments (i.e. trans arterial chemoebolisation, systemic chemotherapy). The remaining patients with end-stage liver function and ECOG performance status 3–4, are offered with best supportive care as their expected survival is approximately 3 months. Liver resection among patients with sporadic HCC (i.e. in the absence of cirrhosis) or with well compensated liver cirrhosis (i.e. normal bilirubin and the absence of portal hypertension) offers a 5-year survival of approximately 70%. However in the presence of portal hypertension this 5-year survival decreases to 50%, highlighting the impact of liver function on the outcomes of liver resection [7].

Another significant clinical difference between cirrhosis related and sporadic HCC is the difference in age of incidence: cirrhosis related HCC is predominantly encountered among elderly patients, with a peak at the age of 70 years, while sporadic HCC appears to have a bimodal distribution, with the first peak occurring between 20–30 years of age and the second peak at the age of 70 [8]. This earlier peak probably reflects the occurrence of fibrolamelar HCC and a number of inherited diseases such as hereditary hemochromatosis, A1 anti-trypsin deficiency, porphyria, hypercitrullinemia and type I glycogen storage disorder, which are predisposing factors for the development of HCC [8]. However, among patients with sporadic HCC, the healthy background liver parenchyma more often allows extensive resection with curative intent and a reported 5-year survival of up to 81% and disease free survival of up to 58% [8]. HCC has a significant genomic diversity and to date there is a lack of clinically significant genetic biomarkers to predict the outcomes of liver surgery based on the biology of the liver tumour [9]. Significant studies are currently being undertaken worldwide which have managed to identify genetic signatures which are associated with improved disease-free survival following resection of HCC [10].

Cholangiocarcinoma (CCA)

CCA is also an aggressive primary liver malignancy arising from the biliary epithelium of either the intrahepatic or extrahepatic bile ducts. As such CCAs are classified based on their anatomical location to either:

(i) peripheral or intrahepatic (8% of cases)—arising from the intrahepatic biliary ducts,
(ii) hilar (50%)—arising from the common hepatic duct up to 1st order biliary ducts (i.e. right and left hepatic duct) and
(iii) distal (42%)—arising from the distal common bile duct (distally to the origin of the cystic duct) [11].

CCA's represent a surgical challenge, as they typically present late in their course, they tend to extend along the biliary epithelium (multifocal) and for anatomical reasons, they may require extensive resections in order to achieve complete tumor resection.

With the exception of peripheral CCAs which will require only liver resection for complete resection, hilar CCAs usually require extended liver resections and distal CCA's usually require a pancreatoduodenectomy (Whipple's procedure). However, the extent of the resection i.e. hepatectomy only or pancreatoduodenectomy only or hepato-pancreatoduodenectomy, will be determined by the intraoperative histopathological assessment of the bile duct margin. Microscopic invasion of the bile duct margin is associated with inferior survival outcomes [12, 13]. Furthermore hilar CCAs often, due to their anatomical location, require major vascular resection and reconstruction—i.e. of either the right or left portal vein [14], increasing the gravity of the operation. As a consequence, the resectability rates vary between 30–80% and approximately one third of the resected patients will have microscopically infiltrated margins [14]. To this end, it is evident that there is no scope for palliative procedures aiming to debulking, when complete resection is deemed not feasible on preoperative imaging, or the patient is unfit to undergo major intrabdominal resection including the potential resection of the main portal vein.

Following liver resection for peripheral CCAs with clear margins (R0), the reported 5-year survival rate is between 30–35%; this dismal figure occurs despite the fact that an R0 resection is achieved in the majority of cases of intrahepatic CCAs (74%), further demonstrating the aggressiveness of this tumor [15]. The 5-year survival of resected hilar CCAs is reported to be 32.4%, with microvascular invasion, lymph node metastasis, microscopically infiltrated margins and poor tumor differentiation being prognostic indicators of even poorer survival [16]. Survival after complete resection of distal CCAs (pancreatoduodenectomy) is reported to be 35%, with perineural invasion, lymph node metastasis, microscopically infiltrated margins and poor tumor differentiation being prognostic of poorer survival outcomes [13]. Given the poor prognosis, there are a number of studies investigating both the genomic and epigenetic factors impacting cholangiocarcinoma [17–19]. Although no clinically applicable results are available yet, there are promising findings such as the identification of the BRCA-associated CCA and the identification of KRAS and BRAF mutant cases of CCA, which are associated with worse prognosis, allowing for potential targeted/tailored adjuvant therapy.

Metastatic Liver Tumors

Colorectal Liver Metastases (CRLM)

The treatment of colorectal liver metastases (CRLM) is a great example of how radically outcomes of liver surgery have improved during the last two decades. Colorectal cancer (CRC) has a major impact in developed countries and it's the 3rd most commonly diagnosed cancer worldwide [20]. Up to 25% of patients will present with synchronous liver metastases, while a further 25% of patients will develop metachronous liver metastases [21]. As we achieved a better understanding of CRC biology, we were able to transform this understanding to better outcomes for patients by delivering more effective regimes of chemotherapy, resecting metastatic disease when appropriate or using ablative techniques to compliment the effect of chemotherapy or surgery [22]. The overall outcome of these achievements is reflected in the net increase of expected survival; in the early 2000s the anticipated 5-year survival for Stage IV CRC (metastatic disease) was between 10–20% [23] and now can reach up to 74.3% [24].

This significant survival benefit was achieved through the implementation of more effective chemotherapy regimens, with or without targeted therapies, which in turn led to a paradigm shift on what is considered resectable disease within the liver. Until the end of the last decade, factors such as the presence of more than 4 tumour deposits, tumour size >5 cm, inability to achieve more than 1 cm tumour free resection margin etc. were considered features of unresectable disease. However, the later factors were based on the "target" liver to be resected rather than the future liver remnant. Today, although there is significant variability among liver surgeons on their definition of resectable disease, the majority will agree that the three main prerequisites to consider a patient for liver resection are: (1) feasibility to achieve R0 resection both at the primary site and the secondary site, (2) at least two adjacent liver segments to be preserved with intact vascular inflow and outflow, as well as biliary drainage and (3) adequate parenchymal volume of the future liver remnant as a proportion of the patient's body weight [25]. That means for a normal liver a minimal necessary future liver remnant volume is 20%, thus allowing for a formal Right extended hepatectomy or Right trisectionectomy including the caudate lobe. For an "injured" liver (i.e. after prolonged chemotherapy >3 months) a 30% future liver remnant volume is necessary, (i.e. allowing for a modified right hepatectomy including the caudate lobe or of one of segment IVa/b), and for a cirrhotic liver a 40% future liver remnant volume is necessary (i.e. allowing for a right hepatectomy) [26]. Alternatively a more precise approach would be calculating the standardized future liver remnant volume to the patient's body weight ratio, with an acceptable figure of 0.5–0.8% depending on liver parenchymal quality [27].

There has been significant advances in the understanding of tumour biology of CRC. The three oncogenes—KRAS, NRAS and BRAF have been shown to be involved in the tumorigenesis of CRC, and they signify aggressive and/or chemotherapy resistant tumours indicating a poorer prognosis [28–30]. As a consequence, the biological profile of the primary tumour can be extrapolated to the treatment of the metastatic disease of CRC, mainly liver metastases [31]. Evidently the genomic profile of the tumour itself has a uniform impact on the outcomes of treatment i.e. as patients with KRAS or BRAF mutated primary tumours have a poorer prognosis in comparison to patients with wild type status, likewise patients with CRLM and mutant KRAS/BRAF status are expected to have worse long-term oncological outcomes than their counterparts with wild type status for the aforementioned oncogenes [31]. Although current established practice guidelines do not include the mutational status of KRAS, BRAF or any other biomarker of tumour biology in the selection of patients for resection of liver metastases, there are studies that have shown significant differences in survival outcomes [32]. It is a matter of time before our understanding of tumour biology will reflect on patient selection for liver resection in this clinical setting.

Neuroendocrine Liver Metastases (NLMs)

Neuroendocrine tumors (NETs) are a diverse group of tumors arising from neuroendocrine cells of the gastrointestinal tract that can either be functional (i.e. producing hormones and causing specific symptoms—insulin/insulinomas, gastrin/gastrinomas etc.) or non-functional (usually pancreatic NETs). In principle NETs are considered to have a less aggressive course, however 46–93% of patients have liver metastases at the time of diagnosis, being the most common site of metastasis [32]. The biology of these tumors is better described by their proliferation index Ki67%, as well as their pattern of metastasis. Hence tumors are classified as either Grade 1 when Ki67%<2%; Grade 2 when Ki67% is 3–20% and Grade 3 when Ki67% >20% (Neuroendocrine carcinomas—small or large cell) [34]. Furthermore, there are specific patterns of liver metastases in NETs which correlate with the prognosis of the patient, with type I being a restricted type of metastasis, affecting only one lobe, type II being a dominant lesion with bi-lobar liver metastases and type III being a diffuse type of multiple liver metastases. Unfortunately the latter pattern comprises approximately 60% of all cases, while the first two comprise 25% and 15% respectively [35]. The indications for liver resection in NLMs may vary significantly, including curative intent, symptom control or prolongation of survival in the palliative setting, thus sound clinical judgement is imperative.

In principle, the goal remains to achieve an R0 resection in both the primary and secondary sites of disease and this is associated with a 5-year survival rate of up to 85%. However, R1 or even R2 resection may achieve survival rates of 70% and 60% respectively. Furthermore, optimal cytoreductive surgery (i.e. resection of tumor burden by more than 90%) may achieve a survival benefit and prolonged symptomatic relief [35]. The above statements are applicable for those patients with a more indolent NET tumor biology (i.e. Grade I or II); patients with NET tumors of more aggressive biology (Grade III) usually develop high volume metastatic disease which is both refractory to treatment and usually has early recurrence with a 5 year survival of 0% and a median survival of 6 months [33].

Non-colorectal, Non-neuroendocrine Liver Metastases

The presence of metastatic liver disease is a marker of severe disease and dismal prognosis. However, with advances in chemotherapy which may achieve an improved response and control of malignant tumours, the argument can be made to attempt liver resection for metastases from a number of both intrabdominal and extra-abdominal malignancies. There are a large number of case reports of resection of hepatic metastases for melanoma, gastrointestinal stromal tumours (GIST), breast cancer, oesophageal cancer, gastric cancer, pancreatic cancer, small bowel cancer, renal cell cancer, testicular cancer, ovarian cancer, urothelial cancer, lung cancer, adrenocortical tumours and endometrial cancer. The level of evidence for each of the above tumours is at best limited; it follows that the indications for patient selection to be offered liver resection is similarly limited. However, the argument that "among selected patients, liver resection improves survival outcome" remains [37]. Recent studies have demonstrated a 5 year overall survival rate of 30–41% [36] and they are even reports of a 10 year survival of 15% [37]. Despite this, there is a lack of established prognostic factors. Commonly reported factors associated with poorer outcomes include older age (>60 years), synchronous liver metastases or short interval of appearance of metachronous liver metastases and a large burden of liver disease (>4 liver lesions) [38].

However, from a critical standpoint, it needs to be stated that there is a treatment bias in favour of liver resection for these patients, as the alternative is either no treatment, or continuation of a chemotherapy regime without curative intent. Thus, sound clinical judgement is warranted prior to offering a patient liver resection for non-colorectal, non-endocrine metastasis. To this end it is imperative that the decision is made within an appropriately experienced multidisciplinary team, familiar with the natural history and biology of the tumour. This decision should not solely be made on grounds of technical feasibility of the liver resection.

It is the strong opinion of the author that the indications for resection of metastatic liver disease should be further explored. With further advances in chemotherapy and the safety of liver resection, we will be able to identify more patients that might benefit from liver resection. The sceptical reader should reflect upon the fact that approximately 20 years ago colorectal liver metastases was consider a terminal/palliative state of disease.

References

1. NCCN. https://www.nccn.org/professionals/physician_gls/. Accessed on 09 April 2019.
2. Ananthakrishnan A, Gogineni V, Saeian K. Epidemiology of primary and secondary liver cancers. Semin Intervent Radiol. 2006;23:47–63.
3. Kew MC. Hepatic tumors and cysts. In: Felman M, Friedman LS, Sleisenger MH, Scharschmidt BF, editors. Sleisenger and Fordtrans's gastrointestinal and liver disease: pathophysiology/diangosis/management. 7th ed. Philadelphia: Saunders; 2002. p. 1589.

4. Surveillance Eepidemiology and End Results Program (SEER), National Cancer Institute. Cancer Stat Facts: Liver and intrahepatic bile duct cancer 2019. https://seer.cancer.gov/statfacts/html/livibd.html. Accessed on 09 April 2019.
5. Wiesner R, Edwards E, Freeman R, Harper A, Kim R, Kamath P, et al. Model for end-stage liver disease (MELD) and allocation of donor livers. Gastroenterology. 2003;124:91–6. https://doi.org/10.1053/gast.2003.50016.
6. Forner A, Reig M, Bruix J. Hepatocellular carcinoma. Lancet. 2018;391(10127):1301–14. https://doi.org/10.1016/S0140-6736(18)30010-2.
7. Liccioni A, Reig M, Bruix J. Hepatocellular carcinoma. In: Jarnagin WR, editor. Blumgart's surgery of the liver, biliary tract, and pancreas, vol II. 6th ed. Philadelphia, PA 19103-2899: Elsevier; 2017, p. 1333–8.
8. Trevisani F, Frigerio M, Santi V, Grignaschi A, Bernardi M. Hepatocellular carcinoma in non-cirrhotic liver: a reappraisal. Dig Liver Dis. 2010;42:341–7. https://doi.org/10.1016/j.dld.2009.09.002.
9. Niu ZS, Niu XJ, Wang WH. Genetic alterations in hepatocellular carcinoma: an update. World J Gastroenterol. 2016;22:9069–95. https://doi.org/10.3748/wjg.v22.i41.9069.
10. Lim HY, Sohn I, Deng S, Lee J, Jung SH, Mao M, et al. Prediction of disease-free survival in hepatocellular carcinoma by gene expression profiling. Ann Surg Oncol. 2013;20:3747–53. https://doi.org/10.1245/s10434-013-3070-y.
11. DeOliveira ML, Cunningham SC, Cameron JL, Kamangar F, Winter JM, Lillemoe KD, et al. Cholangiocarcinoma: thirty-one-year experience with 564 patients at a single institution. Ann Surg. 2007;245:755–62. https://doi.org/10.1097/01.sla.0000251366.62632.d3.
12. Ercolani G, Dazzi A, Giovinazzo F, Ruzzenente A, Bassi C, Guglielmi A, et al. Intrahepatic, peri-hilar and distal cholangiocarcinoma: three different locations of the same tumor or three different tumors? Eur J Surg Oncol. 2015;41:1162–9. https://doi.org/10.1016/j.ejso.2015.05.013.
13. Wellner UF, Shen Y, Keck T, Jin W, Xu Z. The survival outcome and prognostic factors for distal cholangiocarcinoma following surgical resection: a meta-analysis for the 5-year survival. Surg Today. 2017;47:271–9. https://doi.org/10.1007/s00595-016-1362-0.
14. Govil S, Reddy MS, Rela M. Surgical resection techniques for locally advanced hilar cholangiocarcinoma. Langenbecks Arch Surg. 2014;399:707–16. https://doi.org/10.1007/s00423-014-1216-4.
15. Mavros MN, Economopoulos KP, Alexiou VG, Pawlik TM. Treatment and prognosis for patients with intrahepatic cholangiocarcinoma: systematic review and meta-analysis. JAMA Surg. 2014;149:565–74. https://doi.org/10.1001/jamasurg.2013.5137.
16. Kimura N, Young AL, Toyoki Y, Wyatt JI, Toogood GJ, Hidalgo E, et al. Radical operation for hilar cholangiocarcinoma in comparable Eastern and Western centers: outcome analysis and prognostic factors. Surgery. 2017;162:500–14. https://doi.org/10.1016/j.surg.2017.03.017.
17. Golan T, Raitses-Gurevich M, Kelley RK, Bocobo AG, Borgida A, Shroff RT, et al. Overall survival and clinical characteristics of BRCA-associated cholangiocarcinoma: a multicenter retrospective study. Oncologist. 2017;22:804–10. https://doi.org/10.1634/theoncologist.2016-0415.
18. Maemura K, Natsugoe S, Takao S. Molecular mechanism of cholangiocarcinoma carcinogenesis. J Hepatobiliary Pancreat Sci. 2014;21(10):754–60. https://doi.org/10.1002/jhbp.126.
19. Salati M, Braconi C. Noncoding RNA in cholangiocarcinoma. Semin Liver Dis. 2019;39:13–25. https://doi.org/10.1055/s-0038-1676097.
20. Ferlay J, Soerjomataram I, Dikshit R, Eser S, Mathers C, Rebelo M, et al. Cancer incidence and mortality worldwide: sources, methods and major patterns in GLOBOCAN 2012. Int J Cancer. 2015;136:E359–86. https://doi.org/10.1002/ijc.29210.
21. Gorgen A, Muaddi H, Zhang W, McGilvray I, Gallinger S, Sapisochin G. The new era of transplant oncology: liver transplantation for nonresectable colorectal cancer liver metastases. Can J Gastroenterol Hepatol. 2018;2018:9531925. https://doi.org/10.1155/2018/9531925.

22. Van Cutsem E, Cervantes A, Adam R, Sobrero A, Van Krieken JH, Aderka D, et al. ESMO consensus guidelines for the management of patients with metastatic colorectal cancer. Ann Oncol. 2016;27(8):1386–422. https://doi.org/10.1093/annonc/mdw235.
23. Ponz de Leon M, Benatti P, Di Gregorio C, Fante R, Rossi G, Pedroni M, et al. Staging and survival of colorectal cancer: are we making progress? The 14-year experience of a specialized cancer registry. Dig Liver Dis. 2000;32:312–7. (PMID: 11515629).
24. Hallet J, Sa Cunha A, Adam R, Goere D, Bachellier P, Azoulay D, et al. Factors influencing recurrence following initial hepatectomy for colorectal liver metastases. Br J Surg. 2016;103:1366–76. https://doi.org/10.1002/bjs.10191.
25. Pawlik TM, Schulick RD, Choti MA. Expanding criteria for resectability of colorectal liver metastases. Oncologist. 2008;13:51–64. https://doi.org/10.1634/theoncologist.2007-0142.
26. Shindoh J, Madoff, D, Aloia T, Vauthey JN. Preoperative portal vein embolisation—technique and results. In: Jarnagin WR, editor. Blumgart's surgery of the liver, biliary tract and pancreas, vol II. 6th ed. Philadelphia, PA 19103-2899: Elsevier; 2017, p. 1654–63.
27. Vauthey JN, Chaoui A, Do KA, Bilimoria MM, Fenstermacher MJ, Charnsangavej C, et al. Standardized measurement of the future liver remnant prior to extended liver resection: methodology and clinical associations. Surgery. 2000;127:512–9. https://doi.org/10.1067/msy.2000.105294.
28. Cicenas J, Tamosaitis L, Kvederaviciute K, Tarvydas R, Staniute G, Kalyan K, et al. KRAS, NRAS and BRAF mutations in colorectal cancer and melanoma. Med Oncol. 2017;34:26. https://doi.org/10.1007/s12032-016-0879-9.
29. Van Cutsem E, Kohne CH, Lang I, Folprecht G, Nowacki MP, Cascinu S, et al. Cetuximab plus irinotecan, fluorouracil, and leucovorin as first-line treatment for metastatic colorectal cancer: updated analysis of overall survival according to tumor KRAS and BRAF mutation status. J Clin Oncol. 2011;29:2011–9. https://doi.org/10.1200/JCO.2010.33.5091.
30. Palomba G, Doneddu V, Cossu A, Paliogiannis P, Manca A, Casula M, et al. Prognostic impact of KRAS, NRAS, BRAF, and PIK3CA mutations in primary colorectal carcinomas: a population-based study. J Transl Med. 2016;14:292. https://doi.org/10.1186/s12967-016-1053-z.
31. Tosi F, Magni E, Amatu A, Mauri G, Bencardino K, Truini M, et al. Effect of KRAS and BRAF mutations on survival of metastatic colorectal cancer after liver resection: a systematic review and meta-analysis. Clin Colorectal Cancer. 2017;16:e153–63. https://doi.org/10.1016/j.clcc.2017.01.004.
32. Passot G, Denbo JW, Yamashita S, Kopetz SE, Chun YS, Maru D, et al. Is hepatectomy justified for patients with RAS mutant colorectal liver metastases? An analysis of 524 patients undergoing curative liver resection. Surgery. 2017;161:332–40. https://doi.org/10.1016/j.surg.2016.07.032.
33. Harring TR, Nguyen NT, Goss JA, O'Mahony CA. Treatment of liver metastases in patients with neuroendocrine tumors: a comprehensive review. Int J Hepatol. 2011;2011:154541. https://doi.org/10.4061/2011/154541.
34. Klimstra DS, Modlin IR, Coppola D, Lloyd RV, Suster S. The pathologic classification of neuroendocrine tumors: a review of nomenclature, grading, and staging systems. Pancreas. 2010;39:707–12. https://doi.org/10.1097/MPA.0b013e3181ec124e.
35. Zilbert N, Moulton C-A, Gallinger S. Non-colorectal hepatic metastases. In: Parks RW, editor. Hepatobiliary and pancreatic surgery: a companion to specialist surgical practice. 6th ed. Elsevier; 2019, p. 121–32.
36. Maeda Y, Shinohara T, Katayama T, Futakawa N, Hamada T. Hepatectomy for liver metastases in non-colorectal, non-neuroendocrine cancer patients. The survival benefit in primary unresectable cases. Int J Surg. 2015;22:136–42. https://doi.org/10.1016/j.ijsu.2015.07.716.

37. Sano K, Yamamoto M, Mimura T, Endo I, Nakamori S, Konishi M, et al. Outcomes of 1,639 hepatectomies for non-colorectal non-neuroendocrine liver metastases: a multicenter analysis. J Hepatobiliary Pancreat Sci. 2018;25:465–75. https://doi.org/10.1002/jhbp.587.
38. Adam R, Chiche L, Aloia T, Elias D, Salmon R, Rivoire M, et al. Hepatic resection for non-colorectal nonendocrine liver metastases: analysis of 1,452 patients and development of a prognostic model. Ann Surg. 2006;244:524–35. https://doi.org/10.1097/01.sla.0000239036.46827.5f.

Chapter 19
Anaesthesia for Live Donor Hepatectomy

Khaled Yassen

Live liver donors (LLDs) are healthy individuals who undergo removal of a considerable hepatic mass for use in living donor liver transplantation (LDLT) surgery. LDLT programs increase organ availability, particularly in the Middle East and Asia, where cadaveric liver transplantation is not widely available. However, liver donation is not a complication-free procedure and should only be performed at well-equipped centres experienced in the field of transplantation [1–4]. The anaesthesia principles for LLDs are the same as those for liver resection (LR) for liver tumours. The fact that LLDs are undergoing surgery for the benefit of another individual puts all members of the surgical team under pressure.

Donation Criteria and Pre-assessment

Donors are usually relatives within the third degree of consanguinity with the recipient or their spouse. Unrelated donors may be accepted, but need to be verified and approved by official medical authorities. The criteria for donation vary worldwide and have changed over the years with the accumulation of experience [5].

Clinical examination and assessment of the medical records are useful to assess the donors in terms of remnant liver volume, graft suitability, and psychological capacity [6].

It is preferable for donors to be of an ABO-compatible blood group. However, in rare occasions, preoperative plasmapheresis of recipients who received

K. Yassen (✉)
Anaesthesia Department National Liver Institute, Menoufia University,
Shebeen El Kom City Al Menoufia, Egypt
e-mail: kyassen61@hotmail.com; kyassen@kfu.edu.sa

Surgery Department College of Medicine, Office Room 2040, King Faisal University, 400,
Hofufu Al-Ahsa 31982, Kingdom of Saudi Arabia

Z. Milan and C. Goonasekera (eds.), *Anesthesia for Hepatico-Pancreatic-Biliary Surgery and Transplantation*, https://doi.org/10.1007/978-3-030-51331-3_19

incompatible ABO-incompatible livers provides satisfactory postoperative results [7].

Although the age requirement for donors has recently been increased to over 50 years, a younger donor is beneficial in terms of early graft function, the regenerative capacity and longevity of the donor liver [8].

Donors are expected to be of American Society of Anaesthesiologists class 1 or 2, with negative serology for hepatitis B and C, human immune deficiency virus, cytomegalovirus and Epstein bar virus. Liver function tests, complete blood count, blood urea nitrogen, serum creatinine, fasting and postprandial blood sugar, electrolytes, and coagulation studies are all required. No history of liver disease or previous surgeries that might interfere with the surgery, and no previous organ donations, are also requirements [8].

Chest X-ray, electrocardiography (ECG), echocardiography and pulmonary function tests are mandatory.

Donors at risk of acute myocardial infarction should be excluded from consideration during the pre-assessment period. There have been few case reports of postoperative development of acute myocardial infarction among donors resulting in mortality [9, 10].

Risk of Thromboembolism in Donors

In addition to well-known risk factors, including obesity, oestrogen treatment, older age, presence of varicose veins, smoking and a family history of thrombosis, most centres screen donors preoperatively for factor V Leiden gene mutations, prothrombin gene mutations, thrombophilia, low protein S, low protein C, and low anti-thrombin III levels, and positive anti-phospholipid antibody. Patients with these risk factors have a higher likelihood of developing venous thromboembolic disease. Whether potential donors with a mildly increased risk of thromboembolic disease should be excluded from donation should be discussed between centres [11, 12].

Mohamed et al. monitored the coagulation process for 30 days post-donation via rotational thromboelastometry, and reported no cases of hypercoagulability in the study group, unlike in a study using classical coagulation laboratory tests [13].

Body Weight and Obesity

Donors with a body mass index (BMI) >25 kg/m^2 may have significant hepatic steatosis. Donors with mild steatosis are advised to reduce their body weight by following an exercise and diet program. Individuals a BMI >30 kg/m^2 but no evidence of hepatic steatosis can be donors [14]; no immediate or long-term negative outcomes in these donors, or recipients, have been reported [15].

Evaluation of Graft and Remnant Donor Liver Volume

A graft weight of more than 0.8% of the recipient's body weight (graft to body weight ratio [GBWR] >0.8) is necessary to prevent small-for-size syndrome [16, 17].

Radiology studies are used to assess the potential donor's graft weight, but they can overestimate the volume of the donor's liver.

The postoperative remaining residual liver volume (RLV) of the donors, in relation to their preoperative estimated whole liver volume, should be calculated (RLV % = RLV/estimated whole liver volume × 100) to ensure that sufficient liver tissue remains.

A donor will not be approved if the surgeons are not satisfied with the volume of remnant liver, or the intraoperative gross appearance or anatomy of the donor liver [18].

Anaesthetic Management

Even after a meticulous pre-assessment, donors must be re-assessed prior to the scheduled surgery to ensure that there has been no change in their clinical status.

Packed red blood cells, with or without a cell saver, should be available in the operating suite.

Any available induction and analgesic agents, and muscle relaxants, can be used to induce general anaesthesia (GA). Maintaining GA with a mixture of air, oxygen and volatile anaesthetics is more common than total intravenous anaesthesia (TIVA).

After inducing GA, at least one large-bore peripheral intravenous cannula, an ultrasound-guided central venous catheter (CVC) and a radial arterial cannula should be inserted.

After induction of GA, the donor should be placed in the supine position with both arms tucked by their sides and padded. This will help avoid injury to the peripheral nerves and compression of the brachial plexus between the first rib and the clavicle during surgical traction [3, 19, 20].

GA and subcostal surgical retraction during open LR is known to reduce residual functional capacity. The alveolar recruitment manoeuvre and positive end expiratory pressure (PEEP) can help re-expand peripherally collapsed alveoli, improve lung dynamic compliance, and increase arterial blood oxygen tension with no increase in blood loss [21].

Neither desflurane nor sevoflurane are clinically superior with respect to liver and kidney function, but desflurane better preserves haemodynamic function and enhances recovery [22]. Sevoflurane may be better than intravenous propofol for pharmacological preconditioning [23].

A urinary Foley catheter and an oesophageal temperature probe are placed following induction of GA. Fluid- and forced air-warming devices reduce the incidence of hypothermia.

A nasogastric tube (NG) can be inserted to decompress the patient's stomach and optimize exposure of the surgical field, particularly during laparoscopic and robotic surgery. Two Cochrane systematic reviews demonstrated that prophylactic NG tube insertion during LR should be performed selectively, as it increases pulmonary complications and delays recovery of bowel function post-surgery [24, 25].

The most important risk to the donor during hepatectomy is bleeding, particularly in deeper parts of the liver near the middle hepatic vein. Common measures to reduce intraoperative bleeding include reducing hepatic congestion on the anaesthetic side by using the head-up position, restricting fluid intake, peripheral vasodilatation with epidural analgesia or administration of nitro-glycerine, or diuretics, all with intention to minimize elevation of central venous pressure (CVP) [26–29].

More details of the method used for reducing bleeding during LR surgery are presented in Chapter Strategies for lover central venous pressure in liver resection surgery.

A 1,000 IU aliquot of heparin is given intravenously by the anaesthetist immediately prior to removing the graft to avoid thrombosis in the microvasculature of the graft [30].

At the end of the surgical procedure, donors are extubated in the operating room after reversal of muscle relaxation with either neostigmine-atropine or sugammadex [31].

Following emergence from anaesthesia, all donors are transferred to the post-anaesthesia care unit, and later to the intensive care unit (ICU) or high-dependence unit (HDU), according to the policy of each individual centre for clinical and laboratory monitoring, and to ensure adequate analgesia.

Intraoperative Monitoring

Monitoring consists of standard procedures and tests, such as ECG, pulse oximetry, non-invasive blood pressure, end tidal carbon dioxide, fractioned inspired and expired oxygen, anaesthetic inhalational agents and core temperature. Additionally, continuous invasive blood pressure, continuous CVP, anaesthesia depth and neuromuscular monitoring are performed according to the preferences of each individual centre.

The transoesophageal Doppler (TED) flow time parameter can be used as a minimally invasive alternative to CVP for guiding fluid management. Mahmoud et al. utilized Doppler technology during right lobe living donor hepatotomy to guide fluid therapy. They reported that TED was able to detect haemodynamic changes during and after a right hepatotomy [32].

Ibrahim et al. successfully used a TED probe to guide fluid therapy and monitor systemic haemodynamics in donor recipients during liver transplantation [33]. El Sharkawy et al. demonstrated that TED monitoring reduced the need for colloid administration during LR (post-resection), which resulted in a shorter hospital stay [34].

Other Alternatives to CVP Monitoring

Dynamic preload measures are based on the ‘normal’ physiological effects of positive pressure ventilation on the right and left sides of the heart. During positive pressure inspiration, the increased intrathoracic pressure is associated with a decrease in venous return to the right ventricle (RV). During inspiration, left ventricular (LV) filling increases due to compression of the pulmonary veins, in turn increasing LV stroke volume. LV stroke volume decreases during expiration due to reduced RV filling. These changes in LV stroke volume are most marked when the patient is hypovolemic [35, 36].

A non-invasive alternative to traditional CVP is now available that depends on dynamic parameters. An array of non-invasive monitoring tools, such as the plethysmographic variability index, pulse pressure variation (PPV) and stroke volume variation (SVV) are available for both donors and recipients [37–39].

Choi et al. demonstrated that SVV can be used as a proxy for fluid responsiveness, and that a high SVV (10–20%) reduces blood loss during live donor hepatectomy [40]. The benefit of SVV lies in tracking the changes therein over time rather than relying on isolated readings. Changes in SVV, as a proxy for fluid responsiveness and to guide optimisation thereof, can be useful following the fluid restriction phase associated with liver transection. Dynamic monitoring indices, such as SVV, require tidal volumes of 8–10 ml/kg to achieve sufficient accuracy [40].

Utilizing an already-inserted invasive arterial blood pressure catheter to analyse arterial wave forms and derive more specific measures, such as cardiac output (CO), systemic vascular resistance (SVR) and oxygen delivery (DO2), is an additional benefit. When available, these data can help guide fluid management and maintain haemodynamic stability, particularly in cases of surgical blood loss.

Donations are not routinely performed under continuous CO monitoring. Mahmoud et al. used a minimally invasive TED probe to identify significant increases in CO and heart rate immediately following a right hepatectomy. These changes were significantly less marked with prophylactic intravenous infusion of $MgSO_4$ [32]. These haemodynamic changes may occur due to the release of splanchnic mediators, such as endotoxins, during dissection [41, 42].

Postoperative Pain Management

There is a general belief that LRLDs experience more pain than patients undergoing the same size LR as a curative procedure due to psychological reasons. However, there is no firm evidence to support this view.

Thoracic epidural analgesia (TEA) provides the best postoperative pain relief following LRLD, particularly when there is a clear plan for transitioning from TEA to another method of pain control [43]. Post-LR coagulopathy peaks on days 2–3, according to a significant body of evidence [44, 45]. There is also evidence that LR patients are hypercoagulable, and that the international normalised ratio (INR) and number of platelets are not indicative of the coagulopathy status [46].

Intrathecal morphine plus intravenous opioid patient controlled-analgesia (PCA) has the advantage of better haemodynamic stability, less fluid and opioid consumption, and faster recovery compared with TEA, as well as less morphine consumption than morphine PCA alone [47, 48].

Intravenous opioids and intravenous PCA syringes have been adopted to increase donor safety, albeit at the expense of an increase in opioid consumption and the side-effects thereof [49].

A multimodal approach is currently in favour, such as combining regional blocks (wound catheter analgesia, and transversus abdominis plane [TAP], erector spinae and serratus block) with intravenous opioids and additional boluses of other intravenous analgesics, such as paracetamol, ketamine, non-steroidal antiinflammatory drugs (NSAIDs) or lignocaine [50–52]. An additional catheter can be placed between the rectus abdominis muscle and the posterior wall of the rectal sheath (sub-rectal sheath block), paying particular attention to blood vessels in this space to increase the pain relief efficiency when combined with a TAP block [53].

Intensive Care Unit Management for Donors

Donors are kept in a monitored bed at an intermediate care unit, or in an ICU in hospitals with no intermediate care units. High–volume centres have transplant wards and patients are monitored in the ICU for the first night following surgery, or until early ambulation. Serial ultrasound studies are performed to detect any fluid collection, together with daily Doppler studies of the hepatic vasculature. Standard deep venous thrombosis prophylaxis (low-molecular-weight heparin and intermittent calf compression) is administered over the first 24 hours. Chest physiotherapy, early mobilisation and oral nutrition (clear liquids) is encouraged as tolerated. An antibiotic and an H_2 blocker are provided according to the preference of each individual centre. Serial liver function tests (prothrombin time, renal function, serum electrolytes [mainly phosphate and magnesium] and serum lactate) are performed daily during the first 3 days until discharge. Arterial blood gases and pH, haemoglobin, haematocrit, serum sodium, potassium, chloride, magnesium, phosphate, glucose and ionized calcium, complete blood count, prothrombin, activated partial thromboplastin time and fibrinogen are not routinely monitored, but can be evaluated in the few centres wherein rotational thromboelastometry is available.

Reduced blood levels of magnesium and phosphate are not uncommon during the postoperative period and need to be addressed [54–56]. There appear to be several reasons for the reduced levels, such as hepatic cell regeneration, the stress response, and use of relatively phosphate- and magnesium-free intravenous crystalloids and colloids. Blood levels of lactate, aspartate aminotransferase (AST) and alanine aminotransferase (ALT) increase significantly immediately following LR, but gradually decrease by days 2 and 3 [57].

Donor Morbidity and Mortality

The most frequent postoperative complication of live donor hepatectomy is intra-abdominal fluid collection, which occurs due to a biliary leak and can lead to sepsis caused by Gram-negative bacteria. Injury to the hepatic bile duct requires intraoperative reconstruction and stent placement. A bile leak from the cut surface of the liver can resolve spontaneously, but may require endoscopic retrograde cholangiopancreatography and insertion of a stent [58].

Vascular complications involving the portal vein (PV) have been reported, varying in severity. Pomfret et al. (0.18%) [59], Jianget et al. (3.8%) [60] and Yassen et al. [61] each reported one donor with PV thrombosis, which was managed by relaparotomy and intraoperative infusion of tissue plasminogen activator.

The most life-threatening complications are deep-vein thrombosis and pulmonary embolism. Air pressure devices for massaging both legs should be used during the operation, and until the donor is no longer bedridden; prophylactic low-molecular-weight heparin should also be administered.

Liver donation for LDLT is not a complication-free procedure and should always be done in a specialized transplant centre, and preferably in a high-volume centre. In a study conducted at Johns Hopkins University (USA), all LLDs between April 1994 and March 2011 were followed for a mean of 7.6 years; 1.7 deaths/1,000 donors were reported [62].

A recent French systematic review of published studies concerning donor morbidity and mortality related to LDLT was conducted by Brige et al. [63]. Data retrieved from the Medline database between 2000 and 2017 indicated that the major cause of donor death was sepsis (30%). Morbidity ranged from 10 to 78.3% among different centres [63]. Three donor deaths were reported in Egypt [64, 65].

Reporting donor mortality and morbidity is important to facilitate the development of protocols promoting safer donation procedures and perioperative management, particularly in countries where LDLT is the only option available.

Newly developed protocols for enhanced recovery after liver surgery (ERAS) may lead to significant reductions in morbidity and length of hospital stay [66,

67]. ERAS protocols for LLD volunteers have recently been introduced to promote recovery, minimise postoperative pain and decrease postoperative narcotic use [68, 69].

Laparoscopic Live Donor Hepatotomy

Few transplant centres have accumulated sufficient experience to perform laparoscopic and hepatotomy for donors. In Japan, Takahara et al. (2017) reported the outcomes of pure laparoscopic LR for donors [70]. At the second International Consensus Conference for Laparoscopic Liver Resection, institutional ethical approval and a registry was recommended for the procedure of "adult-to-adult laparoscopic donor surgery". The laparoscopic approach has been in use for longer, results in less blood loss, and allows for early rehabilitation [71].

In addition, robotic hemihepatectomy is gaining popularity and is safe and feasible in selected patients. It has similar perioperative outcomes as laparoscopic liver resection and was better than laparoscopic liver resection regarding estimated blood loss [72].

Acknowledgements I would like to acknowledge the help in revising the text by:

Prof. Fuat H. Saner,
Professor for Critical Care
Essen University Medical Center
Department of General- and Visceral- and Transplant Surgery
Hufelandstr. 55
45147 Essen
Email: fuat.saner@uni-due.de

Dr. Fatimah Salah Danyan
Consultant Anaesthesia and Head of liver Transplant Section
King Fahad Specialist Hospital, Ministry of Health, Dammam, Kingdom of Saudi Arabia.
Email: fatimah.salah@kfsh.med.sa
Prof. Ahmed M. Mukhtar
Professor for Anaesthesia, Cairo University, Kasr AlAiny Hospital, Liver Transplant Unit.
Email: Ahmed.Mukhtar@kasralainy.edu

References

1. Gorgen A, Goldaracena N, Zhang W, Rosales R, Ghanekar A, Lilly L, et al. Surgical complications after right hepatectomy for live liver donations: largest single-center western world experience. Semin Liver Dis. 2018;38:134–44.
2. Dar FS, Zia H, Hafeez Bhatti AB, Rana A, Nazer R, Kazmi R, et al. Short term donor outcomes after hepatectomy in living donor liver transplantation. J Coll Physicians Surg Pak. 2016;26:272–6.

3. Kamel E, Abdullah M, Hassanin A, Fayed N, Ahmed F, Soliman H, et al. Live donor hepatectomy for liver transplantation in Egypt: lessons learned. Saudi J Anaesth. 2012;6:234–41.
4. Abdullah K, Abdeldayem H, Hali WO, Sakran A, Yassen K, Abdulkareem A. Twenty cases of adult-to-adult living-related liver transplantation: single center experience in Saudi Arabia. Transplant Proc. 2005;37:3144–6.
5. Gordon EJ, Mullee J, Skaro A, Baker T. Live liver donors' information needs: a qualitative study of practical implications for informed consent. Surgery. 2016;160:671–82.
6. Parikh ND, Lander D, Abecassis M, Butt Z. Quality of life in donors after living donor liver transplantation: a review of the literature. Liver Transpl. 2010;16:1352–8.
7. Kim JM, Kwon CH, Joh JW, Han SB, Sinn DH, Choi GS, et al. Case-matched comparison of ABO-incompatible and ABO-compatible living donor liver transplantation. Br J Surg. 2016;103:276–83.
8. Broering DC, Sterneck M, Rogiers X. Living donor liver transplantation. J Hepatol. 2003;38(Suppl 1):S119–35.
9. Soin AS, Chaudhary RJ, Pahari H, Pomfret EA. A worldwide survey of live liver donor selection policies at 24 centers with a combined experience of 19009 adult living donor liver transplants. Transplantation 2019;103:e39–e47.
10. Polido W Jr, Hoe LK, Siang NK, Chah TK. Acute myocardial infarction after live donor liver surgery. Liver Transpl. 2007;13:154–6.
11. Kamei H, Onishi Y, Kurata N, Ishigani M, Ogura Y. Donor selection and prophylactic strategy for venous thromboembolic events in living donors of liver transplantation based on results of thrombophilia screening tests. Ann Transplant. 2017;22:409–16.
12. Gomathy N, Safwan M, Kota V, Reddy MS, Bharathan A, Dabora A, et al. Donor outcomes in living donor liver transplantation—analysis of 275 donors from a single centre in India. Transplantation. 2016;100:1251–6.
13. Mohammed M, Fayed N, Hassanen A, Ahmed F, Mourad W, El Sheikh M, et al. Rotational thromboelastometry and standard coagulation test for live liver donors. Clin Transplant. 2013;27:E101–8.
14. Andert A, Becker N, Ulmer F, Schoning W, Hein M, Rumek A, et al. Liver transplantation and donor body mass index >30: use or refuse? Ann Transplant. 2016;21:185–93.
15. Knaak M, Goldaracena N, Doyle A, Cattral MS, Greig PD, Lilly L, et al. Donor BMI >30 is not a contraindication for live liver donation. Am J Transplant. 2017;17:754–60.
16. Kiuchi T, Kasahara M, Uryuhara K, Inomata Y, Uemoto S, Asonuma K, et al. Impact of graft size mismatching on graft prognosis in liver transplantation from living donors. Transplantation. 1999;67:321–7.
17. Vasavada B, Chen CL, Zakaria M. Using low graft/recipient's body weight ratio graft with portal flow modulation an effective way to prevent small-for-size syndrome in living-donor liver transplant: a retrospective analysis. Exp Clin Transplant. 2014;12:437–42.
18. Hwang S, Lee SG, Lee YJ, Sung KB, Park KM, Kim KH, et al. Lessons learned from 1000 living donor liver transplantations in a single center: how to make living donations safe. Liver Transpl. 2006;12:920–7.
19. Karna ST, Pandey CK, Pandey VK, Singh A. Brachial plexus injury in live related donor hepatectomy: a chart review. J Postgrad Med. 2014;60:287–9.
20. Dulitz MG, De Wolf AM, Wong H, Wray C, Sherwani S, Herborn J, et al. Compression of the brachial plexus during right lobe liver donation as a cause of brachial plexus injury: a case report. Liver Transpl. 2005;11:233–5.
21. Yassen K, Abuzaid A, Hussain N, Ibrahim E, Khater Y. The respiratory and haemodynamic effects of alveolar recruitment in cirrhotic patient undergoing liver resection surgery. a randomized controlled trial. Am Soc Anesthesiol. 2018;A2167. http://www.asaabstracts.com/strands/asaabstracts/abstract.htm?year=2018&index=19&absnum=4527.

22. Hussein AM, Mahmoud F, Beltagy R, Hasanin A, Yassen K, Attar A. Desflurane compared to sevoflurane for cirrhotic patients undergoing major liver resection. A randomized control study. Middle East J Anaesthesiol. 2015;23:213–23.
23. Beck-schimmer B, Breitenstein S, Urech S, De Conno E, Wittlinger M, Puhan M, et al. A randomized controlled trial on pharmacological preconditioning in liver surgery using a volatile anesthetic. Ann Surg. 2008;248:909–18.
24. Nelson R, Edwards S, Tse B. Prophylactic nasogastric decompression after surgery. Cochrane Database Syst Rev. 2007;3:CD004929.
25. Pessaux P, Regimbeau JM, Dondero F, et al. Randomized clinical trial evaluating the need for routine nasogastric decompression after elective hepatic resection. Br J Surg. 2007;92:297–303.
26. Wang WD, Liang LJ, Huang XQ, Yin XY. Low central venous pressure reduces blood loss in hepatectomy. World J Gastroenterol. 2006;12:935–9.
27. Huntington JT, Royal NA, Schmidt CR. Minimizing blood loss during hepatectomy: a literature review. J Surg Oncol. 2014;109:81–8.
28. Latchana N, Hirpara DH, Hallet J, Karanicolas PJ. Red blood cell transfusion in liver resection. Langenbeck's Arch. Surg. 2019:404 1–9.
29. Sand L, Lundin S, Rizell M, Wiklund J, Stenqvist O, Houltz E. Nitroglycerine and patient position effect on central, hepatic and portal venous pressures during liver surgery. Acta Anaesthesiol Scand. 2014;58:961–7.
30. Kim SH, Kim YK. Improving outcomes of living donor right hepatectomy. Br I Surg. 2013;100:528–34.
31. Abdulatif M, Lotfy M, Mousa M, Afifi MH, Yassen K. Sugammedex antagonism of rocuronium-induced neuromuscular blockade in patients with liver cirrhosis undergoing liver resection: a randomized controlled study. Minerva Anestesiol. 2018;84:929–37.
32. Mahmoud G, Sayed E, Eskander A, ElElsheikh M, Lotfy M, Yassen K. Effect of intraoperative magnesium intravenous infusion on the hemodynamic changes associated with right lobe living donor hepatotomy under transesophageal Doppler monitoring-randomized controlled trial. Saudi J Anaesth. 2016;10:132–7.
33. Ibrahim N, Hasanin A, Allah SA, Saued E, Afifi M, Yassen K, et al. The haemodynamic effects of the perioperative terlipressin infusion in living donor livertransplantation: a randomised controlled study. Indian J Anaesth. 2015;59(3):156–64. https://doi.org/10.4103/0019-5049.153037.
34. El Sharkawy OA, Refaat EK, Ibraheem AE, Mahdy WR, Fayed NA, Mourad WS, et al. Transoesophageal Doppler compared to central venous pressure for perioperative hemodynamic monitoring and fluid guidance in liver resection. Saudi J Anaesth. 2013;7:378–86.
35. Pinsky MR, Payen D. Functional hemodynamic monitoring. Crit Care. 2005;9:566–72.
36. Marik PE, Cavallazzi R, Vasu T, Hirani A. Dynamic changes in arterial waveform derived variables and fluid responsiveness in mechanically ventilated patients: a systematic review of the literature. Crit Care Med. 2009;37:2642–7.
37. Niemann CU, Feiner J, Behrends M, Eilers H, Ascher NL, Roberts JP. Central venous pressure monitoring during living right donor hepatectomy. Liver Transpl. 2007;13:266–71.
38. Kim SH, Hwang GS, Kim SO, Kim YK. Is stroke volume variation a useful preload index in liver transplant recipients? A retrospective analysis. Int J Med Sci. 2013;10:751–7.
39. Gouvea G, Diaz R, Auler L, Toledo R, Marinho JM. Evaluation of the pulse pressure variation index as a predictor of fluid responsiveness during orthotopic liver transplantation. Br J Anaesth. 2009;103:238–43.
40. Choi JM, Lee YK, Yoo H, Lee S, Kim HY, Kim YK. Relationship between stroke volume variation and blood transfusion during liver transplantation. Int J Med Sci. 2016;13:235–9.
41. Niemann CU, Roberts JP, Ascher NL, Yost CS. Intraoperative hemodynamics and liver function in adult-to-adult living liver donors. Liver Transpl. 2002;8:1126–32.
42. Marinangeli F, Ciccozzi A, Angeletti C, Guetti C, Aloisio T, Paladini A, et al. Hemodynamic changes during hepatic vascular exclusion: use of intraoperative transesophageal echocardiography a case series. Anesthesiology. 2011;2011:1–6.

43. Koul A, Pant D, Rudravaram S, Sood J. Thoracic epidural analgesia in donor hepatectomy: an analysis. Liver Transpl. 2018;24:214–21.
44. Stamenkovic DM, Jankovic ZB, Toogood GJ, Lodge JP, Bellamy MC. Epidural analgesia and liver resection: postoperative coagulation disorders and epidural catheter removal. Minerva Anesthesiol. 2011;77:671.
45. Jacquenod P, Wallon G, Gazon M, Darnis B, Pradat P, Virlogeux V, et al. Incidence and risk factors of coagulation profile derangement after liver surgery: implications for the use of epidural analgesia-a retrospective cohort study. Anesth Analg. 2018;126:1142–7.
46. Mallet SV, Sugavanam A, Krzanicki DA, Patel S, Broomhead RH, Davidson BR, et al. Alterations in coagulation following major liver resection. Anaesthesia. 2016;71:657–68.
47. Ko JS, Choi SJ, Gwak MS, Kim MS, Ahn HJ, Kim JA, et al. Intrathecal morphine combined with intravenous patient-controlled analgesia is an effective and safe method for immediate postoperative pain control in live liver donors. Liver Transplant. 2009;15:381–9.
48. Kasivisvanathan R, Abbasi-Ghad N, Prout J, Clevenger B, Fusai GK, Mallet SV. A prospective cohort study of intrathecal versus epidural analgesia for patients undergoing hepatic resection. HPB (Oxford). 2014;16:768–75.
49. Revie EJ, McKeown DW, Wilson JA, Garden OJ, Wigmore SJ. Randomized clinical trial of local infiltration pluspatient-controlled opiate analgesia versus epidural analgesia following liver resection surgery. HPB (Oxford). 2012;14:611–8.
50. Kang R, Chin KJ, Gwak MS, Kim GS, Choi SJ, Kim JM, et al. Bilateral single-injection erector spinae plane block versus intrathecal morphine for postoperative analgesia in living donor laparoscopic hepatectomy: a randomized non-inferiority trial. Reg Anesth Pain Med 2019 Oct 23. pii: rapm-2019-100902. https://doi.org/10.1136/rapm-2019-100902. [Epub ahead of print].
51. Kitlik A, Erdogan MA, Ozgul U, Aydogen MS, Ucar M, Topak HI, et al. Ultrasound-guided transversus abdominis plane block for postoperative analgesia in living liver donors: a prospective, randomized, double-blinded clinical trial. J Clin Anesth. 2017;37:103–7.
52. Dewe G, Steyaert A, De Kock M, Lois F, Reding R, Forget P. Pain management in living related adult donor hepatectomy: feasibility of an evidence-based protocolin 100 consecutive donors. BMC Res Notes. 2018;11:834.
53. Milan ZB, Duncan B, Revari V, Kocarev M, Collin R. Subcostal transversus abdominis plane block for postoperative analgesia in liver transplant recipients. Transplant proc. 2011;43:2687–90.
54. Mahmoud AA, El-Sharaway AM, Mansour MA, Abdelhaq MM, Maher MA, Kamal AM. Perioperative calcium, magnesium, and phosphorus levels in live donors for liver transplant. Exp Clin Transplant. 2015;13:550–5.
55. Yassen K, Tamimi W, Al Abdulkareem A, et al. Hypomagnesaemia and hypophsphataemia during and after right hepatectomy for living donor liver transplantation. Egyptian J Anaesthesia. 2005;21:111–3.
56. Pomposelli JJ, Pomfret EA, Burns DL, Lally A, Sorcini A, Gordon FD, et al. Life-threatening hypophosphatemia after right hepatic lobectomy for live donor adult liver transplantation. Liver Transpl. 2001;7:637–42.
57. Yassen K, Al Abdul Kareem A. Living donor liver transplantation: perioperative experience from Saudi Arabia. Int Anesthesiol Clin. 2006;44:161–70.
58. Woo HY, Lee IS, Chang JH, Youn SB, Bae SH, Choi JY, et al. Outcome of donor biliary complications following living donor liver transplantation. Korean J Int Med. 2018;33:705–15.
59. Pomfret E, Pomposelli J, Lewis WD. Live donor adult liver transplantation using right lobe grafts: donor evaluation and surgical outcome. Arch Surg. 2001;136:425–33.
60. Jiang X, Yan L, Li B. Safety of donor in adult-to-adult living donor liver transplantation using right lobe graft. Transplant Proc. 2007;39:150–2.
61. Yassen K, Geldhof G, AlAbdulkareem A. Perioperative anaesthetic management of living related liver transplant donors: a retrospective analysis of a preliminary series in Saudi Arabia. Eg J Anaesth. 2004;20:377–84.

62. Muzaale AD, Dagher NN, Montgomery RA, Taranto SE, McBride MA, Segev DL. Estimates of early death, acute liver failure, and long-term mortality among live liver donors. Gastroenterology. 2012;142:273–80.
63. Brige P, Hery G, Chopinet S, Palen A, Azoulay D, Gregoire E. Morbidity and mortality of hepatic right lobe living donors: systematic review and perspectives. J Gastrointestin Liver Dis. 2018;27:169–78.
64. Chakravarty DK, Lee WC, Jan YY, Chen YC, Lee PO-Huang. Evaluation of live donors. In: Chakravarty DK, Lee WC, Jan YY, Chen YC, Lee PO-Huang, editors. Liver transplantation. New Delhi, India: Jaypee Broth Medical Publishers; 2010, p. 41–53.
65. El-Meteini M, Hamza A, Abdalaal A, et al. Biliary complications including single-donor mortality: experience of 207 adult-to-adult living donor liver transplantations with right liver grafts. HPB (Oxford). 2010;12:109–14.
66. Melloul E, Hubner M, Scott M, Snowden C, Prentis J, Dejong CHC, et al. Guidelines for perioperative care for liver surgery: enhanced recovery after surgery (ERAS) society recommendations. World J Surg. 2016;40:2425–40.
67. Hughes NJ, McNally S, Wigmore SJ. Enhances recovery following liver surgery: a systematic review and meta-analysis. HPB. 2014;16:699–706.
68. Khalil A, Ganesh S, Hughes C, Tevar AD, Hasche JJ, Esper S, et al. Evaluation of the enhanced recovery after surgery protocol in living liver donors. Clin Transplant. 2018;32:e13342. https://doi.org/10.1111/ctr.13342 Epub 2018 Jul 24.
69. Kim SH, Kim YK, Lee SD, Lee EC, Park SJ. The impact of a surgical protocol for enhanced recovery on living donor right hepatectomy: a single-center cohort study. Medicine (Baltimore). 2016;95:e3227. https://doi.org/10.1097/MD.0000000000003227.
70. Takahara T, Wakabayashi G, Nitta H, Hasegawa Y, Katagiri H, Umemura A, et al. The first comparative study of the perioperative outcomes between pure laparoscopic donor hepatectomy and laparoscopy-assisted donor hepatectomy in a single institution. Transplantation. 2017;101:1628–36.
71. Au KP, Chok KSH. Minimally invasive donor hepatectomy, are we ready for prime time? World J Gastroenterol. 2018;24:2698–709.
72. Wang ZZ, Tang WB, Hu MG, Zhao ZM, Zhao GD, Li CG, et al. Robotic versus laparoscopic hemihepatectomy: a comparative study from a single center. J Surg Oncol. 2019;120:646–53.

Chapter 20
Strategies for Low Central Venous Pressure in Liver Resection Surgery

Aidan Patrick Devlin

Rationale for Low Central Venous Pressure Anaesthesia for Liver Resection

Developments in surgical and anaesthetic techniques have contributed to a decline in the morbidity and mortality associated with liver resection since the 1970s, [1] and the development of techniques to minimise blood loss and transfusion rates have contributed to this decline. Good anaesthetic technique can help to minimise blood loss and thereby improve outcomes for patients undergoing liver resection surgery.

The hepatic veins are valveless and drain directly into the inferior vena cava (IVC). During hepatic parenchymal resection, depending on surgical technique, hepatic inflow from the hepatic artery and hepatic portal vein may be occluded. This leaves back-bleeding from the venous system as the main source of blood loss. By reducing the central venous pressure (CVP), bleeding can be reduced and transfusion can often be avoided.

Low CVP anaesthesia has been shown to reduce bleeding and transfusion rates [2] and is generally defined as maintaining the CVP at less than 5 cm H_2O during parenchymal resection. Although bleeding and transfusion rates are significantly reduced by this technique, evidence of reduced morbidity or length of stay in this population directly attributable to low-CVP anaesthesia remains elusive. However blood transfusion carries well-documented risks such as transfusion reactions, transmission of infection, alloimmunisation and post-operative infection and it may increase the risk of cancer recurrence, especially in the early stages of hepatocellular carcinoma [3, 4]. Blood transfusion is an independent predictor

A. P. Devlin (✉)
Department of Anaesthesia, King's College Hospital, Denmark Hill, London SE5 9RS, UK
e-mail: adevlin1@nhs.net

Z. Milan and C. Goonasekera (eds.), *Anesthesia for Hepatico-Pancreatic-Biliary Surgery and Transplantation*, https://doi.org/10.1007/978-3-030-51331-3_20

of morbidity and mortality following liver resection surgery [4] and in order to minimise these risks, low-CVP anaesthesia has become standard practice for liver resection surgery.

Strategies for Achieving Low CVP

There are numerous strategies for achieving low CVP during liver resection and there is a lack of evidence suggesting benefit of any particular strategy over another, excepting partial IVC clamping, which may be associated with pulmonary embolism [5]. In practice more than one strategy is usually used and this varies between anaesthetists and institutions.

Fluid Management

Restriction of intravenous fluid intake is commonly used to achieve low CVP during liver resection, although there is no consensus on what constitutes fluid restriction. In practice this usually means a small bolus of intravenous fluid at induction, with small amounts or no maintenance fluid until resection is complete. When this approach is used an infusion of vasopressor is usually required to maintain adequate perfusion pressure. If the duration of fasting is excessive or there is brisk bleeding this approach can lead to haemodynamic instability. With prolonged surgery and even moderate fluid restriction patients may develop a metabolic acidosis. Any fluid restriction protocol should be modified by clinical judgement and patients should be selected for this technique according to their comorbidities. There is little evidence for or against fluid restriction to achieve low CVP in liver resection.

Hypovolaemic phlebotomy involves draining whole blood from the patient into a specially designed bag containing anticoagulant before resection begins. In contrast to acute normovolaemic haemodilution, intravenous fluid is not given to replace the lost intravascular volume. The blood is stored and given back to the patient when the resection is completed. This technique successfully lowers CVP and has been shown to reduce bleeding and transfusion requirements [6]. There is currently much less in the literature regarding this technique than fluid restriction and further evidence is required before it is widely adopted.

Pharmacological

Pharmacological treatments focus on either vasodilatation or reducing circulating volume. A reduction in CVP can be achieved with an infusion of glyceryl trinitrate or small boluses of furosemide.

Thoracic Epidural

Insertion of a thoracic epidural for liver resection surgery can lower CVP, due to sympathetic blockade causing increased venous capacitance [5]. Sympathetic blockade can also cause arterial hypotension, which may require an infusion of vasopressor especially if the patient is also fluid restricted. Thoracic epidurals lower CVP and decrease blood loss more successfully than intrathecal blockade but this is at the expense of delayed postoperative mobilisation [7]. Postoperatively patients who receive thoracic epidurals tend to have lower mean arterial pressures, require infusions of vasopressors more often and also receive blood transfusions more often [8]. The benefits of thoracic epidurals in providing prolonged analgesia and low CVP conditions should be weighed against these potential risks when selecting a technique.

The use of thoracic epidurals in liver resection surgery is seen as controversial by some due to the potential for coagulopathy and the risk of epidural haematoma post-operatively; however the evidence in this area is based on case reports only and several case series exist demonstrating the safety of this technique [8, 9].

Physical Manoeuvres

These are some of the simplest and most cost-effective methods to reduce CVP. The reverse Trendelenburg position is effective and safe in reducing CVP and does not significantly reduce systemic arterial pressure [10]. Using low amounts of positive-end expiratory pressure (PEEP) and low airway pressures also reduce CVP and bleeding by keeping intrathoracic pressures low [11].

Surgical Strategies

Clamping of the infrahepatic IVC can successfully reduce CVP and bleeding during liver resection, however it may be associated with an increased risk of pulmonary embolism [5]. This technique can cause haemodynamic instability through reduction of venous return, which may be more pronounced in a fluid restricted patient [12]. IVC clamping is not widely used as part of a low-CVP technique during liver resection.

Laparoscopic Liver Resection Surgery and Low CVP

Adding pneumoperitoneum to the physiological changes and haemodynamic instability of low CVP anaesthesia can be challenging. A major advantage of laparoscopic liver resection is that bleeding is reduced because of positive pressure within the abdomen. There is limited evidence on the value of low CVP anaesthesia in this context but the consensus is that a CVP <5 cm H_2O is desirable in order to minimise venous bleeding [13]. Achieving a low CVP in this situation can be more difficult as the decreased analgesic requirements of laparoscopic procedures mean that epidural analgesia is unlikely to be used, and pneumoperitoneum tends to increase CVP. A mixture of techniques is likely to be needed to achieve the desired CVP.

The combination of an open vascular bed and high intra-abdominal pressure makes CO_2 embolism much more likely in laparoscopic liver resection than in other laparoscopic procedures. In animal models numerous small CO_2 emboli were seen during laparoscopic liver resection but this did not cause clinically detectable haemodynamic changes [14]. This may be due to the high solubility of carbon dioxide in blood. Patients with end stage liver disease and those with right to left shunts are at higher risk of systemic embolism and vigilance is required during these cases.

Safety of Low CVP Anaesthesia in Liver Resection

It is widely agreed that low CVP anaesthesia for liver resection is safe. Despite fluid restriction being a common component of low-CVP techniques, the incidence of clinically relevant renal dysfunction following liver resection with low CVP anaesthesia is low [15–17]. Air embolism during hepatic resection has been reported but the incidence is so low that it cannot be quantified.

Low CVP Anaesthesia Without CVP Monitoring?

Cardiac output monitors calculate the stroke volume variation (SVV) as an indicator of fluid status. An SVV of 18–21% has been found to correlate reliably with a CVP of −1 to 1 cm H_2O in open liver resection [18]. By using low CVP techniques and targeting a high SVV, bleeding is reduced to the same degree as when a low CVP is targeted [19]. This technique has also been demonstrated safely in laparoscopic liver resection [20] and may avoid the requirement for central venous catheterisation in some patients undergoing hepatic resection, and the reduction of morbidity associated with these lines. However SVV monitoring cannot be used in patients with arrhythmias and in frail patients with multiple co-morbidities undergoing extensive surgery, a central venous catheter may be required for infusion of vasopressors and other medications in the perioperative period. Targeting SVV rather than CVP and avoiding central venous catheterisation is likely to be suitable for carefully selected patients only.

Summary

Low CVP anaesthesia reduces bleeding and the requirement for blood transfusion after liver resection. There are numerous techniques to achieve a low CVP and there is little evidence to choose between them. In practice a combination of techniques is usually required, tailored to the patient and the clinical situation.

References

1. Hartog A, Mills G. Anaesthesia for hepatic resection surgery. Contin Educ Anaesthesia, Crit Care Pain. 2009;9:1–5.
2. Hughes MJ, Ventham NT, Harrison EM, Wigmore SJ. Central venous pressure and liver resection: a systematic review and meta-analysis. HPB. 2015;17:863–871.
3. Cheng ESW, Hallet J, Hanna SS, Law CHL, Coburn NG, Tarshis J, Lin Y, Karanicolas PJ. Is central venous pressure still relevant in the contemporary era of liver resection? J Surg Res. 2015;200:139–46.
4. De Boer MT, Molenaar IQ, Porte RJ. Impact of blood loss on outcome after liver resection. Dig Surg. 2007;24:259–64.
5. Rahbari NN, Zimmermann JB, Schmidt T, et al. Infrahepatic inferior vena cava clamping for reduction of central venous pressure and blood loss during hepatic resection. Ann Surg. 2011;253:1102–10.
6. Rekman J, Wherrett C, Bennett S, Gostimir M, Saeed S, Lemon K, Mimeault R, Balaa FK, Martel G. Safety and feasibility of phlebotomy with controlled hypovolemia to minimize blood loss in liver resections. Surg (United States). 2017;161:650–7.
7. Kasivisvanathan R, Abbassi-Ghadi N, Prout J, Clevenger B, Fusai GK, Mallett SV. A prospective cohort study of intrathecal versus epidural analgesia for patients undergoing hepatic resection. HPB. 2014;16:768–775.
8. Page A, Rostad B, Staley CA, Levy JH, Park J, Goodman M, Sarmiento JM, Galloway J, Delman KA, Kooby DA. Epidural analgesia in hepatic resection. J Am Coll Surg. 2008;206:1184–92.
9. Miyazaki M, Takasita M, Matsumoto H, Sonoda H, Tsumura H, Torisu T. Spinal epidural hematoma after removal of an epidural catheter: case report and review of the literature. J Spinal Disord Tech. 2005;18:547–51.
10. Soonawalla ZF, Stratopoulos C, Stoneham M, Wilkinson D, Britton BJ, Friend PJ. Role of the reverse-Trendelenberg patient position in maintaining low-CVP anaesthesia during liver resections. Langenbeck's Arch Surg. 2008;393:195–8.
11. Iguchi T, Ikegami T, Fujiyoshi T, Yoshizumi T, Shirabe K, Maehara Y. Low positive airway pressure without positive end-expiratory pressure decreases blood loss during hepatectomy in living liver donors. Dig Surg. 2017;34:192–6.
12. Yoneda G, Katagiri S, Yamamoto M. Reverse Trendelenburg position is a safer technique for lowering central venous pressure without decreasing blood pressure than clamping of the inferior vena cava below the liver. J Hepatobiliary Pancreat Sci. 2015;22:463–6.
13. Tranchart H, O'Rourke N, Van Dam R, Gaillard M, Lainas P, Sugioka A, Wakabayashi G, Dagher I. Bleeding control during laparoscopic liver resection: a review of literature. J Hepatobiliary Pancreat Sci. 2015;22:371–8.
14. Fors D, Eiriksson K, Arvidsson D, Rubertsson S. Elevated PEEP without effect upon gas embolism frequency or severity in experimental laparoscopic liver resection. Br J Anaesth. 2012;109:272–8.

15. Correa-Gallego C, Berman A, Denis SC, et al. Renal function after low central venous pressure-assisted liver resection: assessment of 2116 cases. HPB. 2015;17:258–64.
16. Melendez JA, Arslan V, Fischer ME, Wuest D, Jarnagin WR, Fong Y, Blumgart LH. Perioperative outcomes of major hepatic resections under low central venous pressure anesthesia: blood loss, blood transfusion, and the risk of postoperative renal dysfunction. J Am Coll Surg. 1998;187:620–5.
17. Wang CH, Cheng KW, Chen CL, et al. Effect and outcome of intraoperative fluid restriction in living liver donor hepatectomy. Ann Transplant. 2017;22:671–6.
18. Kitaguchi K, Gotohda N, Yamamoto H, Kato Y, Takahashi S, Konishi M, Hayashi R. Intraoperative circulatory management using the FloTrac TM system in laparoscopic liver resection. Asian J Endosc Surg. 2015;8:164–70.
19. Choi SS, Jun IG, Cho SS, Kim SK, Hwang GS, Kim YK. Effect of stroke volume variation-directed fluid management on blood loss during living-donor right hepatectomy: a randomised controlled study. Anaesthesia. 2015;70:1250–8.
20. Comotti L, Aldrighetti L, Beretta L, Paganelli M, Cipriani F, Ratti F, Catena M, Reineke R. Intraoperative monitoring of stroke volume variation versus central venous pressure in laparoscopic liver surgery: a randomized prospective comparative trial. HPB. 2015;18:136–44.

Chapter 21
Enhanced Recovery After HPB Surgery

Joe Macmillan

Introduction

Enhanced Recovery After Surgery (ERAS) is a patient centred pathway designed to facilitate the delivery of high-quality perioperative care and interventions by coordinating the input and skills of the multidisciplinary team. The interventions are based on clinical and practice-based evidence.

Hepato- pancreatic -billiary (HPB) is a diverse surgical specialty which may involve a single organ, the liver, pancreas or digestive tract. It is however often multivisceral and may also include vascular resection and/or reconstruction. It is regarded as a high-risk specialty.

The complexity and varied nature of HPB surgery presents difficult questions of healthcare systems. It challenges our ability to provide standardised, reproducible and high-quality care. The problem of delivering high quality care is a wicked one by virtue of the multifactorial nature of hospitals, patients and their disease. Issues may be clinically, human resource or finance related. The aspiration of delivering surgical and patient specific care has led to a rapid expansion of outcome-based research and audit.

The evidence hopefully suggests that there are long strands of standardised care that can be applied despite the heterogeneity and complexity of both the surgery and the patients undergoing HPB surgery.

J. Macmillan (✉)
Anaesthetic Consutant, King's College Hospital, London, UK
e-mail: jmacmillan1@nhs.net

Z. Milan and C. Goonasekera (eds.), *Anesthesia for Hepatico-Pancreatic-Biliary Surgery and Transplantation*, https://doi.org/10.1007/978-3-030-51331-3_21

Incremental improvements in perioperative care over recent decades has resulted in significantly improved outcomes. Financially there are potential cost savings in reducing length of stay (LOS) and curtailing post-operative complications.

ERAS as a strategy has gained increasing momentum and acceptance since the turn of the 21st century. This has been catalysed by the work of Kehlet and colleagues and the subsequent validation of the ERAS strategy in colorectal surgery [1, 2].

ERAS delivers evidence-based practice across a range of care elements to modify and attenuate the stress response thus improving the bodies metabolic response to major surgery.

Surgical insult induces a stress response resulting in a catabolic state. The stress response is manifested by an increased cardiopulmonary demand with relative tissue hypoxia, attenuated gastrointestinal function, increased insulin resistance and impaired coagulation. ERAS pathways have been developed to maintain homeostasis and negate the stress response in the perioperative period thereby optimizing patient outcomes and minimizing postoperative complications.

ERAS for colorectal surgery has reduced postoperative complications, length of stay and cost whilst improving the time to functional recovery [3–5]. Indeed over the past decade nearly 600 studies of ERAS have generated a significant evidence base illustrating decreases in perioperative complication rates and also a decreased length of stay (LOS) or return to functional recovery without compromising the incidence of readmission rates [6]. A recent meta-analysis of 42 ERAS randomised control trials across multiple surgical specialities demonstrated a significant reductions in LOS, total hospital costs, total complications, and earlier return of gastrointestinal (GI) function, with no difference in overall mortality or 30-day readmission rates [7]. This confirms similar findings from previous meta-analyses analyses [8, 9] However it should be noted that whilst a reduction in medical morbidity occurs with ERAS, unfortunately surgical morbidity remains largely static [3, 4, 5, 7, 8, 9].

Improvements in Perioperative Care

The inverse correlation between postoperative mortality in patients undergoing surgically complex procedures and hospital volume and experience is widely recognised. This phenomenon has been investigated and studied in recent years [10–14]. These studies have demonstrated that institutional experience and processes, such as care pathways have a significant impact on outcomes.

The identification and subsequent investigation of this inverse correlation has led to many healthcare systems opting to centralise surgical and perioperative care for complex surgical procedures. The aim and result being to drive the improvement of surgical and perioperative care through experience, expertise and focused resource allocation to ensure the delivery of standardised, reproducible and high-quality care. These so called high volume centres have demonstrated improved outcome and performance metrics and are often referred to as centres of excellence [14–17].

The importance of these improvements is highlighted by the observation that both the number and type of complication has a marked impact on the incidence of postoperative mortality in patients undergoing HPB surgery. A synergistic effect of complications has been observed creating a greater than expected increase in the risk of 30 day mortality [18].

The marked reduction in mortality and improved outcomes in pancreatic and liver surgery over time are in part attributable to serial and evolving improvements in perioperative care [19–21]. These improvements are the result of integrated multi-disciplinary teamworking and the sharing of best practice between institutions and specialties. This approach has informed the development of ERAS pathways and protocols that have been designed and implemented for HPB surgery in particular liver resection and pancreaticoduodenectomy (PD).

Liver Surgery

Historically patients undergoing liver surgery have had to endure high rates of morbidity and mortality. However significant improvements in perioperative mortality have been reported. In the 1980s mortality following liver surgery stood at 10% but today many HPB centres achieve mortality rates below 4% [13, 22, 23].

These improvements are the result of refined patient selection, enhanced perioperative management and the development of high-volume centres. Improved surgical technique has minimised intraoperative liver parenchyma loss which has been rewarded with reductions in intraoperative blood loss, transfusion requirements and postoperative liver failure [24, 25].

Despite these advances over half (56%) of patients undergoing liver resection will experience a postoperative complication [13]. The incidence of major complications (Clavien-Dindo class 3 or 4) remains high and ranges from 17% in benign disease to 27% in malignant (Hepatocellular carcinoma and colorectal metastasis) to 42% for those with biliary malignancy [13]. Pulmonary complications can reach a zenith of 30% whilst thromboembolic events may be as high as 5% [13, 26, 27]. Patient specific factors that increase the risk of perioperative complications are sarcopenia and/or liver dysfunction [13]. Major complications result in a significant health and resource burden for the patient and institution respectively.

Cardiopulmonary, renal and septic complications can result in longer hospital stay, additional healthcare interventions, mortality and costs [13]. For those undergoing liver surgery for malignancy (in the UK the number of liver resections for colorectal metastatic disease was 1600 in 2006 [28]) complications following surgery are associated with a decrease in disease free and overall survival. The reasons for this are unclear but are thought in part to be due to upregulation of pro-inflammatory mediators and subsequent downregulation of the immune response to cancer [29].

Pancreatic Surgery

Surgery remains the treatment of choice for periampullary and pancreatic tumours. Pancreatic surgery and its associated perioperative care have undergone a dramatic step change since it was first performed over a century ago. Pancreatic resection was first performed successfully by Kausch in 1909. Whipple and colleagues were the first to describe the en-bloc resection of the head of pancreas and duodenum in 1935 [30]. However due to the high hospital mortality rates in the region of 25% pancreatic surgery and specifically pancreaticoduodenectomy (PD) fell out of favour and were rarely performed until the 1980s [31].

The technical demands, duration and severity of surgical complications ensures such procedures remain high risk. The 30-day mortality after pancreatic surgery has decreased significantly over time. During the 1970s mortality rates reported ranged from 12.5 to 23% [32–34]. By the late 1980s the mortality ranged from 4.2 to 11% [35, 36].

In recent years with further development and refinement of practice at high volume HPB centres, mortality has continued its downward trend with a 30 day mortality of 5% cited by some researchers [37, 38] and lower still 2.8–3.5% by others [39]. More recently still mortality rates have been quoted as low as 1.9–4.2%, for patients undergoing general pancreatic resections as well as pancreaticoduodenectomy (PD) [14].

Currently perioperative morbidity varies from 30 to 40% [39–42]. Of note the complications characteristic of pancreatic surgery such as delayed gastric emptying (DGE) and postoperative pancreatic fistula (POPF) have until recently failed to demonstrate any improvement [41, 42].

ERAS

ERAS protocols have been increasingly applied to HPB surgery. The evidence across surgical specialties has demonstrated a decreased incidence of postoperative complications, reduced LOS without a reduction in mortality or increase in readmission rates [7].

ERAS principles have been applied across multiple surgical specialties over recent years for example gynae oncology [43], Thoracic [44], Cardiac [45] Liver Surgery [46] and Pancreaticoduodenectomy [47].

ERAS programs are multifaceted and depend on multi-disciplinary teamwork, targeting interventions and care across the three phases of patient care: preoperative, intraoperative and postoperative.

The basic principles of ERAS preoperatively are patient education, nutritional strategies and increasingly prehabilitation exercise. Intraoperatively careful consideration and optimisation of analgesia, fluid balance and maintenance of normothermia. Postoperatively facilitating recovery strategies, such as early mobilization and appropriate thromboprophylaxis. The benefits of ERAS pathways include shorter length of stay, decreased postoperative pain and analgesia requirements, decreased complication and readmission rates, more rapid return of bowel function, and increased patient satisfaction.

The patients ERAS care emphasises key interventions throughout the patient's peri-operative journey and can be considered to promote recovery and minimise complications

ERAS protocols aim to reduce the metabolic stress response and consequently reduce medical complications [4]. The interventions can be broadly summarised as below

- Physiological and psychological preparation: education, assessment, prehabilitation and optimization
- Standards of care: antibiotic prophylaxis, thromboprophylaxis, prevention of postoperative nausea and vomiting, maintenance of normothermia
- Care to minimise the stress response: avoidance of bowel preparation, avoidance of nasogastric tubes, minimally invasive surgery, short-acting anaesthetic agents, TEA in open surgery, no drains, early removal of catheters
- Care to promote maintenance of gut function: avoidance of excessive electrolytes and fluid, minimally invasive surgery, minimising opioid analgesia and use of regional anaesthesia.
- Care to minimise the metabolic response to surgery: avoidance of pro-longed starvation, carbohydrate loading, early return to enteral feeding
- Audit: compliance and outcome

The ERAS Society (http://www.erassociety.org)

The ERAS society was formed at the turn of the century. It has produced a series of ERAS guidelines for a range of surgical specialties. It has been fundamental in raising awareness, driving change and improvement in perioperative care through ERAS.

The ERAS society provides resourceand support to individuals and institutions wanting to engage, implement and embed ERAS principles into their practice.

The mission of the ERAS Society is to develop perioperative care and to improve recovery through research, education, audit and implementation of evidence-based practice.

ERAS and Liver Surgery

There is good evidence demonstrating the negative sequalae of postoperative complications on short and long term survival for patients following liver surgery. It is important to note that in hospital mortality remains relatively resistant to the effects of ERAS [29, 48].

A decrease in complication rates is not always evident or significant in individual studies [6]. As with pancreatic surgery there is a scarcity of high-level evidence to demonstrate the effect ERAS may have on morbidity outcomes.

A meta-analysis by Hughes et al. demonstrated that enhanced recovery pathways for liver surgery were associated with a significant decrease in postoperative complications and length of hospital stay compared to standard care [49]. Overall complication rates were 25.0% (range: 11.5–46.4%) in ERAS patients, and 31.0% (range: 11.8–46.2%) in conventional care patients [49].

A systematic review by Brustia and colleagues analysed recent studies (2016–2018) including two randomised control trials. It showed a significant decrease in post-operative complications from 1–49% in the ERAS groups compared to 10–64% in the conventional care group [6]. A wider analysis of 30 studies by the same group prompted them to suggest there is a morbidity improvement in the ERAS v Conventional care group of 30 v 60% respectively. The severity of complications based on the Clavien-Dindo definition reveals that the effect of ERAS on postoperative morbidity appears weighted toward improving less severe grade I complications than the more severe grade II- IV complications [6, 21].

There is no evidence currently of mortality benefit to be gained from the implementation of ERAS [6]. Why this is the case is unclear given the apparent significant decrease in morbidity. As detailed previously however mortality following liver resection has decreased markedly over the past decades. Mortality now exists as a relatively unusual event. Mortality is not considered a primary endpoint in most studies and there is lack of scale in terms of sample sizes to allow for adequate power to detect a mortality difference between ERAS and conventional care.

The evidence demonstrates consistently across meta-analyses, randomised controlled trials and comparative case studies that ERAS results in a decreased LOS. In a recent European study by Oaevere a reduction of 2.5 days (38%) was observed. This case control study compared ERAS to conventional care. Patients were matched in terms of open and laparoscopic surgery, tumour location and extent of resection [50]. It is important to acknowledge also that despite a decreased LOS there was no effect on morbidity or readmission rates.

A meta-analysis of research conducted by the ERAS society looked at 23 papers in which patients underwent a hepatectomy within an ERAS program. In conjunction with evidence extracted from a meta-analysis, expert opinion was used to help determine the key elements considered most pertinent to delivering an ERAS pathway for liver patients [46]. This has become a standard to which many HPB centres have attempted to work to. The French group Groupe Francophone de Rehabilitation Amelioree apres Chirurgie (GRACE) have also produced guidelines that align closely to those of the ERAS society (Table 21.1).

The use of ERAS in liver surgery should be encouraged and supported to help minimise the general complications whilst recognising that the impact of ERAS on complications specific to surgery itself will be minimal if at all and that a mortality benefit is unlikely.

Table 21.1 Adaptation and summary of Key ERAS recommendations from ERAS society [46] with further recommendations in brackets from GRACE [6]

Element		Summary	Evidence level	Grade of recommendation
Pre-operative				
1	Preoperative counselling	Preoperative Patients should receive routine dedicated preoperative counselling and education before liver surgery	Moderate (*Moderate*)	Strong (*High*)
2	Perioperative nutrition	Patients at risk (weight loss [10–15% within 6 months, BMI<18.5 kg/m^2 and serum albumin<30 g/l in the absence of liver or renal dysfunction) should receive oral nutritional supplements for 7 days prior to surgery. For severely malnourished patients (>10% Weight Loss), surgery should be postponed for at least 2 weeks to improve nutritional status and allow patients to gain weight	High (*High*)	Strong (*High*)
3	Perioperative oral immunonutrition	There is limited evidence for the use of immunonutrition in liver surgery Low	Low (*Low*)	Weak (*Low*)
4	Preoperative fasting	Preoperative fasting does not need to exceed 6 h for solids and 2 h for liquids	Moderate (*Moderate*)	Strong (*High*)
5	Carbohydrate loading	Carbohydrate loading is recommended the evening before liver surgery and 2 h before induction of anaesthesia	Low (*Low*)	Weak (*Low*)
6	Oral bowel preparation	Bowel preparation is not recommended	Low (*Low*)	Weak (*Low*)
7	Pre anaesthetic medication	Long-acting anxiolytic drugs should be avoided. Short-acting medication anxiolytics may be used to perform regional analgesia prior to the induction of anaesthesia	Moderate (*No guidance*)	Strong (*No guidance*)
Intra-operative				
8	Anti-thrombotic prophylaxis	LMWH or unfragmented heparin reduces the risk of thromboembolic complications and should be started 2–12 h before surgery	Moderate (*Moderate*)	Strong (*High*)
9	Anti-thrombotic prophylaxis	Intermittent pneumatic compression stockings should be added to further decrease this risk	Low (*Low*)	Weak (*Low*)

(continued)

Table 21.1 (continued)

Element		Summary	Evidence level	Grade of recommendation
10	Perioperative steroid administration	Steroids (methylprednisolone) may be used in hepatectomy for livers with normal liver parenchyma, since it decreases liver injury and intra-operative stress, without increasing the risk of complications. Steroids should not be given in diabetic patients	Moderate (*Moderate*)	Weak (*Low*)
11	Antibiotic prophylaxis	Single dose Intravenous antibiotics should be administered before skin incision and less than 1 h before hepatectomy. Postoperative "prophylactic" antibiotics are not recommended	Moderate (*Moderate*)	Strong (*High*)
12	Skin preparation	Skin preparation with chlorhexidine 2% is superior to povidone-iodine solution	Moderate (*Moderate*)	Strong (*High*)
13	Incision	The choice of incision is at the surgeon's discretion. Mercedes-type incision should be avoided due to higher incisional hernia risk	Moderate (*Moderate*)	Strong (*High*)
14	Minimally invasive approach	LLR can be performed by hepato-biliary surgeons experienced in laparoscopic surgery, in particular left lateral sectionectomy and resections of lesions located in anterior segments	Moderate (*Moderate*)	Strong (*High*)
15	Prophylactic nasogastric tube	Increases the risk of pulmonary complications after hepatectomy. Its routine use is not indicated	High (*High*)	Strong (*High*)
16	Prophylactic abdominal drains	The available evidence is inconclusive recommendation cannot be given for or against the use of prophylactic abdominal drainage after hepatectomy	Low (*Low*)	Weak (*Low*)
17	Preventing intraoperative hypothermia	Intra-operative normothermia should be maintained for liver resection	Moderate (*Moderate*)	Strong (*High*)
18	Analgesia	Routine TEA cannot be recommended in open liver surgery for ERAS patients. Wound infusion catheter or intrathecal opiates can be good alternatives combined with multimodal analgesia	Moderate (*Moderate*)	Strong (*High*)

(continued)

Table 21.1 (continued)

Element		Summary	Evidence level	Grade of recommendation
19	Fluid management	The maintenance of low CVP (below 5 cm H_2O) with close monitoring during hepatic surgery is advocated. Balanced crystalloid preferred to saline/colloids to maintain intravascular volume and avoid hyperchloremic acidosis or renal dysfunction	Moderate (*Moderate*)	Strong (*High*)
20	Preventing post operative nausea and vomiting (PONV)	Multi modal approach. Two antiemetics advised	Moderate (*Moderate*)	Strong (*High*)
Post-operative				
21	Post-operative early oral intake	Oral intake from day one is recommended	Moderate (*Moderate*)	Strong (*High*)
22	Post-operative glycaemic control	Insulin therapy to maintain normoglycemia is recommended	Moderate (*Moderate*)	Strong (*High*)
23	Prevention of delayed gastric opening (DGE)	An omentum flap to cover the cut surface of the liver reduces the risk of DGE after left-sided hepatectomy	Moderate (*Moderate*)	Strong (*High*)
24	Early mobilisation	Early mobilization after hepatectomy should be encouraged from the morning after the operation until hospital discharge	Low (*Low*)	Weak (*Low*)
25	Preventing post-operative nausea and vomiting (PONV)	Multi modal approach. Two antiemetics advised	Moderate (*Moderate*)	Strong (*High*)
26	Audit	Maintain compliance and track progress	Moderate (*Moderate*)	Strong (*High*)

ERAS and Pancreatic Surgery

Enhanced recovery after surgery protocols for pancreatic surgery have been implemented and studied with increasing frequency over the past 20 years [51–56].

It is notable that nearly all of the pancreatic surgery ERAS studies are founded on weak levels of evidence. The majority of research undertaken are comparative case control studies or retrospective case series studies compared to historical controls.

Importantly however the vast majority of studies demonstrated decreased LOS and significantly no evidence of increased readmission rates [42, 51, 53, 54, 56, 57, 58, 59, 60, 61]. These studies have added further to the ERAS evidence base across specialties and pancreatic surgery. ERAS does not confer any negative morbidity or mortality outcomes compared to standard care.

In what is currently the only randomised control trial by Takagi et al. the effects of ERAS on patients undergoing PD is a significant reduction in post-operative morbidity. The morbidity reduction in the ERAS group compared to the control group was 32.4% versus 56.8%, respectively [42].

A recent meta-analysis by Xiong et al. analysing a total of 14 non randomised comparative studies demonstrated that ERAS results in a significant reduction in LOS, DGE and financial costs [61]. This builds on a previous meta-analysis by Coolsen and colleagues [62] and a systematic review from Kagedan et al. [63]. Thus, supporting the opinion that using an ERAS protocol in pancreatic resections may help to shorten LOS and reduce overall morbidity without affecting readmission rates or mortality.

In a bid to help standardise practice across institutions and facilitate research and evaluation of care the ERAS society in conjunction with the International Association for Surgical Metabolism (IASMEN) and the European Society for Clinical Nutrition (ESPEN) developed a pathway in 2012 [47]. The ERAS Society has published guidelines for perioperative care after pancreaticoduodenectomy making 27 evidence-based recommendations. An adapted version can be seen in Table 21.2. In a recent re-evaluation of the evidence and interventions by Xu et al [64, 65] it is reassuring to see that the recommendations from 2013 remain intact and that further evidence has been added to what existed in 2013.

Further research is required to investigate the effect of ERAS protocols on perioperative outcomes in patients undergoing pancreatic surgery. However, the evidence continues to consolidate the notion that ERAS has a significant benefit to patient and institutional outcomes. Its implementation and evolution are to be encouraged and supported.

Future Developments

The developing role of ERAS programs within HPB surgery will require its expansion to contend with pre- and postoperative adjuvant treatments. Adjuvant interventions inevitably have a health impact cumulative to that of the surgery and the disease itself affecting the immune system and physiological reserve with potential deleterious effects on morbidity and mortality.

Perioperative blood management in HPB ERAS programs requires urgent appraisal. The negative impact of untreated preoperative anaemia for patients including an increase in transfusions, readmissions, morbidity and mortality are increasingly recognised and understood [64].

The use of prehabilitation exercise regimes in preparation for surgical insult as an intervention has gained increasing traction over recent years. Prehabilitation may include preoperative physical, nutritional and psychological optimisation. Preoperative exercise therapy has the potential to reduce postoperative

Table 21.2 Adaptation and summary of Key ERAS recommendations from ERAS society for Pancreaticoduodenectomy

	Element	Summary	Evidence level	Grade of recommendation
Pre-operative				
1	Preoperative counselling	Patients should receive preoperative counselling routinely	Low	Strong
2	Perioperative biliary drainage	Preoperative endoscopic biliary drainage should not be undertaken routinely in patients with a serum bilirubin concentration <250 μmol/l	Moderate	Weak
3	Preoperative smoking	For daily smokers, 1 month of abstinence before surgery is beneficial	Low	Strong
4	Preoperative alcohol consumption	For alcohol abusers, 1 month of abstinence before surgery is beneficial and should be attempted	Moderate	Strong
5	Preoperative nutrition	Routine use of preoperative artificial nutrition is not warranted, but significantly malnourished patients should be optimized with oral supplements or enteral nutrition preoperatively	Moderate	Weak
6	Perioperative immunonutrition	The balance of evidence suggests that immunonutrition for 5–7 days perioperatively should be considered because it may reduce the rate of infectious complications in patients undergoing major open abdominal surgery	Moderate	Weak
7	Oral bowel preparation	Bowel preparation is not recommended	Moderate	Strong
8	Preoperative fasting and intake of clear fluids up to 2 h before	Intake of clear fluids up to 2 h before is recommended before elective surgery. Intake of solids should be withheld 6 h before anaesthesia	Fluid-high Solid low	Strong
9	Carbohydrate loading	Data extrapolation from studies in major surgery suggests that preoperative oral carbohydrate treatment should be given in patients without diabetes	Low	Strong
10	Preanaesthetic medication	Long-acting sedatives, and they should not be used routinely. Short-acting anxiolytics may be used for procedures such as insertion of epidural catheters	Moderate	Weak

(continued)

Table 21.2 (continued)

	Element	Summary	Evidence level	Grade of recommendation
Intra-operative				
11	Anti-thrombotic prophylaxis	LMWH reduces the risk of thromboembolic complications, and administration should be continued for 4 weeks after hospital discharge. Mechanical measures should probably be added for patients at high risk	High	Strong
12	Antimicrobial prophylaxis and skin preparation	Should be used in a single-dose manner initiated 30–60 min before skin incision. Repeated intraoperative doses may be necessary depending on the half-life of the drug and duration of procedure	High	Strong
13	Analgesia Epidural analgesia	Mid-thoracic epidurals are recommended based on data from studies on major open abdominal surgery showing superior pain relief and fewer respiratory complications compared with intravenous opioids	High-Pain Moderate-Respiratory complications Low-Overall morbidity	Weak
14	Analgesia Morphine PCA	Some evidence supports the use of PCA	Very low	Weak
15	Analgesia Intravenous lidocaine	Intravenous lidocaine analgesic methods. There is insufficient information on outcome after PD	Moderate	Weak
16	Wound catheters	Some evidence supports the use of wound catheters	Moderate	Weak
17	Transversus abdominis plane block	TAP blocks in abdominal surgery. Results are conflicting and variable, and mostly from studies on lower gastrointestinal surgery	Moderate	Weak
18	Postoperative nausea and vomiting (PONV)	Multimodal intervention during and after surgery is indicated	Low	Strong
19	Incision	The choice of incision is at the surgeon's discretion, and should be of a length sufficient for adequate exposure	Very low	Strong
20	Avoiding hypothermia	Intraoperative hypothermia should be avoided.	High	Strong
21	Postoperative glycaemic control	Hyperglycaemia should be avoided as far as possible without introducing the risk of hypoglycaemia	Low	Strong

(continued)

Table 21.2 (continued)

	Element	Summary	Evidence level	Grade of recommendation
22	Nasogastric intubation	Pre-emptive use of nasogastric tubes postoperatively does not improve outcomes, and their use is not warranted routinely	Moderate	Strong
23	Fluid balance	Euvolaemia, avoiding overload of salt and water results in improved outcomes. Balanced crystalloids should be preferred to 0.9% saline	High	Strong
24	Perianastomotic drain	Early removal of drains after 72 h may be advisable in patients at low risk (i.e., amylase content in drain\5,000 U/L) for developing a pancreatic fistula. (There is insufficient evidence to recommend routine use of drains, but their use is based only on low-level evidence)	High	Strong
25	Somatostatin analogues	Somatostatin and its analogues have no beneficial effects on outcome after PD	Moderate	Strong
26	Urinary drainage	Transurethral catheters can be removed safely on postoperative day 1 or 2 unless otherwise indicated	Moderate	Strong
Post operative				
27	Delayed gastric emptying (DGE)	There are no acknowledged strategies to avoid DGE. Artificial nutrition should be considered selectively in patients with DGE of long duration	Very low	Strong
28	Postoperative artificial nutrition	Patients should be allowed a normal diet after surgery without restrictions. They should be cautioned to begin carefully and increase intake according to tolerance over 3–4 days. Enteral tube feeding should be given only on specific indications and parenteral nutrition should not be employed routinely	Moderate	Strong
29	Early and scheduled mobilisation	Patients should be mobilized actively from the morning of the first postoperative day and encouraged to meet daily targets for mobilisation	Very low	Strong
30	Audit	Systematic improves compliance and clinical outcomes	Low	Strong

complication rates and accelerate discharge from hospital in patients undergoing cardiac and abdominal surgery [66]. Its application to HPB surgery requires further investigation.

The important issue of postoperative delirium and cognitive dysfunction is another area in which ERAS may have a role to play. The pathogenesis is multifactorial and may result from the systemic inflammatory response to surgery, pain, sleep disturbances and opioid use. Research suggests ERAS programs may lead to a reduction in elderly patients undergoing joint replacement surgery [67]. As such this area requires serious consideration particularly as the age of the HPB population continues to rise.

Areas of Controversy

The appeal of ERAS is not only the clear clinical benefits but also the associated financial benefits and its simplicity. In the beginning ERAS for colorectal surgery was focused on seven basic elements (preoperative counselling, thoracic epidural analgesia, fluid balance, early mobilisation, early oral intake and minimising drains) [1]. Subsequent iterations and adaptations for different surgical specialties has led to for example upwards of 20 elements for both Liver and Pancreatic surgery (Tables 21.1 and 21.2). The increasing layering of additional care elements upon the 7 fundamental elements may help to explain why much work remains in the endeavour to fully embed the practice of ERAS in HPB surgery.

The ERAS society amongst others has played an invaluable role in defining the evidence-based practice and practice-based evidence to enable multi-disciplinary teams to deliver ERAS both in liver and pancreatic surgery. There remains a significant gap between what knowledge and experience tell us we should be doing and what is actually done. This compliance gap is a problem that reminds us of the variation in perioperative care that revealed the inverse care rule. Within colorectal surgery Ahmed et al. noted that, in general, compliance fell during the postoperative period in most of the studies from around 100% to around 20% [68].

In a study by Veziant et al. examining the implementation of and compliance to ERAS it was noted that within colorectal surgery LOS was inversely proportional to the number of ERAS elements successfully applied [69]. In fact, to reduce LOS, adherence to >68% of the care elements was required.

In a systematic review of Liver surgery by Hughes et al. only three of the studies reviewed reported rates of compliance to the protocols and the number of care elements varied markedly [49]. Encouragingly of these, one study the randomised controlled trial by Jones et al. reported a 100% compliance with all 17 care elements of the ERAS program [70]. In a recent review of four RCTs in liver surgery considerable variation in the number of care elements was noted and compliance to care elements was not scrutinised [21].

The number of care elements used in pancreatic surgery within studies ranges dramatically. In a review by Pecorelli et al. the number of care elements ranged from 4 to 17 across seventeen trials comparing ERAS to conventional care from 2000 to 2015 [71]. Of these studies only three reported on compliance to their respective care elements.

In pancreatic surgery the evidence from RCTs is significantly lacking with only one RCT to date [42]. In the RCT ERAS group, 31 patients (84%) were compliant to all preoperative and intraoperative pathways, but only 11 patients (30%) were compliant to all postoperative pathways [42].

Such findings for Liver and Pancreatic surgery ERAS programs are consistent with evidence across other surgical specialties that demonstrates compliance reporting in ERAS studies are approximately 30% [72].

Conclusion

ERAS in HPB surgery has been shown to reduce post-operative complications, LOS and yet it has failed to consistently demonstrate reduced readmission rates or mortality. It is necessary to acknowledge that such conclusions for HPB surgery and ERAS are based on a low number of randomised and cohort investigations. There is a significant heterogeneity in ERAS programs, the number and scope of the care elements as well as the healthcare systems from which they arise (United States, China, Japan and Europe) making interpretation of results and comparison of studies problematic.

Consequently, in order to enhance clinical progress, there is a need for further scientific analysis and implementation of the essential components of ERAS in HPB surgery. This requirement applies especially to the lack of RCTs and meta-analyses and their variable LOS and compliance to the basic ERAS protocols. Currently there is insufficient evidence to enable a definitive interpretation of ERAS programs and the procedure specific role of additional specific components.

There is an urgent need to implement the current established scientific evidence for ERAS practices in HPB in order to bridge the gap between theory and practice.

Whilst RCTs are considered the gold standard for research, their application to ERAS is often impractical and difficult. Perhaps the use of consecutive large and detailed multicentre prospective cohort studies on ERAS developments are more applicable and therefore achievable. The RCT may be better placed when evaluating a single new intervention that is within an existing a fully implemented and compliant ERAS program.

Finally, there are obstacles that have always been present to improving patient care such as financial resources, communication and collaboration between individuals, teams, institutions and nations, lack of multidisciplinary team members and engagement with change that have slowed the rise of ERAS. However, such challenges are in themselves drivers for change and I anticipate that ERAS like centralisation of services previously will continue to erode the levels of mortality and morbidity our patients currently face.

References

1. Kehlet H, Wilmore DW. Evidence-based surgical care and the evolution of fast-track surgery. Ann Surg. 2008;248(2):189–98.
2. Kehlet H. Multimodal approach to control postoperative pathophysiology and rehabilitation. Br J Anaesth [Internet]. 1997;78(5):606–17. http://www.ncbi.nlm.nih.gov/pubmed/9175983.
3. Muller S, Zalunardo MP, Hubner M, Clavien PA, Demartines N. A Fast-track program reduces complications and length of hospital stay after open colonic surgery. Gastroenterology. 2009;136(3).
4. Greco M, Capretti G, Beretta L, Gemma M, Pecorelli N, Braga M. Enhanced recovery program in colorectal surgery: a meta-analysis of randomized controlled trials. World J Surg [Internet]. 2014;38(6):1531–41. http://link.springer.com/10.1007/s00268-013-2416-8.
5. Roulin D, Donadini A, Gander S, Griesser A-C, Blanc C, Hübner M, et al. Cost-effectiveness of the implementation of an enhanced recovery protocol for colorectal surgery. Br J Surg [Internet]. 2013;100(8):1108–14. http://doi.wiley.com/10.1002/bjs.9184.
6. Brustia R, Slim K, Scatton O. Enhanced recovery after liver surgery. J Visc Surg [Internet]. 2019;156(2):127–37. https://linkinghub.elsevier.com/retrieve/pii/S1878788618301528.
7. Lau CSM, Chamberlain RS. Enhanced recovery after surgery programs improve patient outcomes and recovery: a meta-analysis. World J Surg. 2017;41(4):899–913.
8. Nicholson A, Lowe MC, Parker J, Lewis SR, Alderson P, Smith AF. Systematic review and meta-analysis of enhanced recovery programmes in surgical patients. Br J Surg. 2014;101(3):172–88.
9. Greco M, Capretti G, Beretta L, Gemma M, Pecorelli N, Braga M. Enhanced recovery program in colorectal surgery: a meta-analysis of randomized controlled trials. World J Surg. 2014;38(6):1531–41.
10. Nathan H, Cameron JL, Choti MA, Schulick RD, Pawlik TM. The volume-outcomes effect in hepato-pancreato-biliary surgery: hospital versus surgeon contributions and specificity of the relationship. J Am Coll Surg. 2009;208(4):528–38.
11. De Wilde RF, Besselink MGH, Van Der Tweel I, De Hingh IHJT, Van Eijck CHJ, Dejong CHC, et al. Impact of nationwide centralization of pancreaticoduodenectomy on hospital mortality. Br J Surg. 2012;99(3):404–10.
12. Reames BN, Ghaferi AA, Birkmeyer JD, Dimick JB. Hospital volume and operative mortality in the modern era. Ann Surg [Internet]. 2014;260(2):244–51. http://www.ncbi.nlm.nih.gov/pubmed/24368634%0Ahttp://www.pubmedcentral.nih.gov/articlerender.fcgi?artid=PMC4069246.
13. Dokmak S, Ftériche FS, Borscheid R, Cauchy F, Farges O, Belghiti J. 2012 Liver resections in the 21st century: we are far from zero mortality. HPB [Internet]. 2013;15(11):908–15. https://doi.org/10.1111/hpb.12069.
14. Søreide JA, Sandvik OM, Søreide K. Improving pancreas surgery over time: performance factors related to transition of care and patient volume. Int J Surg [Internet]. 2016;32:116–22. http://dx.doi.org/10.1016/j.ijsu.2016.06.046.
15. Bilimoria KY, Talamonti MS, Wayne JD, Tomlinson JS, Stewart AK, Winchester DP, et al. Effect of hospital type and volume on lymph node evaluation for gastric and pancreatic cancer. Arch Surg. 2008;143(7):671–8.
16. Anderson O, Ni Z, Møller H, Coupland VH, Davies EA, Allum WH, et al. Hospital volume and survival in oesophagectomy and gastrectomy for cancer. Eur J Cancer. 2011;47(16):2408–14.
17. Andrianello S, Paiella S, Allegrini V, Ramera M, Pulvirenti A, Malleo G, et al. Pancreaticoduodenectomy for distal cholangiocarcinoma: Surgical results, prognostic factors, and long-term follow-up. Langenbeck's Arch Surg. 2015;400(5):623–8.

18. Merath K, Chen Q, Bagante F, Akgul O, Idrees JJ, Dillhoff M, et al. Synergistic effects of perioperative complications on 30-day mortality following hepatopancreatic surgery. J Gastrointest Surg. 2018;22(10):1715–23.
19. Fernández-Del Castillo C, Morales-Oyarvide V, McGrath D, Wargo JA, Ferrone CR, Thayer SP, et al. Evolution of the Whipple procedure at the Massachusetts General Hospital. Surgery (United States). 2012;152(3 SUPPL.).
20. Ravaioli M, Pinna AD, Francioni G, Montorsi M, Veneroni L, Grazi GL, et al. A partnership model between high- and low-volume hospitals to improve results in hepatobiliary pancreatic surgery. Ann Surg. 2014;260(5):871–7.
21. Rouxel P, Beloeil H. Enhanced recovery after hepatectomy: a systematic review. Anaesth Crit Care Pain Med [Internet]. 2019;38(1):29–34. https://doi.org/10.1016/j.accpm.2018.05.003.
22. Fortner JG, Kim DK, Maclean BJ, Barrett MK, Iwatsuki S, Turnbull AD, et al. Major hepatic resection for neoplasia: Personal experience in 108 patients. Ann Surg. 1978;188(3):363–71.
23. Edwards WH, Blumgart LH. Liver resection in malignant disease. Semin Surg Oncol. 1987;3(1):1–11.
24. Poon RT, Fan ST, Lo CM, Liu CL, Lam CM, Yuen WK, et al. Improving perioperative outcome expands the role of hepatectomy in management of benign and malignant hepatobiliary diseases: Analysis of 1222 consecutive patients from a prospective database. Ann Surg. 2004;240(4):698–710.
25. Jarnagin WR, Gonen M, Fong Y, DeMatteo RP, Ben-Porat L, Little S, et al. Improvement in perioperative outcome after hepatic resection: Analysis of 1,803 consecutive cases over the past decade. Ann Surg. 2002;236(4):397–407.
26. Melloul E, Dondéro F, Vilgrain V, Raptis DA, Paugam-Burtz C, Belghiti J. Pulmonary embolism after elective liver resection: a prospective analysis of risk factors. J Hepatol. 2012;57(6):1268–75.
27. Farges O, Goutte N, Bendersky N, Falissard B. Incidence and risks of liver resection. Ann Surg. 2012;256(5):697–705.
28. Garden OJ, Rees M, Poston GJ, Mirza D, Saunders M, Ledermann J, et al. Guidelines for resection of colorectal cancer liver metastases. Gut. 2006;55(SUPPL. 3).
29. Margonis GA, Sasaki K, Andreatos N, Nishioka Y, Sugawara T, Amini N, et al. Prognostic impact of complications after resection of early stage hepatocellular carcinoma. J Surg Oncol. 2017;115(7):791–804.
30. Whipple AO, Parsons WB, Mullins CR. Treatment of carcinoma of the ampulla of Vater. Ann Surg [Internet]. 1935;102(4):763–79. https://insights.ovid.com/crossref?an=00000658-193510000-00023.
31. Cameron JL, Riall TS, Coleman J, Belcher KA. One thousand consecutive pancreaticoduodenectomies. Ann Surg. 2006;244(1):10–5.
32. Braasch JW, Gray BN. Considerations that lower pancreatoduodenectomy mortality. Am J Surg. 1977;133(4):480–4.
33. Nakase a, Matsumoto Y, Uchida K, Honjo I. Surgical treatment of cancer of the pancreas and the periampullary region: cumulative results in 57 institutions in Japan. Ann Surg [Internet]. 1977;185(1):52–7. http://www.pubmedcentral.nih.gov/articlerender.fcgi?artid=1396263&tool=pmcentrez&rendertype=abstract.
34. Gilsdorf RB, Spanos P. Factors influencing morbidity and mortality in pancreaticoduodenectomy. Ann Surg [Internet]. 1973;177(3):332–7. https://www.ncbi.nlm.nih.gov/pmc/articles/PMC1355536/pdf/annsurg00253-0084.pdf.
35. Grace PA, Pitt HA, Tompkins RK, DenBesten L, Longmire WP. Decreased morbidity and mortality after pancreatoduodenectomy. Am J Surg. 1986;151(1):141–9.
36. Jones BA, Langer B, Taylor BR, Girotti M. Periampullary tumors: which ones should be resected? Am J Surg. 1985;149(1):46–52.

37. Del Castillo CF, Rattner DW, Warshaw AL. Standards for pancreatic resection in the 1990s. Arch Surg. 1995;130(3):295–300.
38. Trede M, Schwall G, Saeger HD. Survival after pancreatoduodenectomy. 118 consecutive resections without an operative mortality. Ann Surg [Internet]. 1990;211(4):447–58. https://www.ncbi.nlm.nih.gov/pubmed/2322039.
39. Yoshioka R, Yasunaga H, Hasegawa K, Horiguchi H, Fushimi K, Aoki T, et al. Impact of hospital volume on hospital mortality, length of stay and total costs after pancreaticoduodenectomy. Br J Surg. 2014;101(5):523–9.
40. Kimura W, Miyata H, Gotoh M, Hirai I, Kenjo A, Kitagawa Y, et al. A pancreaticoduodenectomy risk model derived from 8575 cases from a national single-race population (Japanese) using a web-based data entry system: the 30-day and in-hospital mortality rates for pancreaticoduodenectomy. Ann Surg. 2014;259(4):773–80.
41. Cameron JL, He J. Two thousand consecutive pancreaticoduodenectomies. J Am Coll Surg. 2015;220(4):530–6.
42. Takagi K, Yoshida R, Yagi T, Umeda Y, Nobuoka D, Kuise T, et al. Effect of an enhanced recovery after surgery protocol in patients undergoing pancreaticoduodenectomy: a randomized controlled trial. Clin Nutr [Internet]. 2019;38(1):174–81. https://doi.org/10.1016/j.clnu.2018.01.002.
43. Nelson G, Altman AD, Nick A, Meyer LA, Ramirez PT, Achtari C, et al. Guidelines for postoperative care in gynecologic/oncology surgery: Enhanced Recovery After Surgery (ERAS®) Society recommendations—part II. Gynecol Oncol [Internet]. 2016;140(2):323–32. https://linkinghub.elsevier.com/retrieve/pii/S0090825815302225.
44. Batchelor TJP, Rasburn NJ, Abdelnour-Berchtold E, Brunelli A, Cerfolio RJ, Gonzalez M, et al. Guidelines for enhanced recovery after lung surgery: recommendations of the Enhanced Recovery after Surgery (ERAS®) Society and the European Society of Thoracic Surgeons (ESTS). Eur J Cardio-Thoracic Surg. 2019;55(1):91–115.
45. Engelman DT, Ben Ali W, Williams JB, Perrault LP, Reddy VS, Arora RC, et al. Guidelines for perioperative care in cardiac surgery: enhanced recovery after surgery society recommendations. JAMA Surg. 2019.
46. Melloul E, Hübner M, Scott M, Snowden C, Prentis J, Dejong CHC, et al. Guidelines for perioperative care for liver surgery: Enhanced Recovery After Surgery (ERAS) society recommendations. World J Surg. 2016;40(10):2425–40.
47. Lassen K, Coolsen MME, Slim K, Carli F, De Aguilar-Nascimento JE, Schäfer M, et al. Guidelines for perioperative care for pancreaticoduodenectomy: enhanced recovery after surgery (ERAS®) society recommendations. World J Surg [Internet]. 2013;37(2):240–58. http://dx.doi.org/10.1016/j.clnu.2012.08.011.
48. Matsuda A, Matsumoto S, Seya T, Matsutani T, Kishi T, Yokoi K, et al. Does postoperative complication have a negative impact on long-term outcomes following hepatic resection for colorectal liver metastasis? A meta-analysis. Ann Surg Oncol. 2013;20(8):2485–92.
49. Hughes MJ, McNally S, Wigmore SJ. Enhanced recovery following liver surgery: a systematic review and meta-analysis. HPB [Internet]. 2014;16(8):699–706. http://dx.doi.org/10.1111/hpb.12245.
50. Ovaere S, Boscart I, Parmentier I, Steelant PJ, Gabriel T, Allewaert J, et al. The effectiveness of a clinical pathway in liver surgery: a case-control study. J Gastrointest Surg. 2018;22(4):684–94.
51. Balzano G, Zerbi A, Braga M, Rocchetti S, Beneduce AA, Di Carlo V. Fast-track recovery programme after pancreaticoduodenectomy reduces delayed gastric emptying. Br J Surg. 2008;95(11):1387–93.
52. Di Sebastiano P, Festa L, De Bonis A, Ciuffreda A, Valvano MR, Andriulli A, et al. A modified fast-track program for pancreatic surgery: a prospective single-center experience. Langenbeck's Arch Surg. 2011;396(3):345–51.
53. Abu Hilal M, Di Fabio F, Badran A, Alsaati H, Clarke H, Fecher I, et al. Implementation of enhanced recovery programme after pancreatoduodenectomy: a single-centre UK pilot study. Pancreatology [Internet]. 2013;13(1):58–62. https://linkinghub.elsevier.com/retrieve/pii/S1424390312005443.

54. Kennedy EP, Rosato EL, Sauter PK, Rosenberg LM, Doria C, Marino IR, et al. Initiation of a critical pathway for pancreaticoduodenectomy at an academic institution—the first step in multidisciplinary team building. J Am Coll Surg. 2007;204(5):917–23.
55. Berberat PO, Ingold H, Gulbinas A, Kleeff J, Müller MW, Gutt C, et al. Fast track-different implications in pancreatic surgery. J Gastrointest Surg. 2007;11(7):880–7.
56. Coolsen MME, Van Dam RM, Chigharoe A, Damink SWMO, Dejong CHC. Improving outcome after pancreaticoduodenectomy: experiences with implementing an Enhanced Recovery After Surgery (ERAS) program. Dig Surg. 2014;31(3):177–84.
57. Vanounou T, Pratt W, Fischer JE, Vollmer CM, Callery MP. Deviation-based cost modeling: a novel model to evaluate the clinical and economic impact of clinical pathways. J Am Coll Surg. 2007;204(4):570–9.
58. Kennedy EP, Grenda TR, Sauter PK, Rosato EL, Chojnacki KA, Rosato FE, et al. Implementation of a critical pathway for distal pancreatectomy at an academic institution. J Gastrointest Surg. 2009;13(5):938–44.
59. Nikfarjam M, Weinberg L, Low N, Fink MA, Muralidharan V, Houli N, et al. A fast track recovery program significantly reduces hospital length of stay following uncomplicated pancreaticoduodenectomy. J Pancreas. 2013;14(1):63–70.
60. Porter GA, Pisters PWT, Mansyur C, Bisanz A, Reyna K, Stanford P, et al. Cost and utilization impact of a clinical pathway for patients undergoing pancreaticoduodenectomy. Ann Surg Oncol. 2000;7(7):484–9.
61. Xiong J, Szatmary P, Huang W, de la Iglesia-Garcia D, Nunes QM, Xia Q, et al. Enhanced recovery after surgery program in patients undergoing pancreaticoduodenectomy. Medicine (Baltimore). 2016;95(18):e3497.
62. Coolsen MME, Van Dam RM, Van Der Wilt AA, Slim K, Lassen K, Dejong CHC. Systematic review and meta-analysis of enhanced recovery after pancreatic surgery with particular emphasis on pancreaticoduodenectomies. World J Surg. 2013;37(8):1909–18.
63. Kagedan DJ, Ahmed M, Devitt KS, Wei AC. Enhanced recovery after pancreatic surgery: a systematic review of the evidence, vol. 17, HPB. Blackwell Publishing Ltd; 2015. p. 11–6.
64. Munting KE, Klein AA. Optimisation of pre-operative anaemia in patients before elective major surgery—why, who, when and how? Anaesthesia. 2019;74:49–57.
65. Xu X, Zheng C, Zhao Y, Chen W, Huang Y (2018) Enhanced recovery after surgery for pancreaticoduodenectomy: review of current evidence and trends. Int J Surg [Internet] 50:79–86. Available from: https://doi.org/10.1016/j.ijsu.2017.10.067
66. Valkenet K, Van De Port IGL, Dronkers JJ, De Vries WR, Lindeman E, Backx FJG. The effects of preoperative exercise therapy on postoperative outcome: a systematic review. Clin Rehabil. 2011;25(2):99–111.
67. Kehlet H. Fast-track hip and knee arthroplasty. Lancet. 2013;381(9878):1600–2.
68. Ahmed J, Khan S, Lim M, Chandrasekaran TV, Macfie J. Enhanced recovery after surgery protocols—compliance and variations in practice during routine colorectal surgery. Color Dis. 2012;14(9):1045–51.
69. Veziant J, Raspado O, Entremont A, Joris J, Pereira B, Slim K. Large-scale implementation of enhanced recovery programs after surgery. A francophone experience. J Visc Surg. 2016;154(3):159–66.
70. Jones C, Kelliher L, Dickinson M, Riga A, Worthington T, Scott MJ, et al. Randomized clinical trial on enhanced recovery versus standard care following open liver resection. Br J Surg. 2013;100(8):1015–24.
71. Pecorelli N, Nobile S, Partelli S, Cardinali L, Crippa S, Balzano G, et al. Enhanced recovery pathways in pancreatic surgery: state of the art. World J Gastroenterol. 2016;22(28):6456–68.
72. Day RW, Fielder S, Calhoun J, Kehlet H, Gottumukkala V, Aloia TA. Incomplete reporting of enhanced recovery elements and its impact on achieving quality improvement. Br J Surg. 2015;102(13):1594–602.

Chapter 22
Postoperative Analgesia in Liver Resection Surgery

Nick Schofield and Marta Campbell

Introduction

Liver resection surgery has evolved considerably over the past two decades and can be carried out with relatively low mortality and morbidity. Up to 70% of the liver can be resected with a mortality of less than 5% [1].

Traditionally, surgical access is through transverse and vertical (reverse L shaped) incision in the right upper quadrant, which can be extended with a left transverse extension if greater exposure is required (Mercedes-Benz incision). It may also sometimes be possible to perform the surgery through a single upper midline vertical incision, which may result in less postoperative pain. A larger number of hepatic resections are now being performed laparoscopically or robotically, which may reduce the analgesic needs in the post-operative period. A published survey of laparoscopic liver resection shows evidence of varied perception of the intensity of postoperative pain following laparoscopic liver resection and, consequently, variety in postoperative analgesia techniques [2].

Basic Principles of Postoperative Analgesia

The cause of pain following liver resection is multi-factorial and results from the skin incision, muscle trauma, visceral dissection, capsular distension, and often referred shoulder tip pain from blood or other irritants in the peritoneal cavity. Irritation of the diaphragm is signalled by the phrenic nerve as pain in the area above the clavicle, this is because the supraclavicular nerves have the same cervical nerves origin as the phrenic nerve, C3 and C4.

N. Schofield (✉) · M. Campbell
Consultant Anaesthetist, Royal Free London NHS Foundation Trust, London, UK
e-mail: n.schofield@nhs.net

Z. Milan and C. Goonasekera (eds.), *Anesthesia for Hepatico-Pancreatic-Biliary Surgery and Transplantation*, https://doi.org/10.1007/978-3-030-51331-3_22

Postoperative analgesia for liver surgery is most effective when a multimodal approach is used [3]. Traditionally epidural analgesia and opioid based patient controlled analgesia have been the most commonly used mode of analgesia [4]. However, other techniques are gaining popularity, such as intrathecal opioids, rectus sheath and transversus abdominis plane catheters, erector spinae plane blocks and intravenous lidocaine and ketamine [4–10]. Optimal postoperative pain control is necessary for early mobilisation and improved respiratory function, and this forms part of the 'enhanced recovery' programme (ERP) [11]. Preoperative planning is tailored to the individual patient's liver function, respiratory and coagulation function, comorbidities and extent of hepatic resection.

Simple Analgesics

Paracetamol

Paracetamol is often used as an analgesic following liver resection. Due to a reduction in liver volume and function there is often a reduction of paracetamol metabolism with increased paracetamol levels, which are generally not in the toxic range, but caution should be taken with prolonged use. Therapeutic paracetamol is considered safe after major liver resection provided liver function is adequate [12].

NSAIDs

Non steroidal anti inflammatory drugs (NSAIDs) are often avoided following liver surgery due to their effects on platelet and renal function, however it may be possible to use with caution if the platelet and renal function are normal and monitored closely, and the extent of resection is not too extensive. NSAIDs inhibit platelet cyclooxygenase (COX), which prolongs the bleeding time by impairing thromboxane-dependent platelet aggregation, whilst reversible inhibition of renal prostaglandins via COX1 and COX2 inhibition, can lead to acute kidney injury [13]. Studies have shown that the extend of liver resection has a strong and independent correlation with development of coagulopathy, due to a decrease in hepatocyte count and function causing decrease in clotting factors and platelets count [14, 15].

Opioids

Opioids are commonly given as part of the analgesic strategy following liver resection. These can be given intravenously if 'nil by mouth' or orally once enteral intake has been established. The most commonly used opioids are morphine and fentanyl [13]. Side effects include sedation, respiratory depression, nausea, vomiting, constipation, itching, and worsening of hepatic encephalopathy [13].

Cirrhotic and patients undergoing extensive hepatic resections have increased bioavailability due to decreased drug metabolism in the liver resulting in drug accumulation [13]. Morphine is poorly excreted in renal failure leading to further accumulation, in the presence of post-operative acute kidney injury, which may occur after liver resection surgery. Fentanyl is less affected by renal impairment and is a better choice in patients with impaired renal function following liver resection [16]. Assessment for signs of accumulation should always be performed in patients undergoing major liver resection or in patients undergoing liver resection with a cirrhotic liver [16, 17].

Opioids such as morphine, fentanyl or oxycodone are usually given through a 'patient controlled analgesia' (PCA) pump to allow better titration of pain control [18]. Some of the downsides of PCA are that this form of analgesia can lead to poor pain relief when the patient is sleeping, and often results in poor sleep in the postoperative period. Background PCA infusion might be required during the immediate postoperative period to overcome this. In our institution some patients are given opioids as a continuous infusion in the early postoperative period, when the patient is in a higher dependency ward, where side effects can be closely monitored. In our hospital, we use intravenous fentanyl PCA prescription includes a bolus of 25 micrograms with a 5 min lockout, for 48 h, or until oral absorption has resumed. Examples from other UK centres include postoperative PCA regimens with intravenous oxycodone PCA, (50 mg/50 ml, 1 mg demand, lockout 5 min), or subcutaneous morphine PCA, (2 mg demand, 10 min lockout interval). Once the PCA is ceased, an oral opioid regime can be established on an 'as required basis', for example using Oxycodone Immediate Release IR 5–10 mg. A reduced Oxycodone IR dose should be considered in the elderly and in patients with renal impairment [19].

IV Lidocaine

As an amide local anaesthetic, lidocaine is well placed to modulate pain pathways and there is a growing body of evidence to suggest intravenous lidocaine has a role to play as an adjuvant analgesic agent in the perioperative setting [20]. It is effective in reducing post-operative pain scores, opioid consumption and postoperative nausea and vomiting, with a wide safety margin [21]. It has a well-established therapeutic role in managing chronic pain.

The exact mechanism of action remains unclear, however the proposed theories include inhibition of the nerve impulses via blockade of sodium channels, N-methyl-d-aspartate receptors and G protein-coupled receptors [22]. This results in a suppression of nerve impulses generated from injured peripheral nerve fibres and the proximal dorsal root ganglion. This latter effect reduces central hyperexcitability that leads to neuropathic pain [22].

There have been a number of systematic reviews published recently looking at the efficacy and safety of IV lidocaine [23–28]. It was shown to be useful as a potent anti-inflammatory, anti-hyperalgesic and gastrointestinal pro-peristaltic and, as such, its role in enhanced recovery in the postoperative period [19]. Systematic review showed that pain scores were significantly lower in the lidocaine group compared to the control group in the first 24 h, and opioid consumption was less in the lidocaine group in the first 48 h [9].

The pharmacological half-life of lidocaine in a healthy adult is 2 h. The concentration of free lidocaine in the plasma depends on the patient's plasma protein concentration and acid-base balance. It has a high hepatic extraction ratio and clearance is primarily limited by hepatic blood flow. Avoidance of lignocaine infusion is advised in patients with liver dysfunction affecting hepatic blood flow, including cirrhosis defined as moderate or severe [28, 29]. Lignocaine metabolites are excreted renally and caution should be taken in those patients with severe renal dysfunction with creatinine clearance <30 mL/min/1.73 m^2 (unless on renal dialysis) and in patients with cardiac failure or history of active dysrhythmias [22].

A slow IV bolus of 1–2 mg/kg (ideal body weight if BMI>30) 1% lidocaine should be administered followed immediately by a 1% lidocaine infusion running at a rate between 0.5–2 mg/kg/hour. The maximum bolus dose is 100 mg. Typically the starting rate for the infusion is 1 mg/kg/hour and the infusion is discontinued at close of surgery. This usually forms part of a multimodal analgesic regimen.

Ketamine

Ketamine is a non-opioid N-methyl-D-aspartate receptor antagonist and effective adjunct to opioids for improving postoperative analgesia following major surgery [29].

Low-dose of intravenous ketamine has been shown to improve pain management and decrease opioid requirements during major surgical procedures [30]. There is also some evidence that intraoperative ketamine inhibits early inflammatory markers (i.e. interleukin-6) during major surgery [31].

Ketamine is an analgesic that is most effective when used alongside a low-dose opioid; because, while it does have analgesic effects by itself, the doses required for adequate pain relief when it is used as the sole analgesic agent are considerably higher and far more likely to produce disorienting side effects. Using ketamine as an adjunct may reduce perioperative opioid rescue requirements, and improve postoperative analgesia following liver resection [10].

Small doses intravenously (for example 0.5 mg/kg before skin incision and at hourly interval subsequently) have been shown to reduce opioid requirements as part of a multi-modal approach [32]. Ketamine has also been added to opioid PCA in patients with chronic pain. It can also be given epidurally in small doses (e.g.: 0.2 mg/ml) as an adjunct to opioids, with some studies reporting benefit in analgesic control [10, 32].

Regional Anaesthesia

Safety

Regional anaesthesia in the form of neuraxial block (spinal or epidural) has been shown to be a safe form of analgesia for major abdominal surgery. Data from the National Audit Project of the Royal College of Anaesthetists was the largest study to date looking at complications arising following neuraxial blockade. The national audit produced a denominator of around 700,000 central neuraxial blockade procedures. Of these, 46% were spinals and 41% epidurals, and 45% were performed for obstetric indications and 44% for perioperative analgesia. The incidence of permanent injury due to Central Neuraxial Blockade (CNB) (expressed per 100,000 cases) was 'pessimistically' 4.2 (95% confidence interval 2.9–6.1) and 'optimistically' 2.0 (95% confidence interval 1.1–3.3). These are equivalent to 1 in 24,000 and 1 in 54,000, respectively. This national audit looked at all types of surgery and there is minimal safety data specific to hepatic surgery [33].

Coagulopathy

Derangements in conventional coagulation tests such as Prothrombin Time/International Normalised Ratio (PT/INR), Activated Partial Thromboplastin Time APTT and platelet count are common after hepatic resection and correlate with the extent of resection [14, 31]. This has led to problems in removing epidural catheters in the face of raised INR. However the coagulopathy of liver disease is complex, and as well as a reduction in procoagulants, there is also a reduction in anticoagulants resulting in a more balanced coagulation system, with minimal bleeding risk. Work by Mallett et al. showed a peak PT/INR on postoperative day 1 and nadir in platelet count at day 1 [31]. However despite this apparent coagulopathy, thrombin generation and coagulation measured by viscoelastic tests, was normal suggesting that bleeding risk is minimal, and epidural catheters could potentially be safely removed [31]. Indeed, until clotting factors are below 30% there are adequate levels for haemostasis and this correlated with an INR of around 2 [31].

Data suggests that preoperative cirrhosis, increased INR, low platelet count and presence of massive transfusion lead to increased risk of coagulopathy postoperatively, and a non-neuraxial strategy may be more suited in such cases [13].

Epidural Anaesthesia

Epidural anaesthesia is frequently used for postoperative analgesia for liver resections in many countries [34, 35]. The epidural space is a potential space that lies between the dura and the periosteum lining the inside of the vertebral canal. The anterior and posterior nerve roots in their dural covering pass across this potential space to unite in the intervertebral foramen and form segmental nerves [36]. Epidural analgesia, often placed at a lower thoracic level, has been shown to effectively suppress surgical stress, reduce the incidence of postoperative pneumonia and shorten postoperative ileus [37, 38].

Continuous infusion of local anaesthetic solution and other adjuncts such as opioids is achieved by leaving a flexible catheter in this space. Infusion contents vary between organisations, commonly including bupivacaine, levobupivacaine or ropivacaine, sometimes including additives, such as opioids. In our institution, we use an epidural infusion of 0.125% bupivacaine with 4mcg/ml of fentanyl. Blockage of the sympathetic plexus leads to vasodilatation of resistance and capacitance vessels, causing relative hypovolaemia, with a resultant drop in blood pressure [38]. This is exacerbated by blockade of the sympathetic nerve supply to the adrenal glands, preventing the release of catecholamines. This relative hypotension often requires treatment with intravenous fluids and/or vasopressors [37]. There is conflicting evidence but it is likely true that the use of epidural analgesia may lead to increased use of intravenous fluids and vasopressors, possibly increasing intensive care length of stay [4, 38].

Although considered to be the gold standard form of analgesia for open abdominal surgery, there is an associated failure rate, with some groups reporting up to 25% [39]. This may be: inadequate block and analgesia; increased need for vasopressors; or requirement for rescue analgesia. Often an inadequate or patchy block can be improved with repositioning the catheter or further bolus of local anaesthetic, however in some cases analgesia is inadequate and an alternative is required [40].

Thoracic epidural analgesia has been the mainstay of most multimodal analgesia packages in Enhanced Recovery Programmes (ERP) for hepatic resection surgery [5]. Due to the absence of large scale trials there is a state of clinical equipoise as to whether alternative forms of analgesia can provide better outcomes for patients undergoing liver resection.

The largest randomised trial to date is the MASTER trial, which compared epidural analgesia with PCA opioid in open abdominal surgery. There was no difference between the groups in the primary outcome of death at 30 days or major post-operative morbidity, however there was a reduction in respiratory complications in the epidural group [40]. A randomised trial comparing intrathecal diamorphine and epidural analgesia, HERALD, is currently underway and will report results of this soon [41].

Intrathecal Opioids

Due to some of the risks associated with epidural catheter removal following liver resection, a number of centres now use intrathecal opioids such as, morphine or diamorphine, as a primary source of analgesia [41]. There is some evidence that the combined use of intrathecal opioid with a PCA opioid following surgery, has fairly consistent good analgesia, although probably inferior to epidural [41]. Intrathecal morphine (ITM) and PCA has been shown to be an effective alternative to epidural analgesia and hepatic resection, and may offer advantages in the context of an enhanced recovery programme [41]. A number of studies have shown a reduction in the amount of supplementary parenteral opioid requirement, along with increased time to first opioid rescue analgesia when compared to PCA alone [41]. Some studies have also shown a reduction in intravenous fluid administration and reduction in length of hospital stay [41]. Intrathecal morphine (ITM) with PCA for hepatic resection has been shown to offer equivalent analgesia to epidural analgesia and reduce postoperative opiate consumption [42]. In colorectal surgery, when compared to epidural analgesia, ITM with PCA has been associated with improved outcomes, including decreased postoperative morbicity, reduced resource allocation and shorter length of stay (4 versus 5 days; $P < 0.001$) [42]. However to date there aren't any large prospective controlled trials showing benefit of this technique over alternative analgesic techniques.

As there is still systemic absorption with this technique, patients' are prone to the systemic side effects of opioids, and in our centre we run intravenous opioid either as an infusion or PCA alongside intrathecal opioid technique. General side effects of opioids are seen, and itching can be problematic in this group of patients [43, 44].

Due to the reduced lipid solubility of morphine compared to diamorphine or fentanyl, there is a theoretical risk of late respiratory depression with this technique. Although preservative free morphine has been used successfully in many centres, diamorphine would generally be the opioid of choice. In our centre, intrathecal opioids are either given mixed with saline or with a low dose of local anaesthetic. The diamorphine dose ranges from 300mcg to 1 mg and have been used successfully with minimal side effects.

Transversus Abdominis Plane Block and Quadratus Lumborum Blocks

Ultrasound-guided transversus abdominis plane (TAP) block has become a common analgesic method after abdominal surgery. The transversus abdominis plane is the fascial plane superficial to the transversus abdominis muscle, below external oblique and internal oblique muscles.The effectiveness of TAP blockade is highly dependent on interfascial spread, providing somatic anaesthesia to T6–L1 dermatomes (Fig. 22.1) [45].

A newer technique, quadratus lumborum block (QLB), has gained popularity, as a more consistent method at achieving both somatic and visceral analgesia for many surgeries, including liver resection. The quadratus lumborum (QL) muscle lies in the posterior abdominal wall, dorsolateral to the psoas major muscle [45]. QLB is relatively easy to perform, thanks to clear ultrasound anatomic landmarks.

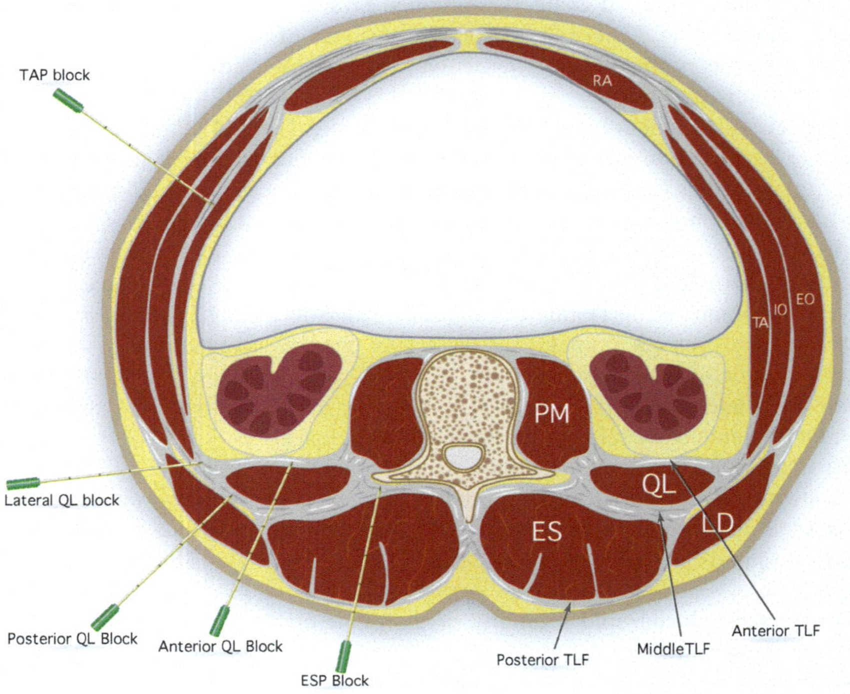

Fig. 22.1 Different regional blocks that can be used as a part of multimodal analgesia for postoperative analgesia in liver resection surgery

It has been shown to provide effective analgesia and facilitate enhanced recovery, following variety of abdominal surgeries, including liver resections, as well as orthopaedic hip surgery [45].

A recent randomised control trial found that continuous QLB (without PCA) significantly improved the pain after open liver resection, whilst shortening the time to first out-of-bed activity and flatus, promoting postoperative recovery; in comparison with IV PCA analgesia [46].

Transversus Abdominis Plane Catheter

A recent multicentre randomized controlled trial, comparing Medial Open Transversus Abdominis Plane (MOTAP) catheters and IV PCA to standard care (IV PCA alone) in patients undergoing subcostal incision for liver resection, demonstrated superior analgesia in patients receiving MOTAP catheters. Patients in the MOTAP group additionally benefited from less opioid use and shorter length of hospitalization. In the treatment group two catheters were placed following liver resection, one in the transversus abdominis plane and another in the posterior rectus space [7].

Erector Spinae Plane Blocks

Erector spinae plane (ESP) block is an interfascial plane block which has grown in popularity as an effective and safe analgesic regional technique [47]. It has wide variety of applications ranging from control of acute postoperative pain to chronic pain [47]. ESP was first described by Chin et al. CHIN [32]. Anatomical and radiological investigation in fresh cadavers indicates that its likely site of action is at the dorsal and ventral rami of the thoracic spinal nerves [48]. This block is usually performed under ultrasound guidance, and involves identifying the transverse process of a lower thoracic vertebrae. The probe is placed in a vertical alignment and the erector spinae muscles are visualised, lying underneath the trapezius muscle. A needle is placed under ultrasound visualisation, underneath the fascia of the erector spinae muscle [49]. Local anaesthetic solution can be given either as a bolus or with an indwelling cathether technique [49]. The block provides some visceral and somatic analgesia, and although this block was only first described in 2016, and the evidence of analgesic benefits are mainly from case series. A recent review found that it is commonly used as part of multimodal analgesia, and that around a third of studies showed a reduction in opioid requirements [50, 51]. There is currently little evidence in hepatic resection surgery, but it may be useful as part of a multimodal technique [47].

Rectus Sheath Catheter

More recently there has been an increased use of rectus sheath catheters for analgesia after laparotomy. The rectus sheath encloses the rectus abdominis muscles and is formed by the aponeuroses of the three flat abdominal muscles; the external oblique, internal oblique and the transversus abdominis muscles. The external oblique aponeurosis and the anterior layer of the internal oblique aponeurosis form the anterior wall of the rectus sheath. The transversus abdominis aponeurosis and the posterior layer of the internal oblique aponeurosis form the posterior wall of the sheath. The fibres of the anterior and posterior walls of the sheath interlace in the mid-line to form the linea alba [52].

The aim of this technique is to block the terminal branches of the 9th 10th, and 11th intercostal nerves which run in between the internal oblique and transversus abdominis muscles to penetrate the posterior wall of the rectus abdominis muscle and end in an anterior cutaneous branch supplying the skin of the umbilical area [52]. Local anaesthetic solution can be injected as a bolus or infused via a catheter into the rectus sheath. There is limited published evidence supporting their effectiveness in liver surgery, however there is promising results in a number of other surgical specialties [31].

Rectus sheath catheters are placed intraoperatively, prior to closure of the laparotomy wound. A Tuohy needle is placed through the layers of the anterior abdominal wall, just lateral to the midline wound, until the tip lies within the rectus sheath [53]. This depth is judged by feel and as such, it is essential for the surgeon to palpate the needle from within the abdomen. The catheter is fed through the needle into the rectus sheath. If sited correctly, it will feed in with little resistance. Once placement is achieved, the needle can be withdrawn, leaving the catheter in place [53]. Usually bilateral blocks are performed for optimal analgesia. Alternatively, the catheters can be placed by the anaesthetic team prior to surgery. Performed under ultrasonography guidance, this allows visualisation of the fascial layers of the abdominal wall and rectus sheath, enabling accurate placement of the catheters [5]. With the Tuohy needle placed, the catheters are sited in a similar fashion to that described above.

In a retrospective study published in 2013, Godden et al. demonstrated that rectus sheath catheters provide effective postoperative pain relief equivalent to epidural in open colorectal cancer surgery [6]. Complications appear to be relatively infrequent compared with epidural analgesia but include visceral injury and local anaesthetic toxicity [6].

Wound Catheter

When using the surgical wound catheter technique, local anaesthetic can be infused either as: an intermittent bolus; using a pump; or through an elastometric pump [54]. There are some safety concerns with regards to inadvertent vascular injection with the intermittent bolus technique, however strict local protocols should avoid this. The elastometric pumps show promise in delivering local anaesthetic at a constant rate in the postoperative period, and avoid the need for a patient to be attached to a pump, which can often interfere with mobilisation and enhanced recovery. An example local anaesthetic infusion regime might include 0.25% bupivacaine, delivered at a constant rate of 4 ml/hour (2 ml/hour for each catheter if a dual connector is used) for up to 72 h [54].

The use of local anesthetic infusions via an elastometric pump system placed in the musculofascial layer of the subcostal wound combined with PCA decreased total morphine consumption and improved pain at rest and after spirometry, when compared to PCA alone in patients who underwent open hepatic resection [55]. An infusion of no more than 0.25% ropivacaine or duration of infusion of less than 3 days is recommended due to increased plasma levels post hepatectomy [12]. More comparative studies are needed, however studies appear to show non-inferior results compared to epidural analgesia [10, 57].

Conclusion

There is a large number of analgesic techniques available for post-operative pain control following hepatic resection surgery, each having advantages and disadvantages over the others. A multimodal technique with good protocols and procedures, will lead to the most effective analgesia following surgery. An evidence based enhanced recovery protocol enables standardisation of practice around perioperative analgesia. Analgesia choices include thoracic epidural, intrathecal opioids, insertion of surgical wound infiltration catheters or the use of QL of ESP blocks, catering to the individual patient's clinical needs and preference. Multidisciplinary team collaboration and continuous measurement and assessment of pain quality indicators ensures delivery of best outcomes and experience to our patient cohort.

References

1. Novell R, Baker D, Goddard N, Davidson, BR. Kirk's general surgical operations. 6th ed. London: Elsevier; 2011.
2. Manu-Priya S, Cubas G, Cottam S, Gill J, Kunst G, Milan Z. Postoperative analgesia in laparoscopic liver resection: an international survey. Edorium J Anesth 2016;2:14–21.
3. Brown EN, Pavone KJ, Naranjo M. Multimodal general anesthesia: theory and practice. Anesth Analg. 2018;127:1246–58.
4. Tzimas P, Prout J, Papadopoulos G, Mallett S. Epidural anaesthesia and analgesia for liver resection. Anaesthesia. 2013;68:628–35.
5. Sakowska M, Docherty E, Linscott D, Connor S. A Change in Practice from Epidural to Intrathecal Morphine Analgesia for Hepato-Pancreato-Biliary Surgery. World J Surg. 2009;33:1802–8.
6. Godden AR, Marshall MJ, Grice AS, Daniels IR. Ultrasonography guided rectus sheath catheters versus epidural analgesia for open colorectal cancer surgery in a single centre. Ann R Coll Surg Engl. 2013;95:591–4.
7. Karanicolas P, Clarke H. Response to the comment on medial open transversus abdominis plane (MOTAP) catheters reduce opioid requirements and improve pain control following open liver resection. Ann Surg. 2019;269:e37–8.
8. Zubair T, Niraj G. Continuous erector spinae plane (ESP) analgesia in different open abdominal surgical procedures: a case series. J Anesthesia Surg. 2018, ISSN: OPEN ACCESS.
9. Marret E, Rolin M, Beaussier M, Bonnet F. Meta-analysis of intravenous lidocaine and post-operative recovery after abdominal surgery. Br J Surg. 2008;95:1331–8
10. Bell RF, Dahl JB, Moore RA, Kalso E. Perioperative ketamine for acute postoperative pain. Cochrane Database Syst Rev. 2006 CD004603. https://doi.org/10.1002/14651858.cd004603.pub2.
11. Melloul E, Hübner M, Scott M, Snowden C, Prentis J, Dejong C, et al. Guidelines for perioperative care for liver surgery: enhanced recovery after surgery (ERAS) society recommendations. World J Surg. 2016;40:2425–40.
12. Hughes M, Harrison E, Jin Y, Homer N, Wigmore S. Acetaminophen metabolism after liver resection: a prospective case–control study. Digest Liver Dis. 2015;47:1039–46.
13. Wrighton LJ, O'Bosky KR, Namm JP, Senthil M. Postoperative management after hepatic resection. J Gastroint Oncol. 2012;3:41–7.
14. Jacquenod P, Wallon G, Gazon M, Darnis B, Pradat P, Virlogeux V, et al. Incidence and risk factors of coagulation profile derangement after liver surgery. Anesth & Analg. 2018;126:1142–7.

15. Stamenkovic DM, Jankovic ZB, Toogood GJ, Lodge JP, Bellamy MC. Epidural analgesia and liver resection: postoperative coagulation disorders and epidural catheter removal. Minerva Anestesiol. 2011;77:671–9.
16. Kuip EJM, Zandvliet ML, Koolen SLW, Mathijssen RHJ, van der Rij CCD. A review of factors explaining variability in fentanyl pharmacokinetics; focus on implications for cancer patients. Br J Clin Pharmacol. 2017;83:294–313.
17. Gomes AR, Milan Z. Perioperative risk factors for acute kidney injury following liver resection surgery. Edori J Anesthesia 2019;5.
18. Yassen K, Lofty M, Miligi A, Sallam A, Hegazi EAR, Afifi M. Patient-controlled analgesia with and without transversus abdominis plane block and rectus sheath space block in cirrhotic patient undergoing liver resection. J Anaesthesiol Clin Pharmacol. 2019;35:58–64.
19. Conway BR, Fogarty DG, Nelson WE, Doherty CC. Opiate toxicity in patients with renal failure. BMJ. 2006; 332: 345–6.
20. Dunn L, Durieux M. Perioperative use of intravenous lidocaine. Anesthesiology. 2017;126:729–37.
21. Sun Y, Li T, Wang N, Yun Y, Gan TJ. Perioperative systemic lidocaine for postoperative analgesia and recovery after abdominal surgery: a meta-analysis of randomized controlled trials. Dis Colon Rectum. 2012;55:1183–94.
22. Daykin H. The efficacy and safety of intravenous lidocaine for analgesia in the older adult: a literature review. British J Pain. 2016;11:23–31.
23. Eipe N, Gupta S, Penning J. Intravenous lidocaine for acute pain: an evidence-based clinical update. BJA Educ. 2016;16:292–8.
24. Weibel S, Jokinen J, Pace N, Schnabel A, Hollmann MW, Hahnenkamp K et al. Continuous intravenous perioperative lidocaine infusion for postoperative pain and recovery in adults. Cochrane Database Syst Rev. 2015; 7:CD009642.
25. McCarthy G, Megalla S, Habib A. Impact of intravenous lidocaine infusion on post-operative analgesia and recovery from surgery; a systematic review of randomised controlled trials. Drugs. 2010;70:1149–63.
26. Weibel S, Jokinen J, Pace N, Schnabel A, Hollman MW, Hahnenkamp K, et al. Efficacy and safety of intravenous lidocaine for post-operative analgesia and recovery after surgery: a systematic review with trial sequential analysis. Br J Anaesth. 2016;116:770–8.
27. Earls B, Bellil L. Systemic lidocaine: an effective and safe modality for postoperative pain management and early recovery. Off J Anesthesia Patient Saf Found. 2019;33.
28. Benowitz N, Meister W. Clinical pharmacokinetics of lignocaine. Clin Pharmacokinet. 1978;3:177–201.
29. Loftus RW, Yeager MP, Clark JA, Brown JR, Abdu WA, Sengupta DK, et al. Intraoperative ketamine reduces perioperative opiate consumption in opiate-dependent patients with chronic back pain undergoing back surgery. Anesthesiology. 2010;113:639–46. https://doi.org/10.1097/ALN.0b013e3181e90914.
30. Dale O, Somogyi AA, Li Y, Sullivan T, Shavit Y. Does intraoperative ketamine attenuate inflammatory reactivity following surgery? A systematic review and meta-analysis. Anesth Analg. 2012;115:934–43. https://doi.org/10.1213/ANE.0b013e3182662e30.
31. Brinck ECV, Tiippana E, Heesen M, Bell RF, Straube S. Moore RA, Kontinen V. Perioperative intravenous ketamine for acute postoperative pain in adult. Cochrane Syst Rev Int Version. 2018 https://doi.org/10.1002/14651858.CD012033.pub4.
32. Sethi M, Sethi N, Jain P, Sood J. Role of epidural ketamine for postoperative analgesia after upper abdominal surgery. Indian J Anaesthesia. 2011;55:141.
33. Cook T, Mihai R, Wildsmith J. A national census of central neuraxial block in the UK: results of the snapshot phase of the third national audit project of the royal college of Anaesthetists*. Anaesthesia. 2008;63:143–6.
34. Mallett S, Sugavanam A, Krzanicki D, Patel S, Broomhead R, Davidson B, et al. Alterations in coagulation following major liver resection. Anaesthesia. 2016;71:657–8.
35. Matot I, Scheinin O, Eid A, Jurim O. Epidural anesthesia and analgesia in liver resection. Anesth Analg. 2002;95:1179–81.

36. Jonathan R, Gerbrand JG. Applied epidural anatomy. Cont Educ Anaesthesia Critic Care Pain. 2005;5:98–100.
37. Moraca RJ, Sheldon DG, Thirlby RC. The role of epidural anesthesia and analgesia in surgical practice. Ann Surg. 2003;238:663–73.
38. Sanford DE, Hawkins WG, Fields RC. Improved peri-operative outcomes with epidural analgesia in patients undergoing a pancreatectomy: a nationwide analysis. HPB (Oxford). 2015;17:551–8.
39. Motamed C, Fayezi F, Remerand F, Stephanazzi J, Laplanche A, Jayr C. An analysis of postoperative epidural analgesia failure by computed tomography epidurography. Anesth Analg. 2006;103(1026–32):1026–32.
40. Rigg JRA, Jamrozik K, Myles PS, Silbert BS, Peyton PJ, Parsons RW, et al. Epidural anaesthesia and analgesia and outcome of major surgery: a randomised trial. Lancet, April 2002; 359 (9314):1276–82.
41. Kasivisvanathan R, Abbassi-Ghadi N, Prout J, Clevenger B, Fusai GK, Mallett SV. A prospective cohort study of intrathecal versus epidural analgesia for patients undergoing hepatic resection. HPB Off J Int Hepato Pancreato Biliary Assoc. 2014;16:768–75.
42. Koea JB, Young Y, Gunn K. Fast track liver resection: the effect of a comprehensive care package and analgesia with single dose intrathecal morphine with gabapentin or continuous epidural analgesia. HPB Surgery 2009:1–8.
43. Ko JS, Choi SJ, Gwak MS, Kim GS, Ahn HJ, Kim JA, et al. Intrathecal morphine combined with intravenous patient-controlled analgesia is an effective and safe method for immediate postoperative pain control in live liver donors. Liver Transplant. 2009;15:381–9.
44. Slappendel R, Weber EW, Benraad B, Van Limbeek J, Dirksen R. Itching after intrathecal morphine. Incidence and treatment. Eur J Anaesthesiol, 2000 Oct;17(10):616–21.
45. Ultrasound-Guided Transversus Abdominis Plane and Quadratus Lumborum Blocks - NYSORA [Internet]. NYSORA. 2019 [cited 15 June 2019]. Available from: https://www.nysora.com/regional-anesthesia-for-specific-surgical-procedures/abdomen/ultrasound-guided-transversus-abdominis-plane-quadratus-lumborum-blocks/.
46. Zhu Q, Li L, Yang Z, Shen J, Zhu RF, Wen YP, Cai W, Li L. Ultrasound guided continuous Quadratus Lumborum block hastened recovery in patients undergoing open liver resection: a randomized controlled, open-label trial. BMC Anesthesiol. 2019;19:23. https://doi.org/10.1186/s12871-019-0692-z.
47. Jaiswal V, Jain K, Puri A. Erector spinae plane block: relatively new block on horizon with a wide spectrum of application—a case series. Indian J Anaesthesia. 2018;62:809.
48. Forero M, Adhikary SD, Lopez H, Tsui C, Chin KJ. The erector spinae plane block: a novel analgesic technique in thoracic neuropathic pain. Reg Anesth Pain Med. 2016;41:621–7.
49. Hamilton DL, Manickam B. Erector spinae plane block for pain relief in rib fractures. Br J Anaesth. 2017;118:474–5.
50. Tsui BCH, Fonseca A, Munshey F, McFadyen G, Caruso TJ. The erector spinae plane (ESP) block: a pooled review of 242 cases. J Clin Anesth. 2019;53:29–34.
51. Thoracic and Abdominal Wall Blocks Archives—NYSORA [Internet]. NYSORA. 2019 [cited 15 June 2019]. Available from: https://www.nysora.com/truncal-and-cutaneous-blocks/.
52. Yarwood J, Berrill A. Nerve blocks of the anterior abdominal wall. Contin Educ Anaesthesia Critical Care & Pain. 2010;10:182–6.
53. McDermott F, Wilson I, Boorman P. Surgically placed rectus sheath catheters. Updates in anaesthesia, 2010;26: 9–11.
54. Whiteman A, Hasan M. Novel techniques of local anaesthetic infiltration. *Continuing* Education in Anaesthesia Critical Care & Pain, 2011; 11:167–71. Dalmau A, Fustran N, Camprubi I, Sanzol R, Redondo S, Ramos E et al. Analgesia with continuous wound infusion of local anesthetic versus saline: Double-blind.
55. Ventham NT, Hughes M, O'Neill S, Johns N, Brady RR, Wigmore SJ. Systematic review and meta-analysis of continuous local anaesthetic wound infiltration versus epidural analgesia for postoperative pain following abdominal surgery. Br J Surg. 2013;100:1280–9.

Part IV
Pancreas

Chapter 23
Surgical Aspects of Hepato-Pancreato-Biliary Surgery

Evangelia Florou, Joe Macmillan and Andreas Prachalias

Introduction

Hepato-Pancreato-Biliary (HPB) surgery is considered today as a separate subspecialty of General Surgery requiring not only surgical but also anesthetic insight. The anatomical and functional complexity of the liver, pancreas and biliary tree require an in-depth knowledge to enable understanding and appreciation of the challenges within this surgical field. A high level of surgical skill is required in order to achieve and maintain acceptable oncologic outcomes.

This chapter summarizes the indications for surgery on the liver, pancreas and biliary tree. Focus is given to familiarizing the reader with the basics of surgical practices, emphasizing the points of anesthetic outcomes.

Liver Surgery

Much has changed since 1958 when the "finger fracture technique" was used to dissect liver parenchyma by "melting" the tissue by surgeon's fingers in order to isolate and identify the vessels [1]. Even though the anatomical infrastructure of

E. Florou (✉)
Clinical Fellow in Hepato-Pancreato-Biliary Surgery
and Liver Transplantation, King's College Hospital, London, UK
e-mail: e.florou@nhs.net

J. Macmillan
Consultant Anaesthetist, King's College Hospital, London, UK
e-mail: jmacmillan1@nhs.net

A. Prachalias
Consultant Surgeon in Hepato-Pancreato-Biliary Surgery
and Liver Transplantation, King's College Hospital, London, UK
e-mail: andreas.prachalias@nhs.net

Z. Milan and C. Goonasekera (eds.), *Anesthesia for Hepatico-Pancreatic-Biliary Surgery and Transplantation*, https://doi.org/10.1007/978-3-030-51331-3_23

the liver was studied by Couinaud in 1950s, it was only in the late 1980s that this knowledge of vascular and biliary anatomy began to truly find its application in liver surgery [1].

The introduction of ultrasonography allowed the early diagnosis of small liver masses leading to a more limited hepatectomies. Later on, the experience gained from liver transplantation and cadaveric liver splitting provided surgeons with a thorough understanding of intrahepatic liver anatomy [1].

Preoperative assessment and anesthetic practices have also contributed to improvements in results following liver surgery [2, 3]. Close monitoring and manipulation of fluid balance has helped to minimize intraoperative blood loss [2, 3]. Further technological advances provided surgical instruments specialized in liver parenchyma dissection, minimizing further intraoperative blood loss [1].

Cross-sectional imaging studies and radiological interventions allowed procedure planning, preparation and assessment of future liver remnant before major liver resections. Today liver surgery is considered safe and mortality for major hepatectomies does not exceed 5% in HPB centers [4, 5].

Indications of Liver Surgery and Outcomes

Liver resections are performed for benign or malignant pathologies, summarized in Table 23.1.

Table 23.1 Main indications for liver resection

Malignant
Primary liver cancers • Peripheral/Hilar Cholangiocarcinoma • Hepatocellular carcinoma
Gallbladder cancer
Liver Metastases from primary cancer of other organs • Colorectal cancer
• Neuroendocrine tumors of gastrointestinal (GI) tract
• Selected cases metastatic renal breast, and melanoma
Benign
Cystic liver lesions; simple liver cyst, biliary cystadenoma, hydatid cyst
Focal Nodular Hyperplasia (FNH)
Hepatocellular Adenoma (HCA)
Hepatectomy for Living Liver Donation
Trauma

Primary Liver Cancers

The most common primary malignancies are hepatocellular carcinoma (HCC) and cholangiocarcinoma (CCA). Liver resection constitutes the only treatment modality available to date which has curative intent, whilst the role of chemotherapy and other treatment modalities is gradually increasing [6].

Cholangiocarcinoma (CCA)

Cholangiocarcinoma is a malignancy arising from the epithelium of the bile ducts. CCA is an aggressive malignancy with poor survival rate often limited to a few months without liver resection [7–9]. Only 20% of patients diagnosed with CCA will be offered surgery, as the tumors are often locally advanced or have distant spread at presentation [7, 8]. Depending on the site of development of the tumor across the biliary tree, CCA is classified as [6, 9]:

- Peripheral: tumor is located in the liver parenchyma away from main right and left bile ducts, also referred to as intrahepatic cholangiocarcinoma
- Hilar: tumors arise from the main right and left bile duct and at their bifurcation, also known as Klatskin tumors
- Distal: tumors arising from the mid portion of the common bile duct extending downwards to the ampulla

Preoperative work up includes cross sectional imaging to exclude distal disease spread. Often diagnostic laparoscopy needs to be performed to exclude peritoneal disease prior to the main operation [8, 9]. The extent and type of liver resection depends on the tumor's location. A formal right or left hepatectomy may be needed for peripheral CCAs while hilar CCA is one of the main indications for extended liver resection in order to achieve a negative tumor margin and thus acceptable oncologic result [9]. Pre-operative planning for extended hepatectomy is discussed later in this chapter (see section Extended Liver Resections). The 5 year survival rate depends on tumor location, histological involvement of lymph nodes and involvement of resection margins and varies between 10–50% [7–9].

Hepatocellular Carcinoma (HCC)

Hepatocellular carcinoma is a tumor arising from the hepatocytes of the liver. This type of tumor develops on the background of chronic liver disease in 80% of the cases with or without established liver cirrhosis [10, 11]. The most commonly encountered predisposing risk factors of background liver disease are viral hepatitis, alcoholic liver disease and non-alcoholic fatty liver disease (NAFLD) [10, 11]. The available treatments to date are liver resection, trans-arterial chemoembolization (TACE), ablation and liver transplantation [12–15]. Systemic chemotherapy (sorafenib) treatment is reserved for metastatic or otherwise non-resectable tumors [16, 17].

Liver resection is the first line treatment for HCC when it develops on the background of a healthy liver or in patients with well compensated chronic liver disease (CLD) [12, 14]. The Milan criteria need also to be met; presence of one tumor<5 cm or not more than three tumors each one of them<3 cm. A multidisciplinary approach is required where resection outside Milan criteria is considered. CLD is assessed using Child-Pugh and MELD scoring systems (Table 23.2) [14, 15]. The Milan criteria are widely accepted, however, a universal staging system for HCC is lacking and treatment plans are decided by the multidisciplinary team.

The Barcelona Clinic Liver Cancer (BCLC) staging and treatment strategy has been widely accepted for the treatment of HCC. BCLC stratifies HCC patients with CLD into four categories; very early/early stage, intermediate, advanced and end stage. The very early/early stage includes patients that fall into category A or B in Child-Pugh score and meet the Milan criteria. These patients may be offered, liver resection or liver transplantation. Perioperative mortality is<3% and 5-year survival rate is 50–70% [14]. The intermediate stage includes patients that fall into category A or B in Child-Pugh score, have comorbidities and do not meet the Milan criteria. These patients are offered chemoembolization as a definitive or bridging intervention before being offered liver transplantation. This approach has been found to offer 5 year survival benefit that reaches 50% [17]. Patients in the advanced stage have significantly impaired liver function and median survival is limited to months, thus treatment plan includes chemotherapy, chemoembolization or palliative care [14, 17].

Preoperative assessment of liver function reserve is an important factor when liver resection is planned. Hepatectomy may cause decompensation of CLD and be life-threatening in patients with a Child-Pugh score B. It is also known that in the context of cirrhosis, a Child-Pugh score of A may not be a true indicator of homogenous liver function. Moreover, resection may accelerate the course of chronic liver disease more than any other treatment modality [14].

Table 23.2 Child-Pugh Scoring System

Parameter	Scoring		
	1	2	3
Total Bilirubin (μmol/L)	<34	34–50	>50
(mg/dL)	<2	2–3	>3
Serum Albumin (g/dL)	>3.5	2.8–3.5	<2.8
Prothrombin Time prolongated (sec)	<4	4–6	>6
INR (International Normalised Ratio)	<1.7	1.7–2.3	>2.3
Ascites	none	mild	moderate to severe or refractory
Encephalopathy	none	Gr I-II	Gr III-IV

Category A:5–6, B: 7–9, C>10 points
1 year survival rates 100%, 80% and 45% respectively

Metastatic Liver Disease

Liver resections form a key part of the oncological management of cancer patients. The vast majority of cases being hepatectomies for liver metastases of primary colonic cancer. Liver resection is the only treatment modality that can offer cure for patients with colorectal liver metastases (CRLM) with a 5 year survival 35–60% [18].

Liver parenchyma resection margins should be free of tumor. Histologically positive margins predispose to recurrence and affect overall survival [18, 19]. Extrahepatic metastatic disease, recurrence within the liver and disease-free time periods in between treatments (including resections and chemotherapy courses), all affect prognosis [18, 19]. In cases with oligometastatic liver disease, liver resection varies from non-anatomical liver resections to formal right or left hepatectomy [18, 19].

Cases with multiple liver metastases extending in both right and left liver lobes require a multidisciplinary approach. From an oncological point of view, tumor burden within the liver, extrahepatic disease and tumor biology are taken into account [20]. Surgical approach is considered when resection margins free of tumor can be obtained and remnant liver is of adequate volume and function [20]. Hepatic resection in this setting can happen in one or two stage procedure and often involve major extended liver resection. (See section Extended Liver Resections).

Neuroendocrine tumors of GI tract and pancreas commonly metastasize to the liver. Liver resection contributes significantly to achieving longer survival rates in this group of patients [21]. For this particular group, liver resection can be offered with the aim of "maximum debulking".

Hepatectomy for metastatic disease from other organ primaries have also been found to provide survival benefit. These are selected cases of breast, lung, renal cancer and melanoma, rarely gastric cancer, reproductive system tumors and sarcomas [22, 23].

Gallbladder Cancer (GBC)

Gallbladder cancer has a poor prognosis and tumors are usually locally advanced or metastatic at presentation [24]. Risk factors are gallstone disease, porcelain gallbladder, primary sclerosing cholangitis, gallbladder polyps and choledochal anomalies [24–26]. Usual scenarios with treatment options available are:

1. Abnormal appearance of gallbladder (GB) incidentally discovered on imaging studies performed for other reasons. Disease is expected to be in its early stages and surgery is offered
2. GBC which is incidentally discovered on histological examination after laparoscopic GB resection [26].

In both scenarios, work up includes cross-sectional imaging studies to exclude distant metastatic spread and upon negative results patients are offered surgical exploration [24, 25]. The procedure aims to clear the tumor by removal of the GB (if still present) and additional GB liver bed resection along with regional lymphadenectomy. The procedure is known as a 'radical cholecystectomy' [26]. The extent of liver resection can vary from non anatomical resection of segments IV/V to central hepatectomy [26, 27]. More extensive liver resections in the form of right hepatectomy may be required provided that negative resections margins can be obtained [26, 27]. Cystic duct margins are examined by frozen section at the time of laparotomy and if positive for tumor infiltration, the procedure is extended to include resection of the extrahepatic biliary tree [26, 27].

Presence of peritoneal disease precludes any resection and the procedure is abandoned [26].

Types of Liver Resection

Terminology of liver resections is described in Table 23.3 (Fig. 23.1a).

The Liver Resection

The standard incision used for left, right or segmental hepatectomies is the reversed L. A midline incision is also common for limited liver resections. Extension of the incision to an inverted T (Mercedes incision) may also be needed when an extended liver resection is planned [6].

The laparotomy starts with organ inspection to exclude peritoneal disease, followed by assessment of the tumor/s to confirm concordance with preoperative

Table 23.3 Terminology of Liver Resection

Type of Hepatectomy	Resection of Segments
Left lateral segmentectomy	II, III
Left hepatectomy	I, II, III, IV
Left extended hepatectomy	I, II, III, IV, V, VIII
Right hepatectomy	V, VI, VII, VIII
Right extended hepatectomy	IV, V, VI, VII, VIII (with or without I)
Central Hepatectomy	IV, V, VIII
Anterior Sectionectomy	V, VIII
Posterior Sectionectomy	VI, VII
Segmental resection	Individual segment
Non anatomical liver resection	Partial resection of one or more segments that does not follow the anatomical infrastructure

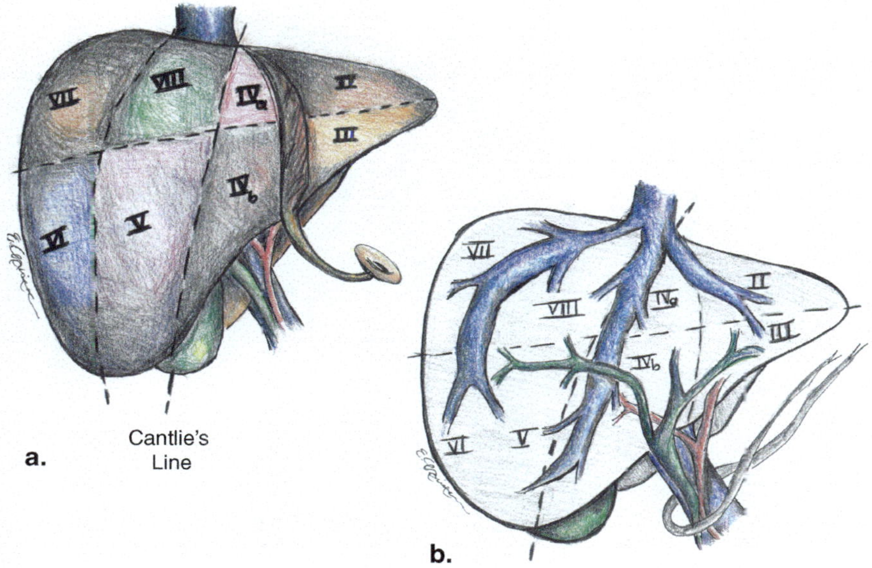

Fig. 23.1 **a** Cantlie's line marks the division of liver in right and left lobes. Arterial, portal and biliary anatomy (portal triads) follow segmental liver anatomy within the liver parenchyma defining surgical division of the liver in eight segments I-VIII. Saegment I, the caudate lobe. **b** The portal vein (PV), bile duct and hepatic artery are the structures contained in the hepatoduodenal ligament. Encirclement by tape facilitates intermittent inflow control, the "Pringle maneuver"

assessment and radiological findings. Intraoperative Ultrasound (IOUS) is used to locate and mark tumor margins as well as assess liver lesions in relation to vascular structures [28].

The liver is considered to be a blood reservoir due to its highly vascularized parenchyma. Anesthetic manipulation of fluid balance and maintenance of low central venous pressure as well as use of special instruments for dissection of liver parenchyma, liver inflow control and meticulous surgical technique, all result in minimizing intraoperative blood loss [6, 29].

Liver parenchyma dissection is performed using specific equipment. The Cavitron Ultrasonic Surgical Aspirator (CUSA) emits ultrasound waves that destroy water rich tissue (liver parenchyma) whilst sparing collagen rich structures (blood vessels, bile ducts) (Fig. 23.2) [30, 31]. A variety of other parenchymal dissectors have been proposed and used.

The 'Pringle Maneuver' is a surgical method that allows intermittent liver inflow occlusion. The hepatoduodenal ligament is surrounded by a tape which is subsequently passed through a plastic tube. The tape can be tightened or loosened causing occlusion of liver inflow by this snugging mechanism (Fig. 23.1b). The maneuver can be applied in an intermittent pattern with duration of ten to fifteen minutes on and five to ten minutes off [32–35]. The maneuver is well tolerated

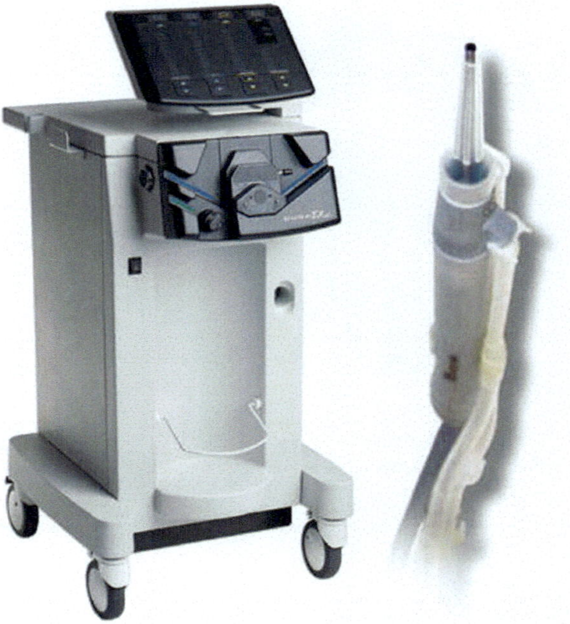

Fig. 23.2 The Cavitron Ultrasonic Surgical Aspirator (CUSA). The liver parenchyma is dissected by ultrasound waves, leaving vascular and biliary structures intact; these are sealed with metal clips or suture ligation

by normal and cirrhotic livers and has been found to reduce intraoperative blood loss, parenchyma transection times and the need for blood transfusion [33, 36, 37]. However, nowadays, it is not always a necessity during hepatectomy.

'Ischemic preconditioning' of the liver is achieved by a single Pringle maneuver prior to the commencement of liver resection. This has been found to have a beneficial effect on the ischemia-reperfusion injury that follows liver resection [34, 38].

Upon completion of parenchymal transection, meticulous hemostasis of the cut surface of the liver is performed aided by hemostatic agents and Argon beam coagulation (Fig. 23.3).

Liver surgery is constantly evolving. Anatomical and non-anatomical segmental resections as well as Right or Left hepatectomies are performed by laparoscopic approach in high volume centers [39–41]. The benefits of a laparoscopic approach are quicker postoperative recovery, shorter length of hospital stay, and less postoperative pain. The oncologic results are comparable to those achieved by the open approach with similar morbidity and mortality rates [39–41].

Extended Liver Resections

The main indications for major hepatectomies are primary liver malignancies.

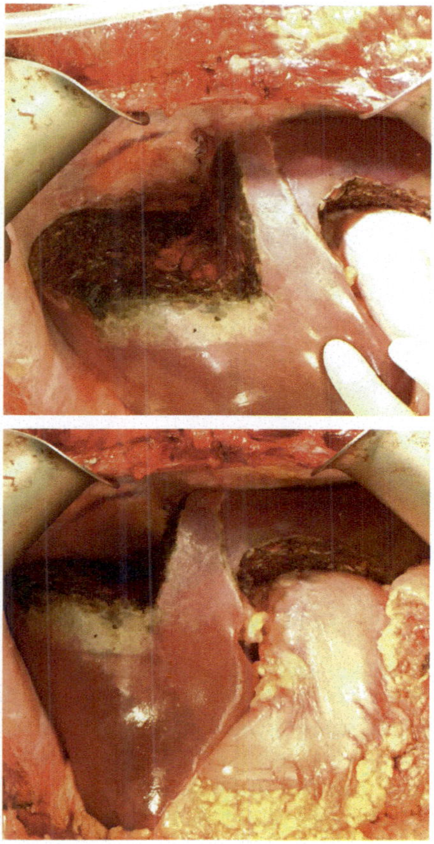

Fig. 23.3 Anatomical resection of segments III and VII/VIII of the liver for metastatic insulinoma

Extended liver resections run the risk of post hepatectomy liver failure (PHLF). The volume of remnant liver mass is a contributing factor, however, is not the only one [6, 42]. The patient's age, performance status, presence of background liver pathology e.g. steatosis, cirrhosis or chemotherapy induced liver injury as well as metabolic disorders are all recognized as risk factors for clinically evident liver failure in the postoperative setting [5, 43]. Chemotherapy induced sinusoidal injury and steatohepatitis reduce the liver's regenerative capacity and predispose to post-operative liver dysfunction [6, 43]. An interval time period of four to six weeks from the last chemotherapy session is often required to allow for parenchymal recovery prior to planned liver surgery [6].

In the setting of chronic liver disease, liver function qualitative studies need to be performed prior to hepatectomy [5]. These include portal pressure measurements, fibroscan and liver biopsy to further assess the status of the background liver parenchyma [5]. Liver function scoring systems are an integral part of the assessment of cirrhosis (MELD/Child Pugh score).

Preoperative surgical assessment is completed by imaging studies. Focus is made now on the quantitative assessment of the future liver remnant (FLR) which is estimated by computed tomography. In terms of liver volume mass, an extended right hepatectomy constitutes resection of 60–80% of standard liver volume. It is generally considered that a FLR of 20–30% in an otherwise healthy liver can safely serve the metabolic needs of an adult. In contrast, in the context of previous chemotherapy or steatosis, a FLR of more than 30% is required. In cirrhotic livers a minimum FLR of 40% of the standard liver volume should remain.

In cases of planned extended liver resections where inadequate FLR is anticipated and/or risk factors are present, one or more surgical strategies are applied to prevent PHLF. All strategies are based on portal flow modulation [44, 45]. The aim is to induce liver regeneration and thus improve functional reserve of the FLR [44, 45] (Table 23.4).

Right Portal Vein Embolisation (RPVE)
Following segmental portal vein embolization compensatory hypertrophy to the contralateral liver occurs [44, 46]. FLR volume increases on average about 25% and reaches its peak in the first 3 weeks [44]. Repeat imaging preoperatively is needed to confirm volume augmentation of FLR. Hepatic vein embolization can also be performed radiologically in cases where there is an inadequate response to RPVE [44–46], as it has been shown to increase the effect of RPVE.

Two-stage Hepatectomy
In the first procedure, the left side of the liver is cleared of disease and the right portal vein is ligated [47]. The left liver regenerates and a second procedure follows 4–6 weeks later. The regenerated FLR is assessed radiologically as adequate and free of disease and a second procedure follows in the form of extended right hepatectomy [48, 49].

Associating Liver Partition and Portal vein ligation for Staged hepatectomy (ALPPS)
Of a similar concept is the ALPPS procedure. In this procedure the right portal vein is ligated, while the right hepatic artery and right hepatic vein remain intact. The hepatic parenchyma is transected completely but left in situ [50]. The stimulus of transecting the parenchyma along with portal ligation has been found to trigger rapid regeneration of the contralateral liver. Left liver hypertrophy reaches 75% within 10 days post operatively, confirmed by repeat imaging. In the second procedure the remaining vascular structures are ligated and the diseased lobe is removed [50].

Table 23.4 Surgical strategies for Prevention of PHLF

Surgical strategies for Prevention of PHLF
1. Right Portal Vein Embolization
2. Two-Stage Hepatectomy
3. Portal ligation and in situ liver splitting (Associating Liver Partition and Portal vein ligation for Staged hepatectomy ALPPS)
4. Splenic artery ligation
5. Porto-Caval Shunt

Splenic Artery Ligation (SAL)
SAL is performed at the time of liver resection in order to prevent the 'hepatic artery buffer response' (HABR). The portal flow decreases alleviating the small in volume remnant liver from the deleterious effects of portal hyper-perfusion [51, 52].
Portocaval Shunt is a communication between the portal vein and the inferior vena cava. This is another surgical maneuver to reduce high portal flow within the remnant liver and prevent PHLF. This anastomosis is fashioned either directly using the stump of the right portal vein which is anastomosed to the IVC or by using a cadaveric or other interpositional graft to connect the two structures [53, 54].

Post Hepatectomy Liver Failure (PHLF) and Small-for-Size Syndrome (SFSS)

PHLF on a normal liver background has an incidence of 1–5% in the literature with higher rates amongst cirrhotic patients 5–15% [5]. Risk factors for postoperative liver failure are related to the patient, the liver and the surgery per se [5] (Table 23.5).

There is no consensus for the definition of PHLF. A definition for PHLF was proposed by the International Study Group of Liver Surgeries (ISGLS) in 2011; "A post-operatively acquired deterioration in the ability of the liver (in patients with normal and abnormal liver function) to maintain its synthetic, excretory and detoxifying function, characterised by increase in the INR and hyperbilirubinemia on or after post-operative day 5" [56].

Attempts at predicting PHLF are based on laboratory markers. A commonly used system suggested by Balzan et al. is the "50–50" criteria. A serum bilirubin>50umol/L and Prothrombin Time<50% of normal on day 5 post-surgery is predictive of 60-day mortality in 59% of cases [55].

Table 23.5 Risk factors for Postoperative Hepatic Failure

Risk factors for Postoperative Hepatic Failure
Patient
Age>65years old
Metabolic factors: Insulin depletion, malnutrition, sepsis
Miscellaneous; hyperbilirubinemia, renal impairment, cardiopulmonary compromise
Liver
Steatosis
Chemotherapy: duration of treatment and chemotherapeutic agent
Background liver pathology
Extent of fibrosis/cirrhosis
Surgery
Intraoperative blood loss
Vascular compromise/dissection/reconstruction
Remnant Liver Volume

Small-For-Size Syndrome (SFSS) is a term used mainly in liver transplantation. SFSS is defined as 'the dysfunction of a "small" partial liver graft during the first postoperative week after the exclusion of other causes' [58]. Dysfunction is presence of two of the following on three consecutive days; bilirubin > 100umol/L, INR > 2, encephalopathy grade 3 or 4. 'Small for size non function' is a more severe form of the syndrome that leads to re-transplantation or recipient 's death [57].

The pathophysiological mechanisms and clinical picture of SFSS observed in liver transplantation with partial grafts are similar to that of PHLF after extended liver resections. Intractable ascites is not included to the current definition of either SFSS or PHLF, though it is a very common clinical finding encountered after extended hepatectomies.

Pancreatic Surgery

Pancreatic pathologies have always represent a significant surgical challenge. The organ lies in a strategic anatomical position in the retroperitoneal space and is surrounded by major vessels (superior mesenteric artery (SMA), hepatic artery (HA), superior mesenteric vein (SMV), portal vein (PV) [41]. Surgical resection of the pancreas requires a high level of surgical skill and experience [6].

The vast majority of pancreatic procedures are indicated for suspected or proven malignant disease (Table 23.6).

Pancreatic Surgery for Tumors Located in the Head of the Pancreas

Tumors located on the right side of the PV/SMV axis are treated with pancreaticoduodenectomy. There is a close proximity and complex anatomical interface between the pancreatic head and the second part of the duodenum which involves

Table 23.6 Main indications for Pancreatic Resection

Malignant
Pancreatic cancer (adenocarcinoma, acinar cell carcinoma, squamous cell carcinoma, neuroendocrine tumors)
Ampullary adenocarcinoma
Duodenal adenocarcinoma
Distal cholangiocarcinoma
Metastatic lesions from other organ primaries; melanoma, renal cell cancer, lung cancer
Benign/Premalignant conditions
Complex cystic lesions/neoplasms that are premalignant or have malignant potential (intraductal papillary mucinous neoplasm (IPMN), mucinous cystadenoma, pseudopapillary neoplasm)
Chronic pancreatitis

the ampulla and surgical separation of the two is not feasible. Thus, the term 'pancreaticoduodenectomy' always involves resection of the duodenum, the very first part of the jejunum and the pancreatic head along with the uncinate process. The common bile duct is also incorporated into the resection Fig. 23.4a and b [6]. The aim of the procedure is to obtain negative tumor margins.

If the distal stomach is included in the resection, the procedure is called a classic Whipple's [6]. If the gastric antrum is spared and pylorus is preserved, the procedure is called pylorus preserving pancreatico-duodenectomy (PPPD) [6] (Fig. 23.4b). Restoration of the GI tract requires anastomosis with the pancreas, bile duct and stomach (Fig. 23.5a, b).

The surgical approach can be via a bilateral subcostal rooftop or midline incision. The initial assessment is to confirm the tumor's resectability and exclude peritoneal disease.

Tumors located in the head of the pancreas can involve the PV/SMV axis and vascular reconstruction is required. In high volume centers, these tumors can be resected provided that the relevant surgical experience exists. Portal vein resection is followed by primary reconstruction or by using inter-positional cadaveric vein or synthetic graft. In such cases, complete occlusion of portal inflow to the liver is required during fashioning the anastomosis [6].

Post-surgical complications are related to anastomotic leak, with the most serious being a pancreatico-jejunostomy leak [58, 60]. This anastomosis is the Achilles heel of the procedure contributing significantly to the 5% mortality rate for this procedure [58, 59].

Several risk factors have been identified such as soft pancreas, non-malignant underlying pathology and small diameter of the pancreatic duct and poor surgical technique [61]. Alternative methods of anastomosing the pancreas have been proposed e.g. with stomach, however, results did not demonstrate a benefit [58].

Distal Pancreatectomy and Splenectomy

This type of pancreatectomy and is performed when the tumor is located on the left of the PV/SMV axis [6] (Fig. 23.4a).

A limited left transverse or left subcostal incision is required. After a negative assessment for evidence of peritoneal or distant disease, the distal part of the pancreas and the spleen are both mobilised from the retroperitoneal space. The splenic artery and vein are ligated and divided and the specimen is removed completing the resection. The pancreatic stump is assessed for any leak and occasionally it is oversewn.

Depending on the underlying pathology, a spleen preserving distal pancreatectomy is also feasible.

Postoperative complications include pancreatic leak from the remnant pancreas that can be self-limiting or lead to development of pancreatic fistula [6].

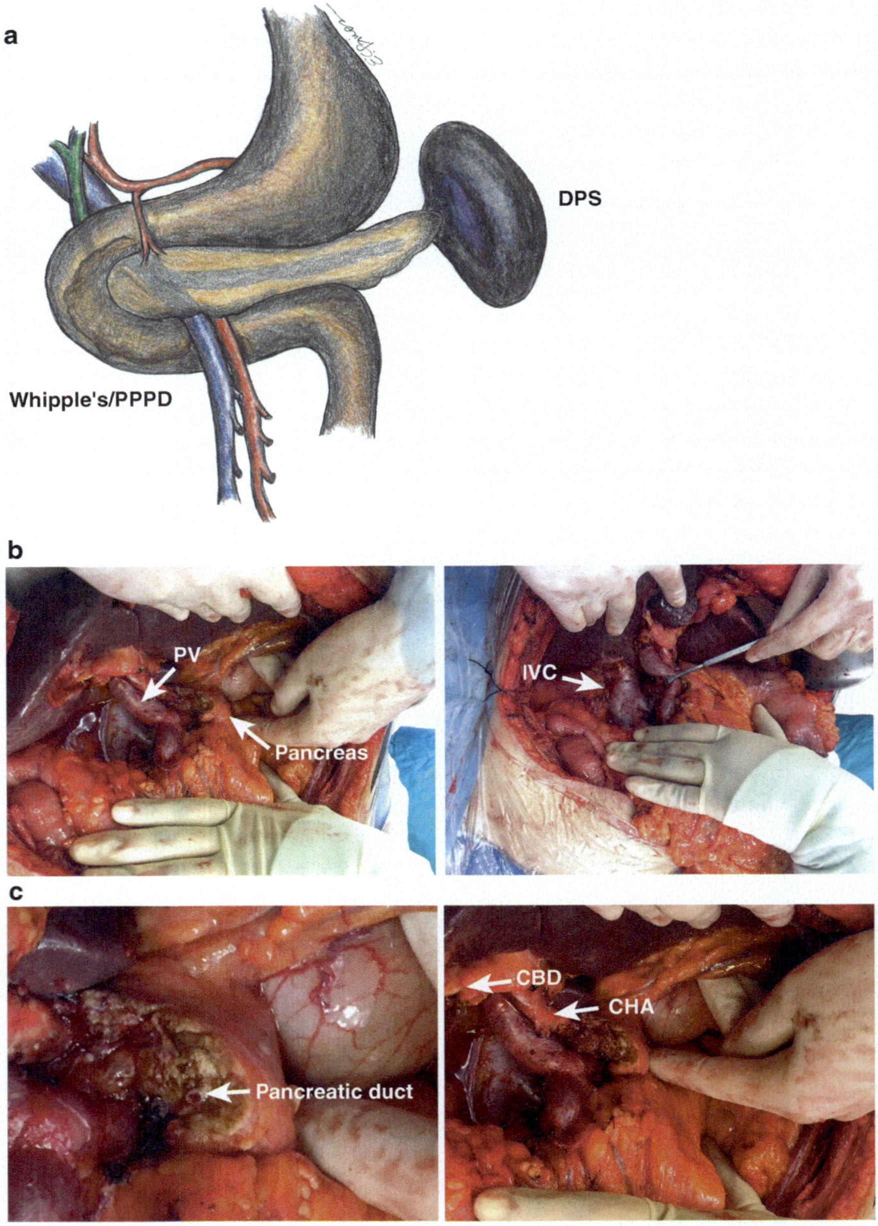

Fig. 23.4 **a**. Anatomy of the pancreas. The extent of pancreatic resection is defined by the location of the tumor in relationship to PV/SMV axis. The figure demonstrates the extent of both Pancreaticoduodenectomy (Whipple's and PPPD) and Distal pancreatectomy and Splenectomy (DPS) procedures. **b**. Right; Pancreaticoduodenectomy completed. Left; Specimen has been removed. PV/SMV axis retracted with vein retractor. IVC and left renal vein lying underneath. **c**. Pancreatic stump; pancreatic duct

Total Pancreatectomy

A total pancreatectomy is indicated for benign or malignant conditions. Tumors of the pancreatic head can extend from the head to the body of the gland. After pancreaticoduodenectomy for a head of pancreas tumor, a positive tumor margin at the pancreatic stump obtained intraoperatively is an indication for total pancreatectomy [6]. The anesthetic management should consider the need for diabetic control. The GI reconstruction phase includes only two anastomoses, the bile duct with the jejunum and the jejunum with the stomach.

Biliary Surgery

Gallbladder Resection

Resection of the gallbladder (GB) is the commonest procedure of the biliary tree. Indications for GB resection are calculi, cholecystitis and its complications, polyps that measure more than 1 cm and porcelain GB [6].

The procedure is usually performed laparoscopically and the open approach is reserved for complex cases or when complications are present. Complications following laparoscopic GB resection can be severe. Injury of the bile duct or of the vascular structures in liver hilum can have potentially fatal outcomes. HPB centers should be involved in the care of patients with complications following laparoscopic GB resection [62, 63].

The most common injury is an incomplete or complete bile duct division. This requires surgical intervention on a semi urgent basis depending on the patient' s clinical condition [64, 65].

The clinical picture of the patient with bile duct injury is variable; vague abdominal pain and mild derangement of liver function tests or severe sepsis and biliary peritonitis [64, 65]. Surgery involves resection of extrahepatic biliary tree and reconstruction of GI tract with hepatico-jejunostomy via Roux loop.

Extrahepatic biliary tree

Choledochal anomalies or choledochal cysts are hereditary anatomical dilatations of the biliary tree. Classification is made depending on the level of the biliary tree involvement. Surgical intervention is required to avoid complications e.g. lithiasis, pancreatitis, malignant transformation of the biliary epithelium within the cyst [6, 66, 67]. Surgery involves resection of the extrahepatic biliary tree and reconstruction with hepaticojejunostomy. Very rarely pancreaticoduodenectomy is indicated [6].

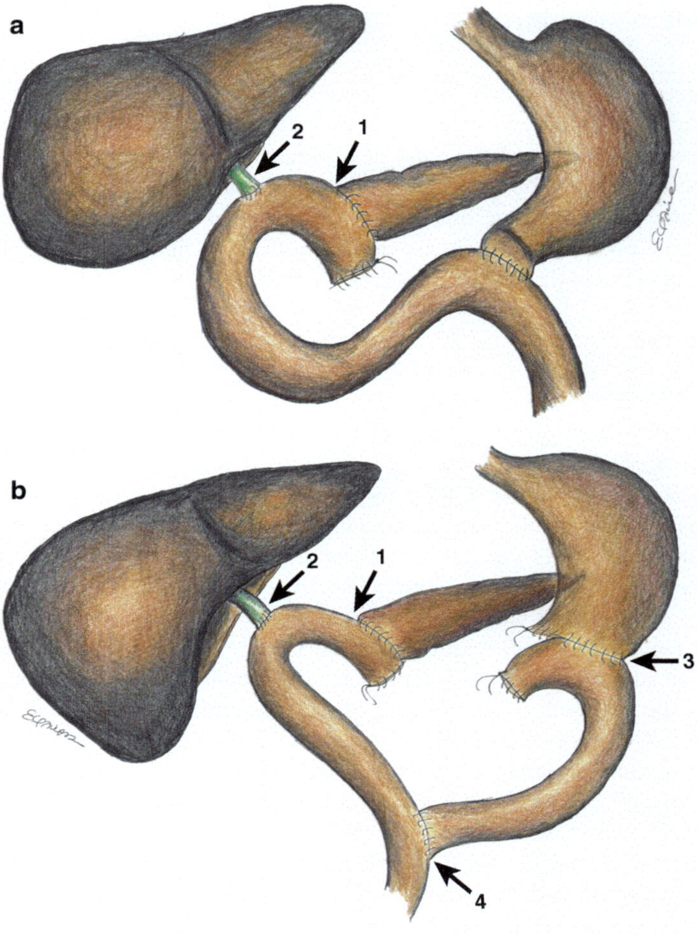

Fig. 23.5 **a.** Pylorus Preserving Pancreatico-Duodenectomy (PPPD). GI tract reconstruction on a 'C shape' configuration. The first anastomosis is the pancreatico-jejunostomy (1), followed by the hepatico-jejunostomy (2) and finally the gastro-jejunostomy (3). **b.** Whipple' s procedure. GI tract restoration can be fashioned in various ways. The example given here is GI reconstruction via Roux en Y. Jejunojejunostomy (4)

References

1. Bismuth H, Eshkenazy R, Arish A. Milestones in the evolution of hepatic surgery. Rambam Maimonides Med J. 2011;2:e0021.
2. Gasteiger L, Eschertzhuber S, Tiefenthaler W. Perioperative management of liver surgery—review on pathophysiology of liver disease and liver failure. Eur Surg. 2018;50:81–6.
3. Wang CH, Chang KA, Chen CL, et al. anesthesia management and fluid therapy in right and left lobe living donor hepatectomy. Trans Proc. 2018;50:2654–6.

4. Zheng Y, Yang H, He L, et al. Reassessment of different criteria for diagnosing post-hepatectomy liver failure: a single-center study of 1683 hepatectomy. Oncotarget. 2017;8:89269–77.
5. Ray S, Mehta NN, Golhar A, Nundy S. Post hepatectomy liver failure—a comprehensive review of current concepts and controversies. Ann Med Surg. 2018;34:4–10.
6. William R. Blumgart's Surgery of the liver, biliary tract and pancreas. 5th Edition, Elsevier Medical Books; 2012.
7. Guglielmi A, Ruzzenente A, Campagnaro T, et al. Intrahepatic cholangiocarcinoma: prognostic factors after surgical resection. World J Surg. 2009;33:1247–54.
8. Wang Y, Li J, Xia Y, Gong R, et al. Prognostic nomogram for intrahepatic cholangiocarcinoma after partial hepatectomy. J Clin Oncol. 2013;31:1188–95.
9. Ito F, Cl. Cho CS, Rikkers LF, Weber SM. Hilar Cholangiocarcinoma: current management. Ann Surg 2009;250: 210–8.
10. Calvet X, et al. Prognostic factors of hepatocellular carcinoma in the west: a multivariate analysis in 206 patients. Hepatology. 1990;12:753–60.
11. Balogh J, David Victor D, Asham EH, et al. Hepatocellular carcinoma: a review. J Hepatocell Carcinoma. 2016;3:41–5.
12. Bruix J, Sherman M, Llovet JM, Beaugrand M, Lencioni R, Burroughs AK et al. Clinical management of hepatocellular carcinoma: conclusions of the Barcelona-2000 EASL conference. European Association for the Study of the Liver. J Hepatol 2001; 35:421–30.
13. Llovet JM, Brú C, Bruix J. Prognosis of hepatocellular carcinoma: the BCLC staging classification. Semin Liver Dis. 1999;19:329–38.
14. Llovet JM, Schwartz M, Mazzaferro V. Resection and liver transplantation for hepatocellular carcinoma. Semin Liver Dis. 2005;25:181–200.
15. Llovet JM, Bruix J. Systematic review of randomized trials for unresectable hepatocellular carcinoma: chemoembolization improves survival. Hepatology. 2003;37:429–42.
16. Keating GM, Santoro A. Sorafenib: a review of its use in advanced hepatocellular carcinoma. Drugs. 2009;69:223–40.
17. Forner A, Reig ME, de Lope CR, Bruix J. Current strategy for staging and treatment: the BCLC update and future prospects Semin Liver Dis. 2010;30:61–74.
18. House MG, Ito H, Gönen M, Fong Y, Allen PJ, DeMatteo RP, et al. Survival after hepatic resection for metastatic colorectal cancer: trends in outcomes for 1,600 patients during two decades at a single institution. J Am Coll Surg. 2010;210:752–5.
19. Tomlinson JS, Jarnagin WR, De Matteo RP, et al. Actual10-year survival after resection of colorectal liver metastases defines cure. J Clin Oncol. 2007;25:4575–80.
20. Chow FC, Chok KS. Colorectal liver metastases: an update on multidisciplinary approach. World J Hepatol. 2019;11:150–72.
21. Pavel M, O'Toole D, Costa F, Capdevila J, Gross D, Kianmanesh R, et al. ENETS consensus guidelines update for the management of distant metastatic disease of intestinal, pancreatic, bronchial neuroendocrine neoplasms (NEN) and NEN of unknown primary site. Neuroendocrinology. 2016;103:172–8.
22. Adam R, Chiche L, Aloia T, Elias D, et al. Hepatic resection for noncolorectal nonendocrine liver metastases: analysis of 1,452 patients and development of a prognostic model. Ann Surg. 2006;244:524–35.
23. Adam R, Aloia T, Krissat J, Bralet MP, Paule B, Giacchetti S, et al. Is liver resection justified for patients with hepatic metastases from breast cancer? Ann Surg. 2006;244:897–907.
24. Reid KM, De la Medina AR, Donohue JH. Diagnosis and surgical management of gallbladder cancer: a review. J Gastrointest Surg. 2007;11:671–81.
25. Krell RW, Wei AC. Gallbladder cancer: surgical management. Chin Clin Oncol 2019;8:36. www.nccn.org/professionals/physician_gls/default.aspx. Accessed on 4th December 2019.
26. Zaidi MY, Abou-Alfa GK, Ethun CG, Shrikhande SV, et al. Evaluation and management of incidental gallbladder cancer. Chin Clin Oncol. 2019;8:37.

27. D'Angelica M, Dalal KM, Dematteo RP, et al. Analysis of extent of resection for adenocarcinoma of gallbladder. Ann Surg Oncol. 2009;16:806–16.
28. Yahya AI. Use of intraoperative ultrasound (IOUS) in liver surgery. Intech Open. May 2019. http://org.doi.10.5772/intechopen.81175.
29. Bhattacharya S, Jackson DJ, Beard CI, Davidson BR. Central venous pressure and its effects on blood loss during liver resection. Br J Surg. 1999;86:282–3.
30. Fasulo F, Giori A, Fissi S, Bozzetti F, Doci R, Gennari L. Cavitron ultrasonic surgical aspirator (CUSA) in liver resection. Int Surg. 1992;77:64–6.
31. Bodzin AS, Leiby BE, Ramirez CB, Frank AM, Doria C. Liver resection using cavitron ultrasonic surgical aspirator (CUSA) versus harmonic scalpel: a retrospective cohort study. Int J Surg. 2014;12:500–3.
32. Pringle JHV. Notes on the arrest of hepatic hemorrhage due to trauma. Ann Surg. 1980;48:541–9.
33. Chouker A, Schachtner T, Schauer R, Dugas M, Lohe F, Martignoni A, et al. Effects of Pringle manoeuvre and ischaemic preconditioning on haemodynamic stability in patients undergoing elective hepatectomy: a randomized trial. Br J Anaesth. 2004;93:204–11.
34. Clavien PA, Yadav S, Sindram D, Bentley RC. Protective effects of ischemic preconditioning for liver resection performed under inflow occlusion in humans. Ann Surg. 2000;232:155–62.
35. Horiuchi T, Muraoka R, Tabo T, et al. Optimal cycles of hepatic ischemia and reperfusion pedicle clamping during liver surgery. Arch Surg. 1995;130:754–8.
36. Man K, Fan ST, Ng I et al. Prospective evaluation of Pringle manoeuvre in hepatectomy for liver tumours by a randomised trial. Annals of Surg 226;6: 704–13.
37. Sugiyama Y, Ishizaki Y, Imamura H, Sugo H, Yoshimoto J, Kawasaki S. Effects of intermittent Pringle's manoeuvre on cirrhotic compared with normal liver. Br J Surg. 2010;97:1062–9.
38. Maurer CA, Walensi M, Käser SA, et al. Liver resections can be performed safely without Pringle maneuver: a prospective study. World J Hepatol. 2016;8:1038–46.
39. Jia C, Li H, Wen N, Chen J, Wei Y, Li B. Laparoscopic liver resection: a review of current indications and surgical techniques. Hepatobiliary Surg Nutr. 2018;7:277–88.
40. Nguyen KT, Gamblin TC, Geller DA. World review of laparoscopic liver resection—2,804 patients. Ann Surg. 2009;250:831–41.
41. Cai X. Laparoscopic liver resection: the current status and the future. Hepatobiliary Surg Nutr. 2018;7:98–104.
42. Schindl MJ, Redhead DN, Fearon KC, et al. The value of residual liver volume as a predictor of hepatic dysfunction and infection after major liver resection. Gut. 2005;54:289–96.
43. Grice PT, Isherwood J, Arshad A, Issa E, Garcea G, Dennison AR. Liver failure after major hepatic resection, a persistent clinical conundrum. J Hepato Gastroenterol. 2018;2:19–26.
44. Hung ML, McWilliams JP. Portal vein embolization prior to hepatectomy: techniques, outcomes and novel therapeutic approaches. Gastrointestinal Int. 2018;7:2–8.
45. Azoulay D, Castaing D, Krissat J, Smail A, Hargreaves GM, Lemoine A, et al. Percutaneous portal vein embolization increases the feasibility and safety of major liver resection for hepatocellular carcinoma in injured liver. Ann Surg. 2000;232:665–72.
46. Kahn D, Kajani M, Zeng Q, Lai HS, et al. Effect of partial portal vein ligation on hepatic regeneration. J Invest Surg. 1988;1:267–76.
47. Homayounfar K, Liersch T, Schuetze G, Niessner M, Goralczyk A, Meller J, et al. Two-stage hepatectomy (R0) with portal vein ligation—towards curing patients with extended bilobular colorectal liver metastases. Int J Colorectal Dis. 2009;24:409–18.
48. Aussilhou B, Lesurtel M, Sauvanet A, Farges O, Dokmak S, Goasguen N, et al. Right portal vein ligation is as efficient as portal vein embolization to induce hypertrophy of the left liver remnant. J Gastrointest Surg. 2008;12:297–303.
49. Adam R, Laurent A, Azoulay D, et al. Two-stage hepatectomy: a planned strategy to treat irresectable liver tumors. Ann Surg. 2000;232:777–85.

50. Schnitzbauer AA, Lang SA, Goessmann H, Nadalin S, Baumgart J, Farkas SA, et al. Right portal vein ligation combined with in situ splitting induces rapid left lateral liver lobe hypertrophy enabling 2-staged extended right hepatic resection in small-for-size settings. Ann Surg. 2012;255:405–14.
51. Carrapita J, Abrantes AM, Campelos S, Goncalves AC, Cardoso D, et al. Impact of splenic artery ligation after major hepatectomy on liver function, regeneration and viability. Sci Rep. 2016;6:34731.
52. Lo CM, Liu CL, Fan ST. Portal hyperperfusion injury as the cause of primary nonfunction in a small-for-size liver graft-successful treatment with splenic artery ligation. Liver Transpl. 2003;9:626–8.
53. Troisis R, Riccaiardi S, Smeets P, Petrovic M, Van Maele G, Colle I, et al. Effects of hemi-portocaval shunts for inflow modulation on the outcome of small-for-size grafts in living donor liver transplantation. Am J Transplant. 2005;5:1397–404.
54. Troisi R, Cammu G, Militerno G, et al. Modulation of portal graft inflow: a necessity in adult living-donor liver transplantation? Ann Surg. 2003;237:429–36.
55. Balzan S, Belghiti J, Farges O et al. The "50–50 Criteria" on postoperative day 5. an accurate predictor of liver failure and death after hepatectomy. Ann Surg 2005; 242: 824–9.
56. Rahbari NN, Garden OJ, Padbury R, Brooke-Smith M, et al. Post hepatectomy liver failure: a definition and grading by the international study group of liver surgery (ISGLS). Surgery. 2011;149:713–24.
57. Dahm F, Georgiev P, Clavien PA. Small-for-size syndrome after partial liver transplantation: definition, mechanisms of disease and clinical implications. Am J Trans. 2005;11:2605–10.
58. He T, Zhao Y, Chen Q, Wang X, Lin H, Han W. Pancreaticojejunostomy versus Pancreaticogastrostomy after pancreaticoduodenectomy: a systematic review and meta-analysis. Dig Surg. 2013;30:56–69.
59. Trede M, Schwall G. Complications of pancreatectomy. Ann Surg. 1988;207:39–47.
60. Cullen JJ, Sarr MG, Ilstrup DM. Pancreatic anastomotic leak after pancreaticoduodenectomy: incidence, significance, and management. Am J Surg. 1994;168:295–8.
61. Nahm CB, Connor SJ, Sarma JS, Mittal A. Postoperative pancreatic fistula: a review of traditional and emerging concepts. Clin Exp Gastroenterol. 2018;11:105–18.
62. Strasberg SM, Helton WS. An analytical review of vasculobiliary injury in laparoscopic and open cholecystectomy. HPB (Oxford). 2011;13:1–14.
63. Pulitano C, Parks RW, Ireland H, Wigmore SJ, Garden OJ. Impact of concomitant arterial injury on the outcome of laparoscopic bile duct injury. Am J Surg. 2011;201:238–44.
64. Clavien PA, Sanabria JR, Strasberg SM. Proposed classification of complications of surgery with examples of utility in cholecystectomy. Surgery. 1992;111:518–26.
65. Lau WY, Lai EC, Lau SH. Management of bile duct injury after laparoscopic cholecystectomy: a review. ANZ J Surg. 2010;80:75–81.
66. Ando H, Ito T, Kaneko K, Seo T. Congenital stenoses of the intrahepatic bile ducts associated with choledochal cysts. J Am Coll Surg. 1995;181:426–30.
67. Ando H, Keneko K, Ito T, Watanabe Y, Seo T, Harade T, et al. Complete excision of the intrapancreatic portion of choledochal cysts. J Am Coll Surg. 1996;183:317–21

Chapter 24
Perioperative Anaesthetic Considerations for the Whipple Procedure and Other Pancreatic Surgeries

K. Lankester and T. Hughes

Pancreatic Surgery

Introduction

Pancreatic surgery is high risk with significant levels of perioperative mortality and morbidity. Generally, patients presenting for surgery have a malignancy or pancreatitis, both are debilitating and deconditioning diseases with intrinsically high mortality. Furthermore, surgical resections or debridement are a complex undertaking on a friable and enzyme rich tissue. Resulting in surgery more prone to complications and causing significant postoperative morbidity.

Approximately 90% of exocrine pancreatic cancer is diagnosed as adenocarcinoma [1] and the majority of pancreatic surgery involves resection to remove tumours. Due to late presentation only 15–20% of patients have disease which is resectable at presentation [2] and the large majority do not survive, 5-year survival remains at 5% [3]. Patient selection for surgery can be difficult and should involve a multidisciplinary team (MDT) approach encompassing technical feasibility of intervention, functional status and patient views and expectations.

The anaesthetist has an important role over the perioperative period as part of the MDT in patient selection, preoperative assessment and optimisation, careful intraoperative management and within the initial postoperative period. They are also best placed to develop enhanced recovery pathways and guidelines to optimise outcomes for a high risk patient group.

K. Lankester · T. Hughes (✉)
Anaesthetic Department, King's College Hospital, London, UK
e-mail: t.hughes1@nhs.net

Z. Milan and C. Goonasekera (eds.), *Anesthesia for Hepatico-Pancreatic-Biliary Surgery and Transplantation*, https://doi.org/10.1007/978-3-030-51331-3_24

Anatomy and Physiology

The pancreas is divided into head, neck, body and tail anatomically. It is a secretory organ with both endocrine and exocrine functions and the parenchyma of the gland is made up of acinar cells. Arterial supply is from branches of celiac and superior mesenteric arteries and venous drainage following the arteries to the portal vein. Sympathetic nervous supply is from the splanchnic nerves and parasympathetic fibres are received from the vagus nerve.

90% of pancreas gland is formed of exocrine acinar cells secreting digestive proteolytic enzymes into a tubular system which eventually forms the main pancreatic duct. 2000 mL of enzymes in alkaline fluid are produced per day; it is regulated by the neuroendocrine system and modulated by endocrine pancreas to breakdown nutrients ready for absorption.

The endocrine cells form the Islets of Langerhans, the functional units of the endocrine pancreas. Adult pancreas has around one million islets, accounting for 1–2% of the gland and distributed evenly throughout. Islets consist of B (β) cells secreting insulin, A (α) cells secreting glucagon, D (δ) cells and F cells secreting pancreatic polypeptide (PP). The vital role of islets of Langerhans is glucose haemostasis.

Pancreatic Conditions Requiring Surgery

Broadly, indications for elective pancreatic surgery can be classified into management of neoplasms and pancreatitis. Rarely, emergency surgery involving the pancreas is performed for a variety of indications, most commonly abdominal trauma.

The majority of neoplasms (approximately 95%) involve adenocarcinoma of the head, tail or whole pancreas. Occasionally the primary disease is of the pancreatic duct and this is called intraductal pancreatic medullary neoplasia (IPMN). Around 3–5% of neoplasms involve a diverse group of neuroendocrine tumours (NETs) that arise from the GI tract and may spread to pancreas, liver or other adjacent organs. Surgical management involves resection, most often by pancreaticoduodenectomy (PD) also known as the Whipple procedure.

Surgery is indicated in acute pancreatitis for the management of symptomatic pseudocyst and infected necrosis. With chronic pancreatitis surgical resection is used where less invasive pain control methods have failed and for the management of ductal obstruction from stenosis or pseudocyst formation. Abdominal trauma occasionally involves the pancreas and may require surgical resection as part of damage control or function restoring surgery.

Neoplasms

Adenocarcinoma

Epidemiology

Pancreatic adenocarcinoma inflicts a significant healthcare burden with 8000 new cases reported in the UK and 57,000 new cases in USA each year [4]. It is aggressive and lethal ranking as the 7th most common cause of cancer death, despite being only the 13th most common cancer overall [3]. This is often due to symptoms appearing once the disease has advanced beyond curative intervention.

Clinical Features

Tumours often present with nonspecific abdominal pain and/or jaundice. Courvoisier's sign described as a palpable gallbladder in the presence of painless jaundice occurs in less than 25% of patients [5]. Unexplained weight loss, steatorrhoea and gastric outlet obstruction due to tumour compressing the duodenum or stomach may result in nausea and satiety.

Risk factors for developing pancreatic cancer include age, smoking, alcohol, raised BMI, diabetes mellitus, chronic pancreatitis and family history. It is also associated with familial cancer syndromes, inflammatory bowel disease, peptic ulcer and periodontal disease.

Full blood count may reveal normochromic anaemia or thrombocytosis or both. Patients presenting with obstructive jaundice have significant elevations in serum bilirubin (conjugated and total), alkaline phosphatase and G-glutamyl transferase. The tumour marker CA19–9 has a sensitivity of 80% and specificity of 73% for pancreatic cancer [6]. Imaging is the most important diagnostic tool in the detection of pancreatic tumours. Ultrasound, CT scans and endoscopic ultrasound (EUS) are used in the diagnosis and prognostication of PC. Positron emission tomography (PET) scanning can image primary tumours and also detect metastatic disease and is increasingly used in the context of staging of the condition. Staging laparoscopy is reserved for those cases with a large primary tumour or initial CA19–9 > 100units/ml, these patients have a higher chance of radiologically occult metastasises [7].

Management

Where surgery is not deemed feasible of appropriate palliative measures include: systemic chemotherapy, chemo-radiotherapy, surgical bypass, ablative therapies, gastrointestinal and biliary stenting. Biliary stenting is sometimes performed preoperatively in patients with jaundice.

Surgical resection is the only treatment with curative potential for pancreatic adenocarcinoma, but it is high risk surgery with prolonged recovery and high morbidity. Median survival after surgery is 11–23 months and 5-year survival is 10–15% [8–10]. Therefore, accurate prognostication with MDT decision making is required for appropriate patient selection. The most important post resection prognostic factor is tumour stage and nodal involvement. Five-year survival with resected node-negative disease is 30% compared with 10% if one or more nodes are positive [11]. Other important factors include tumour differentiation, lymphatic invasion, pre and post-operative CA19–9 levels. Smoking history, functional and nutritional status of the patient are also important determinants of patient survival.

Disease limited to pancreas or with limited node involvement has the highest chance of cure. Pancreatic tumours involving the major blood vessels have increased perioperative risk and evaluation of such patients requires recognition of anatomical variability with extensive pre-operative planning and counselling. Evidence of any metastases or tumour invading aorta, vena cava or coeliac axis are contraindications to surgery.

There maybe a role for neoadjuvant chemotherapy to shrink tumours in localised unresectable and borderline resectable disease. Also, because adjuvant chemotherapy is often delayed due to an extended recovery period, preoperative chemotherapy may reduce reoccurrence improving outcomes with no increased perioperative risk; this is an emerging area of research [12, 13].

Intraductal Papillary Mucinous Neoplasm (IPMN)

IPMNs tumours are composed of mucin producing cells, with varying degrees of dysplasia and potential to become malignant. Seventy percent of IPMNs located within the main pancreatic duct convert to carcinoma in 10 years, those within duct branches have a much lower conversion rates at 20% in ten years [14, 15]. Management involves surveillance, if there is evidence of malignancy or pancreatitis from obstruction surgical resection is indicated. 3-year survival following surgery for carcinoma insitu is 60–80% [16].

Pancreatic Neuroendocrine Tumours (PNETS)

Epidemiology

These are rare tumours arising from endocrine pancreatic tissue, they account for 3% of pancreatic neoplasms. The majority (75%) are non-functioning and the remaining 25% secrete a variety of peptide hormones most commonly insulin and gastrin. Classification and staging of PNETs is difficult because they are a heterogeneous group and though generally survival rates are good there is a wide variability in individual outcome according to cell differentiation and tumour grade, there is no association between functionality and rates of tumour growth or spread.

Clinical Features

Functioning PNETs exhibit signs and symptoms associated with excess hormone production. Insulinomas cause paroxysmal and postprandial hypoglycaemia. Gastrinomas present with features of Zollinger-Ellison syndrome; gastric acid hypersecretion causing peptic ulceration, heartburn, weight-loss and diarrhoea. Glucagonomas present with weight loss, diabetes and neurolytic migratory erythema an erythematous papular rash on face perineum and extremities. Only 10% of somatostatinomas produce any symptoms from the triad of diarrhoea/steatorrhea, cholelithiasis and diabetes. Vasoactive intestinal peptide secreting tumours (VIPomas) are very rare, patients have high volume watery diarrhoea causing hypokalaemia and dehydration with associated symptoms. Non-functioning PNETs generally present much later with symptoms from extrinsic compression or metastasises. They are often diagnosed as an incidental finding on imaging for unrelated conditions.

PNETs are mostly incidental but can be associated with genetic endocrinopathies. Multiple endocrine neoplasia type 1(MEN 1), Neurofibromatosis type 1, von Hippel-Lindau syndrome (VHL) and tuberous sclerosis should be excluded in patients where PNETs are diagnosed.

Management

Optimal management decisions are complex, the balance of medical and surgical management is based upon tumour histology, rate of growth, potential or actual metastases, functionality and symptoms. Management with the inclusion of surgical resection offers the only complete cure with tumour removal, yet complete cure is rarely achieved with one treatment modality. Tumour de-baulking surgery can improve quality of and prolong life in selected cases where large masses are unresectable and residual disease including metastasises can be controlled with adjuvant therapies such as ablation, embolisation, chemotherapy and hormone therapy. In general, prognosis is favourable even with disseminated disease. But it is also highly variable and dependent upon tumour histology, growth rate and site of tumour.

Pancreatitis

Acute Pancreatitis

Incidence of acute pancreatitis in UK is 15–42 per 100,000 [17]. Inflammation and organ ischaemia causes pancreatic necrosis which occurs in up to 20% of cases [18]. Most of these patients are managed conservatively or with radiological guided drainage. The PANTER trial showed 35% of cases resolve with percutaneous catheter drainage alone [19]. Debridement surgery is indicated in very few cases but may be required in the management of infected necrosis for symptomatic sterile necrosis or for persisting collections. UK guidelines suggest patients with 30% necrosis should have a fine needle aspiration (FNA) to obtain sample for culture. Patients with positive cultures will require a drainage or surgical debridement procedure [17].

When indicated surgery should be delayed to allow patient stabilisation and reduction of retroperitoneal inflammation. More than 4 weeks after presentation is needed for optimisation. Open necrosectomy has been largely superseded by a variety of minimally invasive techniques which have improved outcomes [19]. Mortality from acute pancreatitis complicated by collections remains high at up to 25% [20].

Chronic Pancreatitis

Chronic pancreatitis is characterised by chronic pancreatic inflammation and scarring, causing irreversible loss of both exocrine and endocrine function. Incidence is 40–50 per 100,000 [21] Clinical presentation is of severe abdominal pain. Diabetes and exocrine insufficiency present later in the course of the disease. Patients have an increased risk of developing pancreatic cancer.

Long term complications include duodenal stenosis, biliary stricture, pseudocyst and portal hypertension secondary to portal or splenic vein occlusion. These complications and most commonly control of refractory pain are indications for endoscopic or surgical intervention. The aims of intervention are to improve pancreatic duct drainage, remove extrahepatic biliary obstruction or exogenous venous obstruction. The coeliac plexus may be targeted to control pain.

Generally, less invasive endoscopic techniques are utilised before considering surgical intervention, however surgical procedures are superior to endoscopy at providing long term pain relief according to Cochrane review [22]. The choice of surgical intervention is dependent upon pancreatic ductal and parenchymal morphology. For dilated ducts a ductal drainage procedure such as lateral pancreatico-jejunostomy (LPJ) is considered. With ductal stenosis a pancreatic resection is required.

Emergency Surgery

Emergency pancreatic surgery is rare accounting for just 0.5% of procedures in one observational study [23]. Mortality is high in this group (35%). More frequent indications include duodenal perforation, control of GI bleeding, trauma and pseudocyst complications.

Trauma

Pancreatic injury is rare occurring in 3–5% of severe abdominal trauma [24]. Diagnosis is by CT. Ductal injury requires early repair and the integrity is should be assessed with contrast MRCP. Laparotomy and pancreatic drainage is recommended for parenchymal injuries. For ductal injuries, resection with distal pancreatectomy, or rarely, staged pancreaticoduodenectomy is required. Mortality is approximately 20% and complications such as fistulas, pancreatitis and pseudocysts are common.

Surgical Techniques

Resections

Pancreaticoduodenectomy—The Whipple Procedure

Pancreaticoduodenectomy (PD) was first described by Kausch in 1912, and later popularised by Whipple in 1935. The procedure involves resection of the proximal pancreas, along with distal stomach, duodenum, distal bile duct, gall bladder and lymph nodes as an en-bloc specimen. Reconstruction is with biliary, pancreatic and finally gastric anastomosis. Intestinal continuity is restored via a pancreatico-jejunostomy or pancreatico-gastrostomy.

The most common indication for the Whipple procedure is in the management of adenocarcinoma associated with the pancreatic head, neck and uncinate process. Other indications are: pancreatic neuroendocrine tumours (PNET), Intraductal papillary mucinous neoplasm (IPMN), ampullary tumours, duodenal tumours, cholangiocarcinoma, chronic pancreatitis and pancreatic or duodenal injury.

This complex procedure requires a median operating time of 5.5 h and has 30-day mortality of less than 5% in high volume centres. Significant causes of post-operative morbidity include the development of a pancreatic fistula seen in 15% of cases, [25] delayed gastric emptying in 17% [26] and bile leak from choledochal-jejunal anastomosis in 1–2% (Fig. 24.1).

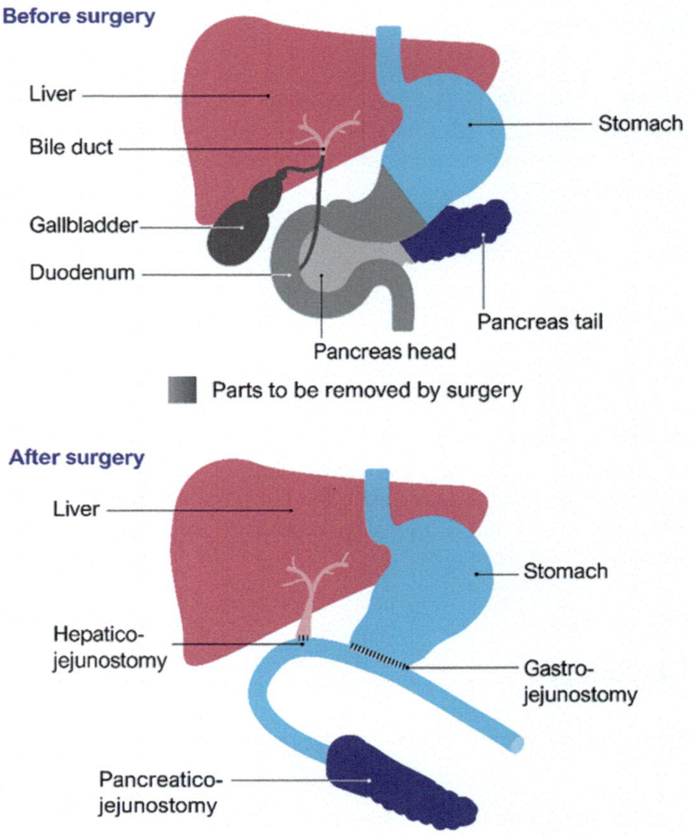

Fig. 24.1 Whipple procedure

Pylorus–Preserving Pancreaticoduodenectomy

Pylorus–Preserving Pancreaticoduodenectomy (PPPD) was first described by Watson in 1942. It is similar to the Whipple procedure; however, the pylorus is not resected with the theoretical advantage of maintaining gastrointestinal function and reducing the risk of delayed gastric emptying and dumping syndrome. Recent Cochrane review comparing PPPD with Classical PD found similar morbidity and survival. PPPD had shorter operation time and less blood loss but paradoxically it had higher incidence of delayed gastric emptying [27].

Subtotal stomach-preserving pancreaticoduodenectomy (SSPPD) has been developed in an attempt to reduce incidence of delayed gastric emptying with good results but increased intraoperative blood loss in one meta-analysis [28]. The choice of technique is based on institution and surgeon preference and on oncological factors such as proximity of the tumour to the duodenum.

Distal Pancreatectomy

25% of resections are distal pancreatectomy. it is performed for malignant and benign lesions of the body and tail of pancreas. It can be performed open or laparoscopically with comparable survival at 3 years [29, 30]. The spleen is removed along with the tail of the pancreas as it lies in close proximity to the tail. Patients post splenectomy will require lifelong antibiotics alongside vaccinations for encapsulated bacteria (Fig. 24.2).

Central Pancreatectomy

The role of central pancreatectomy (CP) is rare and limited due to a narrow spectrum of indications. The procedure is historically reserved for patients with chronic pancreatitis and traumatic injuries. Some centres advocate this resection for neoplasms in the pancreatic neck. The advantages of preserved endocrine and exocrine pancreatic function need to be balanced against increased rates of anastomotic leak.

Total Pancreatectomy

This is an extensive and difficult operation resulting in postoperative endocrine and exocrine insufficiency. It is reserved for patients unsuitable for less invasive resections. The most common indications are for adenocarcinoma, IPMN and for treatment of severe refractory pain in chronic and hereditary pancreatitis. If possible, pancreatic islet auto-transplantation should be performed to reduce the severity of diabetes postoperatively, although 30–40% of patients remain insulin independent after islet transplantation [31, 32]. Exocrine insufficiency is managed with enzyme replacement and nutritional counselling (Fig. 24.3).

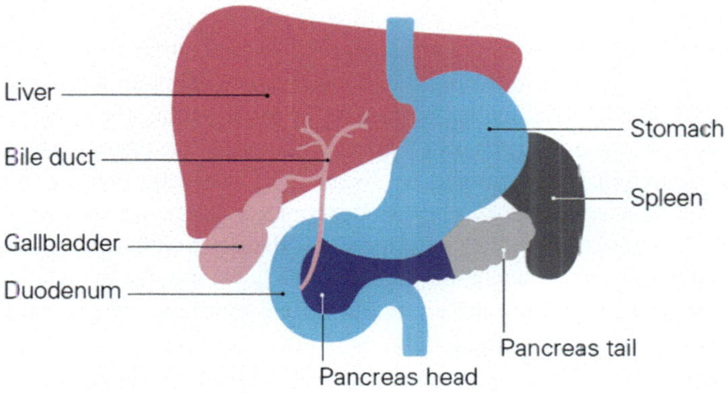

Fig. 24.2 Distal Pancreatectomy

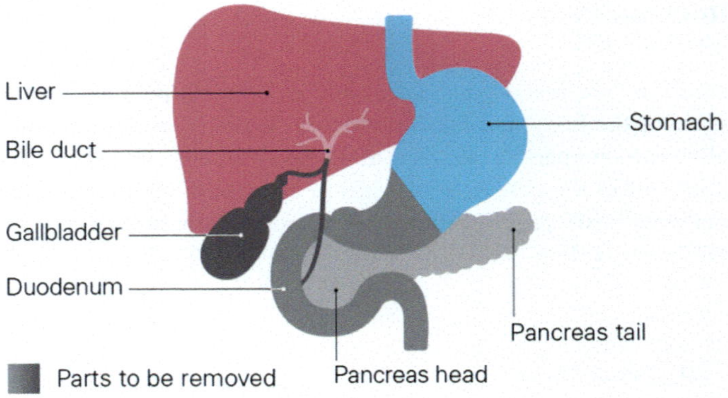

Fig. 24.3 Total pancreatectomy

Enucleation

Local excision can be used for small lesions sited away from ductal structures. Most common indications include PNETs or mucinous cystic tumours. It can be performed as an open or laparoscopic procedure and avoids complications of anastomosis, has shorter operating time and length of stay but carries higher rates of pancreatic fistula formation, though they are less severe than resection fistulas [3, 33].

Debridement

Indications for pancreatic debridement are the acute pancreatitis complications of septic necrosis or symptomatic sterile necrosis. The aim of surgery is to remove necrotic tissue and preserve functional pancreas, whilst limiting fistula formation and damage to other organs. Debridement is preferably performed a minimum of 3 weeks after the episode of acute pancreatitis. Delayed surgery allows for the retroperitoneal inflammation to decrease and enables discrimination between healthy and devitalised tissue. Medically the patient is more stable and with the resolution of end organ damage, the risks of surgery and anaesthesia are reduced. Choice of surgical approach is determined by location of necrosis. Percutaneous drains can be placed as a bridge to surgery. Endoscopic or laparoscopic debridement is appropriate for selected walled off necrosis. Patients with biliary pancreatitis should undergo simultaneous cholecystectomy to prevent recurrence. Debridement is a high risk procedure with many complications; fluid collections and bile leaks requiring reoperations, bleeding, fistula formation, pancreatic insufficiency leading to malnutrition and diabetes lead to high rates of mortality and morbidity.

Lateral Pancreato-Jejunostomy (LPJ) and Frey Procedure

LPJ is indicated as a pancreatic drainage procedure in patients with chronic pain and a dilated main pancreatic duct as a complication of chronic pancreatitis. A limited resection can be performed in conjunction with LPJ to rectify poor drainage to the duct secondary to fibrotic parenchyma and this is known as the Frey procedure. This procedure relieves chronic pain in 60–90% of chronic pancreatitis cases [35, 36].

Laparoscopic Surgery

Pancreatic resection can be approached laparoscopically and is usually carried out for small tumours and tumours of distal pancreas. It remains one of the most challenging minimally invasive operations. Laparoscopic pancreaticoduodenectomy has similar overall survival rates but significantly lower wound infection, blood loss, pancreatic fistula rates, and reduced hospital stay when compared to open surgery [37]. Laparoscopic distal pancreatic resection is currently the most frequently performed minimally invasive pancreatic procedure. Other types of resection and debridements and drainage procedures are increasingly performed laparoscopically and robotically.

Perioperative Management

Preoperative

All pancreatic surgery is high risk with significant mortality, complication rates and a long recovery phase, many patients will not return to their previous level of function after surgery. Patients with adenocarcinoma in particular face dismal 5-year survival rates even after surgery. When we also consider adenocarcinoma is a highly aggressive cancer the challenges of assessment, optimisation and patient preparation are constrained by a limited timeframe. For many patient's conservative treatment is the right option either because they are not fit enough to tolerate surgery or they may choose, given the risks, to accept a shorter life expectancy with better quality of life rather than marginally extended life expectancy with high possibility of limited function.

Assessment

Soon after diagnosis a specialist MDT meeting should plan each individual management strategy. Patients must be fully informed of their diagnosis and the treatment options so they may a take active role in their management decisions. Their views should be given the utmost consideration. Once a treatment plan has been decided patients should have the opportunity to attend a preoperative assessment with an anaesthetist. At this appointment a thorough assessment, examination and any additional investigations can be obtained. It presents an opportunity to initiate pre-optimisation interventions. Furthermore, an in-depth discussion around the patient's perceptions, preferences and expectations with communication of risks can help prepare the patient for surgery.

A detailed anaesthetic history should be recorded and a focused systems examination undertaken. Appropriate investigations will provide accurate information and application of a risk scoring system can aid the patient consultation. Assessment of functional capacity and nutritional status are important and recent weight loss with reduced appetite and reduced exercise tolerance are indicators of compromised nutrition and frailty. Clearly, the risks of morbidity and mortality are increased in such patients.

Risk Scoring

Scoring systems such as P-POSSUM and SORT are useful predictors of morbidity and mortality in the general surgery setting. However, they have not been successfully validated in pancreatic surgery [38]. The preoperative pancreatic resection score (PREPARE) has recently been developed to aid preoperative decision making and has shown promising results [39]. The ACS-NQIP database provides a comprehensive calculation of mortality and morbidity risks, giving individual risk calculations for common complications. It provides invaluable information to enable the accurate communication of risk to patients.

Investigations

Baseline blood testing, group and save and ECG are required for all patients. More specific investigations are dependent upon the history. Pulmonary events account for 40% of postoperative complications and 20% of deaths [40] and those with pulmonary co-morbidities have increased risk. Patients will have CT images to review and recent spirometry is indicated with a significant smoking history or history of pulmonary disease.

Cardiovascular Risk Assessment

Cardiovascular complications are common in elderly cohorts and when they occur, they result in high mortality. Accurate assessment of function and diagnosis of valvular pathology, ischaemia, diastolic dysfunction and arrhythmia is needed to properly inform the patient and plan anaesthetic, surgery and postoperative care.

NT-pro-BNP is a useful screening test to identify patients at risk of developing functional heart failure. Raised NT-pro-BNP levels are associated with increased risk of myocardial injury after non-cardiac surgery (MINS) and can be used to guide further investigations such as echocardiography and post-operative troponin. Guidelines suggest measuring NT-pro-BNP in patients who are 65 years of age or older, or are 45–64 years of age with significant cardiovascular disease, or have a Revised Cardiac Risk Index ≥ 1 [41].

A resting echocardiogram should be considered if the patient has a heart murmur and cardiac symptoms (including breathlessness, pre-syncope, syncope or chest pain) or signs or symptoms of heart failure. Dobutamine stress echocardiography may be indicated in patients unable to exercise due to musculoskeletal impairment.

Functional Capacity and Frailty

Frailty is a syndrome of physical decline characterised by weight loss, sarcopenia, reduced walking speed, fatigue and reduced activity. Frail patients respond poorly to medical interventions and have up to 5 times risk of mortality compared to robust individuals [42]. An assessment of frailty is therefore vital and there are many scoring systems available, the frailty index and Edmonton frail scale are examples.

Reduced exercise tolerance is also a potent predictor of bad outcomes. It can be quantified from the history in metabolic equivalents (METS). For borderline cases or where there is uncertainty the gold standard test is cardio pulmonary exercise testing (CPET). It is a well-tolerated, non-invasive and cost-effective way to provide a global assessment of cardiovascular, respiratory and skeletal muscle systems [43]. Selected CPET variables have a predictive value in determining postoperative complications and length of hospital stay in intra-abdominal surgery. Studies have shown an Aerobic threshold (AT) of less than 10 ml/kg/min is associated with increased morbidity for pancreatic surgery [44].

Optimisation

Enhanced Recovery After Surgery (ERAS)

Enhanced recovery programmes are multimodal strategies that aim to attenuate the loss of functional capacity after surgery and improve its restoration. Morbidity is reduced and recovery enhanced by reducing surgical stress, by optimal control of pain, early oral diet and early mobilisation. Overall pathway adherence is paramount in achieving successful outcomes after pancreatic surgery [45].

Preoperative counselling may diminish anxiety and help to enhance postoperative recovery and discharge. Information leaflets or multimedia information may contribute to early mobilisation, feeding and pain management. Smoking and alcohol cessation for at least a month prior to PD has been shown to be beneficial. There is increasing evidence that improving or maintaining fitness in the perioperative period leads to improved outcomes. Preoperative carbohydrate drinks are recommended in patients without diabetes. Adequate thrombo-prophylaxis should be considered for 4 weeks after hospital discharge [45].

Anaemia

Anaemia is common in patients undergoing pancreatic surgery and can be related to nutritional deficiency and/or anaemia of chronic disease. If anaemia is detected on preoperative full blood count, haematinics should be performed (B12, folate, ferritin and transferrin saturation TSAT). If ferritin <100 ug L^{-1} and/or TSAT less than 20% iron supplementation should be considered. Intravenous iron (i.e. Ferric Carboxymaltose) is usually indicated in view of the urgency of surgery and need to increment haemoglobin rapidly. Folic acid and Vitamin B12 can be supplemented if patients are found to be deficient. Further referral to haematology may be indicated.

Nutrition

Almost all patients with pancreatic disease and especially those with adenocarcinoma are malnourished. Malnutrition is associated with impaired immunity with reduced muscular and respiratory function and results in a much higher incidence of post-operative complications [48]. Malnutrition is reversible though difficult given time constraints. Therefore, nutritional status should be assessed early using a systematic screening tool. The malnutrition universal screening tool (MUST) for adults has been validated by several studies and is easy and rapid to use [46, 47]. This tool can prompt implementation of preoperative nutritional interventions such as calorific foods, oral supplements, vitamins, enteral nutrition and in some cases parenteral nutrition.

Optimisation of Co-morbidities

Medical management of co-morbidities should be optimised. For example, diabetic control, control of AF, or COPD management should be assessed and improved as appropriate. Medications should be reviewed and changes made if required.

Exercise Prehabilitation

Improving aerobic fitness prior to surgery is an expanding area of research with improved outcomes from programs aimed at increasing aerobic threshold (AT) and Oxygen delivery (VO2max). It may be difficult for those requiring pancreatic surgery to benefit from a formal exercise program due to time constraints. However, simple exercises aimed at maintaining muscle strength and cardiovascular fitness will be of benefit.

Intraoperative Strategies

Pancreatic procedures are complex major abdominal surgeries with extensive dissection and prolonged operating times. There is potential for blood loss, fluid and electrolyte imbalances, cardiovascular instability and ongoing respiratory compromise. These factors need due consideration prior to induction so from the setup the anaesthetist is provided with favourable ergonomics and monitoring for cardiac output, CVP, and blood gases with the ability to give rapid blood and fluid boluses. Depth of anaesthesia monitoring is a useful adjunct to titrate amount of anaesthetic drug delivery especially in the higher risk cohorts. The patient must be well protected from injury with mindfulness of positioning, monitoring and infusion line placement, eye protection, temperature measurement and warming.

Analgesia

Effective analgesia in pancreatic surgery is important for postoperative respiratory function, compliance with physiotherapy, mobilisation and prevention of complications.

Mid-thoracic epidurals remain the gold standard for postoperative analgesia and are widely used in open pancreatic surgery; for upper transverse incisions, epidural catheters should be inserted between T5 and T9 root levels. In addition to superior postoperative analgesia epidurals reduce the stress response and improve respiratory mechanics and coronary perfusion hence decreasing the incidence of pulmonary or cardiac complications. With improved anastomotic perfusion and reduced opiate requirements intestinal function is supported and the incidence of thromboembolic events reduced [48]. However, thoracic epidurals can also have significant risks and side-effects prompting some practitioners to move to alternative analgesia options especially in the higher risk patients. Two important issues are: Firstly, a high proportion of epidurals don't work effectively (1 in 8 in some studies). Physiological responses under anaesthesia for example, reduced heart rate and BP in response to epidural drug administration do not accurately predict the epidural's analgesic potential post-operatively and often the anaesthetist has to judge alternative opiate analgesic administration with limited objective information. Secondly, epidurals cause vasodilation with a tendency for lower intraoperative blood pressures, increased vasopressor requirements and fluid volumes administered. Postoperatively, epidurals may delay time to mobilisation.

Alternative regional analgesia techniques include single-shot spinal opioid administration combined with Patient controlled analgesia (PCA), it can provide adequate analgesia for both laparoscopic and open pancreatic surgery [49]. There is evidence supporting the use of wound catheters. The POP-UP study demonstrated that continuous wound infiltration is non-inferior to epidural analgesia in HPB surgery [50]. Paravertebral or erector spinae blocks and catheters are increasingly utilized in major abdominal surgery. Placement of bilateral catheters for pancreatic surgery provides excellent long term analgesia with less complications, contraindications and side-effects than neuroaxial techniques.

PCA with opioids remains the most common modality used as an alternative the epidural. It is used in conjunction with or as an alternative to regional anaesthesia. It is used as rescue in the event of failed regional anaesthesia and for step-down analgesia.

Multimodal analgesia agents including Ketamine, Clonidine or Dexmedetomidine, magnesium, IV Lignocaine infusions and Paracetamol can be routinely employed. Nonsteroidal anti-inflammatory drugs can be used but are often contraindicated.

Goal Directed Fluid Therapy (GDT)

Adverse consequences of hypervolemia include cardiac, pulmonary and renal complications, electrolyte imbalance, coagulopathy, ileus and anastomotic breakdown [51]. In pancreatic surgery there is some evidence that excess fluid administration may also contribute to the development of pancreatic fistulas [52] contributing to the significant morbidity associated with this surgery. Judgement of individual fluid requirements is difficult and GDT provides an evidenced-based method for achieving optimal fluid status. However, clear evidence of improved outcomes is lacking and the optimal application of GDT is still debated. Repeated meta-analyses have reported improved outcomes using GDT including reduced risk of respiratory, GI, renal and wound related complications. However most, failed to demonstrate significant improvements in mortality [53–55]. A small multicentre RCT of patients undergoing pancreaticoduodenectomy showed reduced complications and length of stay using a GDT algorithm [56]. Ongoing trials such as OPTMISE II and FLOELA aim to provide strong evidence of improved outcomes from using GDT. With the increasing volume of evidence showing goal directed fluid management reduces complications we would advocate its utilisation for pancreatic surgery.

Ventilation

Intraoperative use of a protective ventilation strategy with the application of PEEP and limited tidal volume of 6–7 ml/kg, for prolonged surgery, improves respiratory function and reduces postoperative pulmonary complications, especially in susceptible individuals and those who remain ventilated for delayed extubation in ITU.

Prevention of Infection

Surgical site infections make up 17% of hospital acquired infection so antibiotic prophylaxis is essential and repeated dosing during prolonged surgery may be required (NNIS). Meticulous attention to sterility with central venous catheter and epidural placement is important. Avoidance of hypothermia, tight glycaemic control and optimal fluid management all reduce risk of postoperative infection.

Other Considerations

A nasogastric tube (NGT) is placed after induction, for the Whipple procedure this is replaced intraoperatively with a surgically guided nasojejunal tube (NJT). In line with patient blood management protocols Hb should be maintained above 70 g/L and above 80 g/L in the context of ischaemic heart disease with single unit transfusion if required. Intraoperative thromboprophylaxis is provided with intermittent pneumatic compression devices and graduated compression stockings which should be continued until low molecular weight heparin can be recommenced.

Specific Considerations for PNETs

Functional PNETs hypersecreting hormones with systemic effects need careful anaesthetic management. Patients often receive somatostatin analogue infusions perioperatively for cardiovascular stability and symptom relief. These patients may not respond or conversely may have an exaggerated response to vasoactive drugs which should be titrated carefully. A Remifenanil infusion will help to modulate cardiovascular responses. Periods of hypertension can be treated with 20–50mcg Ocreotide boluses and/or short acting antihypertensive infusions such as Esmolol or GTN [57].

Postoperative Strategies

Sixty four percent of the large cohort of patients with pancreatic cancer who undergo pancreatic surgery have more than 10% weight loss preoperatively [58]. Malnutrition in this group increases the risk of complications associated with major surgery including bleeding, chest infection, wound infection and thromboembolism. Therefore, morbidity remains high with reported complications ranging between 35–50% [59].

Pancreatic resection also has a unique set of conditions including three different anastomoses giving rise to other complications such as anastomotic leak, pancreatic fistula formation, delayed gastric emptying, endocrine and exocrine insufficiency. Mortality from pancreatic surgery is related to systemic complications, including sepsis and multi organ dysfunction syndrome (MODS). This is mostly driven by anastomotic leaks causing pancreatic fistula, abscesses and collections. All patients should be considered for postoperative high dependancy care because early recognition is the most important determinant of the successful treatment of complications and up to 18% of patients require ICU admission with complications after pancreaticoduodenectomy [60]. Certainly patients who are preoperatively assessed as high risk should initially be managed in intensive care. The majority of cases will be extubated at end of surgery unless there is significant respiratory disease, or an intraoperative complication necessitating ongoing level 3 management. Ideally, lower risk patients should be managed on a specialist surgical HDU for 24–48 h but for many specialist surgical wards are sufficient.

Ongoing assessment and management of pain is important for patient wellbeing and to minimise complications. Epidurals need ongoing assessment for effectiveness and to exclude complications. Where epidurals or other regional techniques have failed to provide adequate analgesia, pain must be managed aggressively with multimodal opiate based medication. Morphine and ketamine boluses titrated to response and ongoing PCA is one available strategy.

With good pain control early mobilisation can be encouraged from first postoperative day to meet daily targets as a part of ERAS. Delay to mobilisation can be avoided by removal of drains, feeding tubes and epidurals at the earliest opportunity when no longer clinically indicated.

Enteral feeding should be commenced as soon as 12 h following surgery. Chest physiotherapy and deep breathing exercises helps to prevent pulmonary complications. Maintenance of patient diary helps to monitor progress and accomplish individual goals.

Postoperative Complications

Pancreatic Fistula

Friable pancreatic tissue is prone to anastomotic leak leading to pancreatic fistulae, collections and abscesses. Pancreatic fistula is defined as: measurable drain output on postoperative day 3, with amylase content greater than three times that of normal serum amylase. It is the most common and significant complication after pancreatic surgery occurring after 15% of Whipple procedures [25] and 30–40% of distal and central pancreatectomy [51, 62]. Collections and abscesses occur in another 5- 15% of cases [61, 62]. Signs are non-specific and include abdominal pain, nausea, tachycardia, and fever; a high index of suspicion should be consistently maintained. Prevention strategies using somatostatin analogues have produced equivocal results. Perioperative Octreotide infusions have not reduced incidence of complications [8] but the newer agent Pasireotide has shown promising results with a significant decrease in pancreatic fistula, leak, or abscess [64].

Conservative management of fistula requires avoiding oral intake. Jejunal enteral nutrition via a nasojejunal tube, sited distal to surgical site, is preferred but parenteral nutrition maybe indicated. Somatostatin analogues are administered to reduce pancreatic enzyme release. Endoscopic management includes drainage of collections and abscesses and pancreatic duct stenting to improve drainage.

Delayed Gastric Emptying

Unobstructed gastroparesis is known as Delayed gastric emptying (DGE) and it is a common complication of GI tract surgery, Incidence after pancreatic surgery is particularly high and is often associated with abscesses or fistula. After Whipple procedure the incidence is 10–20% [25, 61] and it results in significantly increased costs and length of stay [65]. DGE can be classified by severity into grades A, B, and C according to need for nasogastric tube (NGT), tolerance of oral intake, and need for prokinetic therapy [66].

Obstruction is first excluded via upper GI contrast series or endoscopy, then management of DGE is supportive. Gastric decompression with a nasogastric tube, stopping oral intake and administration of prokinetics reduce symptoms and recovery times. Secondary causes of DGE should be excluded and enteral or parenteral nutrition commenced.

Haemorrhage

Major haemorrhage occurs after 1% to 8% of pancreatic resections but is implicated in 11% to 38% of mortality [68]. Onset may be early (<24 h) or late (>24 h) after surgery. Early bleeding is likely to have a technical surgical source and require return to theatre, it has a better prognosis. Late bleeding is more likely to be secondary to a complication such as fistula, abscess or pseudoaneurysm eroding a vessel. Late blood loss can be massive and catastrophic with a mortality of 10% compared to 1% with early haemorrhage [60].

Exocrine Insufficiency

Pancreatic exocrine insufficiency can occur post pancreatic resection, causing fat malabsorption with a requirement for supplemental pancreatic enzymes (Pancreatin).

Management of Diabetes

Diabetes after pancreatic resection surgery is different to type 1 and type 2diabetes. It rarely produces ketoacidosis as in type 1 and patients are sensitive to exogenous insulin in comparison to type 2 diabetes. It is more common in patients with total pancreatectomy unless an islet cell transplant has been performed simultaneously.

Summary

All surgery on pancreas is complex and debilitating with high complication and morbidity rates. The majority of procedures are resections to treat pancreatic adenocarcinomas. This aggressive cancer continues to have dismal rates of survival even after resection.

The perioperative role of the anaesthetist is central to the MDT in improving outcomes for patients. Preoperatively in patient selection, optimisation and preparation by accurately conveying the risks involved.

Intraoperative techniques are continually advancing and we are gaining more evidence supporting the contribution of anaesthetic management in improving outcomes and reducing complications. The importance of optimised fluid management and maintaining normal blood pressure has become clear. Novel regional anaesthetic techniques with fewer complications are increasingly utilised in place of thoracic epidurals, enabling reduced fluid administration and earlier mobilisation.

Post operative complication rates remain high and patients benefit from high dependancy care with anaesthetic input in the early postoperative period to optimise recovery, reducing the frequency and impact of complications with early recognition and management.

References

1. Li D. Jiao L Molecular epidemiology of pancreatic cancer. Int J Gastrointest Cancer. 2003;33:3–14 PMID: 12909734.
2. Cancer research UK. Pancreatic cancer mortality: UK incidence statistics 2011. Available from http://www.cancerresearchuk.org/health-professional/cancer-statistics-for-the-uk.
3. WHO International agency for research on cancer: Cancer today report 2018. Available from http://gco.iarc.fr/today/data/factsheets/cancers/39-All-cancers-fact-sheet.pdf.

4. Siegel RL, Miller KD, Jemal A. Cancer statistics, 2019. CA Cancer J Clin. 2019;69:7.
5. Bond-Smith G, Banga N, Hammond TM, Imber CJ Pancreatic adenocarcinoma. BMJ 2012; 344 e2476.
6. Vallas C, Andia E, Sanchez A, Fabregat J, Pozuelo O, Quintero JC, et al. Dual phase helical CT of pancreatic adenocarcinoma: assessment of resectability before surgery. AJR Am K Roentgenol. 2002;178:821–6.
7. Doucas H, Sutton CD, Zimmerman A, Dennison AR, Berry DP. Assessment of pancreatic malignancy with laparoscopy and intraoperative ultrasound. Surg Endosc. 2007;21:1147–54.
8. Yeo CJ, Cameron JL, Sohn TA, Lillemoe KD, Pitt HA, Talamini MA, et al. Six hundred fifty consecutive pancreaticoduodenectomies in the 1990s: pathology, complications, and outcomes. Ann Surg. 1997;226:248–60.
9. Benassai G, Mastrorilli M, Quarto G, Cappiello A, Giani U, Mosella G. Survival after pancreaticoduodenectomy for ductal adenocarcinoma of the head of the pancreas. Chir Ital. 2000;52:263–70.
10. Millikan KW, Deziel DJ, Silverstein JC, Kanjo TM, Christein JD, Doolas A, Prinz RA. Prognostic factors associated with resectable adenocarcinoma of the head of the pancreas. Am Surg. 1999;65:618–23.
11. Allen PJ, Kuk D, Castillo CF, Basturk O, Wolfgang CL, Cameron JL, et al. Multi-institutional Validation Study of the American Joint Commission on Cancer (8th Edition) Changes for T and N Staging in Patients With Pancreatic Adenocarcinoma. Ann Surg 2017; 265:185–91.
12. Van Tienhoven G, Versteijne E, Suker M, Groothuis KBC, Busch OR, Bonsing BA, et al. Preoperative chemoradiotherapy versus immediate surgery for resectable and borderline resectable pancreatic cancer (PREOPANC-1): a randomized, controlled, multicenter phase III trial (abstract). J Clin Oncol 36, 2018 (suppl; abstr LBA4002). Abstract available online at https://meetinglibrary.asco.org/record/160063/abstract.
13. Murphy JE, Wo JY, Ryan DP, Jiang W, Yeap BY, Drapek LC, et al. Total neoadjuvant therapy with FOLFIRINOX followed by individualized chemoradiotherapy for borderline resectable pancreatic adenocarcinoma: a phase 2 clinical trial. JAMA Oncol. 2018;4:963–9.
14. Longnecker DS, Adsay NV, Fernandez-del CC, Hruban RH, Kasugai T, Klimstra DS, et al. Histopathological diagnosis of pancreatic intraepithelial neoplasia and intraductal papillary-mucinous neoplasms: interobserver agreement. Pancreas. 2005;31:344–9.
15. Hruban RH, Takaori K, Klimstra DS, Adsay NV, Albores-Saavedra J, Biankin AV, et al. An illustrated consensus on the classification of pancreatic intraepithelial neoplasia and intraductal papillary mucinous neoplasms. Am J Surg Pathol. 2004;28:977–87.
16. Kobari M, Egawa S, Shibuya K, Shimamura H, Sunamura M, Takeda K, et al. Intraductal papillary mucinous tumors of the pancreas comprise 2 clinical subtypes: differences in clinical characteristics and surgical management. Arch Surg. 1999;134:1131–6.
17. Working Party of the British Society of Gastroenterology; Association of Surgeons of Great Britain and Ireland; Pancreatic Society of Great Britain and Ireland; Association of Upper GI Surgeons of Great Britain and Ireland. UK guidelines for the management of acute pancreatitis. Gut. 2005;54 Suppl 3(Suppl 3):iii1–iii9.
18. Whitcomb DC. Clinical practice. Acute pancreatitis. N Engl J Med. 2006;354:2142–50.
19. Besselink MG, van Santvoort HC, Nieuwenhuijs VB, Boermeester MA Bollen TL, Buskens E, et al. Minimally invasive 'step-up approach' versus maximal necrosectomy in patients with acute necrotising pancreatitis (PANTER trial): design and rationale of a randomised controlled multicenter trial [ISRCTN13975868]. BMC Surg. 2006;6:6.
20. Gupta R, Wig JD, Bhasin DK, Singh P, Suri S, Kang S, et al. Severe acute pancreatitis: the life after. J Gastrointest Surg. 2009;13:1328–36.
21. Yadav D, Timmons L, Benson JT, Dierkhising R, Chari S. Incidence, prevalence, and survival of chronic pancreatitis: a population-based study. Am J Gastroenterol. 2011;106:21946280.

22. Ahmed Ali U, Pahlplatz JM, Nealon WH, van Goor H, Gooszen HG, Boermeester MA. Endoscopic or surgical intervention for painful obstructive chronic pancreatitis. Cochrane Database Syst Rev 2015; CD007884.
23. Strobel O, Schneider L, Philipp S, Fritz S, Büchler MW, Hackert T. Emergency pancreatic surgery—demanding and dangerous. Langenbecks Arch Surg. 2015;400:837–41.
24. Heuer M, Hussmann B, Lefering R, Taeger G, Kaiser GM, Paul A, Lendemans S. Pancreatic injury in 284 patients with severe abdominal trauma: outcome, course, and treatment algorithm. Langenbecks Arch Surg. 2011;396(1067–1076):21847623 PMID: 21847623.
25. Cameron JL. He J Two thousand consecutive pancreaticoduodenectomies. J Am Coll Surg. 2015;220:530–6 PMID: 25724606.
26. van Berge Henegouwen MI, van Gulik TM, DeWit LT, Allema JH, Rauws EAJ, Obertop H, Gouma JH. Delayed gastric emptying after standard pancreaticoduodenectomy versus pylorus-preserving pancreaticoduodenectomy: an analysis of 200 consecutive patients. J Am Coll Surg. 1997;185:373–9.
27. Huttner FJ, Fitzmaurice C, Schwarzer G, Seiler CM, Antes G, Büchler MW, Diener MK. Pylorus-preserving pancreaticoduodenectomy (pp Whipple) versus pancreaticoduodenectomy (classic Whipple) for surgical treatment of periampullary and pancreatic carcinoma. Cochrane Database Syst Rev. 2; 2016: CD006053 26905229.
28. Huang W, Xiong JJ, Wan MH, Szatmary P, Bharucha S, Gomatos I, et al. Meta-analysis of subtotal stomach-preserving pancreaticoduodenectomy vs pylorus preserving pancreaticoduodenectomy. World J Gastroenterol. 2015;21(6361–73):26034372 PMID: 26034372.
29. Wade TP, Virgo KS, Johnson FE. Distal pancreatectomy for cancer: results in U.S. Department of Veterans Affairs hospitals, 1987–1991. Pancreas 1995; 11:341–4.
30. Brennan MF, Moccia RD, Klimstra D. Management of adenocarcinoma of the body and tail of the pancreas. Ann Surg. 1996;223:506–12.
31. Chinnakotla S, Beilman GJ, Dunn TB, Bellin MD, Freeman LM, Radosevich DM, et al. Factors predicting outcomes after a total pancreatectomy and islet autotransplantation lessons learned from over 500 cases. Ann Surg. 2015;262:610–22.
32. Wilson GC, Sutton JM, Abbott DE, Smith MT, Lowy AM, Matthews JB, et al. Long-term outcomes after total pancreatectomy and islet cell autotransplantation: is it a durable operation? Ann Surg. 2014;260:659–67.
33. Pitt SC, Pitt HA, Baker MS, Christians K, Touzios JG, Kiely JM, et al. Small pancreatic and periampullary neuroendocrine tumors: resect or enucleate? J Gastrointest Surg. 2009;13:1692–8.
34. DiNorcia J, Lee MK, Reavey PL, Genkinger JM, Lee JA, Schrope BA, et al. One hundred thirty resections for pancreatic neuroendocrine tumor: evaluating the impact of minimally invasive and parenchyma-sparing techniques. J Gastrointest Surg. 2010;14:1536–46.
35. Keck T, Wellner UF, Riediger H, Adam U, Sick O, Hopt UT, Makowiec F. Long-term outcome after 92 duodenum-preserving pancreatic head resections for chronic pancreatitis: comparison of Beger and Frey procedures. J Gastrointest Surg. 2010;14:549–56.
36. Negi S, Singh A, Chaudhary A. Pain relief after Frey's procedure for chronic pancreatitis. Br J Surg. 2010;97:1087–95.
37. Delitto D, Luckhurst CM, Black BS, Beck JL, George JA, Sarosi GA, et al. Oncologic and perioperative outcomes following selective application of laparoscopic pancreaticoduodenectomy for periampullary malignancies. J Gastrointest Surg. 2016;20:1343–9.
38. Tamijmarane A, Bhati CS, Mirza DF, Bramhall SR, Mayer DA, Wigmore SJ, Buckels JAC. Application of Portsmouth modification of physiological and operative severity scoring system for enumeration of morbidity and mortality (P-POSSUM) in pancreatic surgery. World J Surg Onc. 2008;6:39–45.
39. Uzunoglu FG, Reeh M, Vettorazzi E, Ruschke T, Hannah P, Nentwich MF, et al. Preoperative pancreatic resection (PREPARE) score, a prospective multicentre- based morbidity risk score. Ann Surg. 2014;260:857–64.

40. Canat J, Gallart L. Predicting postoperative pulmonary complications in the general population. Curr Opin Anaesthesiol. 2013;26:107–15.
41. Duceppe E, Parlow J, MacDonald P, Lyons K, McMullen M, Srinathan S, et al. Canadian cardiovascular society guidelines on perioperative cardiac risk assessment and management for patients who undergo noncardiac surgery. CJC. 2017;33:1–16.
42. Theou O, Brothers TD, Mitnitski A, Rockwood K. Operationalization of frailty using eight commonly used scales and comparison of their ability to predict all-cause mortality. J Am Geriatr Soc. 2016;621:1537–51.
43. Ridgway ZA, Howell SJ. Cardiopulmonary exercise testing: a review of methods and applications in surgical patients. Eur J Anaesthesiol. 2010;27:858–65.
44. Moran J, Wilson F, Guinan E, McCormick P, Hussey J, Moriarty J. Role of cardiopulmonary exercise testing as a risk assessment method in patients undergoing intra-abdominal surgery: a systemic review. BJA. 2016;116:177–91.
45. Lassen K, Coolsen MM, Slim K, Carli F, de Aguilar-Nascimento JE, Schäfer M, et al. European Society for Clinical Nutrition and Metabolism. International Association for Surgical Metabolism and nutrition. Guidelines for perioperative care for pancreaticoduodenectomy: Enhanced Recovery after Surgery (ERAS) Society recommendations. World J Surg 2013; 37: 240–58.
46. La Torre M, Ziparo V, Nigri G, Cavallini M, Balducci G, Ramacciato G. Malnutrition and pancreatic surgery: prevalence and outcomes. J Surg Oncol. 2013;107:702–8.
47. Cooper C, Brierly ER, Burden ST. improving adherence to a care plan generated from the malnutrition universal screening tool. Eur J Clin Nutr. 2013;67:174–9.
48. Popping DM, Elia N, Van Aken HK, Marret E, Schug S, Kranke P, et al. Impact of epidural analgesia on mortality and morbidity after surgery: systematic review and meta-analysis of randomized controlled trials. Ann Surg. 2014;259(6):1056–67.
49. Kasivisvanathan R, Abbassi-Ghadi N, Prout J, Clevenger B, Fusai GK, Mallett SV. A prospective cohort study of intrathecal versus epidural analgesia for patients undergoing hepatic resection. HPB (Oxford). 2014;16(8):768–75.
50. Mungroop T, Veelo D, Busch OR, van Dieren S, van Gulik TM, Karsten TM, et al. Continuous wound infiltration versus ep idural analgesia after hepato-pancreato-biliary surgery (POP-UP): a randomised controlled, open-label, non-inferiority trial. Lancet Gastroenterol Hepatol. 2016;1:105–13.
51. Holte K, Sharrock NE, Kehlet H. Pathophysiology and clinical implications of perioperative fluid excess. Br J Anaesth. 2002;89:622–32.
52. Bruns H, Kortendieck V, Raab HR, Antolovic D. Intraoperative fluid excess is a risk factor for pancreatitic fistulas after partial pancreaticoduodenectomy. HPB Surg 2016 e1601340.
53. Pearse RM, Harrison DA, MacDonald N, Gillies MA, Blunt M, Ackland G, et al. Effect of a perioperative, cardiac output-guided hemodynamic therapy algorithm on outcomes following major gastrointestinal surgery: a randomized clinical trial and systematic review. JAMA. 2014;311:2181–90.
54. Corcoran T, Rhodes JE, Clarke S, Myles PS, Ho KM. Perioperative fluid management strategies in major surgery: a stratified meta-analysis. Anesth Analg. 2012;114:640–51.
55. Grocott MP, Dushianthan A, Hamilton MA, Mythen MG, Harrison D, Rowan K. Perioperative increase in global blood flow to explicit defined goals and outcomes following surgery. Cochrane Database Syst Rev 2012; 11:CD004082.
56. Weinburg L, Ianno D, Churilov L, Chao I, Scurrah N, Rachbuch C, et al. Restrictive intraoperative fluid optimisation algorithm improves outcomes in patients undergoing pancreaticoduodenectomy: a prospective multicentre randomized controlled trial. PLoS ONE. 2017;12(9):e0183313.
57. Powell B, al Mukhtar A, Mills GH. Carcinoid: the disease and its implications for anaesthesia. CEACCP 2011; 11:9-13.

58. Bozzetti F, Mariani L, Le Vullio S, Amerio ML, Biffi M, Caccialanza R, et al. The nutritional risk in oncology: a study of 1,453 cancer outpatients. Support Care Cancer. 2012;20:1919–28.
59. DeOliveira ML, Winter JM, Schafer M, Cunningham SC, Cameron JL, Yeo CJ, Clavien PA. Assessment of complications after pancreatic surgery: a novel grading system applied to 633 patients undergoing pancreaticoduodenectomy. Ann Surg. 2006;244:931–7.
60. Welsch T, Degrate L, Zschäbitz S, Hofer S, Werner J, Schmidt J. The need for extended intensive care after pancreaticoduodenectomy for pancreatic ductal adenocarcinoma. Langenbecks Arch Surg. 2011;396::353–362 PMID: 20336311.
61. Nathan H, Cameron JL, Choti MA, Schulick RD, Pawlik TM. The volume-outcomes effect in hepato-pancreato-biliary surgery: hospital versus surgeon contributions and specificity of the relationship. J Am Coll Surg. 2009;208:528–38 PMID: 19476786.
62. Crippa S, Bassi C, Warshaw A, Falconi M, Partelli S, Thayer SP, et al. Middle pancreatectomy: indications, short- and long-term operative outcomes. Ann Surg. 2007;246:69–76 PMID: 17592293.
63. Yeo CJ, Cameron JL, Lillemoe KD, Sauter PK, Coleman J, Sohn TA, et al. Does prophylactic octreotide decrease the rates of pancreatic fistula and other complications after pancreaticoduodenectomy? Results of a prospective randomized placebo-controlled trial. Ann Surg. 2000;232:419–29 PMID: 10973392.
64. Allen PJ, Gönen M, Brennan MF, Bucknor AA, Robinson LM, Pappas MM, et al. Pasireotide for postoperative pancreatic fistula. N Engl J Med. 2014;370:2014–22 PMID: 24849084.
65. Beane JD, House MG, Miller A, Nakeeb A, Schmidt M, Zyromski NJ, et al. Optimal management of delayed gastric emptying after pancreatectomy: an analysis of 1,089 patients. Surgery. 2014;156:939–46 PMID: 25151555.
66. Wente MN, Bassi C, Dervenis C, Fingerhut A, Gouma DJ, Izbicki JR, et al. Delayed gastric emptying (DGE) after pancreatic surgery: a suggested definition by the International Study Group of Pancreatic Surgery (ISGPS). Surgery. 2007;142:761–8 PMID: 17981197.

Chapter 25
Anaesthetic Management for Patients Undergoing Pancreas Transplantation

Lakshmi Kumar and Ramachandran N. Menon

Abbreviations

SPKTx	Simultaneous pancreas kidney transplant
PAKTx	Pancreas after kidney transplant
PTx	Pancreas transplant alone
BMI	Body mass index

Introduction

Options for pancreas transplantation (PTx) offer new hope to insulin-dependent diabetics. Advances in surgical skills and the availability of improved drugs for immunosuppression have improved the availability of PTx for diabetic patients. Simultaneous pancreas-kidney transplantation (SPKTx) offers a solution to patients with diabetes and renal impairment. Pancreas transplants were originally indicated for type I diabetics with hypoglycaemia unawareness, uncontrolled and brittle diabetes, and renal failure [1]. Today, the scope has increased to include adult diabetics, as well as various options for transplanting only the pancreas, renal transplantation as a bridge until pancreatic graft availability, and even islet cell transplantation in select situations [2]. Knowledge of the indications, potential concerns, and patient comorbidities are essential for the effective management of anaesthesia.

L. Kumar (✉) · R. N. Menon
Amrita Institute of Medical Sciences, Kochi, India
e-mail: lakshmi.k.238@gmail.com

Z. Milan and C. Goonasekera (eds.), *Anesthesia for Hepatico-Pancreatic-Biliary Surgery and Transplantation*, https://doi.org/10.1007/978-3-030-51331-3_25

Indications and Types of Pancreatic Transplantation

Insulin-dependent diabetes mellitus (IDDM) is believed to occur due to genetic, environmental, and autoimmune factors. IDDM diabetics with poor glucose control are ideal candidates for PTx. The benefits of PTx include better glucose control, prevention of the progression of diabetic complications, and even a regression of some of the complications [1].

There are several surgical options for PTx, presented in Table 25.1.

The following chapter will discuss challenges in the preoperative evaluation and preparation and anaesthetic management of PTx.

Indication of Patients for Pancreas and Kidney Transplantation

Patients are considered eligible for a pancreas transplant if they have or are at high risk of developing secondary complications of diabetes, or if they have disabling hypoglycaemia. Candidacy for SPK transplantation is based upon IDDM with C peptide levels <2 ng/ml or a C peptide level >2 ng/ml and a glomerular filtration rate <20 ml/kg/m^2 [3].

If a patient is being considered for PTx or pancreas transplantation after a kidney transplant (PAKTx), then the United Network of Organ Sharing criteria require at least one of three conditions: an exocrine deficiency of the pancreas, diabetes, or a need for the pancreas as a part of multi-organ transplant requirements. To be confirmed for inclusion on the transplantation list, the candidate should not have secondary complications related to diabetes and must be compliant with treatment protocols [4].

Table 25.1 Surgical options for pancreatic transplantation

Simultaneous pancreas and kidney transplant (SPKTx) is the most common operation (>70%), mainly indicated in IDDM patients with renal failure
Pancreas alone transplant (PTx) is indicated in IDDM patients with hypoglycaemia unawareness is much less common (<10%) Pancreas after kidney transplant (PAKTx) (<20%)
Simultaneous deceased donor pancreas and live donor kidney transplant (rare operation)
Total pancreatectomy and islet cell auto transplant
Laparoscopic live donor distal pancreatectomy for pancreas or islet cells allotransplant and pancreas kidney transplant
Islet cell allotransplant

Absolute contraindications for transplantation include active infection, malignancy, substance abuse, and psychiatric disorders [5]. Medical conditions that contraindicate transplantation are advanced coronary artery disease, severe respiratory illness, peripheral vascular disease, poor ejection fraction from cardiomyopathy, liver disorders, and positive serology results for HIV and hepatitis B [6].

Relative contraindications include age (>55 years), symptomatic cerebrovascular and peripheral vascular disease, and severe aortoiliac disease [6]. Body mass index (BMI)>30 has just been removed from the list of contraindications for PTx [7].

Preoperative Evaluation

A thorough history and physical examination are mandatory. Routine preoperative evaluation includes haematological, biochemical, renal, and liver function tests (Table 25.2). Specific tests for the pancreas include insulin C peptide, islet antibody (ICA), glutamic acid decarboxylase 65 (GAD65) antibody, and T cell autoreactivity testing.

Table 25.2 Preoperative evaluation: laboratory tests

System	Tests performed	Interpretation
Haematology	CBC, Differentials, CRP	Rule out incidental Infection
Liver	Total protein, Albumin, Globulin	Hypoalbuminemia in renal disease
	AST, ALT, ALP	Coexistent hepatic conditions and as baseline
Coagulation tests	Prothrombin time, aPTT, INR	vWF, factor VII deficiencies
Lipid profile	Total cholesterol, LDL-C, HDL-C, triglycerides	Renal failure can be associated with elevated triglycerides
Pancreas	Insulin, pro-insulin, split pro-insulin, C peptide	
	Islet cell antibody, GAD antibody	
Viral Screening	EBV, HSV, VZV, Hepatitis B and C, HIV, CMV	Rule out and identify concurrent infections
Blood	ABO Grouping and Rh tying	
	HLA typing and HLA antibody screen	
Tuberculosis (endemic countries)	Mantoux Text, C x R, sputum AFB,	Active infection contraindicates transplant
	QuantiFERON: immune gamma release assay for latent TB	

Cardiac Testing for Pancreas with/without Kidney Transplantation

There is significant heterogeneity in the cardiac screening process for patients with end-stage renal disease being evaluated for kidney and/or SPK transplantation. There is little evidence to suggest that current conservative strategies are effective in mitigating future cardiovascular events [8].

In our current practice, an initial cardiac evaluation includes an ECG and transthoracic echocardiography. Additional non-invasive diagnostic procedures are recommended for patients who have three or more of the following risk factors: diabetes, age>60 years, prior coronary artery disease, history of smoking, obesity, dyslipidaemia, dialysis>1 year, and left ventricular hypertrophy [9].

Cardiopulmonary exercise testing (CPEX) is gaining popularity for the preoperative assessment of all high-risk surgeries, including SKPTx [10]. Both CPEX and dobutamine stress echocardiography have negative predictive value [11].

Coronary angiography should be performed in high-risk patients. Sometimes, coronary stents have to be fitted before proceeding with major surgery [12].

Evaluation of Other Systems

Diabetes and renal disease may predispose patients to chest infections. Tuberculosis is endemic in India, and tests to rule out tuberculosis must be performed (Table 25.2) [13]. Anaemia is a common finding in PTx candidates [14]. Interstitial oedema and evidence of volume overload in the lungs and incidental pleural or pericardial effusion must be evaluated. These can be corrected by regular dialysis if patients are on dialysis. Endocrine abnormalities coexist in patients with chronic kidney disease. Modifications of hormonal feedback mechanisms and abnormal production, transport and metabolism, as well as uremic toxins and concomitant medications, impact endocrine function [15].

Airway difficulties are encountered more often in diabetics because of collagen crosslinking due to non-enzymatic glycosylation in connective tissues following chronic hyperglycaemia [16]. Given the evolving profiles of patients listed for SPKTx, elderly diabetics may be included. Vascular complications can coexist in elderly diabetics, and severe peripheral vascular disease and aortoiliac disease are contraindications for transplantation.

Autonomic dysfunction can coexist in elderly patients with long-standing diabetes, making them prone to hypotension and blood pressure fluctuations during surgery [17]. Gastroparesis can also predispose patients to aspiration during the induction of anaesthesia [5].

Pre-anaesthetic Management

Once a potential donor is available, a preliminary crossmatch is performed to assess suitability. The recipient is called to the hospital and blood investigations are repeated. To optimise fluids and electrolytes during the waiting period, dialysis is initiated upon admission if the patient is on dialysis awaiting SKPTx. Anaesthetic concerns for potential recipients are listed in Table 25.3.

Induction of immunosuppression is achieved with anti-thymocyte globulin (ATG) or alemtuzumab (Campath). ATG prepared from rabbit serum is associated with allergic reactions. Paracetamol and pheniramine maleate injections are given prior to the infusion of ATG at a dose of 1.0–1.5 mg/kg over 4 hours [17]. Allergic reactions, flushing, itching, and hypotension warrant temporarily stopping the infusion and treating with hydrocortisone. The duration of administration can be prolonged to minimise reactions.

Alemtuzumab is an anti-CD52 monoclonal antibody with lymphocyte-depleting potential [18, 19]. Alemtuzumab is well-tolerated with minimal reactions upon administration. Injection hydrocortisone (200 mg IV), oral tacrolimus (2 mg), and mycophenolate (1 mg) are also administered with sips of water.

Table 25.3 Anaesthetic concerns

System	Manifestations	Implications	Interventions to prevent / manage
Cardiovascular	Cardiomyopathy, coronary artery disease, pericardial effusions	Hypotension following induction Ischemic events	Cardiomyopathy improved by Regular dialysis? Role for intervention in coronary artery disease versus Medical management
Respiratory	Infections, pulmonary edema, pleural effusions	Postoperative pulmonary complications	Evaluate and treat infections Regular dialysis
Endocrine	Sex hormones, growth hormones and thyroid hormone		Correction/replacements started preoperatively
Autonomic dysfunction (AD)	Precipitate hypotension following anaesthesia Suboptimal response to direct and indirect sympathomimetics Impaired vasodilation	Predisposition to MACE Graft dysfunction Hypothermia	Identify AD preoperatively
Airway	Atlanto-occipital joint stiffness	Difficult intubation	Videolaryngoscopy
Vascular access	Difficult intravenous lines, Thrombosis in IJV/subclavian		USG screening prior to access
Electrolyte abnormalities	Hyperkalemia, hypocalcemia	Arryhthmia	Management of hyperkalemia and use of non potassium containing fluids

Methylprednisolone (7.5 mg/kg) is administered at the time of pancreatic graft implantation.

Patients usually have 4–6 hours of notice, which provides enough time for fasting requirements to be fulfilled. Clear fluids can be administered orally until 2 hours before the procedure, except in patients with symptoms of delayed gastric emptying and obesity. Anxiolytics such as midazolam are usually administered at 0.02–0.05 mg/kg, and metoclopramide is given as aspiration prophylaxis along with proton pump inhibitors. An intravenous line is secured in the non-fistula arm, and a balanced salt solution such as Ringer's lactate or Plasmalyte is started at a rate of 50 ml/h.

Surgical Procedure

Pancreatic Graft Implant

A midline incision extending from above the umbilicus to the pubic symphysis is performed for SPKTx. Bench work for the pancreatic graft may take about an hour and involves the connection of the graft superior mesenteric and splenic artery to the recipient common iliac artery (Fig. 25.1). The donor portal vein is anastomosed to the recipient inferior vena cava for venous drainage. Exocrine drainage is performed by the anastomosis of the C-shaped duodenal graft from the donor by a Roux-en-Y jejunal loop (Fig. 25.2). Pancreatic transplantation is a relatively long surgical procedure, and may take more than 7 h.

Kidney Graft Implant

In SPK transplantation, implant of the kidney begins after the pancreas, since the kidney can tolerate longer cold ischaemia times. The kidney is implanted in the extraperitoneal space, usually on the left iliac fossa, when a pancreatic implant is

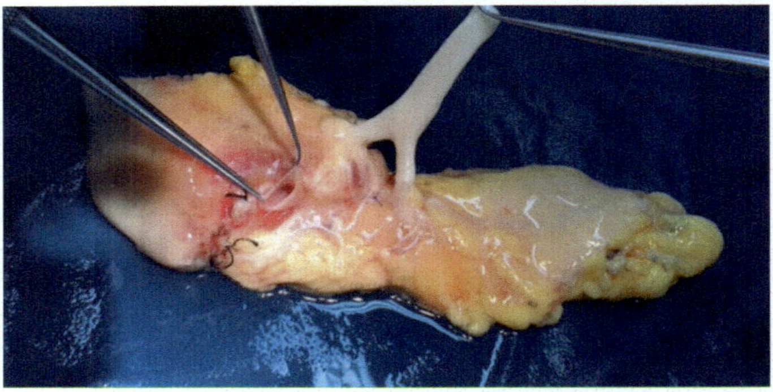

Fig. 25.1 Graft pancreas with Y shaped arterial graft and portal vein

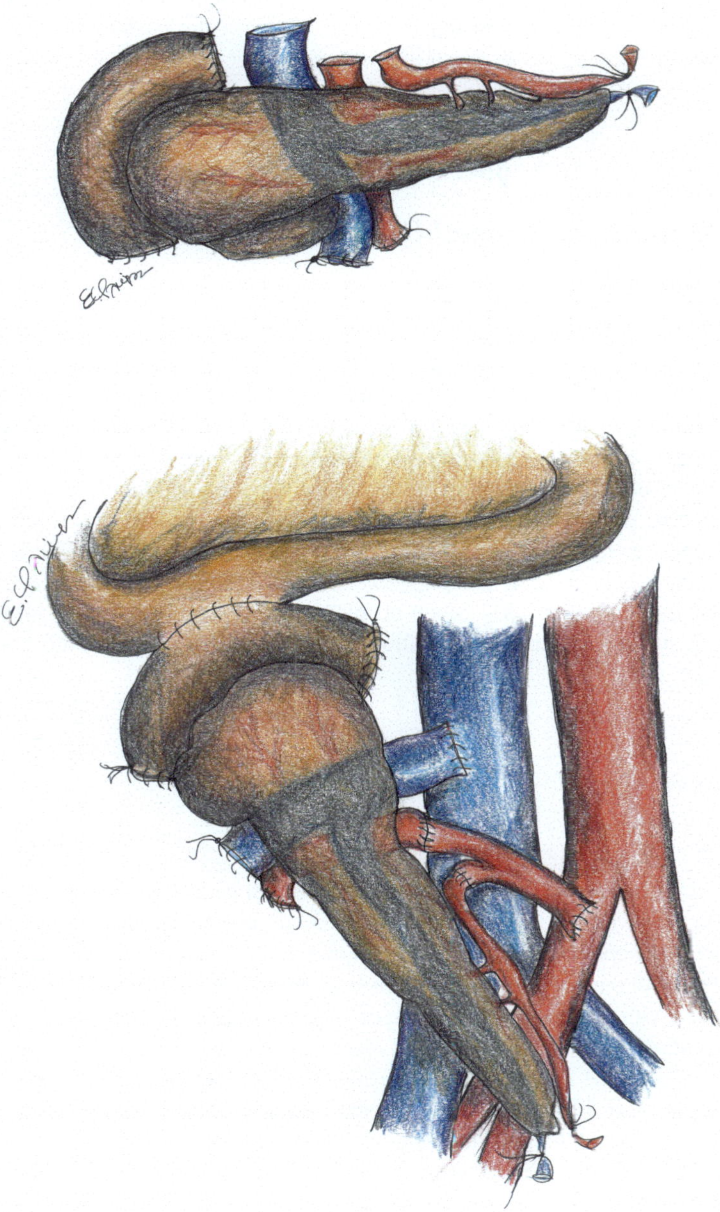

Fig. 25.2 On top the pancreatic graft; The donor's duodenum (D) is attached to the pancreas. The spleen has been removed. On the posterior surface of the gland are lying the vascular structures. Superior mesenteric vein (SMV), splenic vein (SV) and their confluence the portal vein (PV). Superior mesenteric artery (SMA), splenic artery (SA). Distal end of SMV, SV, SA are all ligated. On the bottom; the pancreatic graft implanted. The PV is directly implanted to the recipient's inferior vena cava (IVC). The proximal SMA and SA are implanted via cadaveric iliac graft to the recipient's right common iliac artery (RCIA). The donor's D is anastomosed to recipient's small bowel

being performed simultaneously. Anastomosis is begun with the renal vein to the external iliac vein, and reperfusion is completed with the perfusion of the renal artery anastomosis with the external iliac artery.

Anaesthesia and Intraoperative Management

Patient Position and General Care

The patient is positioned with attention to pressure points, care of the fistula (if present) arm, and intravenous access. The fistula arm is protected by soft padding and can be kept abducted to allow monitoring of the thrill during surgery to ensure patency.

Patients are provided with thromboembolic deterrent stockings during surgery. Intermittent pneumatic compression devices can be applied since surgery may take 6–8 hours for completion. Deep venous thrombosis prophylaxis is continued postoperatively for up to 6 hours after surgery until the patient is ambulant.

Heparin-free dialysis or regional anticoagulation in the dialysis circuit should be performed during pre-transplant dialysis to avoid anticoagulant effects during surgery.

Particulate antacid and H_2 receptor blockers are given prior to intubation. Warming blankets and warmers for intravenous fluids maintain normothermia during surgery.

Anaesthetic Agents

A modified rapid sequence induction with fentanyl (2–3 μg/kg), and propofol titrated to loss of verbal response followed by intubation with *cis*-atracurium or rocuronium (0.8–1.2 mg/kg) with cricoid pressure is practiced. The metabolism of propofol is dependent upon hepatic blood flow, and less than 0.3% is excreted unchanged by the kidneys. Propofol may be the ideal induction agent in renal failure patients.

In patients with preoperative cardiomyopathy, etomidate at 0.3 mg/kg can be used as it has minimal myocardial-depressant effects. The pharmacokinetics of etomidate are unaffected in renal failure, although protein binding may be reduced [20].

Neuromuscular blockade: The pharmacokinetics and duration of action of atracurium are unaffected by renal failure. The elimination half-life of laudanosine, the principal metabolite of atracurium, increases in renal failure, although the levels are insignificant. *Cis*-atracurium is superior, since 77% of its metabolism occurs through Hoffman elimination, versus 50% with atracurium. Furthermore, histamine release is low or negligible with *cis*-atracurium, reducing allergic reactions during intubation [21].

Inhalational agents are useful in patients with renal failure since they are not eliminated by the kidneys and can control haemodynamic responses. Accelerated induction and emergence has been reported in patients with severe anaemia and chronic kidney disease due to alterations in blood gas partition coefficient or minimum alveolar concentration. Isoflurane and desflurane are tolerated well in these patients [22]. Sevoflurane is reportedly nephrotoxic due to the formation of compound A in soda lime when used in flows less than 2 l/min, but no reports of nephrotoxicity in humans have emerged thus far [23]. Inhaled anaesthetics cause a transient reversible depression in renal function, glomerular filtration rate, renal blood flow, and urine output [24]. Data suggest that renal blood flow is maintained with halothane, isoflurane, and desflurane, but is decreased with enflurane and sevoflurane [25].

Perioperative analgesic options: Central neuraxial blockade provides excellent analgesia, but the safety of an indwelling epidural catheter with ongoing low molecular weight and the use of unfractionated heparin for graft vascular patency remains a cause for concern [26]. Opioid infusions, including fentanyl (0.5–0.8 μg/kg/h) or remifentanil (0.2–0.5 μg/kg/min), are commonly used. Ultrasound guided tranverse abdominus plane blocks are emerging as supplemental analgesic options that has opioid sparing benefits.

Invasive Lines

A central venous catheter is essential despite questions regarding its utility [27]. The optimal site is the right internal jugular vein on account of its more straight course and is lesser predisposition to thrombosis in comparison with the subclavian vein. Since jugular lines are often used as vascular access for haemodialysis preoperatively, ultrasound screening of the venous anatomy to rule out stenosis or thrombosis is ideal.

An arterial line in the radial artery of the non-fistula arm facilitates blood pressure monitoring and sampling for blood sugars and metabolic status. Arterial lines in the foot, dorsalis pedis, or posterior tibialis may be occluded during vascular anastomosis of the pancreas or the kidney and should be avoided.

Haemodynamic Monitoring

Most centres use central venous pressure and direct arterial blood pressure measurement as the only variables for haemodynamic monitoring during PTx or SKPTx. Haemodynamic changes during reperfusion for a pancreatic transplant can be significant. Although the magnitude is less than that of liver transplantation it can be more than changes during kidney transplantation. However, bleeding during pancreas transplantation is a common occurence; therefore, advanced haemodynamic monitoring may be required in more challenging cases.

Cardiac output (CO) monitoring using minimally invasive CO monitors may be useful in assessing volume status during surgery. These systems are derived from arterial pulse contour analysis, where the CO derived from the integrity of the arterial trace and vascular compliance can serve as an index of systemic vascular resistance [28]. The technology varies between different monitors, including Flotrac Vigileo (Edward Lifesciences, Irvine, CA, USA), which can be calibrated using patient demographics, and pulse contour analysis LiDCO (LiDCO Ltd., London, UK).

Fluid administration is guided by pulse pressure variation and stroke volume variation (SVV), which is based upon the principle that the SVV with respiration is dependent upon fluid deficit, and that correction of this deficit will increase CO within physiological limits. Additional advantages of the monitors mentioned above are data storage and reproducibility, which are becoming increasingly important in current medical practice.

Transoesophageal echocardiography can help with volume assessment and perioperative ischaemia assessment. As the parameters are objective, its reliability is very high; however, equipment availability and the need for technical training have limited its use in non-cardiac theatres [29].

Anaesthetic Management of Blood Sugars and Metabolic Abnormalities During Surgery

Intense blood sugar monitoring is required for PTx. Readings are taken hourly until pancreatic graft reperfusion, and then half-hourly until sugar levels stabilise. The aim is to keep blood sugars within 120–150 mg/dl (a higher value of 180 mg/dl may be acceptable for those prone to hypoglycaemia). An infusion of 5% dextrose at 50 ml/h is started during surgery. An infusion of insulin 1 IU/ml is connected to the patient and titrated according to the algorithm (Table 25.4). A number of protocols are available for blood sugar management [30], but it is prudent to begin with a conservative approach and incrementally increase the dosage. Insulin infusions are stopped immediately upon pancreatic graft reperfusion. Blood sugars will immediately normalise and dextrose administration can be adjusted accordingly.

Metabolic Abnormalities

Fluids in Pancreas Transplant Surgery

Generally, PTx surgery patients should be normovolaemic to maintain adequate blood pressure and transplanted organ perfusion and avoid kidney damage, since diabetic patients are prone to acute deterioration of already fragile kidneys. For SKPTx, a fluid replacement protocol for kidney transplantation should be followed.

Table 25.4 Perioperative Blood Sugar management protocol

Algorithm 1		Algorithm 2		Algorithm 3		Algorithm 4	
Blood sugar mg/dL	Insulin Units/h	Blood sugar mg/dL		Blood sugar mg/dL	Insulin Units/h	Blood sugar mg/dL	Insulin Units/h
70–99	–	70–99	–	70–99	–	70–99	–
100–124	0.2	100–124	1	100–124	1.5	100–124	2
125–149	0.5	125–149	2	125–149	3	125–149	4
150–175	1	150–175	3	150–175	4	150–175	6
176–200	1.5	176–200	4	176–200	5.5	176–200	8
201–225	2	201–225	5	201–225	7	201–225	10
226–250	2.5	226–250	6	226–250	8.5	226–250	12
251–275	3	251–275	7	251–275	10	251–275	14
276–300	3.5	276–300	8	276–300	11.5	276–300	16
301–325	4	301–325	9	301–325	13	301–325	18
326–350	4.5	326–350	10	326–350	14.5	326–350	20
350–375	5	350–375	11	350–375	16	350–375	22
>375	5.5	>375	12	>375	17.5	>375	24
276–300	3.5	276–300	8	276–300	11.5	276–300	16
301–325	4	301–325	9	301–325	13	301–325	18

[a]If the blood sugar is more than 200 mg/dL or has not dropped by>60 mg/dL in the previous hour: higher algorithm
[b]If blood sugar remains above 150 mg/dL for more than 2 hours: higher algorithm
[c]If the blood sugar is lower than 100 mg/dL for 2 readings: lower algorithm

Postoperative Care

At the end of surgery, most patients are extubated. A decision to extubate on the table is determined by the presence of haemodynamic stability on low or no vasopressor support, functioning grafts as witnessed by normalisation of blood sugars and urine output, a normal metabolic profile with no acidosis or dyselectrolytemia, normothermia, and adequacy of neuromuscular blockade reversal. Absence of bleeding or coagulopathy and euvolemic status may factor into the decision to extubate. Vascular complications are a common cause for concern in the immediate postoperative period and are typically due to technical issues rather than rejection [31] (Fig. 25.3).

Postoperative analgesia: Visceral pain may be greater with PTx than with many other abdominal procedures [32]. Analgesia for PTx has traditionally been managed with intravenous opioids. The side effects of opioid use can be reduced with reduced opioid dosage that can be facilitated with regional blocks.

Recently, the use of ultrasound-guided transversus abdominal plane (TAP) blocks have improved the scope for analgesia [32]. Bilateral TAP blocks involve the deposition of 15 ml of local anaesthetic solution on each side in the plane

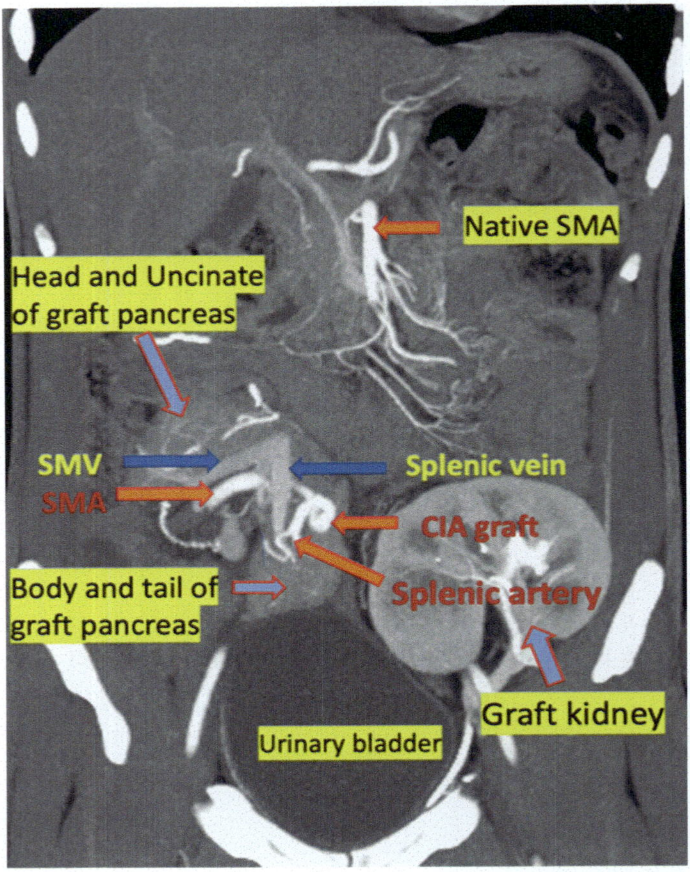

Fig. 25.3 SPK with vascular details. HOP: head of pancreas, SMV: Superior mesenteric vein, SMA: Superior mesenteric artery

between the internal oblique and transversus abdominis muscle. This provides analgesia in the ventral branches of T10–L1 [33]. Indeed, a recent study reported reduced use of morphine and faster intestinal function with a TAP block [34].

Rectus abdominis sheath block and bilateral erector spinae plane blocks can also be performed safely concurrent with low-molecular-weight heparin usage since it is a superficial block and the placement of catheters can provide continuous analgesia. This may not provide visceral analgesia, but it can treat the somatic pain from long surgical incisions [35, 36].

The addition of other peripheral analgesics as a part of a multimodal analgesia approach to postoperative analgesia is gaining popularity and is part of enhanced recovery.

Anaesthetic Management of Islet Transplantation (ITx) Patients

The indication for pancreatic ITx are the same as for PTx: IDDM patients with conservatively intractable hypoglycaemia unawareness syndrome [37]. Islets are isolated according to protocol, purified, cultured, and diluted for injection via the portal vein. The procedure consists of the injection of processed pancreatic islets transhepatically into the portal vein under local anaesthesia and radiological control, or under general anaesthesia through laparoscopy or laparotomy [38].

Immunosuppression is required for this procedure and consists of anti-T lymphocyte globulin treatment pre-transplant and a single dose one day post-transplant, methylprednisolone, and one dose of entanercept (followed by maintenance treatment based on sirolimus and low-dose tacrolimus) [39].

Complications and Outcomes of PTx

The results of PTx are continually improving. Graft and patient survival rates increase in every three-year report. However, numerous complications are still reported in the literature. Intraoperative bleeding is a relatively common perioperative complication during PTx. Other surgical complications include infection and duodenal graft complications requiring duodenotomy [40]. Acute rejection and chronic graft rejection are standard complications associated with all transplant surgeries. Another recently published and unusual complication (incidence: 1:400) is the risk of spinal cord ischaemia [41]. Hypotension intraoperatively and postoperatively is a prominent risk factor for spinal cord ischaemia.

In SPK transplantation, systemic complications such as acute myocardial infarction, atrial fibrillation, chronic heart failure (CHF), and transient ischaemic attack/stroke are present in 4.9% of patients [42]. Significantly higher rates of stroke and CHF are found in SPKTx compared with PAKTx/PTX. Based on the latest results from the US national database, intrahospital mortality does not significantly differ between SPKTx and PACTx/PTx recipients [42]. Uraemia is a well-known independent risk factor for stroke.

Lower survival rates are reported in NIDDM in all types of PTx, likely secondary to this group's older age and comorbidities [42].

Complications Following ITx

Although ITx appears much less invasive than PTx, postoperative complications are still present. Acute rejection is the most feared complication [37, 43]. Other rare complications include graft infection, intrahepatic haematoma, portal vein thrombosis, orthostatic hypotension, sepsis, cholecystitis, urinary tract infection, pneumonia, thrombocytopaenia, and leucopoenia [44].

Allograft thrombosis is responsible for most cases of early graft failure. Early postoperative anticoagulation regimes include the following: none, subcutaneous heparin/aspirin, and heparin infusion [44].

Conclusions

PTx has the potential to improve the quality of life for diabetic patients while preventing end organ complications. Advances in immunosuppression and expansion of the graft pool may improve graft function in the future. The anaesthesiologist plays a crucial role in supporting the surgical process, and a thorough understanding of these technical advances will ensure optimal care for the patient. Newer anaesthetic agents with faster recovery, optimal haemodynamic management, and improved analgesic options will enable further progress in anaesthesia care in the future.

References

1. Dholakia S, Mittal S, Quiroga I, Gilbert J, Sharples EJ, Ploeg RJ, Friend PJ. Pancreas Transplantation: Past, Present Future. Am J Med. 2016;129:667–73.
2. Stites E, Kennealey P, Wiseman AC. Current status of pancreas transplantation. Curr Opin Nephrol Hypertens. 2016;25:563–9.
3. Bhargava R, Mitsides N, Saif I, MacDowall P, Woywodt A. C-peptide and combined kidney-pancreas transplantation. NDT Plus. 2009;2:489–92.
4. https://unos.org/wp-content/uploads/unos/Pancreas_Brochure.pdf Accessed 22 Jan 2020.
5. Macnab WR, Pichel AC. Anesthesia for pancreas transplant. Contin Educ Anaesth Crit Care Pain. 2005;5:149–52.
6. Scalea JR, Redfield RR III, Arpali E, Leverson G, Sollinger HW, Kaufman DB, Odorico JS. Pancreas transplant in older patients is safe but patient selection is paramount. Transplant Int. 2016;29:810–8.
7. Kandaswamy R, Stock PG, Gustafson SK, SkeansMA, Urban R, Fox A et al. OTPN/SRTR 2018 Annual Data Report: Pancreas. Am J Surg 2020;20 Suppl s1:131–92.
8. Mathur AK, Stemper-Bartkus C, Engholdt K, Thorp A, Dosmann M, Khamash H, et al. Identifying patterns of adverse events of solid organ transplantation through departmental case reviews. Mayo Clin Proc Innov Qual Outcomes. 2019;3:335–43.
9. Lentine KL, Costa SP, Weir MR, Robb JF, Fleisher LA, Kasiske BL et al. Cardiac disease evaluation and management among kidney and liver transplantation candidates. A scientific statement from the American Heart Association and the American College of Cardiology Foundation and on behalf of the American Heart Association Council on the kidney in cardiovascular disease and council on peripheral vascular disease. Circulation. 2012;126:617–63.
10. Chakkera HA, Angadi SS, Heilman RL, Kaplan B, Scott RL, Bollempalli H, et al. Cardiorespiratory fitness (Peak Oxygen Uptake): Safe and effective measure for cardiovascular screening before kidney transplant. J Am Heart Assoc. 2018;7(11). pii:e008662.
11. Bates JR, Sawada SG, Segar DS, Spaedy AJ, Petrovic O, Fineberg NS, et al. Evaluation using dobutamine stress echocardiography in patients with insulin-dependent diabetes mellitus before kidney and/or pancreas transplantation. Am J Cardiol. 1996;77:175–9.

12. Mann DM, Fernandez S, Mondal Z, Laskow D, Osband A, Debroy M, et al. Role of coronary angiography in the assessment of cardiovascular risk in kidney transplant candidates. Am J Cardiol. 1996;77:175–9.
13. Abad CL, Razonable RR. Prevention and treatment of tuberculosis in solid organ transplant recipients. Expert rev Anti Infect Ther. 2020;18:63–73.
14. Gomez MF, Aljure O, Ciancio G, Lynn M. Hemoglobin-based oxygen carrier rescues double-transplant patient from life-threatening anaemia. Am J Transplant. 2017;7:1941–4.
15. Singh A.K, Raed A, Kari J. Endocrine complications of chronic kidney disease. In: Kimmel PL, Rosenberg ME, editors. Chronic kidney disease. Chapter 26. 1st ed. Academic Press is an imprint of Elsevier.
16. Warner ME, Contreras MG, Warner MA, Schroeder DR, Munn SR, Maxson PM. Diabetes mellitus and difficult laryngoscopy in renal and pancreatic transplant patients. Anaesthesia Analgesia. 1998;86:516–9.
17. Khurana A, McCuskey CF, Slavcheva EG. Orthostatic hypotension in kidney pancreas transplant patients and it's relation to pre-existing autonomic neuropathy. Exp Clin Transplant. 2008;6:127–31.
18. Mohty M, Bacigalupo A, Saliba F, Zuckermann A, Morelon E, Lebranchu Y. New directions for rabbit antithymocyte globulin (Thymoglobulin(®)) in solid organ transplants, stem cell transplants and autoimmunity. Drugs. 2014;74:1605–34.
19. Bösmüller C, Messner F, Margreiter C, et al. Good results with individually adapted long-term immunosuppression following Aemtuzumab versus ATG induction therapy in combined kidney-pancreas transplantation: a single-centre report. Ann Transplant. 2019;24:52–6.
20. Morgan, Mikhail. Anaesthesia for patients with kidney disease. In: Butterworth JF, Mackey DC, Wasnick JD, editors. Clinical anaesthesiology, Chapter 30. 5th ed. McGraw Hill Education. p. 653–669.
21. Noranee N, Fathi M, Golestani Eraghi M, Dabbagh A, Massoudi N. The effect of intraoperative alkali treatment on recovery from atracurium-induced neuromuscular blockade in renal transplantation: a randomized trial. Anesth Pain Med. 2017;7:e42660.
22. Steadman R.H, Wray C.L. Anesthesia for solid organ transplantation. In: Ronald D. Miller, editor. Miller's anesthesia, Chapter 74. 8th ed. Associate Editors: Cohen NH, Eriksson LI, Fleischer LA, Weiner-Kornish JP, Young WL. p. 2262–89.
23. Savran Karandez M, Senturk Ciftci H, Tefk T, Oktar T, Nane I, Turkmen A, et al. Effect of different volatile anaesthetics on cytokine and chemokine production after ischaemia-reperfusion injury in patients undergoing living donor kidney transplant. Exp Clin Transplant. 2019;17:68–74.
24. Wu Y, Jin S, Zhang L, Cheng J, Hu X, Cheng H, et al. Minimal alveolar concentration-awake of sevoflurane is decreased in patients with end-stage renal disease. Anesth Analg. 2019;128:77–82.
25. Iguchi N, Kosaka J, Booth LC, Iguchi Y, Evans RG, Bellomo R, et al. Renal perfusion, oxygenation, and sympathetic nerve activity during volatile or intravenous general anaesthesia in sheep. Br J Anaesth. 2019;122:342–9.
26. Sadowski SM, Andres A, Morel P, Schiffer E, Frossard JL, Platon A, et al. Epidural anesthesia improves pancreatic perfusion and decreases the severity of acute pancreatitis.World J Gastroenterol. 2015;21:12448–56.
27. Marik PE, Baram M, Vahid B. Does central venous pressure predict fluid responsiveness? A systematic review of the literature and the tale of seven mares. Chest. 2008;134:172–8.
28. Marik PE. Noninvasive cardiac output monitors: a state-of the-art review. J Cardiothorac Vasc Anesth. 2013;27:121–34.
29. Bubenek-Turconi ŞI, Hendy A, Băilă S, Drăgan A, Chioncel O, Văleanu L et al. The value of a superior vena cava collapsibility index measured with a miniaturized transoesophageal monoplane continuous echocardiography probe to predict fluid responsiveness compared to stroke volume variations in open major vascular surgery: a prospective cohort study. J Clin Monit Comput. 2019 July 5. https://doi.org/10.1007/s10877-019-00346-4. [Epub ahead of print].

30. Riou M, Renaud-Picard B, Munch M, Lefebvre F, Baltzinger P, Porzio M, et al. Organized Management of Diabetes Mellitus in Lung Transplantation: Study of Glycemic Control and Patient Survival in a Single Center. Transplant Proc. 2019;51:3375–84. https://doi.org/10.1016/j.transproceed.2019.07.019 (Epub 2019 Nov 14).
31. Surowiecka-Pastewka A, Matejak-Górska M, Frączek M, Sklinda K, Walecki J, Durlik M. Endovascular interventions in vascular complications after simultaneous pancreas and kidney transplantations: A Single-Center Experience. Ann Transplant. 2019;24:199–207.
32. Yeap YL, Fridell JA, Wu D, Mangus RS, Kroepfl E, Wolfe J, et al. Comparison of methods of providing analgesia after pancreas transplant: IV opioid analgesia versus transversus abdominis plane block with liposomal bupivacaine or continuous catheter infusion. Clin Transplant. 2019;33:e13581.
33. Milan Z, Tabor D, McConnell P, Pickering J, Kocarev M, du Feu F, Barton S. Three different approaches to Transversus abdominis Plane Block: a cadaveric study. Med Glas (Zenica). 2011;8:181–4.
34. Jankovic ZB, Pollard SG, Nachiappan MM. Continuous transversus abdominis plane block for renal transplant recipients. Anesth Analg. 2009;109:1710–1.
35. Hausken J, Rydenfelt K, Horneland R, Ullensvang K, Kjøsen G, Tønnessen TI, et al. Experience with rectus sheath block for postoperative analgesia after pancreas transplant: a retrospective observational study. Transplant Proc. 2019;51:479–84. https://doi.org/10.1016/j.transproceed.2019.01.065 (Epub 2019 Jan 28).
36. Kelava M, Anthony D, Elsharkaway H. Continuous erector spinae block for postoperative analgesia after thoracotomy in a lung transplant recipient. J Cardiothorac Vasc Anaesthesia. 2018;32:e9–11.
37. Bachul PJ, Gołębiewska JE, Basto L, Gołąb K, Anteby R, Wang LJ, et al. BETA-2 score is an early predictor of graft decline and loss of insulin independence after pancreatic islet allotransplantation. Am J Transplant. 2019:1–8.
38. Movahedi B, Keymeulen B, Lauwers MH, Goes E, Cools N, Delvaux G. Laparoscopic approach for human islet transplantation into a defined liver segment in type-1 diabetic patients. Transpl Int. 2003;16:186–90.
39. Voglova B, Zahradnicka M, Girman P, Kriz Jan, Berkova Z, Koblas T, et al. Benefits of islet transplantation as an alternative to pancreas transplantation: retrospective study of more than 10 years of experience in a single center. Rev Diabet Stud. 2016;14: 10–21.
40. Pieroni E, Napoli N, Lombardo C, Marchetti P, Occhipinti M, Cappelli C, et al. Duodenal graft complications requiring duodenectomy after pancreas and pancreas-kidney transplantation. Am J Transplant. 2018;18:1388–96.
41. Phillips BL, Papadakis G, Bell R, Sinha S, Callaghan CJ, Akyol M, et al. Spianal cord ischemia in pancreas transplantation. Transplantation. 2019. https://doi.org/10.1097/TP.0000000000003028. [Epub ahead of print].
42. Zerillo J, Smith NK, Sakai T. Noteworthy literature published in 2017 for abdominal organ transplantation. Seemin Cardiothorac Vasc Anaesth. 2018;22:67–80.
43. Raveh V, Ciancio G, Burke GW, Figueiro J, Chen L, Morsi M, et al. Susceptibility-directed anticoagulation after pancreas transplantation: A single-center retrospective study. Clin Transplant. 2019;33:e13619.
44. Bertuzzi F, Colussi G, Lauterio A, De Carlis L. Intramuscular islet allotransplantation in type 1 diabetes mellitus. Eur Rev Med Pharmacol Sci. 2018;22:1731–6.

Part V
Paediatric

Chapter 26
Anaesthesia for Paediatric HPB Surgery

James Gill and Anish Gupta

Introduction

Anaesthesia for paediatric hepatico-pancreatico-biliary (HPB) surgery is complex, diverse, and challenging. The role of the anaesthetist involves preassessment, optimisation, choice of anaesthesia for the procedure, and postoperative analgesia and care. Knowledge of a plethora of liver conditions and the multifaceted organ dysfunction that accompanies serious liver disease is essential.

This chapter focuses on the anaesthetist's roles in preassessment and the provision of intra- and postoperative analgesia and care for children undergoing HPB surgery.

Kasai Portoenterostomy for Biliary Atresia

Biliary atresia (BA) is a rare congenital anomaly in which an absence of intra- and extrahepatic bile ducts leads to cholestasis, hepatic fibrosis, and cirrhosis [1]. It has an incidence of about 1 in 14,000 live births in the United Kingdom and is the most common indication for paediatric liver transplantation (LT) [2]. About 25% of cases have associated anomalies, including polysplenia, abdominal situs inversus, and atrial septal defect [2, 3]. Affected babies appear normal, but signs of cholestasis, such as failure to thrive, malabsorption, pale stools, and jaundice (conjugated hyperbilirubinaemia), appear soon after birth. The Kasai portoenterostomy (PE) is a surgical procedure used to establish bile drainage and halt the

J. Gill (✉) · A. Gupta
Consultant Anaesthetist, King's College Hospital, London, UK
e-mail: James.gill@nhs.net

A. Gupta
e-mail: anish.gupta@nhs.net

Z. Milan and C. Goonasekera (eds.), *Anesthesia for Hepatico-Pancreatic-Biliary Surgery and Transplantation*, https://doi.org/10.1007/978-3-030-51331-3_26

progression to hepatic fibrosis and cirrhosis. The overall survival of children with BA is excellent, although most patients ultimately require liver transplantation (LT) [2, 4].

The main anaesthetic challenges, apart from the very young age of the patient at the time of surgery, are intermittent interruption of venous drainage via the inferior vena cava (IVC) by surgical retraction, fluid loss and replacement, and provision of postoperative analgesia [5]. Coagulopathy is unlikely once the baby has been given vitamin K [1]. Central venous catheters (CVCs) are often used and may be retained after the operation for fluid and drug administration and blood sampling. In the absence of an associated cardiac abnormality or other significant indication, no invasive blood pressure measurements are required. There is some evidence that sevoflurane anaesthesia may have protective effects on hepatic blood flow in infants with obstructive jaundice who have reduced portal blood flow and a compensatory increase in hepatic artery blood flow [5]. Epidural analgesia can usually be offered safely [6]. Patients with epidurals have lower pain scores, are more likely to be extubated in the operating theatre, and have a shorter hospital stay [6]. Alternatively, nurse-controlled analgesia (NCA) utilising a morphine pump provides good analgesic results and mitigates patient discomfort due to remaining nil by mouth for up to 4 days due to bile duct-to-bowel anastomosis.

Approximately one third of PE procedures are partially successful for various periods of time. Another one third initially reduce jaundice but cause persistent problems, such as recurrent cholangitis, leading to the development of liver cirrhosis. The final third never achieve a significant decrease in serum bilirubin and require early LT [2, 4]. Total bilirubin and albumin levels and variceal bleeding 3 months after a PE procedure are predictive of the need for LT [2–4].

Most patients with BA typically require LT before reaching adulthood [7]. Those who reach adulthood with their own liver are still at risk of needing LT [7]. The most common indications for LT listing are refractory cholangitis (31%), synthetic failure (21%), and variceal bleeding (14%) [8]. Patients listed for LT by an adult team wait longer than patients listed by a paediatric team but are more likely to require intensive care at the time of listing and have a poorer outcome of LT [8].

Choledochal Cyst Resections and Other Hepatico-Entero Anastomosis Surgeries

These rare abnormalities of the biliary tree are cystic dilations that may be asymptomatic or cause pain, obstructive jaundice, or an abdominal mass [9]. A choledochal cyst perforation is a very rare event, with symptoms, such as abdominal pain and biliary peritonitis, that usually occur at an early age and may result in biliary peritonitis and a fatal outcome [9, 10]. Surgery, laparoscopic or open, is conducted to excise the cyst, as there is potential for perforation or later malignancy [11]. The anaesthetic technique is similar to that used for BA. Laparoscopic and robotic surgery for a choledochal cyst or any other biliary-entero anastomosis is less invasive than open surgery [12]. Consequently, analgesia is adapted to the smaller surgical incision, and recovery is faster than for open surgery [13].

Liver Tumour Resection

Hepatoblastoma, the most common paediatric liver tumour with an incidence of about 1 per million, usually presents in the first 3 years of life [14]. Liver function is usually normal. Clinical symptoms are discrete, and a diagnosis may be made when the tumour is already very advanced. Treatment is chemotherapy (doxorubicin, anthracycline, or cisplatin) followed by surgical resection, if possible; if surgical resection is not possible, LT can be curative if there is no extrahepatic disease [14]. Doxorubicin can cause cardiomyopathy, which requires an echocardiographic assessment [15]. The timing of the surgery must be carefully planned between cycles of chemotherapy to ensure minimal disruption. Resection may be considered 2 weeks after completing a chemotherapy cycle assuming any neutropenia has recovered above 0.5×10^9/L, followed by a further 2-week recovery from surgery before the start of subsequent chemotherapy cycles as dictated by tumour staging [14].

Other rare malignant liver tumours seen in paediatric populations are cholangiocarcinoma, hepatocellular carcinoma, paediatric hepatic sarcoma, and other malignant tumours involving the liver, including liver metastases [16].

There are essentially three important perioperative challenges for the anaesthetist for any liver tumour in the paediatric population: haemorrhage, air embolus, and post-resection liver insufficiency [17].

Major haemorrhage is an ever-present risk during liver tumour resection. A low central venous pressure (CVP) strategy that reduces perioperative bleeding in adult patients should be used in the paediatric population. Unlike adults, who rarely require a blood transfusion, one third to one half of paediatric patients undergoing liver resection require a perioperative blood transfusion (PBT) [17]. Patients who require a PBT are more likely to have preoperative risk factors, including ventilatory dependence, haematological disorders, chemotherapy, sepsis, transfusion before surgery, and American Society of Anaesthesiologists class $\geq$3 [17].

Because of the risk for massive bleeding, venous access should include a large-bore CVC to facilitate rapid transfusion, the administration of drugs, and CV pressure monitoring. Vascular access should be in the upper body to ensure drainage into the superior vena cava, as the IVC may be occluded at some point during the surgery. A large proportion of patients already have Hickman catheters. These are not ideal for intraoperative use and should generally not be used to minimise the risk for sepsis. However, if there is no adequate vascular access before the induction of anaesthesia, a Hickman line can be used to induce anaesthesia. Rapid transfusion and fluid warming devices appropriate to the size of the child are necessary, as is timely access to large volumes of blood products. The use of intraoperative red cell salvage for cases of malignant tumour resection in older children is controversial; the benefits of avoiding allogenic blood transfusion and potential immunomodulation must be balanced against systemic infusion of malignant cells and possible metastasis [18]. Leucocyte depletion filters appear effective for removing tumour cells from salvaged blood.

Surgery may involve a right or left hemi-hepatectomy. This can expose large hepatic veins held open to the risk for air entrainment and embolus. Relative fluid restriction, which is often used to decrease liver congestion and bleeding, contributes to the high risk for air embolism.

Intermittent clamping of the portal vein and hepatic artery or their branches may be used to reduce bleeding and expedite surgery, but these manoeuvres can lead to cardiovascular instability and dysfunction in the remaining liver. There is no consensus about the use of invasive or noninvasive haemodynamic monitoring during liver resection in the paediatric population.

Hepatic dysfunction may also result from a large-volume resection, which can increase metabolic acidosis, hypoglycaemia, and coagulopathy. Current preoperative imaging techniques allow anaesthetists to predict postoperative complications and choose the surgical option that will prevent their occurrence.

The majority of cases are returned to a high dependency unit after surgery. PBT is associated with a longer postoperative length of stay [17].

Postoperative complications include biliary leakage, bleeding, liver dysfunction, liver failure, acute kidney injury, the need for reoperation, peritonitis, chylous ascites, pneumonia, urinary infection, CVC infection, deep vein thrombosis, and wound dehiscence [19].

Liver insufficiency is one of the most serious postoperative complications in patients undergoing extensive liver resection [19]. Among several strategies for increasing resectability of the liver tumour are portal vein occlusion (embolisation or ligature), bilateral tumour resection in two stages, and resection combined with locoregional therapy [16, 19].

Anaesthesia for Complex HPB Procedures

A two-stage hepatectomy with initial portal vein ligation and in situ splitting of the liver parenchyma is known as ALPPS (associating liver partition with portal vein ligation for staged hepatectomy) [20], and it has been performed in paediatric patients considered inoperable in the past, with good outcomes.

More extensive tumours invade surrounding structures (i.e., lymph nodes and the adrenal gland) and blood vessels, such as the IVC. In the most severe cases, a tumour can invade the vena cava up to the right atrium, or an intra-caval clot can extend up to the right atrium [21]. Several case reports have been published in which cardiopulmonary bypass and controlled hypothermia were used to successfully remove caval and right atrial tumours or blood clots [22]. Combined liver and cardiac surgery for these complex cases requires coordination between teams and hospitals with paediatric cardiac and liver teams.

Another complex extensive liver tumour resection surgery that requires complex anaesthesia in paediatric HPB surgery is ex vivo liver resection and autotransplantation with cardiopulmonary bypass. In one case study, a patient had a massive liver tumour and thrombus in the IVC and right atrium. As it was difficult to achieve complete tumour resection using conventional hepatectomy, *ex vivo* resection with the patient on bypass led to a positive outcome [23].

These complex cases are rare in the paediatric population. They require interdisciplinary skill, such as cardiac and HPB anaesthesia and some planning beforehand.

Anaesthesia for Vascular Radiological Procedures

Vascular radiological procedures, such as the use of transjugular porto-systemic shunts (TIPSS), liver biopsy, portal vein or hepatic artery embolisation, and radiofrequency ablation for liver tumours, may require general anaesthesia. Inserting a Hickman's line in children also requires general anaesthesia. Intubating is advised for all above procedures, to secure the airway. Deranged clotting should not be corrected for the TIPSS procedure, as there is no evidence that a corrected INR will reduce bleeding [24]. Hypervolaemia achieved with transfusion of fresh frozen plasma (FFP) can cause more damage than benefit in these procedures [25].

Anaesthesia for Vascular Surgical Procedures

Vascular surgical procedures called meso-caval shunts and portosystemic venous shunt ligation can be performed in children with portal hypertension or congenital portosystemic venous shunts [26]. When working with vascular shunt procedures, anaesthetists should be prepared for massive bleeding: a good-size intravascular cannula, CVC, and invasive BP monitoring should be employed in situ, and blood and products should be on standby in case they are needed. Postoperative transient acute kidney injury is expected in cases of massive bleeding.

Anaesthesia for Paediatric Pancreatic Surgery

Pancreatic tumours are relatively uncommon in the paediatric population. Anaesthesia for a distal pancreatectomy or the Whipple procedure are similar as for adult pancreatic surgery, with invasive BP monitoring, CVC, and epidural analgesia [27].

Postoperative Analgesia for Paediatric HPB Surgery

Numerous options are available for intra- and postoperative analgesia in this patient population. Patient- and nurse-controlled or patient-controlled analgesia (PCA), with or without background infusion, is the most commonly used [28]. Epidural analgesia provides good pain control when it works and when there is an adequate pain team capable of delivering boluses and dealing with issues such as hyper- or hypofunctional epidural analgesia, hypotension, and reduced urine output [29]. Some paediatric anaesthetists use a caudal approach to the epidural space with a long epidural catheter reaching desired dermatomas up to T7/8 [30, 31]. Multimodal analgesia that includes a transversus abdominis plane block and PCA, paravertebral block and PCA, wound catheter and others is available and used by anaesthetists with special interest in paediatric regional anaesthesia [32–35]. A preoperative discussion with the parents and child about available analgesic options can contribute to a good outcome. Epidural analgesia can be used for liver resection when postoperative extubation is planned, without risk of epidural haematoma [36].

References

1. Bromley P, Bennett J. Anaesthesia for children with liver disease. Continu Educ Anaesthesia, Criti Care Pain. Brit J Anaesthesia. 2014;14:207–12.
2. Ramos-Gonzales G, Ekisofon S, Dee EC, Staffa SJ, Medford S, Lillehei C, et al. Predictors of need for liver transplantation in children undergoing hepatoportoenterostomy for biliary atresia. J Pediatr Surg. 2019;54:1127–31.
3. Harumatsu T, Muraji T, MasuyuaR, Ohtani H, Nagai T, Yano K et al. Microvascular proliferation of the portal vein branches in the liver of biliary atresia patients at Kasai operation is associated with a better long-term clinical outcome. Pediatr Surg Int 2019;35:1437–41
4. Sohn H, Park S, Kang Y, Koh H, Han SJ, Kim S. Predicting variceal bleeding in patients with biliary atresia. Scand J Gastroenterol. 2019;54:1385–90.
5. Zhou ZJ, Wang X, Song Z, Dong KR, Zheng S. Effect of sevoflurane anaesthesia on hepatic blood flow in infants with obstructive hapatobiliary disease. Acta Anaesthesiol Scand. 2016;60:1067–74.
6. Phelps HM, Robinson JR, Chen H, Luckett TR, Conroy PC, Gills LA, et al. Enhancing recovery after Kasai portoenterostomy with epidural analgesia. J Surg Res. 2019;243:354–62.
7. Jain V, Burford C, Alexander EC, Sutton H, Dhawan A, Joshi D, et al. Prognostic markers at adolescence in patients requiring liver transplantation for biliary atresia in adulthood. J Hepatol. 2019;71:71–7.
8. Samyn M, Davenport M, Jain V, Hadzic N, Joshi D, Heneghan M, et al. Young people with biliary atresia requiring liver transplantation: a distinct population requiring specialist care. Transplantation. 2019;103:99–107.
9. Soares KC, Goldstein SD, Ghaseb MA, Kamel I, Hackman DJ, Pawlik TM. Pediatric choledochal cysts: diagnosis and current management. Pediatr SurgInt. 2017;33:637–50.
10. Diao M, Li L, Cheng W. Timing of choledochal cyst perforation. Hepatology. 2019. https://doi.org/10.1002/hep.30902. [Epub ahead of print].

11. Diao M, Li L, Cheng W. Laparoscopic management for aberrant hepatic duct in children with choledochal cyst. Surg Endosc. 2019;33:2376–80.
12. Koga H, Murakami H, Ochi T, Miyano G, Lange GJ, Yamataka A. Comparison of robotic versus laparoscopic hepaticojejunostomy for choledochal cyst in children: a first report. Pediatr Surg Int. 2019;35:1421–5.
13. Edney JC, Lam H, Raval MV, Heiss KF, Austin TM. Implementation of an enhanced recovery program in pediatric laparoscopic colorectal patients does not worsen analgesia despite reduced perioperative opioids: a retrospective, matched, non-inferiority study. Reg Anesth pain Med. 2019;44:123–9.
14. Yuan XJ, Wang HM, Jiang H, Tang MJ, Li ZL, Zou X, et al. Multidisciplinary effort in treating children with hepatoblastoma in China. Cancer Lett. 2016;375:39–46.
15. Prathumsap N, Shinlapawittayatorn K, Chattipakom SC, Chattipakom N. Effects of doxorubicin on the heart. From molecular mechanisms to intervention strategies. Eur J Pharmacol. 2019:172818. https://doi.org/10.1016/j.ejphar.2019.172818. [Epub ahead of print].
16. Aronson DC, Meyers RL. Malignant tumors of the liver in children. Semin Pediatr Surg. 2016;25:265–75.
17. Gonzales DO, Ciooper JN, Mantell E, Minneci PC, Deans KJ, Aldrink JH. Perioperative blood transfusion and complications in children undergoing surgery for solid tumours. J Surg Res. 2017;216:129–37.
18. Elias D, Lapierre V, Billard V. Perioperative autotransfusion with salvage blood in cancer surgery. Ann Fr Anesth Reanim. 2000;19:739–44.
19. Grisotti G, Cowles R. Complications in pediatric hepatobiliary surgery. Semin Pediatr Surg. 2016:25:388–94.
20. Wiederkehr JC, Avilla SG, Mattos E, Coelho IM, Ledesma JA, Conceicao AF, et al. Associating liver partition with portal vein ligation and staged hepatectomy (ALPPS) for treatment of liver tumors in children. J Pediatr Surg. 2015;50:1227–31.
21. Shi Y, Commander SJ, Masand PM, Heczey A, Goss JA, Vasudevan SA. Vascular invasion is a prognostic indicator in hepatoblastoma. J Pediatr Surg. 2017;52:956–61.
22. Sayed S, Prabhu S, Fawcett J, Choo K, Alphonso N. A systematic surgical approach to hepatoblastoma with intracardiac extension. Asian Cardiovasc Thoracic Ann. 2017;25:300–3.
23. Shi SJ, Wang DL, Hu W, Peng F, Kang Q. Ex vivo liver resection and autotransplantation with cardiopulmonary bypass for hepatoblastoma in children: a case report. Pediatr Transplant. 2018;22:e13268.
24. Rowley MW, Agrawal S, Seetharman AB, Hirch KS. Real-time ultrasound-guided paracentesis by radiologist: near zero risk of hemorrhage without correction of coagulopathy. J Vasc Interv Radiol. 2019;30:259–64.
25. Schepis F, Turco L, Bianchini M, Villa E. Prevention and management of bleeding risk related to invasive procedures in cirrhosis. Semin Liver Dis. 2018;38:215–29.
26. Nobre S, Khanna R, Bab N, Kyrana E, Height S, Karani J, et al. Primary Budd-Chiari syndrome in children: King's college hospital experience. J Pediatr Gastroenterol Nutr. 2017;65:93–6.
27. Cao G, Mendez J, Navacchia D. Pancreatoblastoma in paediatric patient: anatomo-pathological aspects of a case with multiple hepatic metastases. Ecancer. 2018;12:861.
28. Rashed AN, Tomlin S, Aguado V, Forbes B, Whittlesea C. Sources and magnitude of error in preparing morphine infusions for nurse-patient controlled analgesia in UK paediatric hospital. Int J Clin Pharm. 2016;38:1069–74.
29. Warmann SW, Lang S, Fideler F, Blumenstock G, Schlisio B, Kumpf M, et al. Perioperative epidural analgesia in children undergoing major abdominal tumor surgery-a single center experience. J Pediatr Surg. 2014;49:551–5.

30. Singh R, Kumar N, Singh P. Randomized controlled trial comparing morphine or clonidine with bupivacaine for caudal analgesia in children undergoing upper abdominal surgery. BJA. 2011;106:96–100.
31. Simpao AF, Galvez JA, Wartman EC, England WR, Wu L, Rehman MA, et al. The migration of caudally threaded thoracic epidural catheters in neonates and infants. Anesth Analg. 2019;129:477–81.
32. Baeriswyl M, Zeiter F, Piubellini D, Kirkman KR, Albecht E. The analgesic efficacy of transverse abdominis plane block versus epidural analgesia: a systematic review with meta-analysis. Medicine (Baltimore). 2018;97:e11261.
33. Sato M, Lida T, Kikuchi C, Sesakawa T, Kunisawa T. Comparison of caudal ropivacaine-morphine and paravertebral catheter for major upper abdominal surgery in infants. Pediatric Anesthesia. 2017;27:527–30.
34. Page EA, Taylor KL. Paravertebral block in paediatric abdominal surgery-a systematic review and meta-analysis of randomized trials. BJA. 2017;118:159–66.
35. Machoki MS, Millar AJ, Albetyh H, Cox SG, Thomas J, Numanoglu A. Local anesthetic wound infusion versus standard analgesia in paediatric post-operative pain control. Pediatr Surg Int. 2015;31:1087–97.
36. Jacquenood P, Wallon G, Gazon M, Darnis B, Pradat P, Virlogeux V, et al. Incidence and risk factors of coagulation profile derangement after liver surgery: implications for the use of epidural analgesia—a retrospective cohort study. Anesth Analg. 2018;126:1142–7.

Chapter 27
Anaesthesia for Paediatric Liver Transplantation

Gurinder Singh Malhi and Peter Bromley

Background

The first successful paediatric liver transplantation (LT) was performed in 1967 by Thomas Starzl. The 19-month-old recipient survived just 1 year [1]. Poor mortality figures persisted until the introduction of cyclosporin in 1979 [2]. The current one year survival rate in the United Kingdom for paediatric liver only transplants (donor after brain death) is 97% [3], and these children are expected to reach adulthood. The improvement in survival rate is attributable to better immunosuppressive drugs, surgical techniques, graft availability and assessment of end-stage liver disease [2].

The timing of transplantation is a critical decision; progression towards end-stage disease must be balanced against growth and development of the child. The refinement of paediatric hepatology scoring systems has aided this difficult challenge.

A well-validated scoring system exists in adults (Model of End-stage Liver Disease, MELD) to aid in their prioritisation for transplant, using specific criteria to estimate pre-transplant mortality. This has been modified for paediatric use (Paediatric End-stage Liver Disease, PELD), although there are problems in comparing adult and paediatric scores [4].

G. S. Malhi · P. Bromley (✉)
Birmingham Children's Hospital, Birmingham, UK
e-mail: p.bromley@nhs.net

G. S. Malhi
e-mail: gurinder.malhi@nhs.net

Z. Milan and C. Goonasekera (eds.), *Anesthesia for Hepatico-Pancreatic-Biliary Surgery and Transplantation*, https://doi.org/10.1007/978-3-030-51331-3_27

General Indications for Transplantation

Indications for LT are acute or chronic end-stage liver disease. The underlying aetiology of the liver disease can vary depending on the age of the child, but all age groups can be affected (Fig. 27.1). Neonatal haemochromatosis is specific to the neonatal period, whereas biliary atresia typically affects infants. With increasing age, α1-antitrypsin deficiency and autoimmune hepatitis become more common.

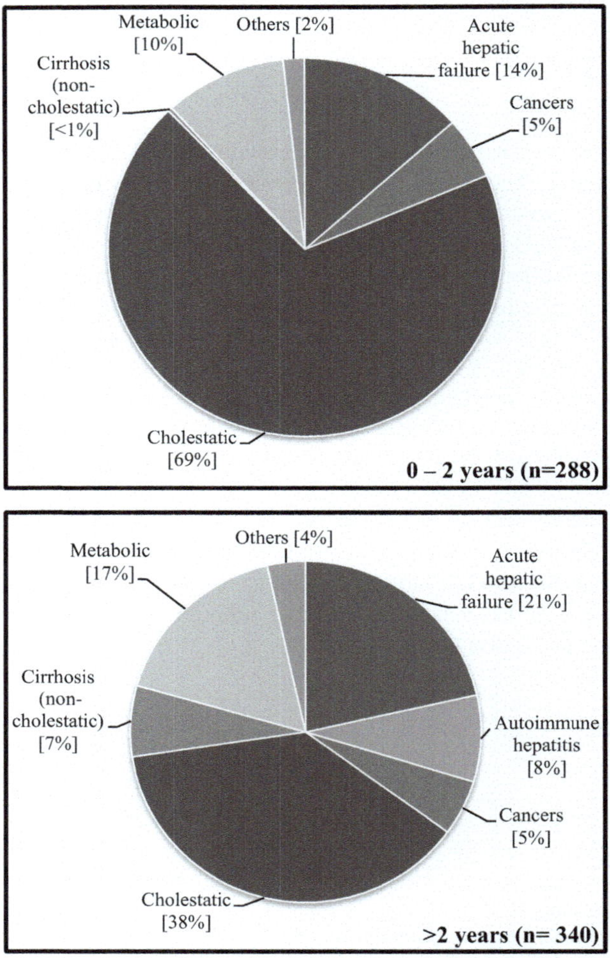

Data provided by Carla Lloyd (Liver Unit, Birmingham Children's Hospital)

Fig. 27.1 Primary indications for liver transplantation in paediatric patients between 1983 and 2013 (Birmingham Children's Hospital and University Hospitals Birmingham). Data provided by Carla Lloyd (Liver Unit, Birmingham Children's Hospital)

Once children reach adolescence, diseases associated with adulthood predominate (Fig. 27.1).

Biliary atresia is the commonest indication for paediatric LT worldwide. Infants with biliary atresia will typically undergo a Kasai portoenterostomy to re-establish bile flow within the first 8 weeks of life [5]. However, despite this intervention many children will go onto develop chronic liver disease requiring transplantation.

Contraindications

The absolute and relative contraindications to paediatric LT continue to evolve, and transplant teams continue to push the boundaries for their patients as they increase their experience and expertise. Absolute contraindications are primarily confined to uncontrolled systemic (bacterial, fungal or viral) infections at the time of transplantation, metastatic extra-hepatic spread of cancer, incurable hepatic tumours and actively replicating hepatitis B or human immunodeficiency virus (HIV) infections [6, 7].

Relative contraindications are variable between different transplant centres. However, children with end-stage liver disease (ESLD) and significant cardiopulmonary disease, multi-organ failure states or HIV infection will require particularly careful multidisciplinary assessment prior to listing [6]. With a limited supply of donor livers, transplant teams have a responsibility to ensure proper utilisation, and it is generally accepted that the anticipated five year survival rate should be in excess of 50% [8].

Preoperative Assessment for Liver Transplantation

The complex medical history frequently encountered in children with liver disease requires a co-ordinated and thorough multidisciplinary assessment. This is best done by an elective hospital admission lasting a few days.

Admission provides an opportunity to evaluate co-morbidities, medication, vascular access, results of investigations, and to seek specialist opinions. This aids the formation of a patient-specific plan for the transplant anaesthetic. LT is major surgery in complex patients; ample time should be allocated to the anaesthetist to meet with the child and parents. Particular areas to address include perioperative anxiety, pre-medication, induction of anaesthesia, venous access and post-operative pain relief.

On the day of surgery, a senior medical doctor will review the children, complete clerking paperwork, confirm consent, repeat bloods, order a chest X-ray (unless performed less than 1 month ago or child asymptomatic), perform urinalysis and measure temperature.

Systemic Manifestations of End-Stage Liver Disease

Progressive liver disease inevitably leads to the involvement and deterioration of other vital organ systems. The clinical implications for the anaesthetist depend on the extent of the liver disease, coupled with the presence and magnitude of the extra-hepatic manifestations. A structured and systems-based approach helps navigate the complex medical histories associated with these patients.

Cardiovascular Function

ESLD is associated with an increased cardiac output and low systemic vascular resistance ('high-output, low-resistance state'). Fluid retention and accumulation of vasoactive compounds including nitric oxide are the likely culprits, but the precise mechanism remains unclear [9]. Thorough cardiac assessment is essential and typically involves history, examination, electrocardiogram (ECG) and transthoracic echocardiogram (TTE). Identification of significant pathology may exclude the child from being listed for transplantation.

Cardiomyopathy is rare in children with liver disease, but can develop as a consequence of immunosuppressive treatment with tacrolimus [10]. Therefore, children listed for retransplantation are particularly susceptible. Additionally, the retransplantation group are prone to developing hypertension; treatment should be optimised and continued during the perioperative period.

Portopulmonary hypertension is very rare in children and presents late, as symptoms remain subtle. ECG and chest X-rays are poor screening tools [11]. Suspicion should arise with the discovery of a new heart murmur, syncope or dyspnoea. Echocardiogram remains the best investigation to assess for this particular complication [11, 12].

The majority of children with minor congenital cardiac abnormalities require no special measures, except where there may be a risk of paradoxical embolus, in which case careful attention is needed to avoid entrainment of air in intravenous lines and surgical anastomoses. More complex cardiac pathology requires multidisciplinary discussions, focused on the timing of cardiac intervention, balancing the risks of performing LT in the presence of an uncorrected cardiac anomaly, against the potential precipitation of hepatic decompensation by performing a cardiac intervention first. Delaying LT while waiting for the optimum time to perform the cardiac intervention also carries a risk of liver disease progression, or death while awaiting LT.

A thorough cardiac assessment is essential in children with Alagille syndrome, who may be considered for LT to treat the complications of chronic cholestasis (severe itching, hypercholesterolaemia, osteodystrophy and failure to thrive). The autosomal dominant disorder is characterised by intrahepatic biliary duct paucity, in association with cardiac, skeletal, ocular and facial abnormalities [13].

Cardiovascular involvement is present in up to 90% of these children, with the most common pathology being peripheral pulmonary artery stenosis or other right sided lesions (including tetralogy of Fallot) [12]. The kidneys, pancreas and vascular systems can be involved, but do not form part of the diagnostic criteria [13].

Respiratory Function

Impaired ventilation and arterial hypoxaemia are commonly encountered in children with advanced liver disease. A reduction in lung volume and basal atelectasis caused by ascites, pleural effusions and hepatosplenomegaly can all contribute to increasing the work of breathing, which may lead to the need for ventilator support and oxygen therapy. Gas exchange can be impaired by concurrent chest infections (encephalopathic, malnourished or debilitated children being particularity at risk) [14].

Children with cystic fibrosis complicated by portal hypertension may be candidates for LT. They are often older, and have well-assessed respiratory function. Respiratory decompensation, sepsis and distal intestinal obstruction syndrome (DIOS) are major post-operative contributors to morbidity in this subgroup [15].

Hepatopulmonary syndrome (HPS) is reported to impact 9–20% of children with liver disease, and can warrant early liver transplantation [16] Abnormal vasodilatation of pulmonary capillary beds and new vessel formation causes right-to-left intra-pulmonary shunting, resulting in arterial hypoxaemia [16, 17]. Nitric oxide (NO) has been implicated in the underlying pathophysiology, which is supported by higher exhaled NO concentrations measured in patients with HPS. Oxygen therapy alone will fail to correct a true intra-pulmonary shunt, but in many cases this simple measure will achieve reasonable oxygen saturations.

Shortness of breath, clubbing and a fall in oxygen levels on standing all support a clinical diagnosis of HPS. The diagnosis can be confirmed by a ^{99m}Tc-radiolabelled albumin scan or agitated saline contrast echocardiography ('bubble echo'). In healthy subjects, 95% of the microaggregated albumin is taken up by the lungs. This percentage declines in HPS, as intra-pulmonary shunting results in greater systemic take-up [17]. In agitated saline contrast echocardiography, intra-pulmonary shunting is suspected upon the detection of 'bubbles' in the left atrium, in the absence of an intra-atrial communication, five heartbeats after the administration of contrast [17].

Warner et al. reported the average duration of supplementary oxygen following liver transplantation was 12 days, in their case series of 20 children with HPS [16]. The delay in reversal of HPS post-transplantation means these interesting children are often extubated whilst still hypoxic, and may be discharged home with domiciliary oxygen therapy.

Severe respiratory failure may exclude a child from urgent liver transplantation. Case reports of extracorporeal membrane oxygenation (ECMO) therapy in the context of paediatric liver transplantation have been reported, but its use remains controversial and not without risk [18].

Renal Function

Renal dysfunction is common in chronic liver disease. It is associated with drug toxicity, sepsis and hypovolaemia. Immunosuppressive drugs are nephrotoxic, and children listed for retransplantation remain vulnerable throughout the perioperative period.

Children with primary hyperoxaluria type 1 (PH1) or autosomal recessive polycystic kidney disease (ARPKD) may be in established renal failure and on renal replacement therapy prior to combined liver and kidney transplantation (CLKT) [19].

Hepatorenal syndrome is less frequently encountered in paediatric patients with liver disease, compared to adults. It is characterised by a circulatory imbalance between renal vasoconstriction and splanchnic vasodilatation, leading to a reduction in the glomerular filtration rate (GFR) [20]. Intravascular filling with albumin and administration of terlipressin are two treatment measures that have some degree of support.

Serum cystatin C has been described as an alternative marker to serum creatinine for assessing renal function in patients with liver failure [13, 21]. The role of cystatin C as a prognostic indicator continues to be explored.

Neurological Function

Impaired neurological function requires urgent assessment, as it can be an ominous sign of end-stage liver disease (ESLD). Easily reversible causes, such as alterations in electrolytes and blood glucose levels, must be ruled out or corrected. Hepatic encephalopathy is a serious and potentially fatal complication of liver disease. It is graded clinically, with grades III and IV often requiring an escalation of care to intensive care and early intubation for airway protection (Fig. 27.2). The precise mechanism is poorly understood, but it is exacerbated by changes in cardiac output, serum ammonia accumulation and neuropeptides acting as false neurotransmitters. The effects of sedatives and general anaesthetics on this group can be profound and varied; post procedural high dependency care may be required.

Fig. 27.2 Clinical grades of hepatic encephalopathy

Grade 0	Normal
Grade 1	Drowsy but orientated
Grade 2	Drowsy and disorientated
Grade 3	Agitated and aggressive
Grade 4	Unrousable to pain

Haematological Function

Coagulopathy is common in liver disease. A reduction in liver synthetic function results in depletion of those clotting factors produced in the liver, coupled with deficiencies specifically in vitamin K dependent factors (II, VII, IX and X) due to insufficient bile acid production. Prothrombin time is a useful indicator of liver synthetic function. Factor V levels are sometimes used as the half-life is short, making it rapidly responsive to changes in synthetic function, and it is unaffected by vitamin K deficiency. Haemostasis may be further impaired by derangement in platelet count (sequestration in splenomegaly secondary to portal hypertension) and function (significantly altered in sepsis). The resultant coagulopathy can be severe.

Anti-thrombin III and proteins C and S levels can be disproportionately reduced compared to the reduction in procoagulant factors, predisposing some children to intravascular thrombosis.

The sequestration of erythrocytes in splenomegaly, malnutrition, and recurrent or chronic gastrointestinal haemorrhage from varices can all lead to anaemia.

Metabolic Function

Glycogen is made and stored in the cells of the liver and skeletal muscle. Impaired glycogen synthesis and gluconeogenesis in end-stage liver disease make patients vulnerable to developing hypoglycaemia. Blood glucose monitoring is essential.

Ammonia is a product of amino acid metabolism. Ammonia crosses the blood brain barrier, and its accumulation can cause life-threatening neurological impairment. Under normal conditions, it is converted to urea in the liver, prior to renal excretion. The capacity of the liver to metabolise ammonia can be further stressed by constipation, a high-protein diet, and the breakdown of blood in the gastrointestinal tract by enteric bacteria. Treatment with neomycin and lactulose aims to reduce bacterial overgrowth and constipation.

Acute Liver Failure

Acute liver failure (ALF) in children is an emergency, has a high mortality and is best managed in specialist centres with access to LT. It is characterised by a severe and rapid decline in liver function, with or without encephalopathy.

Classification systems incorporating hepatic encephalopathy (HE) into their criteria (King's College London), are difficult to apply to paediatric patients, as HE often presents later, is difficult to diagnose in young children and can be rapidly progressive in some patients. Another important difference between adults and paediatric definitions is the requirement for the absence of pre-existing liver disease in adults with ALF, as paediatric acute liver failure can result from the acute decompensation of a previously unknown underlying liver disorder (inherited metabolic disorders) [22].

The aetiology of acute liver failure varies with age. Haemochromatosis is a cause mainly confined to the neonatal period, after which viral hepatitis, drug toxicity and metabolic conditions predominate [14, 23]. In up to half of children aged over 1 year, the cause of their acute liver failure will remain unknown [23].

A methodical and cohesive approach is vital to manage this complex and rapidly changing multisystem disorder. Children should be nursed in a quiet environment, on a ward with staff familiar with managing acute liver failure. Progression to Grade III or IV encephalopathy requires transfer to a paediatric intensive care unit (PICU). Early intubation and ventilation reduces the risk of aspiration pneumonia, ensures adequate oxygenation and helps control intracranial hypertension.

In ALF, there can be total loss of hepatocyte function, removing any possibility of gluconeogenesis, making children prone to hypoglycaemia. Glucose monitoring and supplementation is therefore mandatory. Invasive lines should be sited to allow regular blood sampling and to guide fluid therapy.

Administration of broad spectrum antibiotics and antifungals are usually required as sepsis is common. Hypotension secondary to vasodilatation is initially corrected with intravenous fluid therapy, but noradrenaline infusions are frequently required in addition. Other vasoconstrictors, such as vasopressin, or additional inotropic agents may be added in severe cases. Hemofiltration is commenced if renal dysfunction ensues, or to reduce serum ammonia levels.

Neurological deterioration can be an ominous sign and an indication of life-threatening raised intracranial pressure (ICP). Treatment is mainly supportive, in addition to mechanical ventilation; children should be appropriately sedated, nursed with a 10° head-up tilt, with loose endotracheal tube ties or tape to prevent excessive obstruction to venous drainage from the head. Pupillary changes or cardiovascular signs of intracranial hypertension are treated with boluses of sedation, paralysis agents, transient hyperventilation and administration of hypertonic saline or mannitol. The insertion of invasive ICP monitoring devices to assist clinical teams in maintaining cerebral perfusion pressure in children with severe coagulopathy may cause further harm, mainly as a result of increased risk of intracranial haemorrhage. More commonly now, non-invasive imaging (CT or MRI scan) or electroencephalography (EEG) are used to confirm continuing cerebral viability. Severe intracranial hypertension resistant to treatment may exclude children from transplantation, or cause death before it can be achieved.

Coagulopathy associated with acute liver failure can be challenging to treat, as correction with the administration of fresh frozen plasma, platelets, cryoprecipitate and vitamin K may only partially reverse the coagulopathy, whilst significantly increasing the risk of circulatory overload. Severely coagulopathic children may benefit from the administration of recombinant Factor VIIa, if there is troublesome bleeding, or prior to invasive procedures [23].

The mortality from LT for ALF is significantly greater when compared with chronic liver failure. This difference is attributable to neurological and cardiovascular complications, or sepsis.

Surgical Technique

The transplant operation is classically divided into three phases: dissection, anhepatic and reperfusion.

Dissection Phase

The dissection phase lasts from 'knife to skin' to the occlusion of the hepatic artery and portal vein. The goals are to gain exposure to the native liver and to prepare the major vessels.

This phase can be prolonged in children with previous upper abdominal surgeries, because of dense adhesions. Blood loss can become significant during this early phase. Transfusion is guided by haemodynamics, blood pressure, haematocrit and thromboelastogram. Haematocrit is kept below 25% to minimise the risk of vascular thrombosis. For the same reason, partial correction of coagulation will often suffice. Ionised calcium may fall with the administration of fresh frozen plasma, requiring infusions or boluses of calcium to maintain an ionized calcium of around 1.2 mmol/L [14].

Albumin, synthetic colloid and crystalloid have all been used for intravascular filling, but debate still continues over which is better. Intraoperative volume expansion with human albumin solution has fallen in popularity, and more usually a combination of colloid or crystalloid is used, or fresh frozen plasma if indicated by the thromboelastogram.

Surgical retraction blades may impair diaphragmatic movement, requiring the anaesthetist to pay close attention to ventilatory parameters, or even drag small patients up the operating table, threatening the displacement of lines or monitoring devices. Dissection around the porta hepatis and manipulation of the liver may interfere with venous return, causing sudden but transient hypotension. This responds well to fluid bolus administration and intermittent vasopressor support.

Anhepatic Phase

The anhepatic stage commences when the portal vein and hepatic artery are clamped and lasts until portal vein in-flow to the new transplanted liver is re-established. As there is no liver function in this phase, the anaesthetist should expect a progressive metabolic derangement, decrease in venous return and a fall in core body temperature.

The short and awkwardly placed hepatic veins can prove difficult to isolate. Removing a small segment of cava with the native liver provides a solution, as donor cava attached to the liver graft can be used to restore vessel continuity. Therefore, depending on the surgical technique, the inferior vena cava can be either partially or totally clamped. The compensatory tachycardia is frequently inadequate by itself to correct hypotension, and fluid administration and vasopressor support may be required. Portal vein clamping is better tolerated in the presence of chronic portal hypertension, because blood returns to the heart via large collateral vessels. Splanchnic and renal perfusion may be adversely affected. Liberal use of fluid therapy to correct hypotension may lead to high right atrial pressures at reperfusion (when portal and vena cava clamps are released), which can cause graft congestion and significant bleeding.

Blood glucose levels require close monitoring, and increasing amounts of intravenous dextrose may be required. Despite the profound metabolic acidosis, buffers are usually avoided unless there is haemodynamic instability or hyperkalaemia. Progressive hyperkalaemia during this phase can be managed with calcium, dextrose and insulin, furosemide or bicarbonate. It is desirable that the potassium level is kept reasonably low at the point of reperfusion, when it can rise significantly due to potassium being flushed out of the ischaemic graft.

Reperfusion Phase

The reperfusion phase commences when the inferior vena cava and portal vein are unclamped, restoring flow to the newly transplanted liver, and ends with abdominal wall closure. The reperfusion of a cold and ischaemic organ can provide a considerable challenge to the recipient's cardiovascular reserve.

This phase is characterised by sudden and severe haemodynamic instability, resulting from a decrease in systemic vascular resistance, myocardial stunning, changes in circulating volume (filling the new liver), and blood loss from cut surfaces and vascular anastomoses.

Successfully navigating this phase requires optimisation of the recipient and graft prior to reperfusion, excellent communication with the surgical team and prompt treatment of instability with fluid administration and vasopressor infusion (noradrenaline or adrenaline). The surgical team irrigates the graft with crystalloid or colloid solution, or the recipient's blood, to flush out potassium, cell debris, air, inflammatory mediators and metabolites, which would otherwise be infused into the recipient.

Prior to restoring arterial flow, the graft is inspected for bleeding points. Arterial anastomosis is a critical time and surgeons can be aided by good arterial perfusion and a quiet environment. Reperfusion coagulopathy is common, and thromboelastography is useful in directing clotting factor administration or identifying fibrinolysis, which can be successfully treated with tranexamic acid or aprotinin. A functioning new liver will gradually reduce the base deficit and serum lactate, promote haemodynamic stability and raise core body temperature.

Revascularisation is followed by fashioning a biliary drainage system, often draining the bile duct into a segment of small bowel (Roux-en-Y or Roux loop). For children with large grafts, the abdominal closure may be tight, potentially causing an abdominal compartment syndrome, with graft compression and kinking of blood vessels. The effect of abdominal closure on ventilation is frequently used as an indirect indicator of raised abdominal pressure. Staged abdominal closure with prosthesis may be employed to facilitate a more gradual tightening. This technique can significantly delay time to extubation.

Early Post-operative Phase

The majority of patients are transferred intubated to the paediatric intensive care unit. Figure 27.3 highlights the common causes of acute deterioration following LT. Surgical complications include hepatic artery and portal vein thrombosis, intestinal perforation and bleeding, requiring aggressive transfusion and early surgical exploration. Any acute deterioration will require prompt assessment. However, the majority of children with good graft function will have progressive improvement in biochemical parameters, weaning of inotropic support and be extubated within 24 hours. Fluid balance remains difficult to assess, but desirable parameters might include central venous pressure (CVP) 6–10 cm H_2O, urine output 0.5–1.5 mL/kg/hour and plasma sodium 135–145 mmol/L.

Anaesthetic Management

Anaesthetic care for paediatric liver transplantation is perhaps best provided by a small subset of anaesthetists, who can therefore accumulate experience and familiarity with the procedure, and the local surgeons' usual technique. However, a good working knowledge of the challenges faced in the care of these children will help all anaesthetists who may encounter survivors presenting for perhaps unrelated future surgeries.

Pre-operative Assessment

The benefit of a thorough assessment prior to listing is that most difficulties have been anticipated, investigations completed, expert opinion sought where indicated, culminating in a tailored anaesthetic plan for patients.

Causes of acute deterioration following liver transplantation:

Graft failure: primary non-function

Initial poor function

Vascular problems: kinking or thrombosis of hepatic portal vein or hepatic artery, obstruction of hepatic veins venous outflow

Bleeding: surgical factors, coagulopathy

Sepsis

Abdominal compartment syndrome

Renal failure

Bowel perforation or ischaemia, gastrointestinal bleed

Intracerebral bleed or intracranial hypertension

Seizures, drug-related neurotoxicity

Pulmonary oedema or acute lung injury

Fig. 27.3 Causes of acute deterioration following liver transplantation Figure needs revision

Sedative pre-medication may be used but optimal timing may be difficult, and the effect can be variable. Children may be allowed to drink clear sugar-containing fluids up to 1 h prior to surgery.

Full blood count (FBC), clotting profile, urea and electrolytes (U&Es), glucose, liver function tests (LFT) are repeated and reviewed. Transfusion of platelets and clotting factors prior to surgery can be done in consultation with the anaesthetist, but fluid overload should be avoided. Blood bank and a consultant haematologist should be informed of the transplantation, and blood products reserved according to local guidelines. Serum sodium should ideally be greater than 125 mmol/L prior to theatre, as rapid correction puts the child at risk of central pontine myelinolysis [24].

Intraoperative Care

Anxiety in children undergoing anaesthesia for LT may be significant. Older children may verbally express their concerns regarding mortality, whilst younger children may reveal their anxiety behaviourally. Parental presence in the anaesthetic room might be comforting for the child.

Induction of anaesthesia may be commenced with the child semi-recumbent or in the arms of their parent, following the completion of the World Health Organisation (WHO) pre-anaesthesia induction checklist and the attachment of standard monitoring. As an intravenous cannula is often in situ, a smooth and controlled induction can be achieved with propofol 2–3 mg/kg and fentanyl 2 mcg/kg, without much distress. Alternatively, a gas induction with sevoflurane, carried in a mixture of oxygen and nitrous oxide remains a suitable option.

To rapidly achieve favourable conditions for intubation, non-depolarising muscle relaxants are administered, usually atracurium or rocuronium. However, a larger dose is required to counteract the effects of an increase in volume of distribution and greater binding to acute phase proteins. Vecuronium and rocuronium are both metabolised in the liver and prolonged action is an understandable concern, although the duration of surgery and the use of mechanical ventilation post-operatively mean that this is often not of much practical significance.

In older children, oral intubation is preferred to nasal, especially in the presence of coagulopathy and thrombocytopenia. However, in infants, nasal intubation has the clear advantage of safer fixation. High inflation pressures with positive end-expiratory pressure (PEEP) are required to mitigate the effects of ascites and hepatosplenomegaly on ventilation. Ill-fitting endotracheal tubes, even with the smallest of leaks can be troublesome, and the anaesthetist should opt for a snug fit, or use a cuffed tube. Laryngoscopy for intubation also provides an ideal time for the careful insertion of a nasogastric tube.

Under anaesthesia, children are susceptible to developing hypothermia, which can have a detrimental effect on coagulation, graft function and other organ systems. Strategies which can be employed to limit any reduction in core temperature include: increasing the ambient temperature of the theatre; using a pressure-relieving under-body warming mattress; applying a convective over-body warming system and PVC drapes along the child's flanks to reduce pooling of ascites and blood; and warming all fluids and blood products. By siting invasive lines in theatre, the aforementioned active warming strategies can be commenced without much delay. Should central line insertion prove difficult, placement in theatre provides an additional benefit as an image intensifier can be used to screen the position of the devices.

The size, site and number of intravenous catheters depends on the size of the child and anticipated surgical blood loss. All peripheral cannulae should be firmly secured, especially if they are the main device for rapid volume resuscitation, as access to these devices for inspection or adjustment will be difficult intraoperatively. Commonly a multilumen central venous catheter and a large bore sheath are inserted into a great vein in the distribution of the superior vena cava, under real-time ultrasound guidance. The radial artery is the preferred site for arterial pressure monitoring. The femoral artery is generally avoided as the trace will be damped or obliterated by aortic cross-clamping. The child should be positioned such that access is possible to the endotracheal tube, monitoring equipment and invasive lines. A urethral catheter is passed prior to surgical draping.

Anaesthesia is usually maintained using isoflurane or desflurane in a mixture of oxygen and air, supplemented by infusions of an opioid (remifentanil, fentanyl or morphine) and muscle relaxant (atracurium). Regular measurement of blood gases and electrolytes enables the anaesthetist to identify and treat derangements in ionised calcium, sodium, potassium, lactate and glucose. Coagulation is usually monitored with thromboelastography, often with prothrombin time and activated partial thromboplastin time monitoring in theatre. Blood loss and haemodynamic parameters are used to guide fluid resuscitation. Cardiac output monitoring is sometimes used but is not universally thought to be essential.

Post-operative Care

All patients are transferred to the PICU. A subset of low-risk candidates may be safely extubated immediately [25, 26], but the vast majority will be extubated following an abdominal ultrasound demonstrating good blood flow in the liver vessels, normalising of biochemical parameters and haemodynamic stability with weaning of inotropes. Those children with previous lung disease, reduced respiratory reserve, or complications of transplantation (fluid overload, transfusion related lung injury, HPS and partially closed abdomen with large split graft), may require prolonged ventilation.

The post-operative care will be guided by a standardised protocol that will provide teams with guidance on anti-rejection medication, anti-microbial agents, feed and fluid management, graft function assessment and signs that indicate the development of early complications.

Analgesic management can prove challenging. Non-steroidal anti-inflammatory drugs are avoided, and paracetamol is avoided or used in reduced doses (orally or via nasogastric tube). Morphine or other opioids with or without ketamine via continuous infusion, patient controlled analgesia (PCA) or nurse controlled analgesia (NCA) provide the main method to achieve good postoperative analgesia. Local anaesthetic infusions via wound catheters may improve the quality of analgesia and reduced morphine requirements.

Graft Reduction and Split-Liver Transplantation

The supply of size matched donor livers for paediatric transplantation is limited. The use of either reduced or split liver grafts are two solutions to this obstacle. In the latter technique, the donor liver is split, with the smaller left lateral lobe transplanted into a child and the right lateral lobe transplanted into an adult or larger child. One year survival rates are now over 90% in most centres, but complications are always possible; transplantation remains challenging and risk can never be eliminated completely.

References

1. Starzl TE, Groth CG, Brettschneider L, Penn I, Fulginiti VA, Moon JB, et al. Orthotopic homotransplantation of the human liver. Ann Surg. 1968;168:392–415.
2. McKenna GJ, Klintmalm GBG. The history of liver transplantation. In: Busuttil RW, Klintmalm GB, editors. 3rd ed. Philadelphia: Elsevier Saunders; 2015. p. 2–24.
3. Statistics and Clinical Studies, NHS Blood and Transplant. Organ donation and transplantation activity report 2018/19. https://nhsbtdbe.blob.core.windows.net/umbraco-assets-corp/16469/organ-donation-and-transplantation-activity-report-2018-2019.pdf. Accessed 15 Oct 2019.
4. Freeman RB Jr, Wiesner RH, Roberts JP, McDiarmid S, Dykstra DM, Merion RM. Improving liver allocation: MELD and PELD. Am J Transplant. 2004;4:114–31.
5. Kelly DA, Davenport M. Current management of biliary atresia. Arch Dis Child. 2007;92(12):1132–5.
6. Scott VL, Wahl KM, Soltys K, Belani KG, Beebe DS, Davis PJ. Chapter 28: Anaesthesia for organ transplantation. In: Davis PJ, Cladis FP, Motoyama EK, editors. Smith's anaesthesia for infants and children. 8th ed. Philadelphia: Elsevier Mosby; 2011. p. 905–27.
7. Farkas S, Hackl C, Schlitt HJ. Overview of the indications and contraindications for liver transplantation. Cold Spring Harb Perspect Med. 2014;4:a015602.
8. NHS England. 2013/14 NHS Standard contract for liver transplantation service (Children). https://www.england.nhs.uk/wp-content/uploads/2013/06/e03-liver-trans-child-ad.pdf.
9. Hollenberg SM, Waldman B. The circulatory system in liver disease. Crit Care Clin. 2016;32:331–42.
10. Atkison P, Joubert G, Barron A, Grant D, Paradis K, Seidman E, et al. Hypertrophic cardiomyopathy associated with tacrolimus in paediatric transplant patients. Lancet. 1995;345(8954):894–6.
11. Condino AA, Dunbar D, O'Connor JA, Narkewicz MR, Mengshol S, Whitworth JR, et al. Portopulmonary hypertension in pediatric patients. J Pediatr. 2005;147:20–6.
12. Madan N, Arnon R, Arnon R. Evaluation of cardiac manifestations in pediatric liver transplant candidates. Pediatr Transplant. 2012;16:318–28.
13. Kamath BM, Schwarz KB, Hadzic N. Alagille syndrome and liver transplantation. J Pediatr Gastroenterol Nutr. 2010;50:11–5.
14. Bennett J, Bromley P. Liver, intestine and renal transplantation. In: Bingham R, Lloyd-Thomas AR, Sury MRJ, editors. Hatch and Sumner's textbook of paediatric anaesthesia. 3rd ed. London: Hodder Arnold; 2008. p. 621–8.
15. Dowman JK, Watson D, Loganathan S, Gunson BK, Hodson J, Mirza DF, et al. Long-term impact of liver transplantation on respiratory function and nutritional status in children and adults with cystic fibrosis. Am J Transplant. 2012;12:954–64.
16. Warner S, McKiernan PJ, Hartley J, Ong E, van Mourik ID, Gupte G, et al. Hepatopulmonary syndrome in children: A 20-year review of presenting symptoms, clinical progression, and transplant outcome. Liver Transpl. 2018;24:1271–9.
17. Deep A, Jose B, Dhawan A. Hepatopulmonary syndrome in children-an update. Paediatr Child Health. 2015;25:282–5.
18. Nandhabalan P, Loveridge R, Patel S, Willars C, Best T, Vercueil A, et al. Extracorporeal membrane oxygenation and pediatric liver transplantation, "a step too far?": results of a single-center experience. Liver Transpl. 2016;22(12):1727–33.
19. Grenda R, Kaliciński P. Combined and sequential liver-kidney transplantation in children. Pediatr Nephrol. 2018;33:2227–37.
20. Shah N, Silva RG, Kowalski A, Desai C, Lerma E. Hepatorenal syndrome. Dis Mon. 2016;62:364–75.
21. Amin AA, Alabsawy EI, Jalan R, Davenport A. Epidemiology, pathophysiology, and management of hepatorenal syndrome. Semin Nephrol. 2019;39:17–30.

22. Jain V, Dhawan A. Prognostic modeling in pediatric acute liver failure. Liver Transpl. 2016;22:1418–30.
23. Cochran JB, Losek JD. Acute liver failure in children. Pediatr Emerg Care. 2007;23:129–35.
24. Morard I, Gasche Y, Kneteman M, Toso C, Mentha A, Meeberg G, et al. Identifying risk factors for central pontine and extrapontine myelinolysis after liver transplantation: a case-control study. Neurocrit Care. 2014;20:287–95.
25. Gurnaney HG, Cook-Sather SD, Shaked A, Olthoff KM, Rand EB, Lingappan AM, et al. Extubation in the operating room after pediatric liver transplant: a retrospective cohort study. Paediatr Anaesth. 2018;28:174–8.
26. O'Meara ME, Whiteley SM, Sellors JM, Luntley JM, Davison S, McClean P, et al. Immediate extubation of children following liver transplantation is safe and may be beneficial. Transplantation. 2005;80:959–63.

Chapter 28
Communication Between HPB Anaesthetists: Meetings, Websites and Forums

Naomi Lucas

Despite the lack of a dedicated association of Hepatico-Pancreatic-Biliary (HPB) and transplant anaesthetists worldwide, there are a large number of associated bodies and international organisations relevant to anaesthetists practising within this field. These provide a platform from which to share information and thus improve the delivery of care and outcome for patients undergoing HPB and transplant surgery worldwide. This chapter aims to outline the range of websites, forums and meetings of interest to HPB and transplant anaesthetists.

Anaesthesia and Critical Care Societies

Liver Intensive Care Group of Europe (LICAGE)

<http://licage.org>

LICAGE was founded in 1987 by Dr. JV Farman who worked alongside Professor Sir Roy Calne in Cambridge performing the first ever liver transplantation (LT). The overriding aim of LICAGE was to enable effective communication amongst workers from all disciplines to collaborate, stimulate and share learning to progress the management of patients requiring LT [1]. From its evolution, the society has continued to grow both in numbers and educational activity.

Members of LICAGE receive bi-annual newsletters, have access to online educational and research material and are eligible for significantly reduced registration fees at a range of meetings. The LICAGE Annual Congress is traditionally

N. Lucas (✉)
Consultant Anaesthetist, King's College Hospital, London, UK
e-mail: naomilucas@doctors.org.uk

Z. Milan and C. Goonasekera (eds.), *Anesthesia for Hepatico-Pancreatic-Biliary Surgery and Transplantation*, https://doi.org/10.1007/978-3-030-51331-3_28

located in a historical European city. Every third year, LICAGE, the International Liver Transplant Society (ILTS) and the European Liver and Intestinal Transplantation Association (ELITA) collaborate to form a joint Congress. This is held as either an additional meeting or in place of the annual LICAGE meeting. LICAGE has strong links with ELITA and collaborates to hold joint meetings with them and the Independent Academic Research Studies International Institute (IARS). These meetings have included highly regarded courses such as 'Anaesthesia and Critical Care for liver Transplantation', serving as a thorough introduction for novice liver transplant anaesthetists or a useful refresher for more experienced clinicians.

Liver Transplant Anaesthesia and Critical Care Forum (LiTAC)

<https://ilts.org/education/anes-ccm>

The LiTAC website was created in 2004 by an editorial board within LICAGE, vastly developed by Dr. John Klinck, a former president of LICAGE. It was primarily aimed towards anaesthetists and intensivists involved in the care of patients requiring LT. Authors included a number of internationally renowned authorities within the academic field, providing links to current literature and lecture materials [1]. The website also functioned as a more traditional discussion board, enabling access to expert opinion on specific issues, serving as a valuable tool for information sharing between clinicians across the globe. It proved to be a useful resource for both trainees and more experienced clinicians. LiTAC went on to become a jointly run venture with the International Liver Transplant Society (ILTS), from within ILTS administration. It is now delivered as part of the Anaesthesia/Critical Care Medicine (CCM) section of a reformed ILTS website.

Enhanced Recovery After Surgery Society (ERAS)

<http://erassociety.org>

The ERAS Society stemmed from the 'ERAS Study Group' originated following a meeting between Professor Ken Fearon (UK) and Professor Olle Ljungqvist (Sweden) at a London symposia. Their aim was to progress the ideas expressed in the 1990s by Professor Henrik Kehlet (Denmark) regarding the practice of multi-modal surgical care. The ERAS Study Group examined practices across different centres and found significant discrepancies between actual practice and what was recognised in literature as 'best practice'. This led the study group to initiate a process of change from widely used 'traditional practice' to 'best practice', based upon clinical evidence [2].

The ERAS Society was officially registered in 2010 in Sweden as a 'not for profit' medical society [2]. Their mission was to develop perioperative care and improve patient recovery through education, research, audit and implementation of evidence-based practice. The Society went onto develop a number of implementation programmes. The first National Symposium took place in Milan in 2007. The first International ERAS World Society Congress was hosted in Cannes, France in 2012. This attracted leading investigators interested in Enhanced Recovery from over thirty countries and six continents. Since then, ERAS has grown internationally worldwide, involving a wide range of fields of surgery and anaesthesia.

The ERAS study group initiated the development and publication of evidence-based consensus protocols, initially with patients undergoing colonic surgery. Over time, the society has developed and published a growing number of guidelines, including specific guidelines for Anaesthesia in 2015. Focussed guidelines for the peri-operative care of patients undergoing pancreatoduodenectomy were published in 2013 [2] and peri-operative care for liver surgery in October 2016 [4]. New guidelines continue to be developed and established guidelines are regularly updated in the light of new developments. The implementation of these guidelines have shown a marked reduction in post-operative complications and significantly reduced length of hospital stay [3].

The ERAS website provides links to all published guidelines within surgery and anaesthesia. Access is enabled to a number of associated educational resources, including useful links to expert reviews of recent research undertaken involving ERAS principles within different surgical fields, including liver and pancreas. A web-based interactive software audit tool is available, enabling assessment of compliance with ERAS protocols. In 2016, ERAS Society joined LinkedIn and started a You tube channel. This includes videos from previous World Congresses and Olle Ljungqvist TED talks. It also has an active twitter account, @ErasSociety.

Enhanced Recovery After Surgery, United Kingdom (ERAS UK)

<https://erasuk.net>

ERAS UK was formally adopted as the British chapter of the International ERAS society in 2016. It was developed in 2011, following an International Conference on Enhanced Recovery held in Bristol in 2010 [4]. They agreed that the construction of a UK- based network would be a useful platform from which to share information and best practise, especially as fast-track protocols were rapidly being developed across a range of specialities and distributed throughout the country.

The overall aims of ERAS UK were to improve patient recovery after surgery through promoting knowledge, understanding and research regarding optimal patient outcomes. The organisation hosts one annual conference that is attended by a broad mix of healthcare professionals, from a growing variety of specialties. The website provides links to presentations and abstracts from earlier UK-based meetings, alongside other relevant articles. A 'Knowledge Hub Group' has recently been developed, enabling access to a library of relevant materials, forums and event details.

Evidence Based Perioperative Medicine (EBPOM)

<https://www.ebpom.org>

Since 1997, EBPOM has been a collaborative project between a number of UK and international academic institutions. Together they aim to distribute information and the application of evidence based practise within perioperative medicine. Through research, skill acquisition and knowledge, it is hoped patient outcome will be optimised.

EPBOM host an annual meeting in London in addition to TRIPOM (trainees interested in perioperative medicine). Regular regional and international meetings are also scheduled throughout the year.

It has an active twitter account, @EBPOM.

Transplant Societies

International Liver Transplantation Society (ILTS)

<https://ilts.org>

In 1982, a group of transplant anaesthetists and intensivists at the University of Pittsburgh identified the need for an organisation to promote education and provide a forum for discussion for all those involved in liver transplantation. The first symposium was staged in Pittsburgh in 1984 by the 'Society for Perioperative Care in Liver Transplantation' [5]. A further two symposiums were arranged, with a growing number of invited speakers and attendees from international centres. This included Dr. John Farman, from the team of Sir Roy Calne in Cambridge, who went on to develop the Liver Intensive Care Group of Europe (LICAGE), described earlier.

The First Congress of the 'International Society for Perioperative Care in Liver Transplantation' was held in Pittsburgh in 1990. The society was subsequently renamed the 'International Liver Transplant Society', led by Dr. Yoogoo Kang, who was elected founding president. In 1995, the society held its third Congress in London, alongside LICAGE. Meetings were then scheduled every two years until 2000, when it became an annual event. The Annual International Congress is usually held between May and July with a varied programme comprising of keynote presentations, lectures, topical debates and numerous abstracts. Every three years, the annual Congress is held in Europe, when the ILTC collaborates with LICAGE [5].

The early mission statement of the ILTC emphasised the importance of a multi-disciplinary approach and effective communication between all involved health-care professionals. It was also committed to the publication of a dedicated journal. In order to avoid duplication, the ILTS agreed with the American Association of the Study of Liver Diseases (AASLD) to co-sponsor a single journal. 'Liver Transplantation and Surgery' was first published in January 1995, with a change in editorship and its name in 2000 to 'Liver Transplantation'. The journal's impact factor grew quickly with large numbers of manuscript submissions enabling monthly publications from 2001 onwards.

The ILTS is a non-profit charitable organisation. Its overall mission is to 'promote and disseminate advances in liver transplantation across the world' [5]. In addition to encouraging research and teaching excellence, the society also acts as an advocate for issues and programmes that may impact upon the development of liver transplantation. The society works effectively alongside both public and private organisations to further education and research internationally. Its members include all those working as part of the multi-disciplinary team, in transplant centres across the world.

As of February 2019, Special Interest Groups (SIG) have been introduced within ILTS to bring together clinicians with common interests in more specific aspects of liver transplantation. The approved topics to date include:

- Cardiovascular Topics in Liver Transplantation
- Donors after cardiac death (DCD), Liver Preservation and Machine Perfusion
- Liver Transplant Oncology
- Liver Transplant Immunology
- Infectious Diseases and Liver Transplantation
- Living Donor Liver Transplantation
- Precision Medicine and Biomarkers in Liver Transplantation

Each of Specialist Interest Groups are expected to develop their own online forum, assist with the selection of abstracts submitted to ILTS meetings and develop guidelines within their specific fields.

The ILTS website is a comprehensive resource that is of high quality and easy to navigate. It provides a wealth of information including details of upcoming meetings, recent publications, previous newsletters and access to online forums. It also provides an international directory of transplant centres across the globe and available fellowships for ILTC members. It provides links to 'Congress Resource Platforms', enabling access to the scientific content of recent meetings. Again, this website is easy to navigate and identify specific abstracts, authors or topics.

ILTS Education (https://ilts.org/education) is an excellent online resource for learning surrounding liver transplantation [6]. A large body of material is available to members, comprised of videos, lectures and commentaries. The specialities are split into Anaesthetics/Critical Care Medicine, Hepatology and Surgery. Within each speciality, topics are subdivided with links to relevant journal club reviews, lectures and case discussions with access to expert opinions on specialist topics. Annual scholarships are awarded by the ILTS to assist with the development of clinicians, particularly those in developing countries. The 'Vanguard Committee' and the 'Scholarship Committee' are dedicated to the educational needs of trainees and less experienced clinicians. The Education Committee co-ordinates ILTS educational programs at a number of meetings including the annual Perioperative Care in Liver Transplant course at the American Society of Anesthesiologists meeting, in addition to a variety of symposia and consensus conferences.

Members of ILTS have contributed to major advances in the field of liver transplantation over the years. The initial objectives of the founding members of the ILTC have largely been achieved, with ongoing ILTC leadership and member involvement continuing to facilitate dissemination of new concepts and ideas across the world.

British Transplant Society (BTS)

<http://bts.org.uk>

The BTS represents the breadth of professionals involved in transplantation within the UK.

Its first International Congress of Transplantation was held in 1966. Following this, in September, 1971, the need for a UK-based organisation was discussed and supported by physicians, surgeons and immunologists at a meeting held by the 'London Transplant Club'. The combined transplant and immunology society was then created, with its inaugural meeting held at the Royal Free hospital in April, 1972 [7]. A steering committee was set up and it was decided Spring and Autumn meetings would be associated with the British Society of Immunology (BSI), with an additional separate meeting to be held each year. Throughout the 1970s, meetings were held annually with Spring meetings outside and the others in London, usually hosted between the Wellcome Foundation and other hospitals. Combined meetings were held in France and the Netherlands in 1978 and 1981, with the French and Dutch Transplantation Societies respectively. In 1998, a single three-day Annual Congress was introduced and proved to be extremely popular. Its Annual Congress persists today and includes plenary and parallel sessions to cater for interests in general and associated specialised topics.

Working groups and specialised sub-committees were developed as the need arose. These initially included the Transplant Training and Education Committee and Standards and Ethics Committee, both of which still exist today. Nominations, Standards and Clinical trials committees were later included to complete the five current subcommittees. The separate Chapters of Surgeons and Nurses share a forum for those members of the society, provide a voice for the professionals and consider current issues within their respective fields.

The BTS is described as 'the voice of transplant professionals'. Whilst it contributes to the development of scientific, ethical and clinical practises, it is also actively involved with the development of National Policy and interacting with the media on issues surrounding transplantation. Latest related news releases and statements are easily accessible via the website. The website also provides access to active guidelines and standards alongside resources to information relevant to professionals and the public. Its membership is encouraged for 'everyone in the UK with an interest in transplantation'. To become a member, two sponsors must be provided and approved by the BTS executive. Reduced membership rates are available for students and individuals with existing membership in affiliated organisations.

The Herrick Society

<http://herricksociety.org.uk>

The Herrick Society (formerly the Carrel club) is specifically designed for trainees in transplant surgery in the UK, affiliated with both the BTS and the Association of Surgeons in Training. It aims to bring interested trainees together, providing useful information and support. Its membership benefits include access to training courses, job opportunities, discussion boards, together with collaborative research opportunities and society events.

It has an active twitter account, @herricksociety.

Solid Organ Transplant Pharmacy Association (SOTPA)

<https://sotpa.co.uk>

SOTPA was initiated in 2013 following the recognition of the need of pharmacists working within solid organ transplantation for their own platform to promote education and development within the field. It is affiliated with the British Pharmaceutical Society and BTS. The association's overall aim is to promote excellence in the pharmaceutical care of patients requiring transplantation. Its membership is open to pharmacists within the field (including liver, renal and cardiothoracic transplantation) and does not incur membership fees at present. An educational masterclass event is held annually.

It has an active twitter account, @SOTPA1.

British Liver Transplant Group (BLTG)

<https://www.basl.org.uk/index.cfm/content/page/cid/5>

Launched in 2014, BLTG is one of five subgroups encompassed by the umbrella organisation, British Association for the Study of the Liver (BASL). It represents the professional interests of liver transplantation within the UK. It aims to bring together clinicians and allied personnel whilst working closely with relevant bodies to provide the professional view on aspects regarding planning and delivery of the transplant service within the UK. The BLTG Transplant meeting is linked to the BASL annual meeting, integrating separate meetings arranged by individual transplant centres to provide a central stage for those with an interest in liver transplantation.

European Society for Organ Transplantation (ESOT)

<https://esot.org>

ESOT is the umbrella society under which all European Transplant activities are organised. It collaborates with many other organisations to effectively structure and streamline transplant activity within Europe. There are currently eight 'sections' within ESOT, each of which are specialised groups focusing on a specific organ or aspect of transplantation. Additionally, there are five committees as part of the society. These include the Basic Science Committee, Education Committee, European Transplant Allied Healthcare Professionals (ETAHP) Committee and Young Professionals in Transplantation (YTP) Committee.

The founding assembly meeting of the 'European Society of Transplant Surgeons' took place in April 1982, in Switzerland. The society's name was subsequently changed to ESOT and it sought to include 'all persons actively involved in organ transplantation'. The assembly decided that the society ought to meet every two years, with its first meeting taking place in Zurich in 1983. The Congress continues to gather together the European and International transplant scene, whilst driving progress and learning within the field (esotcongress.org). Each of the five committees also host a number of events throughout the year. These include a range of scientific meetings, educational courses and e-learning modules. ESOT has an extensive educational programme and encourages excellence through a number of awards and grants available to ESOT members. These are allocated at the biennial ESOT Congress and at meetings arranged by associated committees throughout the year. ESOT also endorses initiatives organized by third parties, information on which are accessible via the ESOT website.

'Transplant International' is the official journal of ESOT, ELITA and the German Transplantation Society (DTS). Journals are published monthly and available online only. They are accessible through Wiley online library, or via the

ESOT website for members. 'Transplant International' Application is also available to download.

European Liver and Intestine Transplantation (ELITA)

<https://www.esot.org/ELITA/home>

ELITA, formerly known as 'European Liver Transplant Association', ELTA, is a section of ESOT representing expertise in liver and intestinal transplantation in Europe. It acts as both a scientific forum and an official representative body. ELTA was founded in 1993. Its name was modified in 2005 to 'European Liver and Intestine Transplantation' (ELITA).

ELITA meets every two years, together with ESOT. However, since 2005, ELITA has organised an annual winter meeting with discussions focussed around the European Liver Transplant Registry (ELTR), data management and specific educational topics.

The website provides access to a variety of educational resources, including free research support through the 'Centre for Evidence in Transplantation' and the Transplant Library Database, endorsed by ESOT.

The European Liver Transplant Registry (ELTR)

<http://eltr.org>

ELTR is the official database of ELITA. ELTR was founded in 1985 and now nearly all European transplant centres are contributing to ELTR. The main objectives are to ensure all transplantations performed in Europe are registered, to provide a link between European Liver Transplant centres and to stimulate scientific research and publications centred around the European experience. The website provides access to a wealth of data and publications provided by ELTR. A yearly newsletter is distributed to contributing centres and ELITA members, detailing a summary of the year's activity and new developments within the registry.

The Transplantation Society (TTS)

<https://tts.org>

The transplantation society is a Non-Governmental Organisation (NGO) providing an international forum dedicated to global advancement of organ transplantation. Since its evolution in 1966, just over a decade after the first successful kidney transplant, TTS has grown to include over 6700 members and represent over 105 different countries across the world. The Society's mission is to promote scientific understanding through dissemination of knowledge and education, support global development of professional standards and measure outcomes. It works alongside National Governments, the World Health Organisation (WHO), charitable organisations and collaborates with multiple national and international societies.

Its biennial congresses have been held since 1966, in locations across the world.

Surgical Societies

International Hepato-Pancreato-Biliary Association (IHPBA)

<https://ihpba.org>

The 'International Biliary Association' was founded in Los Angeles in 1978 by Dr. Berci, a clinical professor of surgery at UCLA School of Medicine. The original concept was the formation of a small group of invited international specialists in biliary tract disorders, enabling the facilitation of clinical research protocols. In 1986, a new group was developed, the 'World Association of HPB Surgeons' (WAHPBS). Eventually, in 1991, the 'International Biliary Association' merged with WAHPBS, becoming the IHPBA, an organisation with a much wider membership and clearly defined objectives. The broad objectives of the modern IHPBA is devotion to minimise suffering caused by Hepato-Pancreato Biliary disorders through continuous improvement of education, training, innovation, research and patient care within this field [8].

The association is divided into four regions, including the 'Europe and Africa Middle East: European-African Hepato-Pancreato-Biliary Association'. There are currently over three thousand members from over a hundred different countries. Members are entitled to a number of benefits. These include access to the innovative educational tool and community 'my HPB', membership and fellowship directory, access to the online journal 'HPB', newsletters and discounted fees to world and regional congresses. Active members are also able to interact with other HPB specialists and leaders and have the opportunity to serve on the committee. Allied health professionals and Advanced Practice Practitioners are also welcome to join and enjoy these benefits. The IHPA has also developed an outreach initiative, aiming to assist in the development of care of patients suffering with HPB diseases within developing countries through support of local surgeons and institutions. This work has recently been recognised by the World Health Organisation, with whom they now collaborate on a project-by-project basis. The details of previous and future projects are made available online. This highly functioning website enables rapid and easy navigation through its variety of online tools and resources.

European-African Hepato-Pancreato-Biliary Association (EAHPBA)

<http://eahpba.org>

The EHPBA was founded in 1999 as the European Regional Association of the International Hepato-Pancreato-Biliary Association (IHPBA). The association later expanded to include parts of the Middle East and Africa, thus becoming the EAHPBA. The association serves to expand and support education and research within the field, sets standards and accredited HPB fellowship programmes. It works closely with HPB Regional associations and National Chapters. These include the Americas Hepato-Pancreato-Biliary Association (AHPBA) and the Asian-Pacific Hepato-Pancreato-Biliary Association (A-PHPBA). It aims to work constructively with other speciality organisations to share information whilst continually improving standards of care within the field. Now a paper-free organisation, its communication is optimised through the web-based membership directory, regular e-newsletters and access to the online journal, HPB.

The association conducts a biennial scientific meeting, alternating with the IHPBA World Congress, whilst hosting a number of other educational events annually. As for the IHPBA, it's official journal is HPB. The EAHPBA promotes a multi-disciplinary approach to the treatment of patients with hepato-pancreato-biliary disorders. Its membership is encouraged for qualified interested candidates, including anaesthetists and associated health professionals.

Association of Upper Gastro- Intestinal Surgery of Great Britain and Ireland (AUGIS)

<http://augis.org>

AUGIS is a registered charity that aims to improve the provision, delivery and outcome of patients undergoing surgery involving the oesophagus, stomach, duodenum, pancreas and biliary tract. The association was created in 1996 by a number of senior representatives of academic societies interested in upper gastro-intestinal disease. The British Obesity and Metabolic Surgery Society (BOMSS), the Great Britain and Ireland Hepato Pancreato Biliary Association (GBIHPBA) and the Association of Upper Gastrointestinal Surgeons (Trainees) (AUGISt) were later incorporated.

Over the years, its primary focus has been to improve outcome through implementing a robust audit system. The association also provides comprehensive training objectives to support high quality training programmes within the UK, whilst encouraging progression of academia and education within the field. Its main future goal includes the assistance in the production of guidelines.

AUGIS functions under the umbrella of the ASGBI, (Association of Surgeons of Great Britain and Ireland) alongside the Senate of Surgery, Royal Colleges, the Specialist Advisory Committee (SAC) and associated surgical and academic bodies. It also serves as a forum to share valuable information amongst healthcare professionals and the general population. Although primarily a platform for surgeons, the AUGIS council have made a significant effort to engage with the wider audience involved in patient care. Its membership has opened up to welcome clinical nurse specialists and allied health professionals, who are also now well represented on council.

The inaugural meeting of AUGIS took place in Glasgow in 1996 and has progressed substantially since then. The Annual Scientific Meeting takes place in September each year, providing an opportunity for motivated individuals to share ideas and advance practices within the field. AUGIS also meets each Spring, under the umbrella of the ASGBI.

The AUGIS website itself is a valuable resource, providing accessible links to conferences, guidelines, audits and recent news. The trainee section of AUGIS (AUGISt) has recently been renamed the 'Roux Group'. The Roux group is a trainee-led collaborative representing trainee surgeons from all branches of upper gastrointestinal surgery. The Roux Group website is currently being updated. Additionally, the new AUGIS website allows for social platforms to facilitate case discussion. It also has an active twitter account; @augishealth.

Medical Societies

British Association for the Study of the Liver (BASL)

<https://basl.org.uk>

BASL is the National Association for Hepatology. It is composed of five different sub-groups, including the BLTG, British Liver Nurses' Association (BLNA), British Viral Hepatitis Group (BVHG), British Hepatology Pharmacy Group (BHPG) and HVV-UK. The main aims of BASL include collaboration of research and dissemination of findings, raising awareness of liver disease and interacting with the media. It also provides advice for the formation of policies relating to patients with liver disease. It is a multi-disciplinary, not for profit association with over one thousand members.

The BASL website has links to numerous resources, including information about current clinical trials, research and patient information. It also has links to a number of special interest groups and a variety of bursaries and fellowships that are available to BASL members. The BASL annual meeting takes place over three days in September and has a dedicated website with all relevant information, http://baslannualmeeting.org.uk, and twitter account, @basl_events.

European Association for the Study of the Liver (EASL)

<https://easl.eu>

EASL is a medical association, founded in Europe in 1966, dedicated to promoting excellence in liver research, liver disorders and education in the field. It has become an influential International Organisation attracting members from across the globe. Its membership benefits include online access to the 'Journal of Hepatology', educational tools including LiverTree (the official e-learning portal) and information regarding research grants and fellowships. The International Liver Congress is held annually, with additional educational meetings and summits scheduled throughout the year.

Cancer Based Organisations

Pancreatic Cancer UK

<https://pancreaticcancer.org.uk>

Pancreatic Cancer UK is a charitable organisation that provides information and support, funds innovative research and campaigns for improvements in the care, treatments and outcomes for patients with pancreatic cancer. It has an active medical advisory board and informative website, a valuable resource for patients and relatives in addition to healthcare professionals. A large amount of information and support is available online, including advice for patients regarding treatment options and details surrounding participation in clinical trials. Additionally, the support line provides the opportunity to speak with a pancreatic cancer specialist nurse during daytime hours. Appropriate publications are available to both patients and healthcare professionals, on request.

Information is provided for healthcare professionals involved with treating patients with pancreatic cancer, including how to support patients, access to educational resources and the 'Promoting Innovative Practice' initiative. Health professionals working with patients with pancreatic cancer are eligible to join the 'Health Professional Network'. Members are able to apply for funding to attend study days, request access to relevant publications, apply for funding to support training events and receive the latest bulletins regarding recent pancreatic cancer updates.

Speciality	Society	Web Address/URL	Meeting/Congress	Twitter / Facebook
Anaesthesia & Critical Care	Liver Intensive Care Group of Europe (LICAGE)	http://licage.org	LICAGE Annual Congress 3yrly – LICAGE/ILTS/ELITA	
	Liver Transplant Anaesthesia and Critical Care Forum (LiTAC)	https://ilts.org/education/anes-ccm		
	Enhanced Recovery After Surgery Society (ERAS)	http://erassociety.org	ERAS World Society Congress (Annual)	@ErasSociety
	ERAS UK	http://erasuk.net	ERAS UK Conference (Annual)	@ERASsocietyUK
	Evidence Based Perioperative Medicine (EBPOM)	https://www.ebpom.org	EBPOM London (Annual) TRIPOM (Annual)	@EBPOM
Transplant	International Liver Transplantation Society (ILTC)	http://ilts.org	Annual International Congress	@_ILTS_ ILTS Facebook Page
	British Transplantation Society (BTS)	http://bts.org.uk	BTS Annual Congress	@BTStransplant
	The Herrick Society	http://herricksociety.org.uk		@herricksociety
	Solid Organ Transplant Pharmacy Association (SOTPA)	https://sotpa.co.uk	Annual Masterclass	@SOTPA1
	British Liver Transplant Group (BLTG)	https://www.basl.org.uk/index.cfm/content/page/cid/5	BLTG Transplant meeting (BASL)	
	European Society for Organ Transplantation (ESOT)	https://www.esot.org	ESOT Congress (biennial) http://esotcongress.org	@ESOTtransplant ESOT Facebook Page

Fig. 28.1 Summary Table of Societies, Organisations and Acronyms

	European Liver and Intestine Transplantation (ELITA)	https://www.esot.org/ELITA/home	Annual Winter Meeting Biennial (ESOT Congress)	
	European Liver Transplant Registry (ELTR)	http://eltr.org		@ELTR30
Surgical	International Hepato-Pancreato-Biliary Association (IHPBA)	https://ihpba.org	IHPBA World Congress (biennial)	@IHPBA IHPBA Facebook Page
	European-African Hepato-Pancreato-Biliary Association (EAHPBA)	http://eahpba.org	EAHPBA Biennial Congress	@EAHPBA
	Association of Upper Gastro-Intestinal Surgery of Great Britain and Ireland (AUGIS)	http://augis.org	Annual Scientific Meeting (Sept)	@augishealth
Medical	British Association for the Study of the Liver (BASL)	https://basl.org.uk	BASL Annual Meeting http://baslannualmeeting.org.uk	@basl_events @BASLedu @heppharm
	European Association for the Study of the Liver (EASL)	https://easl.eu	International Liver Congress (Annual)	@EASLnews EASL Facebook Page
Cancer Charitable Organisations	Pancreatic Cancer UK	https://pancreaticcancer.org.uk		@PancreaticCancerUK Pancreatic Cancer UK Facebook Page
	Macmillan Cancer Support	https://macmillan.org.uk		@macmillancancer Macmillan Cancer Support Facebook Page

Fig. 28.1 (continued)

Macmillan Cancer Support

<https://macmillan.org.uk>

Founded by Douglas Macmillan in 1911, who watched his father die of cancer, the originally named 'Society for the Prevention and Relief of Cancer' was created to provide advice and support for patients suffering with cancer. Since then, the charity has grown vastly and adapted to provide necessary support for patients today. This includes emotional, physical and financial support from the moment of diagnosis.

Macmillan Cancer Support provides numerous networking opportunities for healthcare professionals together with links to a variety of resources, including practical tools for those treating patients with cancer. 'Mac Update' is a quarterly e-bulletin for all healthcare professionals and the 'Learn Zone', accessible via the website, provides links to a number of e-learning modules. 'Macvoice' and 'Macmail' provide information and updates for Macmillan professionals, who are also eligible to apply for Learning and Development grants. Healthcare professionals may volunteer and contribute to online patient forums (Fig. 28.1).

References

1. Liver Intensive Care Group of Europe (LICAGE). http://www.licage.org. (Accessed 7th July 2019).
2. Enhanced Recovery after Surgery (ERAS). http://erassociety.org/about/history. (Accessed 7th July 2019).
3. Lasse K., et al. Guidelines for perioperative care for pancreatoduodenectomy: Enhanced Recovery After Surgery (ERAS) Society recommendations. Clin Nutr. 2012;31(6):817–830.
4. Melloul, et al. Guidelines for perioperative care for Liver Surgery: Enhanced Recovery After Surgery (ERAS) society recommendations. World J Surg. 2016;40(10):2425–40.
5. Eskicicoglu F., et al. Enhanced Recovery after Surgery (ERAS) programs for patients having colorectal surgery: a meta-analysis of randomised trials. J Gastrointest Surg. 2009;13(12):2321–9.
6. Francis N., et al. https://www.erasuk.net/about-us.html. (Accessed 8th July 2019).
7. International Liver Transplant Society (ILTS). http://ilts.org/about/history. (Accessed 7th July 2019).
8. International Liver Transplant Society (ILTS). http://ilts.org/education/. (Accessed 7th July 2019).
9. Douglas J (updating version compiled by Professor Mary G. McGeown in 2001 & 2007) 'The History of the BTS'. http://bts.org.uk/about-bts/history-of-the-bts/. (Accessed 7th July 2019).
10. International Hepato-Pancreato-Biliary Association. http://www.ihpba.org. (Accessed 8th July 2019).

Index

A

B

C

Z. Milan and C. Goonasekera (eds.), *Anesthesia for Hepatico-Pancreatic-Biliary Surgery and Transplantation*, https://doi.org/10.1007/978-3-030-51331-3

D

E

F

G

H

The manufacturer's authorised representative in the EU is Springer Nature Customer Service Centre GmbH, Europaplatz 3, 69115 Heidelberg, Germany. If you have any concerns regarding our products, please contact ProductSafety@springernature.com

Printed and bound by CPI Group (UK) Ltd, Croydon, CR0 4YY

30/09/2026

02225240-0009